RIDLEY'S
The Vulva

EN cefte figure font demonfirez les Membres eftant en la femme, quant a la fituatiõ,
liaifon,&entremeſlure. A.demõfire la partie de la veine du foye,aultremēt dicte,caué.
BB.les veines feminales,elles font de coleur blanchaftre: par ces vaines eſt icfte la femence.
CC.font les veines,les ãlles embraffent l'amarri,ou matrice.DD.les couillõs de la femme.
F.l'amarri,matrice.la portiere.GG.les cornes de la matrice.H.l'entree deans la matrice,ou
l'orifice interieux. I. le col de la matrice,aultremēt,la partie honteufe.KK.le tronc de la vei
ne du foye,caué.plante par les cuiffes au bas du genou. LL.ceft le tronc de la plus grãde ar
tere dicte aorte,a caufe qu'elle eſt la fource de toutes les aultres Arteres. M.monfire la veſ
fie. QQ. petiz conduictz par ou paffe l'ourine en la veffie,dictz en grec vriteres.PP.Les
reins,ou roignõs,OO,les veines   defcendãt aux roignõs de couleur blãchatre.

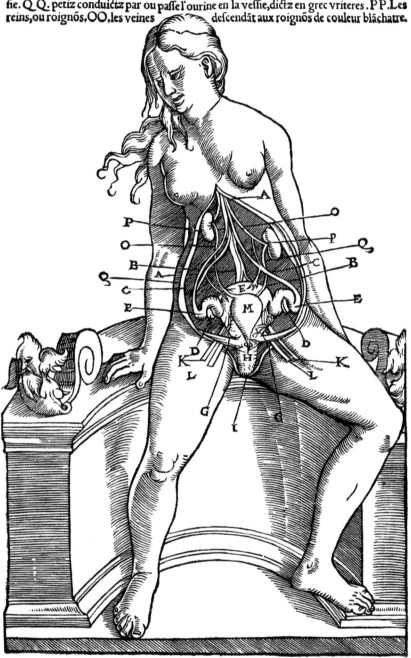

Frontispiece: Seated female showing viscera.
Walter Hermann Ryff (fl. 1539). From the
original in the Wellcome Library by courtesy
of the trustees.

RIDLEY'S
The Vulva

EDITED BY

Sallie M. Neill

AND

Fiona M. Lewis

THIRD EDITION

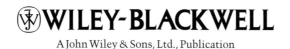

A John Wiley & Sons, Ltd., Publication

This edition first published 1975 (by Churchill Livingstone), 1999 © 2009 by Blackwell Publishing Ltd

Blackwell Publishing was acquired by John Wiley & Sons in February 2007. Blackwell's publishing program has been merged with Wiley's global Scientific, Technical and Medical business to form Wiley-Blackwell.

Registered office: John Wiley & Sons Ltd, The Atrium, Southern Gate, Chichester, West Sussex, PO19 8SQ, UK

Editorial offices: 9600 Garsington Road, Oxford, OX4 2DQ, UK
The Atrium, Southern Gate, Chichester, West Sussex, PO19 8SQ, UK
111 River Street, Hoboken, NJ 07030-5774, USA

For details of our global editorial offices, for customer services and for information about how to apply for permission to reuse the copyright material in this book please see our website at www.wiley.com/wiley-blackwell

Wiley also publishes its books in a variety of electronic formats. Some content that appears in print may not be available in electronic books.

Designations used by companies to distinguish their products are often claimed as trademarks. All brand names and product names used in this book are trade names, service marks, trademarks or registered trademarks of their respective owners. The publisher is not associated with any product or vendor mentioned in this book. This publication is designed to provide accurate and authoritative information in regard to the subject matter covered. It is sold on the understanding that the publisher is not engaged in rendering professional services. If professional advice or other expert assistance is required, the services of a competent professional should be sought.

The contents of this work are intended to further general scientific research, understanding, and discussion only and are not intended and should not be relied upon as recommending or promoting a specific method, diagnosis, or treatment by physicians for any particular patient. The publisher and the author make no representations or warranties with respect to the accuracy or completeness of the contents of this work and specifically disclaim all warranties, including without limitation any implied warranties of fitness for a particular purpose. In view of ongoing research, equipment modifications, changes in governmental regulations, and the constant flow of information relating to the use of medicines, equipment, and devices, the reader is urged to review and evaluate the information provided in the package insert or instructions for each medicine, equipment, or device for, among other things, any changes in the instructions or indication of usage and for added warnings and precautions. Readers should consult with a specialist where appropriate. The fact that an organization or Website is referred to in this work as a citation and/or a potential source of further information does not mean that the author or the publisher endorses the information the organization or Website may provide or recommendations it may make. Further, readers should be aware that Internet Websites listed in this work may have changed or disappeared between when this work was written and when it is read. No warranty may be created or extended by any promotional statements for this work. Neither the publisher nor the author shall be liable for any damages arising herefrom.

Library of Congress Cataloging-in-Publication Data
Ridley's the vulva / edited by Sallie Neill and Fiona Lewis. – 3rd ed.
    p. ; cm.
  Rev. ed. of: Vulva. 2nd ed. 1999.
  Includes bibliographical references.
  ISBN 978-1-4051-6813-7
  1. Vulva–Diseases. 2. Vagina–Diseases. I. Ridley, Constance Marjorie. II. Neill, Sarah M.
III. Lewis, Fiona, 1963– IV. Vulva. V. Title: Vulva.
  [DNLM: 1. Vulva. 2. Vulvar Diseases. WP 200 R546 2009]
  RG261. V85 2009
  618.1′6–dc22

                                                                          2009000402

ISBN: 978-1-4051-6813-7

A catalogue record for this book is available from the British Library.

Set in 9.5/12pt Sabon by Graphicraft Limited, Hong Kong
Printed and bound in Singapore by Fabulous Printers Pte Ltd

1 2009

Contents

Contributors, vii

Preface to the third edition, ix

Preface to the second edition, xi

Chapter 1: Basics of vulval embryology, anatomy and physiology, 1
 S.M. Neill & F.M. Lewis

Chapter 2: Principles of examination, investigation and treatment, 34
 F.M. Lewis & S.M. Neill

Chapter 3: Sexually transmitted diseases of the vulva, 44
 N.C. Nwokolo & S.E. Barton

Chapter 4: Non-sexually transmitted infections of the vulva, 71
 F.M. Lewis & S.M. Neill

Chapter 5: Non-infective cutaneous conditions of the vulva, 85
 S.M. Neill & F.M. Lewis

Chapter 6: Vulvodynia, 145
 F.M. Lewis & S.M. Neill

Chapter 7: Psychological and psychiatric aspects of vulval disorders, 155
 E.R.L. Williams & J. Catalán

Chapter 8: Cysts and epithelial neoplasms of the vulva, 168
 G.W. Spiegel & E. Calonje

Chapter 9: Non-epithelial tumours of the vulva, 199
 E. Calonje & G.W. Spiegel

Chapter 10: Surgical procedures in benign vulval disease, 221
 B.J. Paniel & R. Rouzier

Chapter 11: Management of vulval cancers, 239
 R. Rouzier & B.J. Paniel

Contributors

Simon E. Barton
Clinical Director GU and HIV Medicine
Chelsea and Westminster Hospital NHS Foundation Trust
London, UK

Eduardo Calonje
Director of Dermatopathology
Department of Dermatopathology
St John's Institute of Dermatology
London, UK

Jose Catalán
Consultant Psychiatrist
Psychological Medicine
South Kensington and Chelsea Mental Health Centre
London, UK

Fiona M. Lewis
Consultant Dermatologist
Heatherwood & Wexham Park Foundation Trust Slough
and
St John's Institute of Dermatology
St Thomas' Hospital
London, UK

Sallie M. Neill
Consultant Dermatologist
St John's Institute of Dermatology
St Thomas' Hospital
London, UK

Nneka C. Nwokolo
Consultant Physician
The Victoria Clinic for HIV and Sexual Health
Chelsea and Westminster NHS Foundation Trust
London, UK

Bernard J. Paniel
Professor of Gynaecology
Department of Gynaecology and Obstetrics
Centre Hospitalier Intercommunal de Creteil
40 Avenue de Verdun
94010 Creteil Cedex
France

Roman Rouzier
Professor in Obstetrics and Gynaecology
Department of Gynaecology, Obstetrics
and Reproductive Medicine
Hôpital Tenon
4 Rue de la Chine
75020 Paris
France

Gregory W. Spiegel
Consultant Histopathologist
Department of Histopathology
St Thomas' Hospital
London, UK

Edwina R.L. Williams
Consultant Perinatal Liaison Psychiatrist
The Elizabeth Garrett Anderson & Obstetric Hospital
London, UK

Preface to the third edition

This new edition of Marjorie Ridley's *The Vulva* contains all the topics in the original book but now includes advances that have been made since the last publication. In addition, many of the authors have changed and, therefore, most of the chapters have been extensively revised.

Sadly, since the previous edition of this textbook was published, Marjorie Ridley, who was undoubtedly one of the leading clinicians responsible for the development of vulval skin disease as a specialty, has died. We would like to dedicate this third edition to her and rename it *Ridley's The Vulva* to acknowledge her pioneering work in this field. She was instrumental in encouraging a multidisciplinary approach to the diagnosis and treatment of vulval disorders and brought together the various specialties involved in caring for these patients. She was a generous teacher, inspiring the next generation to continue and develop the specialty.

The last 10 years have seen an enormous increase in interest in genital skin disease along with a much needed expansion in the number of clinics dedicated to the diagnosis and treatment of vulval disorders. These clinics have input from dermatologists, gynaecologists, genitourinary physicians and histopathologists. The increased awareness of the psychosocial and psychosexual impact of vulval disease has led to other specialists being involved, particularly psychiatrists, psychologists and psychosexual therapists. Some of these issues have been addressed in this new edition of the book.

All the illustrations are now in colour, which significantly enhances some of the detail of both the clinical and histological appearances. Clinicopathological correlation is vitally important for an accurate diagnosis.

This book is directed at all those specialists involved in the management of patients with a genital skin problem. The aim of the book is not only to be a reference text, but also to offer up-to-date guidance on diagnosis and management.

Sallie M. Neill
Fiona M. Lewis
2009

Acknowledgements

We thank all our contributors for their dedication and hard work. Our thanks also to the previous authors, John McLean, Harold Fox and Hilary Buckley, who kindly allowed us to use the framework of their original chapters.

We are grateful to those colleagues and patients who have allowed us to use their photographs.

We would like to thank Rebecca Huxley and the editorial staff of Wiley-Blackwell for their infinite patience, encouragement, help and good humour. We would also like to thank Lindsey Williams of Lindsey Williams Publishing Production Services for her unfailing accuracy in the finer detail of the final manuscript and her excellent communication skills.

We are indebted to the publishers for permission to use photographs previously published in the following books:

A Colour Atlas of Diseases of the Vulva (1992) (eds C.M. Ridley, J.D. Oriel & A.J. Robinson). Chapman and Hall Medical, London.

Ricci, J. (1943) *The Genealogy of Gynaecology, 2000 B.C.–1800 A.D.* Blakiston, Philadelphia.

Ridley, C.M. (1975) *The Vulva.* Major Problems in Dermatology, No. 5. W.B. Saunders Co., Philadelphia.

Sawday, J. (1995) *The Body Emblazoned.* Routledge, London.

Wisdom, A. & Hawkins, D. (1997) *Diagnosis in Color: Sexually Transmitted Diseases*, 2nd edn. Mosby-Wolfe, London.

Preface to the second edition

The contents of this new, expanded, multi-author edition range over embryology and development, anatomy and physiology, history, general aspects of management, infections, non-infective cutaneous conditions, pain problems, psychiatric disorders, cysts and non-neoplastic swellings, non-epithelial and epithelial tumours, and surgical procedures applicable to benign and malignant conditions.

The general expansion and considerable revision of content, and the inclusion of new chapters, are, in our opinion, justified by the great increase of interest in vulval disease which has become apparent in the last few years.

There have been significant changes in thought as well as many scientific advances during this period. The relevant material, however, remains scattered in the literatures of the several disciplines involved. This latest edition of *The Vulva* attempts to collate the existing information on the subject and to note its interrelations. We hope that the result will be to facilitate the multidisciplinary cooperation which is so vital in the study and management of vulval disease.

There is of necessity some overlap between the chapters, but we believe that there are no important discrepancies in the views of our contributors.

The book is directed towards those specialists in dermatology, genitourinary medicine, gynaecology and pathology who are involved with vulval problems. It is intended to be a repository of information, interpretation and guidance on management rather than simply an illustrated text; it aims to offer to the reader material which, as a coherent whole, is not readily available elsewhere.

C. Marjorie Ridley
1999

Acknowledgements

We thank all our contributors for their cooperation and hard work. Our thanks go also to the colleagues who have allowed us to use their photographs; that is, those who helped with previous editions and now also Miss Betty Mansell and Dr Jennifer Salisbury.

We are very grateful to the editorial staff of Blackwell Science for their great help and forbearance; in particular to Rebecca Huxley, Dr Stuart Taylor, Audrey Cadogan and Victoria Oddie.

Chapter 1: Basics of vulval embryology, anatomy and physiology

S.M. Neill & F.M. Lewis

Embryology

A basic knowledge of the events in the embryogenesis and organogenesis of the female reproductive tract is important in order to understand the congenital abnormalities that may arise. The female genital tract is closely linked to the development of both the urinary and terminal part of the gastrointestinal tracts, explaining why some congenital abnormalities of the female reproductive tract may be found in association with anomalies of the urinary and gastrointestinal systems.

Sexual determination and differentiation

The term 'determination' describes events that commit cells to a certain course of development, and 'differentiation' describes the processes whereby these cells achieve this development. The differentiating processes are regulated by at least 30 specific genes located on sex chromosomes or autosomes that act through a variety of mechanisms (Grumbach & Conte 1992). Since the genetic sex of an individual is established at fertilization this may be regarded as the point of determination with all that follows being processes of embryonic differentiation. Although the genetic sex is determined at fertilization, the gonads and external genitalia remain sexually indeterminate for the first 6 weeks. A female phenotype develops in the absence of the androgens testosterone, dihydrotestosterone (DHT), anti-Mullerian hormone (AMH) and Mullerian-inhibiting substance (MIS) hormone. However incomplete masculinization can occur when testosterone fails to convert to DHT or when DHT fails to act within the cytoplasm or nucleus of the cells of the external genitalia and urogenital sinus. This can happen despite the presence of testes.

The presence or absence of the Y chromosome determines the sex of the indifferent gonad. Earlier investigation of patients with abnormalities of the sex chromosomes had shown the Y chromosome to be extremely potent in inducing testicular differentiation (Ford *et al.* 1959, Jacobs & Strong 1959). The testis-determining factor (TDF) is a 35 kilobase pair (kbp) sequence on the 11.3 sub-band of the Y chromosome, in an area termed the sex-determining region of the Y chromosome (SRY). When this region is absent or altered, the indifferent gonad develops into an ovary. The *SRY* gene has been found in some cases of Turner's syndrome where there is no detectable Y chromosome in the karyotype. This finding demonstrates that the presence of a single dominant Y chromosomal gene alone is not enough to determine testicular differentiation (Mittwoch 1992). In addition to the Y chromosome, genes on other chromosomes also play a part in testicular development, including Wilm's tumour suppressor (*WT1*) gene, which regulates SRY expression, *DAX1* on the X chromosome, *SF1* on chromosome 9, *SOX9* on chromosome 17 and *AMH* on chromosome 19 (Mittwoch & Burgess 1991).

Hormones also have an important influence on sexual differentiation. The development of the internal ducts is a result of a paracrine effect from the ipsilateral gonad. A female phenotype develops in the absence of testicular tissue owing to the lack of testosterone, MIS or AMH. The level of local testosterone necessary for mesonephric (Wolffian) duct differentiation needs to be high. This is shown as maternal ingestion of androgens does not result in male internal differentiation in a female fetus, nor does this differentiation occur in females with congenital adrenal hyperplasia (CAH). Conversely, high levels of oestrogens can sometimes reduce MIS action, resulting in some paramesonephric (Mullerian) duct development. Two functional X chromosomes are normally required for ovarian development, but female differentiation of the internal and external sexual organs can still occur in the absence of a testis whether or not ovaries are present.

In summary, the genetic sex determines gonadal sex, which then determines the differentiation/regression of the internal ducts (i.e. Mullerian and Wolffian ducts) and the ultimate phenotypic sex. However, the final sexual identity of an individual depends not only on the phenotypic

Ridley's The Vulva, 3rd edition. Edited by Sallie M. Neill and Fiona M. Lewis. © 2009 Blackwell Publishing, ISBN: 978-1-4051-6813-7.

appearance but also on the brain's prenatal and postnatal development.

Early female embryogenesis

In the first 8 weeks of development after ovulation, a system known as Carnegie staging is used to denote the maturity of the embryo. There are 23 Carnegie stages and each stage is based on internal and external physical features of the embryo (O'Rahilly & Muller 1987). The crown–rump length is also included.

Carnegie stage 1: post-ovulatory day 1; approx. size 0.1–0.2 mm

This is the point of fertilization in which the human zygote, with its XX sex chromosome constitution, is conceived in the distal third of the uterine tube. An acellular envelope, the zona pellucida encases the zygote.

Carnegie stage 2: days 2–3; approx. size 0.1–0.2 mm

This stage starts with the first cleavage division, which occurs 24–30 hours after fertilization. The 2 cell zygote increases to 8–16 blastomeres.

Carnegie stage 3: days 4–5; approx. size 0.1–0.2 mm

This is the period of development during which a blastocyst with its fluid-filled cavity forms. There are 16–32 blastomeres, which start to form an inner cell mass (embryonic pole) and outer cell mass (mural and polar trophoblast). The blastocyst eventually comes to lie free within the reproductive tract as the surrounding zona pellucida degenerates (Fig. 1.1).

Carnegie stages 4 and 5: days 6–31; approx. size 0.1–0.2 mm

The blastocyst penetrates and embeds in the uterine endometrium. During this period, the outer envelope of cytotrophoblast, forming the wall of the blastocyst, generates syncytiotrophoblast on its external surface (Enders 1965, Tao & Hertig 1965) and extraembryonic mesoderm on its internal surface (Hertig & Rock 1949). This structure is termed the chorion (Fig. 1.2a).

The primitive amniotic cavity develops at approximately 7–9 days after ovulation (Blechschmidt 1968, Luckett 1973) and its floor forms the primary ectoderm (Fig. 1.2b). The primary endoderm is probably formed from cells that originate from the ectoderm that migrate around the blastocoelic cavity (Heuser & Streeter 1941) and enclose the yolk sac. The ectoderm covering the floor of the amniotic cavity and the endoderm forming the roof of the yolk sac, together in apposition, establish the bilaminar embryonic disc (Fig. 1.2c). A projection of the yolk sac endoderm into the extraembryonic mesoderm forms the allantoic diverticulum, which identifies the caudal end of the bilaminar embryonic disc and the site of the body stalk (Fig 1.2d).

Carnegie stage 6: days 13–15; approx. size 0.2 mm

The primitive streak (Fig. 1.3a) is formed and lies caudally in the midline of the embryonic disc (Heuser & Streeter 1941). The primitive streak subsequently generates intraembryonic mesoderm, which migrates through the bilaminar embryonic disc, in the plane between ectoderm and endoderm (Fig. 1.3b), converting it into a trilaminar disc. The disc remains bilaminar at the caudal and rostral ends. The caudal end forms the cloacal membrane.

Carnegie stage 8: approx. days 17–19; approx. length 1.0–1.5 mm

The primordial germ cells, which are the antecedents of the male and female gametes, are present in the endoderm around the allantoic diverticulum (now a ventral outpouching of the hindgut) and are usually seen in the 17–20 day embryo (Jirasek 1977), although Hertig et al. (1958) identified possible primordial germ cells in a younger 13 day embryo. The primordial germ cells are ectodermal in origin,

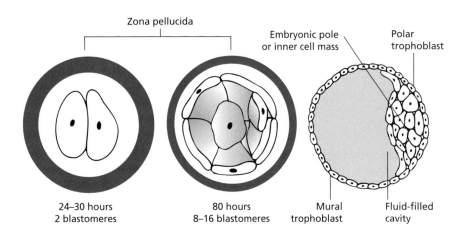

Fig. 1.1 The conceptus is enclosed within an acellular envelope, the zona pellucida. After the formation of the blastocyst and dissolution of the zona pellucida, the characteristic fluid-filled cavity, the embryonic pole or inner cell mass and the mural trophoblast can be identified.

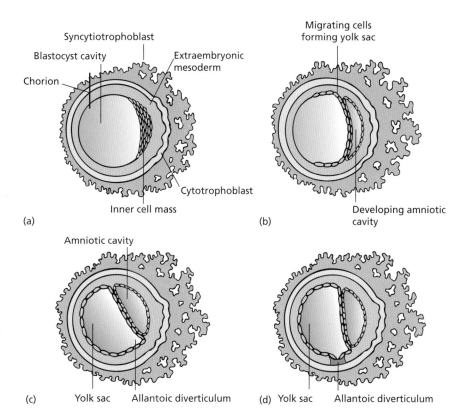

(a)

(b)

Syncytiotrophoblast
Blastocyst cavity
Chorion
Extraembryonic mesoderm
Cytotrophoblast
Inner cell mass

Migrating cells forming yolk sac
Developing amniotic cavity

Amniotic cavity

(c)   Yolk sac   Allantoic diverticulum

(d)   Yolk sac   Allantoic diverticulum

Fig. 1.2 The conceptus continues to differentiate, forming (a) the chorion, (b) the amniotic cavity and (c) the yolk sac. The area of contact between the amniotic cavity and yolk sac is the bilaminar embryonic disc. (d) Projection of yolk sac endoderm into the mesoderm to form the allantoic diverticulum.

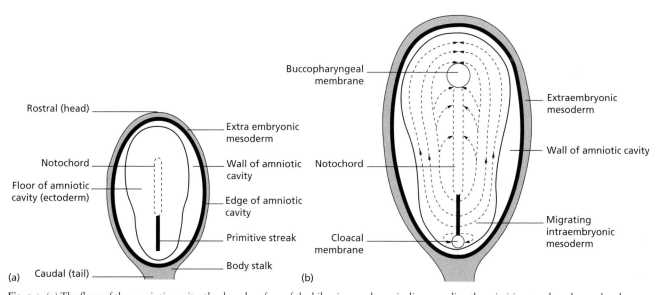

Rostral (head)
Notochord
Floor of amniotic cavity (ectoderm)
Caudal (tail)

Extra embryonic mesoderm
Wall of amniotic cavity
Edge of amniotic cavity
Primitive streak
Body stalk

(a)

Buccopharyngeal membrane
Notochord
Cloacal membrane

Extraembryonic mesoderm
Wall of amniotic cavity
Migrating intraembryonic mesoderm

(b)

Fig. 1.3 (a) The floor of the amniotic cavity, the dorsal surface of the bilaminar embryonic disc, revealing the primitive streak and notochord. (b) Intraembryonic mesoderm, generated by the primitive streak and interposed between the floor of the amniotic cavity and roof of the yolk sac, converts the bilaminar embryonic disc into a trilaminar disc. The buccopharyngeal and cloacal membranes remain bilaminar.

having migrated to the allantoic diverticulum from the epiblast, and they retain two functional X chromosomes in contrast to the somatic cells, which possess only one functional X chromosome (Lyon 1974). From here, they migrate through the mesoderm surrounding the hindgut and into the dorsal mesentery (Hardisty 1978). Their final destination is the medial aspect of the intermediate mesoderm adjacent to the mesonephros, the gonadal ridge, and they begin to reach this area in the human embryo at 35 days (Jirasek 1971) (Fig. 1.4). The primordial germ cells

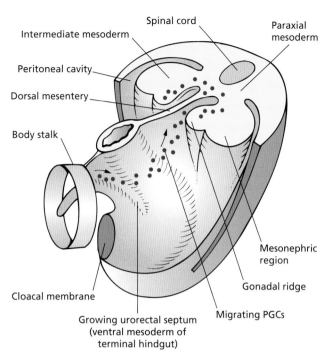

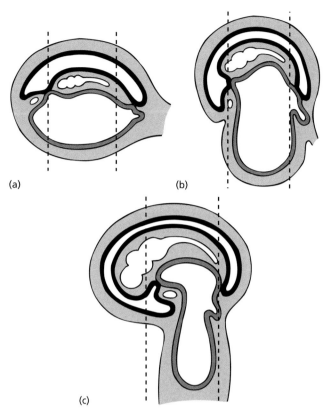

Fig. 1.4 Migration of primordial germ cells (PGCs) into the genital ridge from the body stalk.

Fig. 1.5 (a) As the neural tube is enclosed within the intraembryonic mesoderm it lengthens, and expands rostrally, causing a dorsal convexity and ventral concavity. (b) Further growth of the neural tube increases this curvature in the longitudinal plane, (c) with the eventual formation of the head and tail folds.

migrate to an area known as the indifferent gonad until gonadal sex is established.

Carnegie stage 9: days 19–21; approx. length 1.5–2.0 mm

The neural plate and the longitudinally running neural ridges develop. The embryo undergoes a process of flexion to accommodate the neural tube (Fig. 1.5a–c), and in so doing reorientates the primitive embryonic tissues and their relationship to each other. The endoderm of the dorsal part of the yolk sac is drawn into the ventral concavity of the embryo and is subdivided into foregut, midgut and hindgut (Fig. 1.6a,b). The hindgut appears about the 20th post-ovulatory day and is enclosed within the tail fold of the embryo. In this situation, the hindgut lies caudal to the rostral limit of the allantoic diverticulum and dorsal and rostral to the cloacal membrane. The mesoderm in the mid-embryo region is divided into paraxial, lateral and inter-mediate mesoderm. The paraxial mesoderm surrounds the neural tube and the intermediate mesoderm lies ventrally and lateral to the paraxial mesoderm. The intermediate mesoderm differentiates medially into the gonadal ridge and laterally into the mesonephric region (Fig. 1.7). The intermediate mesoderm at the rostral limit of the allantoic diverticulum extends dorsally then caudally, in line with the curvature of the tail fold, dividing the hindgut into ventral and dorsal parts. As this division proceeds, the two parts of the hindgut remain in continuity with each other caudal

to the advancing mesoderm of the urorectal septum. The caudal end of the hindgut is lined with endoderm and is known as the cloaca. On the ventral aspect of the cloaca there is a membrane which separates the endoderm from the surface ectoderm, the *cloacal membrane*. As development continues a mesenchymal septum, the *urogenital septum*, migrates caudally (Fig. 1.8a–c).

Carnegie stage 11: days 23–25; approx. length 2.5–3.0 mm

At day 24, when the embryo flexion has been completed, the anterior limit of the extensive cloacal membrane abuts on the base of the umbilical cord. On either side of the cloaca are the paired primordia of the genital tubercle (Fig. 1.9a).

Over the next few days the cloaca retracts from the umbilical cord to form an anterior wall and the two primordia of the genital tubercle fuse. Posterior to the tubercle and running laterally by the sides of the cloacal membrane are the cloacal folds, and lateral to these are the genital swellings (Fig. 1.9b).

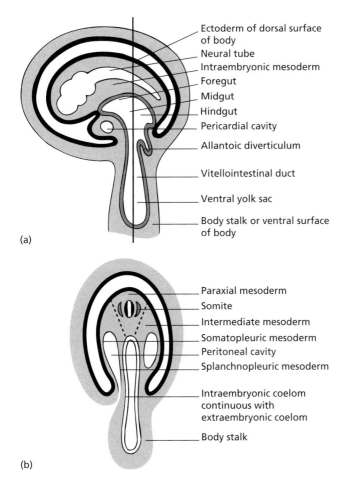

(a)

- Ectoderm of dorsal surface of body
- Neural tube
- Intraembryonic mesoderm
- Foregut
- Midgut
- Hindgut
- Pericardial cavity
- Allantoic diverticulum
- Vitellointestinal duct
- Ventral yolk sac
- Body stalk or ventral surface of body

(b)

- Paraxial mesoderm
- Somite
- Intermediate mesoderm
- Somatopleuric mesoderm
- Peritoneal cavity
- Splanchnopleuric mesoderm
- Intraembryonic coelom continuous with extraembryonic coelom
- Body stalk

Fig. 1.6 (a) Midline section of the embryo after formation of the head and tail folds. (b) A transverse section of the mid-embryo region after formation of the lateral folds.

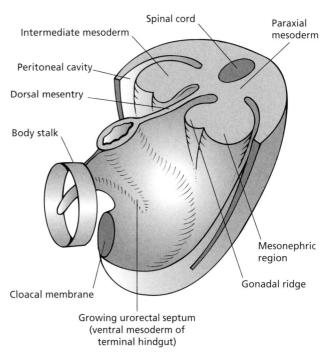

- Spinal cord
- Intermediate mesoderm
- Paraxial mesoderm
- Peritoneal cavity
- Dorsal mesentry
- Body stalk
- Mesonephric region
- Cloacal membrane
- Gonadal ridge
- Growing urorectal septum (ventral mesoderm of terminal hindgut)

Fig. 1.7 The caudal half of the embryo showing the gonadal ridge and mesonephric region of the intermediate mesoderm, which, at its caudal limit, is continuous with the mesoderm investing the hindgut.

Carnegie stages 13 and 14: days 28–35; approx. length 4–7 mm

The urogenital septum reaches the cloacal membrane at 30–32 days (O'Rahilly 1977) and fuses with the cloacal membrane, dividing the embryonic hindgut into the ventral (anterior) urogenital sinus and dorsal (posterior) rectum. Failure of the urogenital septum to reach the cloacal membrane leaves the urethra, vagina and rectum converging into a single channel with a solitary opening on to the perineum.

The cloacal membrane is also divided, the ventral part forming the urogenital membrane and the dorsal part forming the anal membrane. The cloacal membrane will ultimately rupture to form the urogenital and anal orifices. The genital folds develop from the anterior part of the cloacal folds and the anal folds form the posterior component (Fig. 1.9c).

At the same time as the cloaca divides, the two primitive gonadal streaks are proliferating. At the ventral tip of the cloacal membrane, each forms a genital tubercle. The two genital tubercles proliferate further and need to reach a critical mass otherwise only rudimentary structures will be formed. The two tubercles then fuse to form the glans of the clitoris. Labioscrotal swellings and urogenital folds develop on each side of the cloacal membrane. As the urogenital septum reaches the cloacal membrane the labioscrotal folds fuse posteriorly, forming the perineal body which separates the urogenital membrane from the anal membrane. The sexual differentiation at this stage is still indeterminate and remains so until 63–77 days.

Carnegie stages 15 and 16: days 35–42; approx. length 7–11 mm

At 30–32 days cells from cephalic mesonephric vesicles invade the coelomic epithelium on the medial aspect of the adjacent intermediate mesoderm to induce the formation of the indifferent gonad (Wartenberg 1982). At 35 days the indifferent gonad begins to develop on the medial aspect of the mesonephros by the invasion of three other cell types: the primordial germ cells, cells from the overlying coelomic epithelium and the cells from the adjacent mesonephros. All cell types are probably essential to the proper differentiation of the gonad (Byskov 1981).

The paramesonephric ducts (Mullerian ducts) appear at about 40 days. The precursor of each paramesonephric duct extends caudally as a solid rod of cells in the intermediate mesoderm, in close association with, and initially lateral to, the mesonephric (Wolffian) duct. The mesonephric

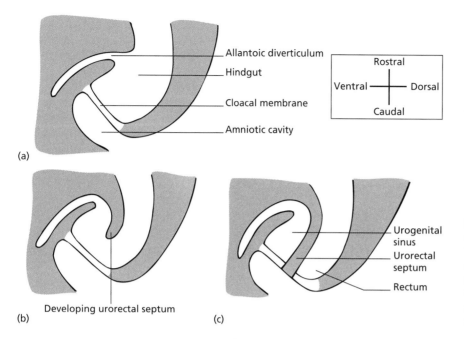

Allantoic diverticulum
Hindgut
Cloacal membrane
Amniotic cavity

	Rostral	
Ventral		Dorsal
	Caudal	

(a)

Developing urorectal septum

(b)

Urogenital sinus
Urorectal septum
Rectum

(c)

Fig. 1.8 (a) The primitive hindgut is enclosed within the embryonic tail fold. (b) The developing urorectal septum grows dorsally and caudally from the rostral limit of the allantoic diverticulum. (c) The fusion of the urorectal septum with the cloacal membrane divides the hindgut into urogenital sinus and rectum.

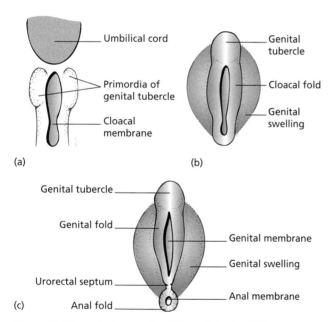

Umbilical cord
Primordia of genital tubercle
Cloacal membrane

(a)

Genital tubercle
Cloacal fold
Genital swelling

(b)

Genital tubercle
Genital fold
Urorectal septum
Anal fold
Genital membrane
Genital swelling
Anal membrane

(c)

Fig. 1.9 (a) The paired primordia of the genital tubercle lie immediately caudal to the umbilical cord. (b) Migration of tissue towards the midline from both sides separates the umbilical cord and cloacal membrane, causes fusion of the primordia to form a midline genital tubercle and establishes bilateral cloacal folds and genital swellings. (c) Fusion of the urorectal septum with the cloacal membrane separates an anterior genital region from a posterior anal region.

duct has been shown experimentally both to induce the paramesonephric duct (Didier 1973a,b) and to guide its descent (Gruenwald 1941). The growing caudal tip of the paramesonephric duct lies within the basement membrane of the mesonephric duct (Frutiger 1969). As they descend, the paramesonephric ducts pass ventral to the mesonephric ducts and, coming into close association with one another, reach the posterior aspect of the urogenital sinus within the urorectal septum (Fig. 1.10). The two paramesonephric ducts begin to fuse even before their growing ends reach the urogenital sinus (Koff 1933). As the urorectal septum reaches the cloacal membrane at 30–32 days the caudal end of the mesonephric duct, having already opened into the urogenital sinus, gives origin to the ureteric bud and begins to be incorporated into the posterior wall of the urogenital sinus (Keith 1948). The portion of each duct incorporated into the urogenital sinus subsequently forms the trigone of the bladder and the posterior wall of the urethra (Fig. 1.11a–d). At 42 days post ovulation there are 300–1300 primordial germ cells within the indifferent gonads destined to become either spermatogonia or oogonia. The close association between the gonad and adrenal at this early stage of development can result in adrenal cells being sequestered in the gonad and maintaining their function in the mature ovary or testis (Grumbach & Conte 1992).

Carnegie stages 17 and 18: days 43–48; approx. length 13–17 mm

The transformation of the indifferent gonad into an embryonic testis occurs in the 43–49 day embryo.

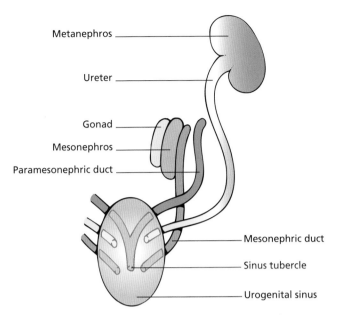

Fig. 1.10 The indifferent human embryo possesses mesonephric and paramesonephric ducts. The terminal paramesonephric ducts fuse within the urorectal septum and reach the urogenital sinus at the sinus tubercle situated between the openings of the two mesonephric ducts.

Carnegie stage 19: days 48–51; approx. length 16–18 mm

The mesonephric ducts terminate in the urogenital sinus on either side of the sinus tubercle at 49 days. At the rostral end of the sinus tubercle, the urogenital sinus is referred to as the vesicourethral canal and from it arise the bladder and the whole of the female urethra (Jirasek 1977). The portion of the urogenital sinus caudal to the sinus tubercle continues to be referred to as the urogenital sinus and is subdivided into pelvic and phallic portions.

Carnegie stage 20: days 51–53; approx. length 18–22 mm

The development of the indifferent gonad into an embryonic ovary occurs gradually in the 45–55 day embryo (Jirasek 1977).

Carnegie stage 23: days 56–60; approx. length 27–31 mm

At this stage the external genital primordium has developed, which is still indeterminate.

End of the female embryonic period

At the end of the embryonic period, the fetus has gonads that are recognizable as ovaries, but still has indifferent external genitalia and both mesonephric and paramesonephric duct systems are still present. Subsequent sexual differentiation of these ducts in the female develops because of a lack of anti-Mullerian hormone. The mesonephric ducts (Wolffian ducts) degenerate but occasionally remnants may be left behind. A remnant of the cephalic mesonephric duct and adjacent vesicles is a constant finding associated with the ovary (Duthie 1925). A more caudal portion of the mesonephros may be encountered in the broad ligament as the paroophoron, while remnants of the terminal mesonephric duct may persist lateral to the uterus and vagina or are incorporated into the cervix (O'Rahilly 1977, Buntine 1979). Remnants of this duct found adjacent to the lower genital tract are referred to as Gartner's ducts.

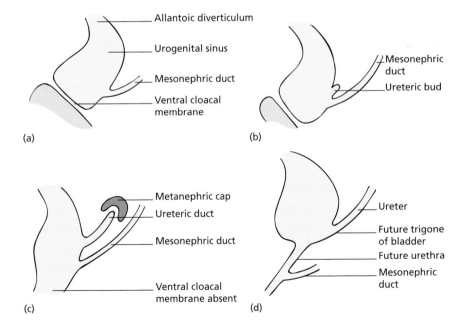

Fig. 1.11 (a) The mesonephric duct, within the urorectal septum, opens into the urogenital sinus. (b) The caudal limit of the mesonephric duct gives origin to the ureteric bud. (c) The metanephric cap forms at the growing end of the ureteric bud or duct. (d) The mesonephric duct gives origin to the ureter and forms the trigone of the bladder and the posterior wall of the urethra.

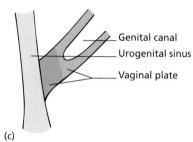

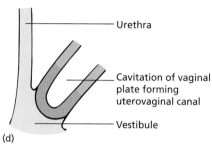

(a)   (b)

(c)   (d)

Fig. 1.12 (a) The fused paramesonephric ducts form the genital canal, the solid caudal end of which abuts on the posterior wall of the urogenital sinus at the sinus tubercle. (b) Cellular proliferation of the sinus epithelium generates the sinuvaginal bulbs, which displace the genital canal dorsally. (c) Further cellular proliferation converts the sinuvaginal bulbs into solid tissue projections, which participate in the formation of the vaginal plate. (d) Extensive caudal growth of the vaginal plate brings its lower surface into the primitive vestibule.

The fallopian tubes develop from upper unfused portions of the paramesonephric ducts and the uterus and vagina from the lower fused portion (Fig. 1.12a). The arrival of the caudal end of the genital canal on the urogenital sinus stimulates cellular proliferation of the sinus epithelium to form three projections (sinuvaginal bulbs) that displace the genital canal dorsally (Fig. 1.12b). Failure of these bulbs to develop results in vaginal agenesis. These sinuvaginal bulbs become solid and together with the solid end of the genital canal form the vaginal plate, which is complete at 19 weeks (Fig. 1.12c). The sinuvaginal bulbs later fuse, but eventually undergo apoptosis to form a lumen. Some time between 14 weeks (Terruhn 1980) and 20 weeks (O'Rahilly 1977) the vagina opens into the pelvic portion of the urogenital sinus converting it into the vaginal vestibule (Fig. 1.12d).

Further feminization of the external genitalia begins be-tween 63 and 77 days, when the genital tubercle lengthens to form the phallus. This then bends caudally to form the glans. During this period the anogenital distance remains unchanged, there is no fusion of the genital folds and the urogenital sinus remains open. The urethral and vaginal openings separate later. The phallus becomes the clitoris, being incorporated within the fused anterior ends of the genital folds, which develop into the labia minora. The genital swellings, lateral to the labia minora, become the labia majora and are continuous with the future mons pubis. The labia minora develop from the genital folds and divide anteriorly into the prepuce and frenulum of the clitoris (Fig. 1.13).

Development of the epithelia
The epidermis of the vulval skin and its appendages – hair

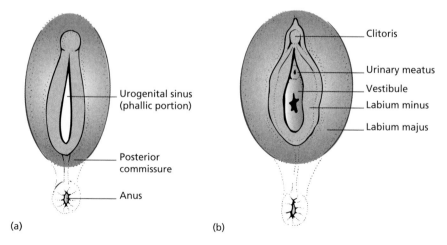

(a)   (b)

Fig. 1.13 (a) The genital and anal membranes rupture. (b) In the female fetus the urogenital sinus remains open as caudal growth of the vaginal plate brings the urethral and vaginal openings into this region converting it into the vestibule.

and sebaceous and sudoriferous glands – is developed from ectoderm. The dermis is developed from mesoderm.

The primitive epidermis is established about the eighth day when ectoderm differentiates within the developing embryo. At this stage the epidermis is a single layer of cells, but over the ensuing 3 weeks specific features develop that set it apart from other epithelia in the body. A second outer layer develops – the periderm – beneath which the primitive epidermis begins the process of stratification. Keratinization occurs at the end of the sixth month, and the periderm is sloughed into the amniotic fluid (Lind *et al.* 1969). Cells that are shed from the stratum corneum combine with sebaceous secretions to form the vernix, which makes the embryo impervious to the amniotic fluid and persists until birth (O'Rahilly & Muller 1992).

Three cell types invade the developing epidermis during the first 6 months of intrauterine life. Melanocytes, derived from neural crests (Niebauer 1968), and Langerhans cells, derived from mesoderm (Breathnach & Wyllie 1965), are present at the end of the third month, while Merkel cells, the origin of which is uncertain, are present by the sixth month (Breathnach 1971).

The dermal–epidermal junction is flat in all parts of the body until hair and glandular primordia reach the dermis. Primary vellus hair follicles begin to form during the third month of gestation and the process proceeds in a cephalocaudal manner. Secondary follicles form in close association with the primary follicles and it is thought that the full complement of hair follicles is present at birth.

Sebaceous glands arise as buds mostly from the hair follicles (O'Rahilly & Muller 1992). They begin to appear during the fourth month and differentiate into sebum-producing cells rapidly. The development and function of sebaceous glands before birth and in the neonatal period is thought to be regulated by maternal androgens and endogenous fetal steroids. At birth the glands are large and well developed over the entire body and display the same regional variation in size as is seen in the adult. Postnatally they involute and remain quiescent until puberty.

Eccrine sweat glands appear during the third month of prenatal life and their ducts are open to the skin surface by the sixth month. The premature infant usually shows an absent or limited sweating response (Sinclair 1972), even though the glands are innervated as soon as they develop. The number of sweat glands, like hair follicles, seems to be complete at birth.

Apocrine development occurs at 6 months of intrauterine life and it has been suggested that their primordia develop in association with each hair follicle but regress in all areas except the areola, axilla, scalp, eyelids, external auditory meatus, umbilicus and anogenital region (Serri *et al.* 1962, Hashimoto 1970). The glandular activity begins during the last trimester but ceases soon after birth, and begins again at puberty.

The dermis originates from the mesoderm in the second month of embryonic life. The mesodermal cells form fibroblasts, macrophages, melanoblasts and mast cells and the matrix is composed of collagen and elastin. The organization of the dermis is progressive throughout gestation and is not complete until some months after birth.

Ambiguous external genitalia

If a female fetus is exposed to significant androgen levels before 84–98 days, complete external virilization will occur at the end of this period of development. Lower levels of testosterone or exposure later will produce variations of incomplete virilization (Grumbach and Ducharme 1960). The sex of the newborn is ascertained from the appearance of the external genitalia but occasionally this may not be possible as the phenotypical appearance may not be characteristic of either male or female.

Classification of these abnormalities has been based on anatomical and aetiological mechanisms. The classification used in this chapter is one based on aetiological mechanisms and clinical syndromes. It is adapted from Grumbach and Conte (1992) and Simpson (1982):
1 disorders of gonadal differentiation
2 female pseudohermaphrodite
3 male pseudohermaphrodite.

Almost all of the affected infants have some degree of phallic enlargement with a small opening for voiding urine on the ventral surface, at its base or on the perineum. A second opening or depression may be identified more posteriorly, while on either side of the midline there is some virilization, ranging from rugose labia majora-like structures to scrotal sacs (Dewhurst 1980).

It is now recognised that there is a need for a reappraisal of these classifications as advances are made in molecular genetics. There are also ethical issues to be considered as well as patient opinion. (Dreger *et al.* 2005, Hughes 2006). Terms such as intersex and hermaphrodite are unacceptable to the patients and can be confusing for the clinician. The new nomenclature proposed would use Disorders of Sex Development in place of intersex and the term hermaphrodite would be dropped completely.

Disorders of gonadal differentiation

Ovarian dysgenesis
Approximately 50% of all patients with ovarian dysgenesis have a chromosomal complement of 45X; a further 25% have sex chromosomal mosaicism without a structural chromosomal abnormality (45X/46XX; 45X/46XY) while

the remainder have either a structurally abnormal X or Y chromosome or no detectable chromosomal abnormality (Simpson 1982).

45X Turner's syndrome
Only a small number of 45X embryos survive intrauterine life (Boue *et al.* 1975, Cockwell *et al.* 1991). Individuals with this karyotype have germ cells which rarely survive meiosis, follicular formation usually fails and the resulting streak gonads are sterile and devoid of endocrine activity (Carr *et al.* 1968). At birth, the genital ducts and external genitalia are entirely female, although clitoral enlargement may occasionally be present (Grumbach & Conte 1992). The ovaries, located in their normal anatomical positions, consist mainly of fibrous stroma and are termed streak gonads. However, almost 25% of girls with Turner's syndrome show some secondary sexual development, 2–5% have spontaneous menses owing to some residual ovarian function (Saenger 1996), and, rarely, they bear children (King *et al.* 1978, Kohn *et al.* 1980). Patients with Turner's syndrome are of short stature and exhibit a range of somatic abnormalities including webbing of the neck, coarctation of the aorta and renal anomalies. Also associated with the condition is a predisposition to develop diabetes mellitus (Engel & Forbes 1965) and other autoimmune diseases, particularly those affecting the thyroid (Elsheikh *et al.* 2001).

45X/46XX mosaicism and X chromosome abnormality
This form of mosaicism is the most common cause of ovarian dysgenesis after Turner's syndrome. One gonad may be of the streak type and the contralateral gonad a normal or hypoplastic ovary; alternatively, both ovaries may be either normal or hypoplastic (Grumbach & Conte 1992). There are fewer of the somatic abnormalities associated with Turner's syndrome, the phenotype is invariably female and some may menstruate and even be fertile.

45X/46XY mosaicism and Y chromosome abnormality
A highly diverse phenotype is encountered in 45X/46XY mosaicism since the presence of a Y-bearing cell line may induce some testicular differentiation. Such individuals may appear typically male or female or may possess ambiguous external genitalia with varied genital duct development. In a series of 60 patients with 45X/46XY mosaicism, two-thirds were reared as females (Zah *et al.* 1975). Several cases of structural abnormality of the Y chromosome have been reported (Davis 1981); the affected individuals are phenotypically female with bilateral streak gonads.

46XX, 46XY
Gonadal dysgenesis may occur in association with apparently normal 46XX or 46XY karyotypes. These individuals are phenotypically female with streak gonads and remain sexually immature. The 46XX form of gonadal dysgenesis appears to be inherited as an autosomal recessive condition and may occur in association with neurosensory deafness, which may also affect otherwise normal male siblings (Pallister & Opitz 1979). The 46XY form of gonadal dysgenesis is again a genetically heterogeneous syndrome, being associated with deletions and/or mutations involving the Y chromosome (Blagowidow *et al.* 1989) and/or the X chromosome (Scherer *et al.* 1989). Clitoral enlargement is not uncommon, but the most important aspect of this condition is the increased incidence of gonadal neoplasms (Simpson 1982). Bilateral gonadectomy is therefore indicated as a prophylactic measure (Dewhurst 1980, Grumbach & Conte 1992). In all forms of ovarian dysgenesis oestrogen replacement therapy is recommended at 12–13 years of age, eventually to be cycled monthly with progesterone (Grumbach & Conte 1992).

Pure gonadal dysgenesis
These patients have a 46XY karyotype but do not possess any gonadal tissue. The condition, variously termed the 'XY gonadal agenesis syndrome' (Sarto & Opitz 1973) or the 'testicular regression syndrome' (Coulam 1979), is characterized by the presence of ambiguous genitalia in association with hypoplastic Mullerian and Wolffian derivatives. A small phallus, ill-developed labia majora and fusion of the labioscrotal folds are features of the external genital appearance (Sarto & Opitz 1973).

True hermaphroditism
True hermaphrodites possess both ovarian and testicular tissue, with an ovary on one side and a testis on the other or, more commonly, with ovotestes situated bilaterally or unilaterally (Grumbach & Conte 1992). The differentiation of the genital tract, the appearance of the external genitalia and the development of secondary sexual characteristics are all variable. The external genitalia are often ambiguous and three-quarters of reported cases have been reared as males because of the size of the phallus (van Niekerk 1976). The majority of the gonads present have oocytes but not spermatozoa, a uterus is almost invariably present and 60% of them have a 46XX karyotype. Four 46XX true hermaphrodites have become pregnant (Tegenkamp *et al.* 1979). In one review (van Niekerk 1976), the remaining 40% of true hermaphrodites were equally distributed between 46XY karyotypes, 46XX/46XY chimeras and sex-chromosome mosaics.

Female pseudohermaphroditism
The chromosomal makeup is 46XX with the ovaries and Mullerian duct derivatives as normal. The external genitalia are abnormal. The clitoris is enlarged, variable degrees of

labial fusion are seen and the urethral opening may not be distinct from the vagina. The external genitalia of the male fetus are completely masculinized by 84–98 days (Jirasek 1977). If a female fetus is exposed to significant androgen levels, in the presence of 5α-reductase, before the end of this period of development, complete virilization will occur (Grumbach & Ducharme 1960). Lower levels or later exposure will produce various forms of incomplete virilization. The source of the virilizing influence may be fetal, maternal or exogenous.

Fetal androgens

Since the adrenal glands begin to function during the third month of intrauterine life, excessive production of adrenal androgens will virilize the fetal female external genitalia. CAH accounts for most of the cases of female pseudohermaphroditism and approximately half of all patients with ambiguous external genitalia. There are several types of CAH and all are transmitted as an autosomal recessive trait (Laue & Rennert 1995). The first, caused by 21-hydroxylase deficiency or 11β-hydroxylase deficiency, limits cortisol production and leads to adrenal overproduction of androgens and their precursors. The second, caused by 3β-ol-dehydrogenase deficiency or 17α-hydroxylase deficiency, reduces cortisol production and also impairs the synthesis of sex steroids by the gonads and adrenals. With 3β-ol-dehydrogenase deficiency the only androgen synthesized is dehydroepiandrosterone (DHEA), which is relatively weak, and females with this deficiency are less virilized than females with 21- or 11β-hydroxylase deficiencies. In 17α-hydroxylase deficiency the female external genitalia are normal at birth but no secondary sexual development occurs at puberty (Simpson 1982).

Maternal androgens

In rare instances, virilization of the female fetus may occur if the mother has certain ovarian or adrenal tumours or if she has unrecognized CAH. The absence of virilization in the mother does not exclude a maternal source of androgens since the level of androgen required to virilize the external genitalia of the early female fetus is much less than would be required to have a virilizing effect on the adult female (Kai et al. 1979).

Exogenous androgens

Virilization of the external genitalia of female infants has been frequently observed following maternal ingestion of testosterone or synthetic progestational agents during the first trimester of pregnancy (Grumbach & Ducharme 1960, Wilkins 1960, Dewhurst & Gordon 1984, Reschini et al. 1985). Administration of such agents between the eighth and 12th week of gestation causes marked virilization, while later in pregnancy their use causes clitoral enlargement.

These agents, as well as stilboestrol, were often prescribed in the past for women with habitual or threatened abortion. Exposure to stilboestrol during intrauterine life is known to cause malformations in the reproductive tracts of both sexes and an increased incidence of cervical and vaginal neoplasia (Herbst et al. 1972, 1974), and it has also been shown to cause female pseudohermaphroditism (Bongiovani et al. 1959). Intrauterine exposure to danazol, used in the treatment of endometriosis, has also been associated with the occurrence of female pseudohermaphroditism (Rosa 1984, Shaw & Farquhar 1984).

Maternal cocaine use during pregnancy has been associated with ambiguous genitalia in both male and female infants, as well as other congenital malformations (Chasnoff et al. 1988).

Structural defects

Lower reproductive tract

Vaginal agenesis

This is the absence of a vagina and occurs in female pseudohermaphroditism and in some cases of 46XX females. Total vaginal agenesis is usually found in association with tubal and uterine agenesis, but occasionally the upper reproductive tract is normal because there has been only a partial Mullerian defect or the vaginal plate has failed to form or cavitate. In a survey of 167 women with total vaginal agenesis, one-third had associated renal tract defects while others had skeletal abnormalities (Evans et al. 1981). The Rokitansky–Kuster–Hauser syndrome (Simpson 1982) describes cases of vaginal agenesis in which there is a very shallow vagina associated with a rudimentary upper reproductive tract.

Vaginal atresia

In this condition the urogenital sinus fails to form the inferior portion of the vagina. The lower vagina is replaced by fibrous tissue above which there is a normal reproductive tract (Simpson 1976).

Vaginal septa

Transverse vaginal septa are said to be located at the junction of the upper one-third and lower two-thirds of the vagina (Simpson 1976). The probable cause of transverse vaginal septa formation is the failure of either the Mullerian or urogenital sinus contributions to the vagina to cavitate completely so the septa can occur at any level. In the Amish community this abnormality is inherited as an autosomal recessive trait (McKusick et al. 1964). Patients with transverse vaginal septa may present at puberty with retained menstrual products or alternatively with a continuous vaginal discharge.

A longitudinal vaginal septum may present in the midline as the result of a fusion defect in the Mullerian system and will be associated with abnormalities of the upper reproductive tract.

Imperforate hymen

This is commonly caused by the failure of the central epithelial cells of the hymenal membrane to degenerate. However, this condition may arise as the result of an inflammatory reaction in the hymen after birth. Presentation is usually at puberty with a haematocolpos.

Vaginal cysts

In the neonatal period vaginal cysts may be found in the anterior or lateral walls of the vagina at the introitus and usually rupture spontaneously (Warkany 1971). Occasionally, one or more of these may enlarge and obstruct the urethra. They are thought to be inclusions from the urogenital sinus epithelium and may persist asymptomatically into adulthood (Robboy et al. 1978). Mucous cysts are found in the same location, interior to the labia minora and external to the hymen, in about 3% of adults attending a vulval clinic (Friedrich & Wilkinson 1973). In addition, the Wolffian ducts, which degenerate in the female, leave caudal remnants in the lateral walls of the vagina. These remnants may undergo cystic degeneration, when they are termed Gartner's cysts.

External genitalia

As detailed above, various abnormalities of the vulva are caused by disturbances of sexual differentiation, which lead to an ambiguous appearance of the external genitalia. Other vulval defects, such as duplication, occur in association with abnormalities of the upper reproductive tract and urinary system. Congenital anomalies of the vulva that occur in isolation involve the clitoris and the labia.

Clitoris

The clitoris may be absent (Falk & Hyman 1971), probably as a result of the genital tubercles remaining hypoplastic or failing to fuse. Enlargement occurs in the rare genetically determined condition of lipoatrophic diabetes (Lawrence–Seip syndrome) (Burton & Cunliffe 1992).

Labia minora

Hypertrophy and/or marked asymmetry of the labia minora may occur without any underlying problem but in rare instances it may be a manifestation of neurofibromatosis (Friedrich & Wilkinson 1985). True hypoplasia of the labia minora occurs infrequently, and may be a sign of defective steroidogenesis. Fusion of the labia minora may occur in association with defective sexual differentiation. This should not be confused with the superficial labial adhesions seen in the neonatal period or in infancy as a result of an inflammatory condition (see Chapter 5).

Vulval and urinary system abnormalities

Kidney

Bilateral renal agenesis is a lethal congenital malformation (Potter 1946), and in the female is frequently associated with anomalies of the external genitalia, absence of the uterus and vagina and abnormalities of other systems (Potter 1965). Unilateral renal agenesis may be associated with malformation of the external genitalia. The incidence of genital anomalies in unilateral renal agenesis is about 40% in females and 12% in males (Warkany 1971).

Ureter

The ureteric bud arises from the Wolffian (mesonephric) duct and separates off when the duct is incorporated into the urogenital sinus to form the trigone of the bladder and urethra. Failure of dissociation between the ureteric bud and Wolffian duct in the female will allow the ureteric orifice to be located at any site along the caudal remnant of the Wolffian duct (Gartner's duct). Secondary rupture of Gartner's duct into the vagina (Weiss et al. 1984) allows for vaginal drainage of urine from the ectopic ureter.

Bladder

Exstrophy of the bladder is caused by a failure of the sub-umbilical portion of the anterior abdominal wall to meet in the midline above the genital tubercles. The genital tubercles remain as paired primordia and the anterior wall of the bladder is either partially or totally absent. This condition may therefore exist as incomplete or complete bladder exstrophy and is always associated with epispadias and other abnormalities of the external genitalia. A more severe form of this structural defect is cloacal exstrophy, in which the urorectal septum fails to divide the hindgut, and the abdominal wall deficit gives access not only to the bladder but also to the terminal gastrointestinal tract (Diamond & Jeffs 1985). Repairing the abdominal defect is possible but the refashioning of the external genitalia must take into account the chromosomal and gonadal sex of the infant (Dewhurst 1980).

Urethra

Congenital abnormalities of the urethra have a much lower incidence in females than in males. Duplication of the urethra is a cause of urinary incontinence in the female. The accessory urethra usually arises from the trigone of the bladder and opens onto the anterior wall of the vagina. Mild forms of epispadias may occur in the female giving rise to disturbance of bladder control and urinary incontinence. In this condition the urethral opening lies deep to the mons between two clitoral elements. Hypospadias in the female occurs in association with female pseudohermaphroditism. In both epispadias and hypospadias, the female urethra is congenitally short (Burbige & Hensle 1985). Meatal stenosis is uncommon in the female but may simulate bladder neck obstruction (Warkany 1971). Prolapse of urethral mucosa occurs only in the female (Capraro *et al.* 1970). Urethral cysts may develop in the Skene's glands which open at the termination of the urethra and may be the cause of recurrent urinary symptoms. Finally, an ectopic ureter may open into the urethra. Any of these urethral abnormalities may present with urinary incontinence, which may cause an irritant contact vulval dermatitis.

Vulval and intestinal abnormalities

In the female an imperforate anus or anal stenosis may be associated with a variety of abnormalities of the genital tract and vulva (Hall *et al.* 1985). An ectopic opening of the lower gastrointestinal tract may be found in the vagina or elsewhere in the perineum. When a rectovaginal fistula is formed there are often urinary tract abnormalities present as well.

Vulval mammary tissue

Originally it was believed that mammary tissue found in the vulva was a result of incomplete atresia of the mammary ridges. It is now thought that the mammary tissue is in fact mammary-like anogenital glands (van der Putte 1994, van der Putte & van Group 1995). However there are rare reports of ectopic mammary glands with associated nipples occurring in the vulva (Green 1936).

Anatomy

The vulva is situated within the perineum, which is the outer area inferior to the sheet of muscle forming the pelvic floor. The perineum is an embryological junctional zone derived from the body wall ectoderm, hindgut endoderm and the intervening mesoderm that surrounded the original cloacal membrane. The perineum furthermore is divided into an anterior urogenital triangle and posterior anal triangle. The vulva lies mainly within the anterior urogenital triangle but extends anteriorly to the pubic symphysis. The anal canal and ischiorectal fossa occupy the posterior anal triangle. The perineal body is a fibromuscular mass which in the female lies between the upper half of the anterior anal wall and the entire posterior portion of the vagina. It is thicker in the female than in the male.

The vulva consists of the mons pubis, the labia majora and minora, the vestibule of the vagina, the hymen, the clitoris and the external urethral orifice (Fig. 1.14).

Mons pubis

The mons pubis (mons) in the adult female is a prominent pad of hair-bearing skin and subcutaneous fat overlying the pubic symphysis. The character of pubic hair varies with ethnic background and age, but its distribution rarely extends more than 2 cm beyond the upper limit of the genitofemoral folds (Lunde 1984). This pattern of distribution produces the horizontal upper margin of female pubic hair.

Arterial supply   Superficial external pudendal artery which is a branch of the femoral artery.
Venous drainage   Via the pudendal veins to the long saphenous.

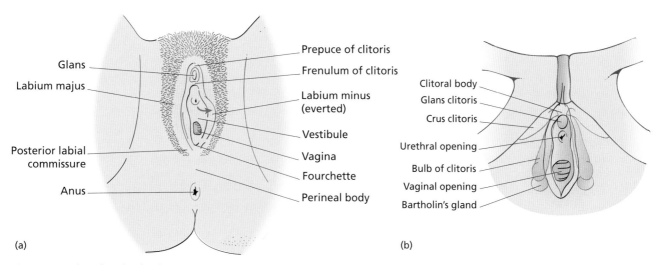

(a)

(b)

Fig. 1.14 (a) The vulva. (b) The clitoris.

Nerve supply   Branches of the perineal nerve.
Lymph drainage   To superficial inguinal nodes and then
                   to deep femoral nodes and pelvic nodes.

Labia majora

The labia majora are two cutaneous folds that form the lateral boundaries of the pudendal cleft. They originate from the mons pubis anteriorly and merge with the perineal body posteriorly (the posterior labial commissure). After puberty there is an increase in pigmentation and hair as well as the deposition of subcutaneous fat. The deposition of fat mainly occurs in the medial aspects and the labia tend to flatten out as they reach the perineal body. The increased pigmentation and hair extends to the perianal area. The lateral surfaces of the labia majora are adjacent to the medial surfaces of the thighs and are separated from them by a deep groove, the genitocrural fold. The medial surfaces may be in contact with each other but may be separated by the labia minora if they are long.

The labia majora have their full complement of adnexal structures, but the inner aspects lack hair in the pilosebaceous unit. An unusual mammary-like gland, the anogenital sweat gland, may also be found at this site (see below).

Arterial supply   Labial branches of the internal
                      pudendal artery.
Venous drainage   Tributaries to the superficial
                      external pudendal vein which then
                      go to the great saphenous vein.
Nerve supply   Labial branches of the perineal
                      nerve.
Lymphatic drainage Superficial inguinal nodes and the
                      inferior aspect to the rectal
                      lymphatic plexus.

Labia minora

The labia minora are two thin folds of cornified skin, again devoid of hair but still possessing sebaceous and eccrine glands. They lack a layer of subcutaneous fat, and lie medial to the labia majora and lateral to the vestibule. The labia minora are separated from the labia majora by interlabial furrows in which the normal secretions from the adjacent skin surfaces may accumulate. Anteriorly, the labia minora divide into lateral and medial parts. The lateral parts unite anterior to the clitoris, in a fold of skin overhanging the glans to form the prepuce of the clitoris. The medial parts unite on the undersurface of the clitoris to form its frenulum. This anterior division of the labia minora in relation to the clitoris is variable. Posteriorly, the labia minora fuse to form a transverse fold behind the vaginal opening, the fourchette.

There is great variation in the size and morphology of the labia minora. Hypertrophy of the labia minora may be associated with local irritation and discomfort in walking and sitting or may interfere with sexual intercourse. Surgical removal of excess labial tissue, leaving the clitoris and fourchette intact, is recommended in such patients (Baruchin & Cipollini 1986). There are two surgical techniques for the simple reduction of the labia minora (see Chapter 12).

The skin of the labia minora is smooth or mildly rugose and pigmented, particularly at the tips. The dermis of the labia minora is composed mainly of elastic fibres and blood vessels and possesses a rich innervation. The arrangement of blood vessels within the labia minora forms erectile tissue similar to that in the penile corpus spongiosus, their embryological counterpart in the male. During sexual excitation the blood supply to the labia minora is increased and causes not only a change in colour but also significant enlargement, sufficient to induce a minimal degree of traction on the clitoris.

Arterial supply   Labial branches of the internal
                      pudendal artery.
Venous drainage   Tributaries to the superficial external
                      pudendal vein which then go to the
                      great saphenous vein.
Nerve supply   Labial branches of the perineal nerve.
Lymph drainage   Superficial inguinal nodes.

The clitoris

The clitoris is a specialized structure covered with a stratified squamous epithelium that is thinly cornified. There are no sebaceous, apocrine or sweat glands present. There has been poor one-dimensional presentation of clitoral anatomy in textbooks (O'Connell *et al.* 1998). Magnetic resonance imaging (MRI) has been used to investigate clitoral function and has complemented the results of anatomical dissection studies (O'Connell & Delancey 2005, Yang *et al.* 2006).

The clitoris has five component erectile tissue parts, most of which lie beneath the skin: the *glans* and *body*, two *crura* and two *clitoral bulbs*. The clitoris is not a flat structure, and therefore not easily represented in a planar diagram. It has a wishbone-like structure; the two arms are the paired crura, which extend forward as the corpora cavernosa and meet in the midline to form the body of the clitoris. The crura are attached to the pubic rami and are covered by the ischiocavernosus muscle. The clitoral body is attached to the pubic symphysis by a suspensory ligament. The tip of the body bends anteriorly away from the pubis forming the glans clitoris, which is the only visible part of the clitoris. The glans is covered by the clitoral hood, which is formed by the labia minora. The clitoral bulbs lie between each clitoral crus and the vaginal opening. The clitoral bulbs were previously termed the vestibular bulbs, but are now more accurately named as anatomically they form part of the clitoris (O' Connell *et al.* 1998, Puppo 2006). They are covered by the bulbospongiosus muscles, which extend from the perineal body, around the vagina and urethra, to the glans clitoris. The whole of the clitoris is composed of similar erectile tissue with the exception of the glans (Yang *et al.* 2006) and is the homologue of the penis.

Arterial supply	Superficial and deep terminal branches of the internal pudendal artery.
Venous drainage	Deep dorsal vein to vesicle plexus, deep external pudendal veins to femoral vein and internal pudendal veins to internal iliac vein.
Nerves	Dorsal nerve of the clitoris, a branch of the pudendal nerve.
Lymph drainage	To deep inguinal and internal iliac nodes.

The vestibule

The vestibule extends anteroposteriorly from the frenulum of the clitoris to the fourchette and laterally from the hymenal ring to a variable position on the inner aspect of each labium minus. The line of demarcation of the vestibule and the labium minus is known as Hart's line. The vulval vestibule is covered by non-cornified stratified squamous epithelium, i.e. a mucosa, and is devoid of any part of the pilosebaceous unit or other adnexal structures. The openings of the vagina, urethra, the ducts of Bartholin's glands and the minor vestibular glands are all localized within the vestibule. That part of the vestibule between the vaginal orifice and the frenulum of the labia minora forms a shallow depression termed the vestibular fossa or fossa navicularis. The clitoral bulbs lie in the superficial perineal pouch adjacent to the lateral wall of the vagina. They are attached to the inferior surface of the urogenital diaphragm by the overlying bulbospongiosus muscle. Thus, the bulbar erectile tissue embraces the vaginal opening and, during sexual arousal, its engorgement narrows the vaginal introitus.

Surrounding the edge of the vestibule and the opening of the vagina is a thin membrane of connective tissue, the *hymen*. The hymen is frequently incomplete but usually ruptures with exercise, the use of tampons or sexual intercourse. The rupture of the hymen will leave an irregular ragged edge around the vaginal opening termed the *hymenal caruncle* or *carunculae myrtiformes*. Occasionally, it may be a more rigid structure which does not rupture spontaneously and this may lead to haematocolpos. In some cases there is a partial division, e.g. a septate hymen, and this will lead to difficulties with tampon use or intercourse.

Arterial supply	Branches of the internal pudendal artery.
Venous drainage	Tributaries to the external pudendal vein.
Nerve supply	Perineal branch of the pudendal nerve.
Lymph drainage	To superficial inguinal nodes.

Major and minor vestibular glands

The openings of the greater and minor vestibular glands can be seen with the naked eye on the lateral part of the vestibule. *Bartholin's glands,* also known as the greater vestibular glands, are situated deeply within the posterior parts of the labia majora. Each gland lies just inferior and lateral to the bulbocavernosus muscle and is normally not palpable. The glandular secretion is clear, mucoid and alkaline and is increased during sexual arousal. Krantz (1977) maintains that these glands 'undergo involution, shrink in size and become atrophic after the thirtieth year of life'. Nevertheless, they may be the site of infection or cyst formation at any age. Bartholin's glands are lobulated and contain multiple acini grouped around the termination of each of the many branching ducts. The acini are lined with cuboidal epithelium and the ducts with stratified transitional epithelium. The main duct of each Bartholin's gland passes deep to the labium minus to open at the lateral margin of the vagina at 5 and 7 o'clock (Fig. 1.15). Argentaffin cells have been described in the epithelial lining of the Bartholin duct system predominantly in the transitional epithelium of the main excretory duct and are similarly found in the paraurethral glands (Fetissof *et al.* 1985). The *minor vestibular glands* are similar in structure to those of the greater

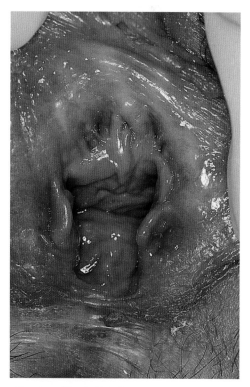

Fig. 1.15 Opening of Bartholin's ducts.

vestibular glands and in postmortem studies vary in number from one to more than 100 (Robboy *et al.* 1978).

The external urethral meatus and urethra

The external urethral orifice lies in the vestibule between the vagina and the clitoris. It is positioned in the midline but its exact location is variable. The orifice is easily seen and on occasions there may be bright red projections of prolapsed mucosa herniating out. The female urethra is 4 cm long and runs from the bladder downwards and forwards, embedded in the anterior wall of the vagina behind the symphysis pubis. After passing through the pelvic floor and perineal membrane it ends at the external urethral orifice. The urethra is fixed at its origin by the pubovesical ligaments and throughout its length by the anterior wall of the vagina. As it enters the perineum it is fixed by the perineal membrane, also known as the urogenital diaphragm or triangular ligament. This is a fibrous membrane that is attached to the pubic rami (Fig. 1.16) and separates the urogenital triangle into superficial and deep perineal pouches. The perineal membrane has three midline breaks, one at the apex of the triangle just below the pubic symphysis where the clitoral vessels and nerves pass from the deep to the superficial perineal pouch and two more posteriorly for the entrances of the urethra and vagina. The pelvic urethra has the same blood and nerve supply as well as lymphatic drainage as the bladder neck. The perineal urethra is supplied by the pudendal vessels and nerves, and the voluntary muscle of the external urethral sphincter is supplied by the perineal branch of the pudendal nerve. The lymphatic drainage of the perineal urethra is to the inguinal nodes.

Arterial supply	Vesical and vaginal arteries which are branches of the anterior internal iliac artery.
Venous drainage	Via plexus around the urethra to vesicle plexus around the bladder neck and into the pudendal veins.
Nerve supply	Pudendal nerve.
Lymph drainage	Urethral lymphatics drain into the internal and external iliac nodes.

The vagina

The vagina is a fibromuscular tube that extends some 7–10 cm from its opening on the vulval vestibule upwards and backwards, to be attached around the periphery of the uterine cervix at some distance above its lower margin. As the long axis of the vagina forms a right angle with the long axis of the normal anteverted uterus, the cervix projects downwards and backwards into the upper vagina. The circumferential vaginal attachment is achieved by the posterior wall of the vagina being some 2 cm longer than the anterior wall. The vaginal fold around the periphery of the cervix is divided into anterior, posterior and lateral fornices. The deep posterior fornix is continuous, via the lateral fornices on either side of the cervix, with the shallow anterior fornix. The anterior and posterior walls of the undistended vagina are in contact with each other throughout most of their length, giving the vagina a crescentic or H-shaped appearance in cross-section.

The vagina is related anteriorly to the base of the bladder and to the urethra, which is embedded in its anterior wall. Posteriorly, the upper part of the vaginal wall is covered with peritoneum. Below the rectouterine pouch the posterior vaginal wall is directly related to the ampulla of the rectum, while in the perineum the fibromuscular perineal body separates it from the anal canal (Fig. 1.17). The upper vagina gives attachment to the uterosacral ligaments posteriorly, the cardinal or transverse ligaments laterally, and the base of the bladder anteriorly, which itself is supported by the pubovesical ligaments. As the vagina passes through the pelvic floor the most medial fibres of the pubococcygeus blend with its walls to form a supporting muscular sling. Below the pelvic floor the vagina is supported by the urogenital diaphragm, the perineal body and the perineal musculature. Thus, the vagina has three compartments:

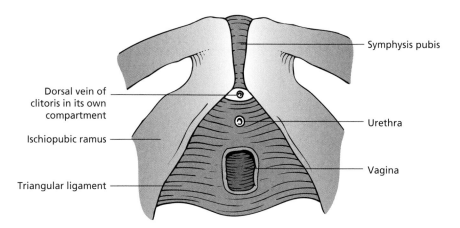

Dorsal vein of clitoris in its own compartment

Ischiopubic ramus

Triangular ligament

Symphysis pubis

Urethra

Vagina

Fig. 1.16 The urogenital diaphragm.

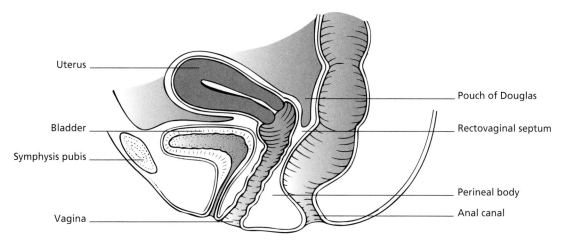

Fig. 1.17 A midline section through the pelvis and perineum.

an upper, which is above the pelvic floor and related to the rectum; a middle, which traverses the pelvic floor and urogenital diaphragm; and a lower, which is in the perineum (Blaustein 1982).

The vagina has an outer adventitial coat of fibroelastic tissue by which it is bound to the urethra and anchored to the pelvic walls by the pelvic ligaments. The intermediate coat of circular and longitudinal smooth muscle is intermingled with striated muscle from the pelvic floor. Between the muscular and inner epithelial layers is a layer of loose fibroelastic tissue in which there is an extensive network of venous channels. This venous network, with distension, changes the vaginal walls into erectile tissue and is the probable source of vaginal secretion during sexual intercourse (Smith & Wilson 1991). The inner aspect of the vagina is lined with non-cornifying stratified squamous epithelium, the cells of which are heavily glycogenated. The vaginal surface of the cervix is covered with stratified squamous epithelium while the cervical canal is lined by columnar epithelium in which there are numerous mucus-secreting cells. The squamocolumnar junction may occur at the external os but more often there is a transformation zone of variable extent situated around the external os, the nature and development of which is described by Singer and Chow (2003).

The outer wall of the vagina accommodates its vascular, lymphatic and nerve supply.

Arteries   The vaginal artery may arise from the internal iliac artery or one of its branches, most commonly the internal pudendal artery (Hollinshead 1971). The uterine artery supplies a descending branch to the upper vagina and there is frequently a vaginal branch from the middle rectal artery. The lower vagina is supplied by branches of the internal pudendal artery. These vessels anastomose with each other in or on the vaginal walls. Vessels from the right and left sides anastomose to form unpaired, midline, anterior and posterior azygos arteries.

Veins   The veins of the vagina drain to the uterovaginal plexus, which itself communicates with the uterine, vesical and rectal venous plexuses, all of which drain mainly to the internal iliac veins.

Nerves   Nerve fibres accompany the vessels as they penetrate the walls of the body of the uterus, cervix and vagina. There is general agreement that almost all of the motor fibres to uterine muscle are sympathetic while afferent innervation of the body is sympathetic and of the cervix is parasympathetic (Swash 1991).

Lymphatics   The upper two-thirds is with the cervix to the internal and external iliac nodes. The lower vessel third drains with the rest of the perineum to the superficial inguinal nodes.

The perineum

The perineum is a diamond-shaped area bounded by the symphysis pubis anteriorly, the ischial tuberosities laterally and the coccyx posteriorly. It is divided into two triangles – the urogenital triangle and the anal triangle. The perineal body is the fibromuscular mass that lies between the vestibule and the anus. It is the central point where muscles attach to the ischial tuberosities. It is supplied by the perineal artery and venous drainage is through the internal pudendal vein. The lymph drainage is to the superficial inguinal glands.

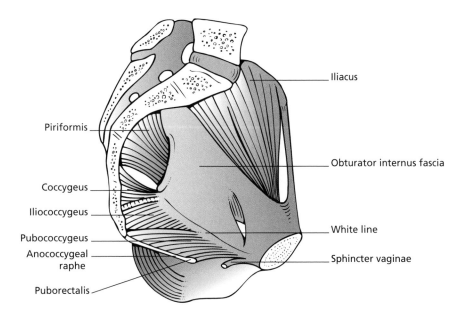

Piriformis

Coccygeus

Iliococcygeus

Pubococcygeus

Anococcygeal raphe

Puborectalis

Iliacus

Obturator internus fascia

White line

Sphincter vaginae

Fig. 1.18 The muscles of the pelvic walls and pelvic floor.

The urogenital triangle and diaphragm

The urogenital triangle is contained within the subpubic arch and is divided into superficial and deep perineal pouches by the tough fibrous membrane attached to the pubic rami, the urogenital diaphragm (also known as the perineal membrane or triangular ligament) (Fig. 1.16). This membrane is attached to the structures of the external genitalia. The deep perineal pouch is bounded above by the pelvic floor and pubovesical ligaments and below by the urogenital diaphragm. On either side lie the pubic rami, while posteriorly it is continuous with the ischiorectal fossae. Passing through the deep perineal pouch, in the midline, are the urethra and vagina. The vessels and nerves pass forwards on either side of the urethra and vagina. The clitoral branches leave the deep perineal pouch through the apical opening in the urogenital diaphragm. The deep pouch also contains voluntary muscle fibres, some of which surround the urethra and vagina while others run transversely into the perineal body behind the vagina.

Anal triangle

The anal triangle is the triangular area bounded by the ischial tuberosities and the coccyx. The anal canal lies within this area. The ischiorectal fossae lie laterally to the anal canal. These are pyramid-shaped areas bounded by ischium and obturator internus laterally, levator ani medially and the perianal skin inferiorly. The fossae contain fat and connective tissue and the nerves to the anus, perineum and external genitalia traverse this space. The anal canal is the terminal 2.5–3.5 cm of the large intestine and passes through the levator ani. It has an internal involuntary sphincter derived from the smooth muscle of the rectum around its upper two-thirds and an external voluntary sphincter muscle around the lower two-thirds. This sphincter muscle blends with the puborectalis muscle (Fig. 1.18).

Muscles of the pelvic floor

The pelvic floor, or pelvic diaphragm, is composed of sheets of muscles arranged around the midline urethra, vagina and anal canal. This sheet of muscle is made up of the ischiococcygeus, iliococcygeus and pubococcygeus, and should be regarded as one morphological entity. Their linear origin, from the white line overlying the obturator fascia on the side wall of the pelvis, extends from the ischial spine posteriorly to the pubic bone anteriorly. From this bilateral linear origin the muscles reach their midline insertion into the sacrum, coccyx, anococcygeal raphe and perineal body, forming a gutter-shaped pelvic floor, which slopes downwards and forwards (Fig. 1.19).

The ischiococcygeus muscle arises from the ischial spine and is inserted into the fifth sacral vertebra and the coccyx. The iliococcygeus and pubococcygeus arise in linear continuity from the ischial spine to the body of the pubis. The iliococcygeus arises from the posterior half of the fibrous linear origin and, overlying the pelvic surface of the ischiococcygeus, it is inserted into the coccyx and anococcygeal raphe. This raphe is the interdigitation of muscle fibres from the right and left sides and it extends from the tip of the coccyx to the anorectal junction.

The pubococcygeus arises from the anterior half of the fibrous linear origin and from the posterior surface of the body of the pubis. The muscle fibres arising from the fibrous linear origin sweep backwards on the pelvic surface of iliococcygeus to be inserted into the anococcygeal raphe. Those fibres arising from the pubic bone form a muscle sling around the anorectal junction, which produces a forward

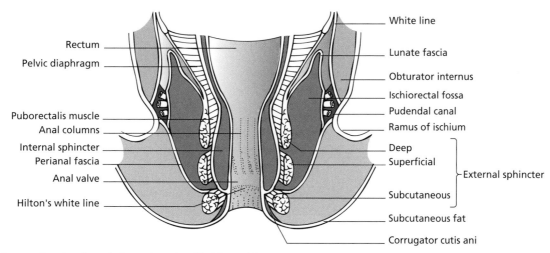

Fig. 1.19 A coronal section through the anal canal and ischiorectal fossa.

angulation of the junction. This part of the pubococcygeus is referred to as puborectalis and it lies beneath the anococcygeal raphe and intermingles with the deep part of the external anal sphincter. The most medial fibres arising from the pubis form a muscle sling around the vagina. This part of the pubococcygeus is the sphincter vaginae and behind the vagina its fibres intermingle with the fibromuscular tissue of the perineal body. The midline gap between the medial edges of the sphincter vaginae is occupied by the pubovesical ligaments and the deep dorsal vein of the clitoris.

The main functions of the pelvic diaphragm are to support the pelvic viscera and to assist in the maintenance of continence when intra-abdominal pressure is raised during episodes of coughing, sneezing and muscular effort. The posterior midline portion of the pelvic diaphragm is an important component of the post-anal plate (Smith & Wilson 1991) upon which the terminal rectum rests.

The nerve supply of the pelvic diaphragm is from the lumbosacral plexus (S2–S4).

The superficial perineal pouch

This lies below the urogenital triangle. The paired clitoral cruri are attached to the lateral margins of the undersurface of the urogenital diaphragm and to the ischiopubic rami. Each is covered by the ischiocavernosus muscle. These cruri extend forward as the corpora cavernosa, which fuse at the subpubic angle to form the body of the clitoris. The clitoral body is attached to the pubic symphysis by a suspensory ligament. Between each clitoral crus and the vaginal opening lies the clitoral bulb (vestibular bulb), which is also attached to the urogenital diaphragm. These bulbs extend forwards beyond the urethra where they fuse to form a slender band of erectile tissue, which is situated on the ventral surface of the clitoris. These bulbs are covered by the bulbospongiosus

muscles, which extend from the perineal body, around the vagina and urethra, to the clitoris. Just behind the vestibular bulbs, also lying on the urogenital diaphragm, are the greater vestibular glands of Bartholin, which open into the vestibule on its lateral aspect. Lying transversely across the base of the urogenital triangle at the posterior margin of the superficial perineal pouch are the superficial transverse perineal muscles (Fig. 1.20). The superficial perineal pouch therefore contains the structural elements of the female external genitalia, which, with their skin covering, exhibit the external appearance characteristic of the vulva.

The inguinofemoral region

The femoral triangle is a gutter-shaped depression below the groin, with its apex situated medially and inferiorly. Its base is formed by the inguinal ligament, the lower free aponeurotic margin of the external oblique muscle of the anterior abdominal wall. The inguinal ligament extends from the anterior superior spine of the iliac bone laterally to the tubercle on the body of the pubic bone medially. Inferiorly, the inguinal ligament gives attachment to the fascia lata, the deep fascia of the thigh. Midway between the pubic symphysis and the anterior iliac spine the external iliac artery becomes the femoral artery as it enters the femoral triangle deep to the inguinal ligament and the fascia lata.

As the external iliac vessels enter the femoral triangle they create a short downward extension of the abdominal fascia, the femoral sheath, which encloses the femoral vessels, with the femoral artery lying lateral to the vein. Medial to the femoral vein is that portion of the femoral sheath termed the femoral canal. The long saphenous vein ascends the leg in the superficial fascia and at the medial end of the inguinal ligament passes through the saphenous opening in the fascia lata to enter the femoral vein.

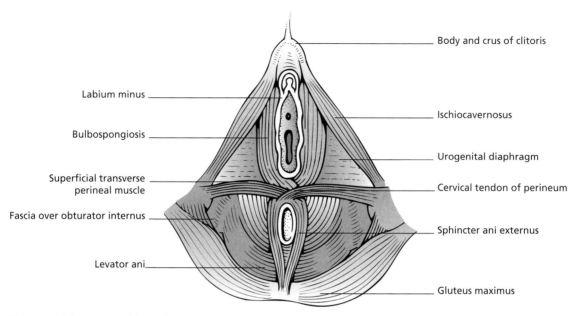

Fig 1.20 The superficial structures of the perineum.

Blood supply

Branches of the internal iliac and femoral artery supply the perineum.

The internal pudendal artery, a branch of the internal iliac artery, leaves the pelvis through the greater sciatic notch below the piriformis muscle. Lying on the tip of the ischial spine it turns forwards through the lesser sciatic foramen to enter the anal triangle posteriorly. Within this triangle it runs forwards on the side wall of the ischiorectal fossa enclosed by the fascia of the pudendal canal. During its course through the ischiorectal fossa it gives off the inferior rectal artery, which arches over the fascial roof of the fossa to reach and supply the anococcygeal raphe, anal canal and perineal body. Entering the urogenital triangle the internal pudendal artery gives off the perineal branch to the perineal body and the structures situated more posteriorly in the superficial perineal pouch. The parent artery enters the deep perineal pouch and supplies the erectile tissue lying in the vestibule, by perforating branches into the superficial perineal pouch, and the clitoris, by way of its deep and superficial terminal branches. The latter vessel reaches the body of the clitoris by entering the superficial perineal pouch through the apical deficit in the urogenital diaphragm.

Within the femoral triangle the femoral artery gives off the superficial and deep external pudendal arteries. The superficial external pudendal artery pierces the deep fascia of the thigh anteriorly, to overlie the round ligament of the uterus. It runs medially to supply the mons pubis and labia of the vulva. The deep external pudendal artery pierces the deep fascia of the thigh medially to enter the labia of the vulva. Within the superficial perineal pouch the terminal branches of the internal and external pudendal arteries anastomose with one another.

The venous drainage of the perineum is similarly arranged and eventually reaches the femoral and internal iliac veins. The internal iliac veins drain a rich venous plexus in the pelvic floor, which, at least in part, drains all the pelvic viscera. Thus, the venous drainage of the terminal gastrointestinal tract is partially to the pelvic plexus but principally to the portal system via the superior rectal and thence the inferior mesenteric vein. The pelvic venous plexus therefore provides a portal systemic anastomosis and portal hypertension predisposes to distension and even thrombosis of the pelvic, rectal, vaginal and vulval veins. Vulvovaginal varices, however, are most common during pregnancy, although they may occur in patients with endometriosis, pelvic inflammatory disease or pelvic tumours. Since many women develop vulval varices during the first trimester of pregnancy, the underlying cause is probably not obstructive but hormonal, and indeed progesterone is known to cause increased venous distensibility (Gallagher 1986). In the non-pregnant patient, particularly those using anovulant contraceptives, vulval varices may undergo cyclic change during the menstrual cycle (Gallagher 1986).

Lymphatic drainage

Lymphatic capillaries arise in the extracellular tissue spaces and form larger channels, which drain to the regional lymph nodes. Efferent vessels leave these regional lymph nodes and the lymph passes through a series of intermediate lymph nodes before returning to the thoracic duct. The regional lymph nodes of the perineum are situated in the groin at the base of the femoral triangle. These superficial lymph nodes subsequently drain to deep nodes in the pelvis and ultimately to para-aortic nodes on the posterior abdominal wall. Any midline structure, and especially an anatomical region as well defined as the perineum, has bilateral lymphatic drainage. Thus, the lymphatic drainage of either labium minus is to both the ipsilateral and contralateral superficial lymph nodes (Iversen & Aas 1983).

The regional lymph nodes of the perineum are arranged in two groups at the base of the femoral triangle. A variable number of lymph nodes lie transversely in the superficial fascia of the thigh, immediately below the medial two-thirds of the inguinal ligament. The superficial femoral or subinguinal lymph nodes, numbering 3–20, lie on both the medial and lateral aspects of the long saphenous vein. Those on the lateral side send efferent lymphatics, through the saphenous opening, to the external iliac group of deep lymph nodes. The superficial lymph nodes of the femoral triangle communicate freely with one another and drain the whole of the perineum, including the lower thirds of the urethra, vagina and anal canal.

The external iliac lymph nodes are described in relationship to the external iliac vessels. The medial group of 3–6 nodes lies on the medial side of the origin of the external iliac vein. Up to three of these nodes may be found in the femoral triangle medial to the femoral vein, and in this situation they are referred to as the deep femoral nodes. If all three are present, the lower one is situated just below the junction of the great saphenous and femoral veins, the medial node in the femoral canal and the uppermost node is known as the node of Cloquet or Rosenmuller. However, this last node is frequently missing (Borgno et al. 1990). The anterior group is variable and when present comprises no more than three nodes lying in the sulcus between the external iliac artery and vein. The lateral group of 2–5 nodes lies on the lateral side of the external iliac artery. The nodes of the external iliac group communicate freely with one another and with the obturator node. This large constant node, so named because of its proximity to the obturator nerve, lies below the external iliac vessels on the side wall of the pelvis and probably belongs to the external iliac group.

The efferent lymphatics from the external iliac group drain to the common iliac nodes situated on the lateral side of the common iliac artery. The external and common iliac nodes drain, either directly or indirectly, the lower limb, the lower anterior abdominal wall, the perineum and some of the pelvic viscera. Many small nodes lie close to each pelvic viscus and these drain into the numerous nodes embedded in the extraperitoneal tissue on the walls of the pelvis. These pelvic nodes are situated alongside the branches of the internal iliac artery and many groups are named according to the vessels with which they are associated. All lymphatics from the pelvis eventually drain to the para-aortic nodes.

Innervation

The perineum has both somatic and autonomic innervation and in each there are sensory and motor components. The perineum having arisen from the most caudal part of the developing embryo derives its somatic innervation from the most caudal segments, S1–S4. The nerve supply of the perineal area anteriorly is supplemented by input from the upper lumbar segments, L1 and L2. The autonomic or visceral innervation of the perineum is entirely from the most caudal elements of both the sympathetic and parasympathetic systems. The sympathetic outflow from and input to the central nervous system are restricted to the region between the first thoracic and second lumbar levels of the spinal cord. The sympathetic innervation of the perineum is located therefore at L1 and L2. It reaches the perineum via postganglionic grey rami communicantes, arising from the first two lumbar and all four sacral ganglia of the sympathetic trunks. These fibres are distributed with the first and second lumbar segmental nerves and the first, second, third and fourth sacral segmental nerves. In addition, other sympathetic fibres from L1 and L2 leave the sympathetic trunk as the hypogastric nerves (lumbar splanchnics, presacral nerves) and descend into the pelvis to be associated with the autonomic pelvic plexuses, which are distributed with the blood vessels. The parasympathetic outflow from and input to the central nervous system consists of cranial and caudal portions. The cranial portion is associated with four of the cranial nerves whereas the caudal portion is associated with the second and third, or third and fourth, sacral segments of the spinal cord as the nervi erigentes. These nerves together with the hypogastric sympathetic nerves form the autonomic pelvic plexuses.

The cutaneous innervation of the perineum conveys all modalities of common sensation – touch, pain, itch, warmth and cold – as well as complex sensations such as wetness. In addition, these cutaneous nerves carry postganglionic sympathetic nerves that are motor to sweat glands, pilomotor units and the adventitia of the microvasculature. No parasympathetic fibres participate in this cutaneous innervation, which is provided by the terminal or perineal branches of several nerves. The anterior part of the perineum is supplied by two nerves that emerge from the superficial inguinal ring just above the body of the pubic bone. These are the ilioinguinal nerve (L1) and the genital branch (L2) of the genitofemoral nerve (L1 and L2). The lateral aspect of the perineum, more posteriorly, is supplied by the perineal branch (S1) of the posterior cutaneous nerve of the thigh (S1–S3). The remainder of the cutaneous innervation of the perineum is supplied by the pudendal nerve (S2–S4) and the perineal branch of the fourth sacral nerve, which also supplies the skin of the anal margin. The pudendal nerve enters the ischiorectal fossa, close to the tip of the ischial spine on the medial side of the pudendal artery. Running anteriorly on the lateral wall of the ischiorectal fossa it gives rise to the inferior haemorrhoidal nerve, which arches over the roof of the fossa to reach the midline, where it supplies the terminal part of the anal canal and the perianal skin. The pudendal nerve then divides into the perineal branch, which supplies the rest of the perineal skin, and the dorsal nerve of the clitoris, which supplies the anterior labia minora and the glans of the clitoris.

These sacral spinal nerves also supply motor innervation to the muscles of the perineum. The pudendal nerve, through its inferior haemorrhoidal branch, supplies the deep and subcutaneous parts of the external anal sphincter and through its perineal branch the muscles of both deep and superficial perineal pouches, as well as the anterior part of the levator ani muscle and the sphincter urethra. The remainder of the levator ani muscle and the superficial part of the external anal sphincter are supplied by the perineal branch of the fourth sacral nerve. Damage to the pudendal nerves may cause loss of muscle tone in the pelvic floor and be associated with problems of incontinence.

The sensory components of the parasympathetic innervation of the perineum mediate the sensation of distension from the anal canal and vagina while its motor component is responsible for the vascular engorgement of vaginal erectile tissue.

Epithelia of the vulva and vagina

The vulva is covered in epithelia that gradually change from normal skin type epithelium on the outer aspects to a mucosa in the vestibule. The vagina is also lined with mucosal epithelium.

Typically cornified stratified squamous epithelium is made up of four layers histologically:
1 a basal layer, or stratum germinativum, the lower border of which rests on the basal lamina
2 a spinous or prickle-cell layer, which forms the bulk of the epidermis
3 a granular layer
4 a horny layer or stratum corneum.

Differentiation is the process that occurs as the keratinocytes move upwards through the spinous layers to form the tough, protective, flexible outer surface of the skin The keratinocytes flatten and lose their nuclei as they progress upwards, ending up as flattened structureless squames at the surface (Fig. 1.21).

The epidermis of the labia majora, labia minora and the frenulum of the clitoris is cornified stratified squamous epithelium. The epithelium on the inner aspects of the labia minora is still cornified, but towards the lower part it merges with the vestibule, which is covered in non-cornified stratified squamous epithelium, i.e. a mucous epithelium. Hart's line may be clearly seen with the naked eye in some patients, marking this transition from cornified to non-cornified epithelium (see Chapter 2).

The mons pubis, the lateral and exposed aspects of the labia majora and the perianal area are covered with hair-bearing skin (Fig. 1.22). The pilosebaceous unit comprises

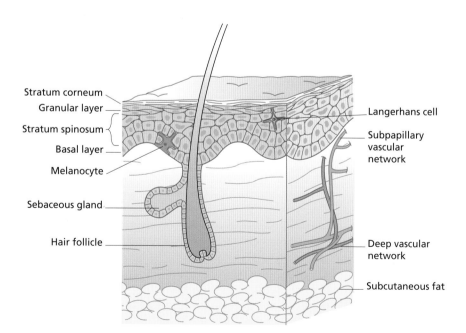

Stratum corneum
Granular layer
Stratum spinosum
Basal layer
Melanocyte
Sebaceous gland
Hair follicle
Langerhans cell
Subpapillary vascular network
Deep vascular network
Subcutaneous fat

Fig. 1.21 Section (diagrammatic) of skin.

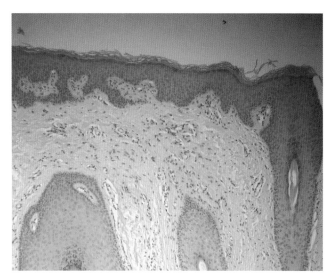

Fig. 1.22 Histological section of skin from labium majus showing hair follicles.

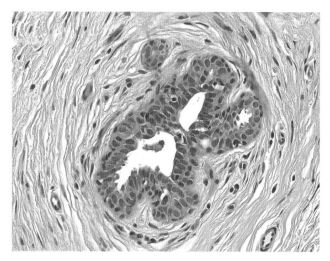

Fig. 1.23 Histological section through lobulated anomammary gland lined with compact columnar epithelium (courtesy of Dr James Scurry).

the hair follicle, the hair, the sebaceous gland and the arrectores pilorum muscle and some are associated with an apocrine gland. Eccrine glands are also present.

The inner aspects of the labia majora, the inner and outer aspects of the labia minora and the frenulum and prepuce of the clitoris are covered with non-hair-bearing skin but the sebaceous glands are still present and they open directly onto the skin. These areas are devoid of apocrine glands and eccrine glands are rarely seen.

A previously undescribed gland – the *anogenital 'sweat' gland* – has been discovered (van der Putte 1991). These glands are found predominantly in the interlabial sulci of the vulva and have distinctive morphological, histological and histochemical features. The glands cannot be categorized as eccrine, apocrine or mammary glands, although they may share some of their morphological features. Interestingly, similar glands have been described in association with hidradenoma papilliferum and on the labia minora of postmortem specimens (Woodworth *et al.* 1971).

The morphology of the glands ranges from a simple wide duct with a few small diverticula to a complicated, convoluted tubular system (Fig. 1.23). Most glands, however, consist of a coiled duct with diverticular extensions at irregular intervals along their length. Some of the diverticula are short and acinar whereas others are more duct-like and have their own acini. The glands all have a straight excretory duct that opens directly onto the skin surface. Occasionally, some of the glands reach a complexity that gives them a lobular appearance reminiscent of the mammary glands of the breast. The anogenital glands extend deeper into the dermis than the eccrine or apocrine glands. They are lined by simple columnar epithelium resting on a layer of myoepithelium. The columnar epithelium extends

into the straight excretory duct until a short distance from the surface and then gives way to non-cornifying, stratified squamous epithelium without a myoepithelial layer. The columnar cells have oval nuclei and a small to moderate amount of cytoplasm with a cytoplasmic 'snout' at the luminal side. Ultrastructurally, these glands are unique with features not seen in other tubular cutaneous glands (van der Putte 1993).

In addition to keratinocytes there are three other cell types in the epidermis: melanocytes, Langerhans cells and Merkel cells.

Melanocytes

Melanocytes are cells of neural crest origin that specialize in the production of melanin pigments, and they are situated in the basal layer of the epidermis. There is a regional variation in the ratio of melanocytes to basal keratinocytes of between 1:10 and 1:5. They appear as rounded cells with clear cytoplasm. Melanocytes convert the amino acid tyrosine to melanin pigments within the melanosomes, which are membrane-bound organelles. These melanosomes are transferred to keratinocytes through the melanocytes' dendritic extensions (Jimbow *et al.* 1993). It is generally assumed that the main purpose of this transfer within the 'epidermal melanin unit' is the protection of keratinocyte DNA from damage by ultraviolet radiation and certain toxins (Slominski *et al.* 1993).

It is now recognized that melanocytes have a considerably wider range of secretory activity than that involved in melanin transfer. Human melanocytes are capable of secreting a number of signal molecules targeting keratinocytes, lymphocytes, fibroblasts, Langerhans cells, mast cells and endothelial cells, all of which express receptors (Slominski *et al.* 1993). Hormones profoundly influence human melanocyte activity, although their precise action at the cellular level is obscure. There is also a marked regional variation in the sensitivity of melanocytes to specific hormones. During pregnancy oestrogens and progestogens stimulate increased melanogenesis in the areola, nipples and perineum, and to a lesser extent in the face and midline of the anterior abdominal wall. The facial hyperpigmentation associated with anovulant contraceptives is accentuated by exposure to ultraviolet light and may not resolve completely after they are discontinued.

Langerhans cells

Langerhans cells are found in the epidermis and are bone marrow-derived dendritic cells, present in all layers of the epidermis. They lack pigment and their unique identifying feature is the presence of Birbeck granules (Birbeck *et al.* 1961) in the cytoplasm best seen using transmission electron microscopy. They represent 1–2% of the epidermal cell population and are located mainly in the suprabasal area. Each cell possesses 5–9 dendritic processes, which extend out in the same horizontal plane, covering 25% of the surface area of the skin (Yu *et al.* 1992). An analysis of the distribution of Langerhans cells in healthy tissue of the genital tract showed there were 19 per 100 basal squamous cells in the vulva, six per 100 basal squamous cells in the vagina, and 13 per 100 basal squamous cells in the cervix (Edwards & Morris 1985).

Langerhans cells play an important immunological role in the skin (Rowden *et al.* 1977), being one of the most potent antigen-presenting cells in the body. They are involved in the sensitization and activation of contact allergic dermatitis as well as participating in the immune surveillance of the skin. These immunological functions are particularly important in the epithelia covering the lower female genital tract as these sites are exposed to a wide range of bacteria, viruses and fungi as well as the antigens of the ejaculate. The oncogenic human papillomaviruses are known to induce changes in the Langerhans cell population in the cervix (Morris *et al.* 1983, Tay *et al.* 1987a,b) and skin (Gatter *et al.* 1984).

Merkel cells

These cells are found throughout the skin, situated singly or in clusters in the basal layer of the epidermis. The dendritic cytoplasmic processes surround adjacent keratinocytes (Winkelmann 1977) and their cell bodies are intimately associated with contiguous nerve fibres (Winkelmann & Breathnach 1973). It had been thought that they were derived from the neural crest and had migrated along the peripheral fibre to the epidermis (Pearse 1969). However, observations on human fetal skin transplanted onto nude mice indicate that Merkel cells arise *in situ* and are derived from epithelial cells (Moll *et al.* 1990). Immunohistochemical studies have shown that Merkel cells in humans, as well as in many other species, contain vasoactive intestinal polypeptide (VIP) (Gould *et al.* 1985). The precise role of Merkel cells in the skin is unknown. Malignant neoplasms of epidermal Merkel cells may occur (see Chapter 8).

The dermis

The dermis lies below the epidermis and is bounded inferiorly by the subcutaneous adipose layer. It has two layers – the papillary dermis and the reticular dermis. The papillary dermis projects upwards into the rete ridges and is composed of fine collagen fibres, running at right angles to the surface, together with reticular and elastic fibres. This arrangement supports vascular and lymphatic channels as well as nerve terminals. The reticular dermis lies below the papillary dermis and is composed of coarse collagen fibres lying parallel with the surface. Accompanying the collagen fibres are thicker elastic fibres that prevent the dermal collagen from being overstretched, and in the perineal area stress-orientated smooth muscle fibres similar to those seen nipple, penis and scrotum are also present. The vascular and lymphatic plexuses that drain the papillary dermis lie within the reticular dermis, which also contains the nerve fibres associated with the papillary nerve terminals.

Cutaneous vascular system

The dermal microvasculature consists of a deep arterial plexus, the *fascial* network. The vessels from this region extend upwards to the border of the subcutaneous fat and the corium and there form a *cutaneous* network. This gives off branches to the appendages and ascending arterioles to a subpapillary plexus, which in turn forms capillary loops in the papillary layer between the dermoepidermal ridges. Blood is drained from these capillaries by venules which drain down to intermediate plexuses.

Cutaneous lymphatic system

The lymphatic system transports fluids such as leaked protein from the extravascular compartment of the dermis. The interconnecting lymphatic spaces arise from the terminal bulbs lying within the papillary dermis. These form the lymphatic network which ultimately drains into the lymph nodes. The vessels have a wide lumen and are lined with a single layer of endothelial cells.

Cutaneous nerve supply

A complex network of neural crest-derived somatic sensory and autonomic nerves supply the skin. The autonomic nerve supply controls the vasculature, adnexae and arrector pili muscles of the hair unit. The cutaneous nerves contain axons with the cell bodies lying in the dorsal root ganglia. The main nerve trunks enter the subcutaneous fat and divide into smaller bundles that form a horizontal network with fibres ascending alongside blood vessels to form a plexus of interlacing nerves in the superficial dermis. A few reach the basement membrane but do not extend far into the epidermis. The hair follicle has a complex nerve network, being an important cutaneous receptor.

Physiology

The epithelia of the vulva differ in their permeability, barrier function and immune responsiveness as they change from skin type epithelium to a mucosa. There is also the variable response to the hormonal changes throughout the different stages of life. During the reproductive years additional cyclic changes occur in the female reproductive tract as a result of sequential alterations in ovarian hormone secretion. These changes will be affected by pregnancy, which creates its own unique hormonal environment, or by the use of anovulatory drugs or hormone replacement therapy.

The principal hormones involved in these changes are oestrogens, progestogens and small amounts of androgens. Immunohistochemical studies have identified receptors for these hormones at different sites within human skin (Pelletier & Ren 2004). Further studies in the female genital skin have mapped out their distribution in the vulva and vagina, showing variation with different stages of the menstrual cycle (Hodgins et al. 1998), with oral contraceptive use (Johannesson et al. 2007) and at the menopause (Schmidt et al. 1990). In one study, the distribution of the oestrogen receptors was lowest in the mons pubis and labia majora but increased in the labia minora and vagina (Schmidt et al. 1990). Androgen receptors on the other hand were greatest in the keratinocytes of the labia majora as well as the adnexal structures and fibroblasts. Progesterone receptors were found only on vaginal epithelium and the distribution of the receptors did not seem to be influenced by the menopause (Hodgins et al. 1998).

Barrier function

The barrier function of skin is dependent on the degree of hydration, the presence of a stratum corneum and an intact surface. Transepidermal water loss (TEWL) is an indicator of the skin's barrier function and varies with the number of cell layers in the epidermis, which in turn vary at different body sites. This number is lowest in the genital area (Ya-Xian et al. 1999). Studies assessing TEWL have shown that water diffuses faster across the stratum corneum of the labium majus than the forearm (Britz & Maibach 1979, Elsner et al. 1990). There is no information, however, on

the variation with the inner aspects of the vulva where the stratum corneum becomes thinner and the area more occluded. In the vestibule there is no stratum corneum as it is a mucosa, and therefore will have physical properties similar to the vagina and mouth. Mechanical friction in the vulva is increased and influenced by occlusion, obesity, immobility and use of sanitary wear. This friction contributes to impairment of the surface integrity with maceration and chafing. All these factors will influence the effect and absorption of topically applied preparations (Britz et al. 1980). In cases of suspected contact irritancy and allergy, routine patch testing may not be sufficient (Wakashin 2007) and additional tests may be needed to allow for the effects of friction and epidermal morphology (Farage & Maibach 2004).

Birth to puberty

During the first few weeks of life the reproductive tract of the female infant is responsive to the sex steroids which she has received transplacentally from her mother. The effects of these hormones are entirely physiological and may be evident for about 4 weeks (Dewhurst 1980). During this period the infant's vagina will be lined with a stratified squamous epithelium rich in glycogen as a direct effect of the maternal oestrogen, and lactobacilli will therefore make up part of the normal flora. There will often be an obvious vaginal discharge, which in some cases will be bloodstained as the result of the infant's endometrium breaking down as oestrogen levels begin to fall. The vaginal epithelium then becomes thinner and the epidermal cells less glycogenated. During the prepubertal years the absence of glycogen from the vaginal epithelium restricts the action of lactobacilli and acidification of the vaginal environment. The resultant neutrality or alkalinity of the vaginal secretions renders all young girls vulnerable to vulvovaginitis and the possibility of lower urinary tract infections.

The physical changes associated with puberty are breast development, hair growth in the axillae, mons pubis and labia majora, and the onset of the menses. The development and growth of pubic hair is described in five stages (Tanner 1962), although during stage 1 there is no pubic hair. In stage 2 sparse hair appears on the labia majora and on the mons pubis in the midline. There is an increase in quantity and coarseness of the hair, particularly on the mons pubis during stage 3. Further increase occurs during stage 4 such that only the upper lateral corners of the usual triangular distribution are deficient. Stage 5 describes the normal adult pubic hair pattern with its extension from the labia on to the medial aspects of the thighs. The adult distribution of pubic hair is usually attained between 12 and 17 years of age. Axillary hair growth is described in three stages: from a stage at which it is absent, through an intermediate stage to full development.

Breast development has been described in five stages (Tanner 1962):

Stage 1   the infantile state, which persists from the time that the effects of maternal oestrogen have regressed until the changes of puberty begin.

Stage 2   the 'bud' stage, during which the breast tissue appears as a small mound beneath an enlarged areola. This is the first sign of pubertal change in the breast.

Stage 3   establishes a small adult breast with a continuous rounded contour.

Stage 4   is associated with further enlargement of the nipple and areola to produce a secondary projection above the contour of the remainder of the breast.

Stage 5   is the typical adult breast with smooth, rounded contour, the secondary projection present in the preceding stage having disappeared.

The first signs of breast development may occur at any age from 8 years onwards, and it is unusual for it not to have begun by 13 years of age. Some girls never show a typical stage 4, passing directly from stage 3 to stage 5, while others persist in stage 4 until the first pregnancy or beyond. Premature breast development seems to occur more often in Afro-Caribbean girls than in any other ethnic group. The enlargement may occur as early as 4–5 years of age but is not accompanied by other evidence of puberty or signs of endocrine disease (Black 1985).

The apocrine glands of the axilla and vulva begin to function at about the time that axillary and pubic hair appears, and the sebaceous glands at all body sites become more active. The growth of any individual is dictated by a number of factors, and Marshall and Tanner (1969) have found that most adolescent girls achieve maximum growth rate between their 10th and 14th birthdays.

The average age of the menarche is 13.0 years in the UK, with a standard deviation of approximately 1 year. Thus, 95% of the adolescent female population have their menarche between their 11th and 15th birthdays. It is unusual for a girl to menstruate before her breasts have reached stage 3 of development, but 25% have done so at this stage. The majority of girls, however, begin to menstruate while they are in stage 4 of breast development, but, in about 10% of girls, menarche is delayed until their breasts have reached stage 5.

During the 2 years preceding the menarche the ovaries increase in size. There is an increase in the number of enlarging follicles, although they subsequently regress. This follicular development is associated with increasing levels of oestrogen production, which is responsible for the thickening of the vaginal epithelium and the glycogenation of the cells. The vagina and cervical canal both begin to lengthen and the cervical glands become active. The vaginal secretions increase in quantity and become more acidic, with a pH of between 4 and 5. Fat deposition increases the size of the labia majora and the prominence of the mons pubis. The labial skin becomes rugose, the clitoris increases in size and the urethral orifice becomes more obvious. Coincidentally, the Bartholin glands become active and the hymenal orifice increases in diameter.

The reproductive years

In addition to ovarian steroids and pituitary gonadotrophins, it is now known that hypothalamic releasing factors, other ovarian hormones and numerous growth factors regulate intraovarian events and the female reproductive system. Ovulation, however, is the significant event of the ovarian cycle and occurs approximately midway between two successive episodes of menstruation. During the preovulatory or follicular phase of the cycle, oestrogen secretion increases to reach a peak before ovulation. Oocyte release probably occurs as a result of coincident surges in the secretion of luteinizing hormone and follicle-stimulating hormone. During the postovulatory or luteal phase of the cycle, progesterone is the predominant hormone, while oestrogen secretion is maintained at a level below that of the preovulatory peak. These cyclic changes in ovarian hormone secretion influence the female reproductive tract so as to create the appropriate environment for internal fertilization and implantation of the embryo.

Cervix

The cervical mucus secretion varies daily from 600 mg at midcycle to 20–60 mg during other phases of the menstrual cycle (Elstein & Chantler 1991). At midcycle the main function of cervical mucus is to facilitate the entry of spermatozoa into the upper reproductive tract, whereas at other times its function is to act as a barrier between the vagina and the upper reproductive tract. The physical character of the cervical mucus together with its specific immunoglobulins provide its barrier function. Any increase in cervical mucus may lead to an irritant vulval eczema.

Vagina

The stratified squamous epithelium of the vagina is extremely responsive to the influence of ovarian steroids. In the absence of oestrogen, the vaginal epithelium is thin and poorly differentiated. Oestrogen causes a thickening of the epithelium and its differentiation into the well-recognized basal, intermediate and superficial layers characteristic of the reproductive years. The percentage of superficial cells present in a vaginal smear is an indicator of the amount of oestrogenic activity. Progesterone produces a relative decrease in the number of superficial cells while increasing the number of intermediate cells.

The normal vaginal flora is mixed, but lactobacilli and corynebacteria, which predominate, utilize the epithelial glycogen to produce lactic acid and therefore lower the vaginal pH. This discourages the overgrowth of *Candida* species, which may be a normal commensal in the vagina. Antibiotics, by inhibiting the growth of lactobacilli and corynebacteria, disturb the equilibrium and allow candidal overgrowth. The acidity of the vaginal environment may be reduced by the alkaline secretions of the cervical glands, particularly in the presence of a large cervical erosion, by the alkaline menstrual flow and by alkaline ejaculate. A more subtle change takes place in the vagina when the effects of oestrogen are moderated by a relative dominance of progesterone, such as occurs during pregnancy and with the use of some oral contraceptives.

Urethra and vulva

The epithelial lining of the urethra is also influenced by the ovarian hormones and the character of exfoliated urethral epithelial cells changes with the phase of the ovarian cycle. Properly stained smears of epithelial cells in fresh urinary sediment reflects cyclic alterations in oestrogen and progesterone levels in sexually mature women. These cells are more accessible than vaginal epithelial cells in young girls and may be examined for diagnostic purposes when excessive oestrogen production is suspected. Changes corresponding to those in the vaginal epithelium may be observed in the epithelium lining the inner aspects of the labia minora (Tozzini *et al.* 1971).

The physiological vulval change that occurs during a woman's reproductive years is the subjective sensation of wetness, which is present about the time of ovulation. This vulval symptom is a consequence of the changes in the quantity and quality of the cervical mucus during the menstrual cycle. During the preovulatory phase of the cycle, the effect of oestrogen on the endometrium is to stimulate mitotic activity and to replace the endometrial lining shed during the previous menstrual flow. The mucus secretion increases and becomes transparent, more viscous and elastic. These changes are most marked just before ovulation when oestrogen secretion is maximal (Ross & Van de Wiele 1981, Elstein & Chantler 1991). After ovulation the endometrium becomes more vascular under the influence of progesterone, which reduces the quantity of mucus produced. Women interpret these changes as a sensation of vulval 'wetness' (Etchepareborda *et al.* 1983), and studies on the enzymatic content of cervical mucus indicate significant changes in the concentration of a number of enzymes (Blackwell 1984, Elstein & Chantler 1991).

Changes related to coitus and pregnancy

Sexual arousal is the end result of physiological changes brought about by neurobiological changes in the central nervous system. Arousal can be divided into three components: *central nervous system arousal*, *non-genital arousal* (nipple erection, increase in blood pressure and heart rate) and *genital arousal* (Graziottin 2004). In genital arousal there is an increase in vaginal lubrication, lengthening and dilatation of the lumen of the distal vagina, uterine elevation from the posterior vaginal wall (vaginal tenting), increase in clitoral length and diameter and engorgement of the labia and clitoral bulbs (Levin 2003).

Release by the efferent nerve fibres of nitric oxide and VIP controls the relaxation of the vascular smooth muscle allowing for the increase in the blood flow to the cavernosal tissues. The role of the epithelium in arousal is through its sensory function of touch, which stimulates release of neurotransmitters (Martin-Alguacil *et al.* 2006). These trigger central nervous system arousal via the pudendal nerve.

There are many conflicting studies on sexual desire and arousal and their relationship to the menstrual cycle. Riley and Trimmer (1991) maintain that in the most reliable studies peaks of sexual interest have been consistently shown to occur in the midfollicular and late luteal phases and that the physiological response is significantly lower during the periovulatory phase than in the immediate postmenstrual and midluteal phases. The difficulties inherent in such studies are that vulval and related problems may make sexual intercourse painful, thus influencing the willingness to engage in sexual activity. In normal circumstances, a minority of women (35–42%) would appear to have very little interest in sexual intercourse (Reader 1991). Low-oestrogen oral contraceptives have also been shown to have an adverse affect on sexual desire and arousal (Caruso *et al.* 2004).

In pregnancy there is a change in the hormonal environment created by the steroid and protein hormones produced by the placenta (Casey *et al.* 1992). Blood flow through the pelvic circulation is increased fivefold during the first 2 months of pregnancy and doubles again during the third month. Progesterone causes an increase of venous distensibility (Gallagher 1986) and in the progesterone-dominant state of pregnancy predisposes to vulval varicosities. In addition, the diminished availability of glycogen from the vaginal epithelium renders the vagina more likely to candidal overgrowth, which is reported to be 10–20 times more common in pregnant than in non-pregnant women (Wallenburg & Wladimiroff 1976). The immune system is downregulated in pregnancy (Toder & Shomer 1990), perhaps to ensure the survival of the fetal allograft, and these alterations appear to make the pregnant woman more susceptible to primary infection, reinfection and reactivated infection (Brabin 1985). Pregnancy may cause hyperpigmentation of the labia majora.

Injury to the genital tract and vulva may occur during delivery, and rupture of vessels outside the wall of the genital tract may lead to paragenital haematoma formation. In these cases, it is important to ascertain whether the haematoma lies above and below the levator ani muscle (Beazley 1981). Infralevator haematomas may occur as the result of an inadequate episiotomy repair, which allows continual ooze into the surrounding tissues. In this way a great quantity of blood can escape into the ischiorectal fossae or paravaginal tissues. Injuries to the vaginal wall and vulva that affect the perineum and may occur spontaneously or as a result of episiotomy are important as they may be associated with functional disturbances later.

The menopause and old age

The menopause is defined by the World Health Organization as the permanent cessation of menstruation resulting from the loss of follicular activity. The term perimenopause is the period beginning with the first menopausal symptoms and menopause is not reached until a full year after the final menstrual period (Burger 1996). Thereafter, oestrogen and progesterone levels remain low while gonadotrophin levels increase and may remain elevated for perhaps 20–30 years (Davey 1981). The median age for the menopause is 50 years for women in Western industrialized societies, but somewhat earlier in non-European women (Ginsberg 1991). The current life expectancy for Western women is now about 80 years, so the menopause will constitute a third of a woman's life.

The postmenopausal changes in the genital and urinary tracts are a result of the fall in oestrogen levels. The vagina becomes less rugose, narrower and drier and the epithelium more fragile and easily damaged (Schaffer & Fantl 1996). Microscopically the epithelial layers are reduced in number as is the intracellular glycogen, and the stroma is infiltrated with lymphocytes and plasma cells. As a consequence of these changes the vaginal environment becomes alkaline (Davey 1981, Utian 1987) and the number of lactobacilli are reduced (Hillier & Lau 1997).

The vulval changes include loss of hair on the labia majora and central part of the mons pubis (Bolognia 1995) owing to a loss in the number of hair follicles. The labia majora become less prominent and slack due to loss of the subcutaneous fat and the introitus may become patulous. Loss of muscle tone contributes to vaginal and uterine prolapse. Urinary incontinence is present in about 12% of women over 65 years of age and in as many as 9% of

younger women (Thomas et al. 1980), and this will have significant clinical effects upon the skin of the perineum.

Changes similar to those in the vaginal epithelium also occur in the vulval vestibule, transitional epithelium of the urethra and bladder with the consequent increased risk of recurrent urethritis and cystitis. These changes may be modified, to an undefined extent, by hormone replacement therapy.

Sexual desire and arousal are also reduced (Berman 1999). A decrease in skin sensitivity to touch and pressure occurs with low oestrogen levels (Romanzi et al. 2001), which may also be a contributory factor. The clitoral erectile tissue also diminishes (O'Connell et al. 1998).

Premature ovarian failure affects approximately 1% of all women under the age of 40 years (Baber et al. 1991). Although premature ovarian failure may be caused by some genetic defect, an autoimmune disorder or following treatment for malignancy, no definite cause can be established in the majority of affected women. It has also been proposed that oestrogen deficiency may follow tubal ligation in some women (Cattanach 1985).

Immune responsiveness

Skin is an important site for antigen presentation and both epidermal Langerhans cells and dermal dendritic cells participate in T-cell-mediated immune responses initiated in the skin (Williams & Kupper 1996). An intact immune surveillance of skin is important in the defence against bacterial, fungal and viral infections. Langerhans cells are important in the immune responses of squamous epithelia and it is interesting that there is a variation in their distribution throughout the genital tract. The vulva has the highest density and the vagina the lowest (Edwards & Morris 1985). There is no change of the Langerhans cell density during the different phases of the menstrual cycle in the vagina and little change in the epithelial thickness (Patton et al. 2000).

An important component of the genital immune system is the cervical mucus, which contains antibodies, in particular secretory immunoglobulin A (IgA). This locally produced antibody is bactericidal in the presence of lysozyme and complement and can agglutinate bacteria and opsonize them for phagocytosis. In addition, secretory IgA can inactivate antigens by forming non-absorbable complexes with them, and can diminish an organism's adhesiveness to mucosa. It also has the capacity to neutralize viruses.

Large numbers of allogeneic spermatozoa enter the female reproductive tract during coitus and some penetrate the tissues of the female host (Zamboni 1971, Hafez 1976). The invading spermatozoa are destroyed by an immune response that generates cytolytic T lymphocytes specifically effective against the alloantigens expressed by the spermatozoa (McLean *et al.* 1980). This coital immune response is limited, by the immunosuppressive function of seminal fluid, to the immediate postcoital period (Thomas & McLean 1984) so that the conceptus, which expresses paternal alloantigens, is not subject to immune attack during implantation. Protection against viral infection also requires an effective cytolytic T-lymphocyte response, and any limitation of this response will increase the possibility of an oncogenic virus in the ejaculate escaping destruction. Seminal fluid, by virtue of its physiological role in reproduction, may limit the antiviral response and thereby predispose the female genital tract to viral infection. An additional factor that may render sexually active young women more vulnerable to such infection is the reduced immune responsiveness associated with anovulant contraceptives (Gerretsen *et al.* 1980). It is also known that pregnancy reduces immunity. Organ transplant recipients are also vulnerable as their therapeutic immunosuppression renders them more susceptible to malignant neoplasia. This has been noted in young women developing vulval squamous cell carcinomas (Caterson *et al.* 1984).

References

Baber, R., Abdalla, H. & Studd, J. (1991) The premature menopause. *Progress in Obstetrics and Gynaecology* **9**, 209–226.

Baruchin, A.M. & Cipollini, T. (1986) Vaginal labioplasty. *British Journal of Sexual Medicine* **13**, 32.

Beazley, J.M. (1981) Maternal injuries and complications. In: *Integrated Obstetrics and Gynaecology for Postgraduates*, 3rd edn (ed. J. Dewhurst), pp. 455–467. Blackwell Scientific Publications, Oxford.

Berman, R., Berman, L.A., Werbin, J.G. *et al.* (1999) Clinical evaluation of female sexual function: effects of age and estrogen status on subjective and physiologic sexual responses. *International Journal of Impotence Research* **1**, S31–S38.

Birbeck, M.S., Breathnach, A.S. & Everall, J.D. (1961) An electron microscopic study of basal melanocytes and high-level clear cells (Langerhans cells) in vitiligo. *Journal of Investigative Dermatology* **37**, 51–63.

Black, J. (1985) Afro-Caribbean and African families. *British Medical Journal* **290**, 984–988.

Blackwell, R.E. (1984) Detection of ovulation. *Fertility and Sterility* **41**, 680–681.

Blagowidow, N., Page, D.C. & Huff, D. (1989) Ullrich–Turner syndrome in an XY female fetus with deletion of the sex determining portion of the Y chromosome. *American Journal of Medical Genetics* **34**, 159–162.

Blaustein, A. (ed.) (1982) *Pathology of the Female Genital Tract*, 2nd edn. Springer-Verlag, New York.

Blechschmidt, E. (1968) *Vom Ei zum Embryo*. Deutsche Verlags-Austalt, Stuttgart.

Bolognia, J.L. (1995) Aging skin. *American Journal of Medicine* **98**, S99–S103.

Bongiovani, A.M., DiGeorge, C. & Grumbach, M.M. (1959) Masculinisation of the female infant associated with estrogen therapy alone during gestation. *Journal of Clinical Endocrinology and Metabolism* **19**, 1004–1010.

Borgno, G., Micheletti, L., Barbero, M. *et al.* (1990) Topographic distribution of groin lymph nodes. *Journal of Reproductive Medicine* **35**, 1127–1129.

Boue, J., Boue, A. & Lazar, P. (1975) Retrospective and prospective epidemiological studies of 1500 karyotyped spontaneous human abortions. *Teratology* **12**, 11–16.

Brabin, B.J. (1985) Epidemiology of infection in pregnancy. *Reviews of Infectious Diseases* **7**, 579–603.

Breathnach, A.S. (1971) Embryology of human skin. *Journal of Investigative Dermatology* **57**, 133–143.

Breathnach, A.S. & Wyllie, L.M. (1965) Electron microscopy of melanocytes and Langerhans cells in human fetal epidermis at 14 weeks. *Journal of Investigative Dermatology* **44**, 51–60.

Britz, M.B. & Maibach, H.I. (1979) Human labia majora skin: transepidermal water loss in vivo. *Acta Dermato-venereologica. Supplementum* **59**, 23–25.

Britz, M.B., Maibach, H.I. & Anjo, D.M. (1980) Human percutaneous penetration of hydrocortisone: the vulva. *Archives of Dermatological Research.* **267**, 313–316.

Buntine, D.W. (1979) Adenocarcinoma of the uterine cervix of probable Wolffian origin. *Pathology* **11**, 713–718.

Burbige, K.A. & Hensle, T.W. (1985) Surgical management of urinary incontinence in girls with congenitally short urethra. *Journal of Urology* **133**, 67–71.

Burger, H.G. (1996) The menopausal transition. *Clinical Obstetrics and Gynaecology* **10**, 347–359.

Burton, J.L. & Cunliffe, W.J. (1992) The subcutaneous fat. In: *A Textbook of Dermatology*, 5th edn (eds R.H. Champion, J.L. Burton & F.J.G. Ebling), pp. 2157. Blackwell Scientific Publications, Oxford.

Byskov, A.G. (1981) Gonadal sex and germ cell differentiation. In: *Mechanisms of Sex Differentiation in Animals and Man* (eds C.R. Austin & R.G. Edwards), pp. 145–164. Academic Press, London.

Capraro, V.J., Bayonet-Rivera, N.P. & Magoss, I. (1970) Vulvar tumors in children due to prolapse of urethral mucosa. *American Journal of Obstetrics and Gynecology* **108**, 572–575.

Carr, D.H., Haggar, R.A. & Hart, A.G. (1968) Germ cells in the ovaries of XO female infants. *American Journal of Clinical Pathology* **49**, 521–526.

Caruso, S., Agnello, C., Intelisano, G. *et al.* (2004) Sexual behavior of women taking low-dose oral contraceptive containing 15 mg ethinylestradiol/60 mg gestodene. *Contraception* **6**, 237–240.

Casey, M.L., MacDonald, P.C. & Simpson, E.R. (1992) Endocrinological changes of pregnancy. In: *Williams' Textbook of Endocrinology*, 8th edn (eds J.D. Wilson & D.W. Foster), pp. 977–981. Saunders, Philadelphia.

Caterson, R.J., Furber, J., Murray, J. *et al.* (1984) Carcinoma of the vulva in two young renal allograft recipients. *Transplantation Proceedings* **16**, 559–561.

Cattanach, J. (1985) Oestrogen deficiency after tubal ligation. *Lancet* **1**, 847–849.

Chasnoff, I.J., Chisum, G.M. & Kaplan, W.E. (1988) Maternal cocaine use and genitourinary tract malformations. *Teratology* **37**, 201–204.

Cockwell, A., MacKenzie, M., Youings, S. & Jacobs, P. (1991) A cytogenetic and molecular study of a series of 45X fetuses and their parents. *Journal of Medical Genetics* **28**, 152–155.

Coulam, C.B. (1979) Testicular regression syndrome. *Obstetrics and Gynecology* **53**, 44–49.

Davey, D.A. (1981) The menopause and climacteric. In: *Integrated Obstetrics and Gynaecology for Postgraduates*, 3rd edn (ed. J. Dewhurst), pp. 592–650. Blackwell Scientific Publications, Oxford.

Davis, R.M. (1981) Localisation of male determining factors in men. *Journal of Medical Genetics* **18**, 161–195.

Dewhurst, J. (1980) *Practical Pediatric and Adolescent Gynecology*. Marcel Dekker, New York.

Dewhurst, J. & Gordon, R.R. (1984) Fertility following change of sex: a follow up. *Lancet* **2**, 1461–1462.

Diamond, D.A. & Jeffs, R.D. (1985) Cloacal exstrophy: a 22 year experience. *Journal of Urology* **133**, 779–782.

Didier, E. (1973a) Recherches sur la morphogenèse du canal de Muller chez les oiseaux. I. Étude descriptive. *Wilhelm Roux Archives* **172**, 271–286.

Didier, E. (1973b) Recherches sur la morphogenèse du canal de Muller chez les oiseaux. II. Étude expérimentale. *Wilhelm Roux Archives* **172**, 287–302.

Dreger, A.D., Chase, C., Sousa, A., Gruppuso, P.A. & Frader, J. (2005) Changing the nomenclature/taxonomy for intersex: a scientific and clinical rationale. *Journal of Pediatric Endocrinology* **18**, 729–733.

Duthie, G.M. (1925) An investigation of the occurrence, distribution and histological structure of the embryonic remains in the human broad ligament. *Journal of Anatomy* **59**, 410–431.

Edwards, J.N.T. & Morris, H.B. (1985) Langerhans cells and lymphocyte subsets in the female genital tract. *British Journal of Obstetrics and Gynaecology* **92**, 974–982.

Elsheikh, M., Wass, J.A. & Conway, G.S. (2001) Autoimmune thyroid syndrome in women with Turner's syndrome-the association with karyotype. *Clinical Endocrinology* **55**, 223–226.

Elsner, P., Wilhelm, D. & Maibach, H.I. (1990) Frictional properties of human forearm and vulvar skin: influence of age and correlation with transepidermal water loss and capacitance. *Dermatologica* **181**, 88–91.

Elstein, M. & Chantler, E.N. (1991) Functional anatomy of the cervix and uterus. In: *Scientific Foundations of Obstetrics and Gynaecology*, 4th edn (eds E. Phillip, M. Setchell & J. Ginsberg), pp. 114–135. Butterworth-Heinemann, Oxford.

Enders, A.C. (1965) Formation of syncytium from cytotrophoblast in the human placenta. *Obstetrics and Gynecology* **25**, 378–386.

Engel, E. & Forbes, A.P. (1965) Cytogenic and clinical findings in 48 patients with congenitally defective or absent ovaries. *Medicine* **44**, 135–164.

Etchepareborda, J.J., Rivero, L.V. & Kesseru, E. (1983) Billings natural family planning method. *Contraception* **28**, 475–480.

Evans, T.N., Poland, M.L. & Boving, R.L. (1981) Vaginal malformations. *American Journal of Obstetrics and Gynecology* **141**, 910–920.

Falk, H.C. & Hyman, A.B. (1971) Congenital absence of clitoris: a case report. *Obstetrics and Gynecology* **38**, 269–271.

Farage, M. & Maibach, H. (2004) The vulvar epithelium differs from the skin: implications for cutaneous testing to address topical vulvar exposures. *Contact Dermatitis* **51**, 201–209.

Fetissof, F., Berger, G., Dubois, M.P. *et al.* (1985) Endocrine cells in the female genital tract. *Histopathology* **9**, 133–145.

Ford, C.E., Jones, K.W., Polani, P.E., de Almeida, J.C. & Briggs, J.H. (1959) A sex chromosome anomaly in a case of gonadal dysgenesis (Turner's syndrome). *Lancet* **1**, 711–713.

Friedrich, E.G. & Wilkinson, E.J. (1973) Mucous cysts of the vulvar vestibule. *Obstetrics and Gynecology* **42**, 407–414.

Friedrich, E.G. & Wilkinson, E.J. (1985) Vulvar surgery for neurofibromatosis. *Obstetrics and Gynecology* **65**, 135–138.

Frutiger, P. (1969) Zur Fruhentwicklung der Ductus paramesenephrici und des Mullerschen Hugels beim Memschen. *Acta Anatomica* **72**, 233–245.

Gallagher, P.G. (1986) Varicose veins of the vulva. *British Journal of Sexual Medicine* **13**, 12–14.

Gatter, K.C., Morris, H.B., Roach, B. *et al.* (1984) Langerhans cells and T cells in human skin tumours: an immunohistological study. *Histopathology* **8**, 229–244.

Gerretsen, G., Kremer, J., Bleumink, K.E. *et al.* (1980) Immune reactivity of women on hormonal contraceptives. *Contraception* **22**, 25–29.

Ginsberg, J. (1991) What determines the age at the menopause? *British Medical Journal* **302**, 1288–1289.

Gould, V.E., Moll, R., Moll, I., Lee, I. & Franke, W.W. (1985) Biology of disease. *Laboratory Investigation* **52**, 334–352.

Graziottin, A. (2004) Sexual arousal: similarities and differences between men and women. *Journal of Men's Health and Gender* **1**, 215–223.

Green, H.J. (1936) Adenocarcinoma of supernumerary breasts of the labia majora in a case of epidermoid carcinoma of the vulva. *American Journal of Obstetrics and Gynecology* **31**, 660–663.

Gruenwald, P. (1941) The relation of the growing Mullerian duct to the Wolffian duct and its importance for the genesis of malformations. *Anatomical Record* **81**, 1–19.

Grumbach, M.M. & Conte, F.A. (1992) Disorders of sex differentiation. In: *Williams' Textbook of Endocrinology*, 8th edn (eds J.D. Wilson & D.W. Foster), pp. 853–951. Saunders, Philadelphia.

Grumbach, M.M. & Ducharme, J.R. (1960) The effects of androgens on fetal sexual development: androgen-induced female pseudohermaphroditism. *Fertility and Sterility* **11**, 157–180.

Hafez, L.S.E. (1976) *Transport and Survival of Spermatozoa in the Female Reproductive Tract*. Mosby, St Louis.

Hall, R., Fleming, S., Gysler, M. & McLorie, G. (1985) The genital tract in female children with imperforate anus. *American Journal of Obstetrics and Gynecology* **151**, 169–171.

Hardisty, M.W. (1978) Primordial germ cells and the vertebrate germ line. In: *The Vertebrate Ovary* (ed. R.E. Jones), pp. 1–45. Plenum Press, New York.

Hashimoto, K. (1970) The ultrastructure of the skin in human embryos. *Acta Dermato-venereologia* **50**, 241–251.

Herbst, A.L., Kurman, R.J. & Scully, R.E. (1972) Vaginal and cervical abnormalities after exposure to stilboestrol *in utero*. *Obstetrics and Gynecology* **40**, 287–298.

Herbst, A.L., Robboy, S.J., Scully, R.E. & Poskanzer, D.C. (1974) Clear-cell adenocarcinoma of the vagina and cervix in girls: analysis of 170 registry cases. *American Journal of Obstetrics and Gynecology* **119**, 713–724.

Hertig, A.T. & Rock, J. (1949) Two human ova of the previllous stage, having a developmental age of about eight and nine days respectively. Carnegie Institution of Washington Publication 583. *Contributions to Embryology* **33**, 169–186.

Hertig, A.T., Adams, E.C., McKay, D.G. *et al.* (1958) A thirteen day human ovum studied histochemically. *American Journal of Obstetrics and Gynecology* **76**, 1025–1043.

Heuser, C.H. & Streeter, G.L. (1941) Development of the macaque embryo. Carnegie Institution of Washington Publication 525. *Contributions to Embryology* **29**, 15–55.

Hillier, S.L. & Lau, R.J. (1997) Vaginal microflora in post-menopausal women who have not received estrogen replacement therapy. *Clinical Infectious Diseases* **25**, S123–S126.

Hodgins, M.B., Spike, R.C., MacKie, R.M. *et al.* (1998) A histochemical study of androgen, oestrogen and progesterone receptors in the vulva and vagina. *British Journal of Obstetrics and Gynaecology* **105**, 216–222.

Hollinshead, W.H. (1971) *Anatomy for Surgeons*, 2nd edn. Harper & Row, New York.

Hughes, I.A., Houk, C., Ahmed, S.F., Lee, P.A. & LWPES/ESPE Consensus Group (2006) Consensus statement on management of intersex disorders. *Archives of Disease in Childhood* **91**, 554–563.

Iversen, T. & Aas, M. (1983) Lymph drainage from the vulva. *Gynecologic Oncology* **16**, 169–179.

Jacobs, P.A. & Strong, J.A. (1959) A case of human intersexuality having a possible XXY sex determining mechanism. *Nature* **183**, 302–303.

Jimbow, K., Lee, S.K., King, M.G. *et al.* (1993) Melanin pigments and melanosomal proteins as differentiation markers unique to normal and neoplastic melanocytes. *Journal of Investigative Dermatology* **100**, S259–S268.

Jirasek, J.E. (1971) Development of the genital system in human embryos and fetuses. In: *Development of the Genital System and Male Pseudohermaphroditism* (ed. M.M. Cohen), pp. 3–23. Johns Hopkins Press, Baltimore.

Jirasek, J.E. (1977) Morphogenesis of the genital system in the human. In: *Morphogenesis and Malformation of the Genital System* (eds R.J. Blandau & D. Bergsma), pp. 13–39. Liss, New York.

Johannesson, U., Blomgren, B., Hilliges, E., Rylander, E. & Bohm-Starke, N. (2007) The vulval vestibular mucosa – morphological effects of oral contraceptives and menstrual cycle. *British Journal of Dermatology* **157**, 487–493.

Kai, H., Nose, O. & Iida, Y. (1979) Female pseudohermaphroditism caused by maternal congenital adrenal hyperplasia. *Journal of Paediatrics* **95**, 418–420.

Keith, A. (1948) *Human Embryology and Morphology*, 6th edn. Arnold, London.

King, C.R., Magenis, E. & Bennett, S. (1978) Pregnancy and the Turner syndrome. *Obstetrics and Gynecology* **52**, 617–624.

Koff, A.K. (1933) Development of the vagina in the human fetus. *Contributions to Embryology* **24**, 59–90.

Kohn, G., Yarkonis, S. & Cohen, M.M. (1980) Two conceptions in a 45X woman. *American Journal of Medical Genetics* **5**, 339–343.

Krantz, K.E. (1977) The anatomy and physiology of the vulva and vagina. In: *Scientific Foundation of Obstetrics and Gynaecology*, 2nd edn (eds E.E. Philipp, J. Barnes & M. Newton), pp. 65–78. Heinemann, London.

Laue, L. & Rennert, O.M. (1995) Congenital adrenal hyperplasia: molecular genetics and alternative approaches to treatment. *Advances in Pediatrics* **42**, 113–143.

Levin, R.J. (2003) Do women gain anything from coitus apart from pregnancy? Changes in the human female genital tract activated by coitus. *Journal of Sex and Marital Therapy* **29**, S59–S69.

Lind, T., Parkin, F.M. & Cheyne, G.A. (1969) Biochemical and cytological changes in liquor amnii with advancing gestation. *Journal of Obstetrics and Gynaecology of the British Commonwealth* **76**, 673–683.

Luckett, W.P. (1973) Amniogenesis in the early human and rhesus monkey embryos. *Anatomical Record* **175**, 375 (abstract).

Lunde, O. (1984) A study of body hair density and distribution in normal women. *American Journal of Physical Anthropology* **64**, 179–184.

Lyon, M.F. (1974) Mechanisms and evolutionary origins of variable X chromosome activity in mammals. *Proceedings of the Royal Society of London Series B* **187**, 243–268.

Marshall, W.A. & Tanner, J.M. (1969) Variation in the pattern of pubertal changes in girls. *Archives of Disease in Childhood* **44**, 291–303.

Martin-Alguacil, N., Schober, J., Kow, L.M. & Pfaff, D. (2006) Arousing properties of the vulvar epithelium. *Journal of Urology* **176**, 456–462.

McKusick, V.A., Bauer, R.L., Koop, C.E. & Scott, R.B. (1964) Hydrometrocolpos as a simply inherited malformation. *Journal of the American Medical Association* **159**, 813–816.

McLean, J.M., Shaya, E.I. & Gibbs, A.C.C. (1980) Immune response to first mating in female rat. *Journal of Reproductive Immunology* **1**, 285–295.

Mittwoch, U. & Burgess, A.M.C. (1991) How do you get sex? *Journal of Endocrinology* **128**, 329–331.

Mittwoch, U. (1992) Sex determination and sex reversal: genotype, phenotype, dogma and semantics. *Human Genetics* **89**, 467–479.

Moll, I., Lane, A.T. & Franke, W.W. (1990) Intraepidermal formation of Merkel cells in xenografts of human fetal skin. *Journal of Investigative Dermatology* **94**, 359–364.

Morris, H.H.B., Gatter, K.C., Sykes, G., Casemore, V. & Masson, D.Y. (1983) Langerhans cells in the human cervical epithelium: effect of wart virus infection and intraepithelial neoplasia. *British Journal of Obstetrics and Gynaecology* **90**, 412–420.

Niebauer, G. (1968) *Dendritic Cells of the Skin*. Karger, New York.

O'Connell, H.E. &. Delancey, J.O.L. (2005) Clitoral anatomy in nulliparous healthy, premenopausal volunteers using enhanced magnetic resonance imaging. *The Journal of Urology* **173**, 2060–2063.

O'Connell, H.E., Hutson, F.M., Anderson, C.R. *et al.* (1998) Anatomical relationship between urethra and clitoris. *The Journal of Urology* **159**, 1892.

O'Rahilly, R. (1977) The development of the vagina in the human. In: *Morphogenesis and Malformation of the Genital System* (eds R.J. Blandau & D. Bergsma), pp. 123–136. Liss, New York.

O'Rahilly, R. & Muller, F. (1987) *Developmental Stages in Human Embryos*. Carnegie Institution of Washington, Washington DC.

O'Rahilly, R. & Muller, F. (1992) *Embryology and Teratology*. Wiley, New York.

Pallister, P.D. & Opitz, J.M. (1979) The Perrault syndrome; autosomal recessive ovarian dysgenesis with non-sex-linked sensorineural deafness. *American Journal of Medical Genetics* **4**, 239–246.

Patton, D.L., Thwin, S.S., Meier, A. *et al.* (2000) Epithelial cell layer thickness and immune cell populations in the normal human vagina at different stages of the menstrual cycle. *American Journal of Obstetrics & Gynecology* **183**, 967–973.

Pearse, A.G.E. (1969) The cytochemistry and ultrastructure of polypeptide hormone producing cells of the APUD series and the embryologic, physiologic and pathologic implications of the concept. *Journal of Histochemistry and Cytochemistry* **17**, 303–313.

Pelletier, G. & Ren, L. (2004) Localization of sex steroid receptors in human skin. *Histology and Histopathology* **19**, 629–636.

Potter, E.L. (1946) Bilateral renal agenesis. *Journal of Paediatrics* **29**, 68–76.

Potter, E.L. (1965) Bilateral absence of ureters and kidneys. A report of 50 cases. *Obstetrics and Gynecology* **25**, 3–12.

Puppo, V. (2006) Re: Clitoral anatomy in nulliparous, healthy, premenopausal volunteers using unenhanced magnetic resonance imaging. *The Journal of Urology* **175**, 790–791.

Reader, F. (1991) Disorders of female sexuality. *Progress in Obstetrics and Gynaecology* **9**, 303–318.

Reschini, E., Giustina, G., D'Alberton, A. & Candiani, G.B. (1985) Female pseudohermaphroditism due to maternal androgen administration: 25 year follow up. *Lancet* **1**, 1226.

Riley, A.J. & Trimmer, E. (1991) Physiology of the human female sexual response. In: *Scientific Foundations of Obstetrics and Gynaecology*, 4th edn (eds E. Phillip, M. Setchell & J. Ginsberg), pp. 179–186. Butterworth-Heinemann, Oxford.

Robboy, S.J., Ross, J.S., Prat, J., Keh, P.C. & Welch, W.R. (1978) Urogenital sinus origin of mucinous and ciliated cysts of the vulva. *Obstetrics and Gynecology* **51**, 347–351.

Romanzi, L.J., Groutz, A., Feroz, F. & Blaivas, J.G. (2001) Evaluation of female external genitalia sensitivity to pressure/touch: a preliminary prospective study using Semmes-Weinstein monofilaments. *Urology* **57**, 1145–1150.

Rosa, F.W. (1984) Virilization of the female fetus with maternal danazol exposure. *American Journal of Obstetrics and Gynecology* **149**, 99–100.

Rowden, G., Lewis, M.G. & Sullivan, A.K. (1977) 1a antigen expression on human epidermal Langerhans cells. *Nature* **268**, 247–248.

Saenger, P. (1996) Turner's syndrome. *New England Journal of Medicine* **335**, 1749–1754.

Sarto, G.E. & Opitz, J.M. (1973) The XY gonadal agenesis syndrome. *Journal of Medical Genetics* **10**, 288–293.

Schaffer, J. & Fantl, J.A. (1996) Urogenital effects of the menopause. *Clinical Obstetrics and Gynaecology* **10**, 401–418.

Scherer, G., Shempp, W. & Baccichetti, C. (1989) Duplication of an Xp segment that includes the Zfx locus causes sex inversion in man. *Human Genetics* **81**, 291–294.

Schmidt, J.B., Lindmaier, A. & Spona, J. (1990) Hormone receptors in pubic skin of premenopausal and postmenopausal females. *Gynecologic and Obstetric Investigation* **30**, 97–100.

Serri, F., Montagna, W. & Mescon, H. (1962) Studies of the skin of the fetus and child. *Journal of Investigative Dermatology* **39**, 199–217.

Shaw, R.W. & Farquhar, J.N. (1984) Female pseudohermaphroditism associated with danazol exposure *in utero*. *British Journal of Obstetrics and Gynaecology* **91**, 386–389.

Simpson, J.L. (1976) *Disorders of Sexual Differentiation*. Academic Press, New York.

Simpson, J.L. (1982) Abnormal sexual differentiation in humans. *Annual Review of Genetics* **16**, 193–224.

Sinclair, J.D. (1972) Thermal control in premature infants. *Annual Review of Medicine* **23**, 129–148.

Singer, A. & Chow, C. (2003) Anatomy of the cervix and physiological changes in cervical epithelium. In: *Haines and Taylor Obstetrical and Gynaecological Pathology*, 5th edn (eds H. Fox and M. Wells), pp. 247–271. Churchill Livingstone, Edinburgh.

Slominski, A., Paus, R. & Schadendorf, D. (1993) Melanocytes as sensory and regulatory cells in the epidermis. *Journal of Theoretical Biology* **164**, 103–120.

Smith, W.C.P. & Wilson, P.M. (1991) The vulva, vagina and urethra and the musculature of the pelvic floor. In: *Scientific Foundations of Obstetrics and Gynaecology*, 4th edn (eds E. Phillip, M. Setchell & J. Ginsberg), pp. 84–100. Butterworth-Heinemann, Oxford.

Swash, M. (1991) Neurology and neurophysiology of the female genital organs. In: *Scientific Foundations of Obstetrics and Gynaecology*, 4th edn (eds E. Phillip, M. Setchell & J. Ginsberg), pp. 110–114. Butterworth-Heinemann, Oxford.

Tanner, J.M. (1962) *Growth at Adolescence*, 2nd edn. Blackwell, Oxford.

Tao, T.W. & Hertig, A.T. (1965) Viability and differentiation of human trophoblast in organ culture. *American Journal of Anatomy* **116**, 315–327.

Tay, S.K., Jenkins, D., Maddox, P. & Campion, M. (1987a) Subpopulations of Langerhans cells in cervical neoplasia. *British Journal of Obstetrics and Gynaecology* **94**, 10–15.

Tay, S.K., Jenkins, D., Maddox, P. & Singer, A. (1987b) Lymphocyte phenotypes in cervical human papillomavirus infection. *British Journal of Obstetrics and Gynaecology* **94**, 16–21.

Tegenkamp, T.R., Brazzell, J.W., Tegenkamp, I. & Labidi, F. (1979) Pregnancy without benefit of reconstructive surgery in a bisexually active true hermaphrodite. *American Journal of Obstetrics and Gynecology* **135**, 427–428.

Terruhn, V. (1980) A study of impression moulds of the genital tract of female fetuses. *Archives of Gynecology* **229**, 207–217.

Thomas, I.K. & McLean, J.M. (1984) Seminal plasma abrogates the post-coital T cell response to spermatozoal histocompatibility antigen. *American Journal of Reproductive Immunology* **6**, 185–189.

Thomas, T.M., Plymar, K.R., Biannan, J. & Meade, T.W. (1980) Prevalence of urinary incontinence. *British Medical Journal* **281**, 1243–1245.

Toder, V. & Shomer, B. (1990) The role of lymphokines in pregnancy. *Immunology and Allergy Clinics of North America* **10**, 65–78.

Tozzini, R., Sobrero, A.J. & Hoovise, E. (1971) Vulvar cytology. *Acta Cytologica* **15**, 57–60.

Utian, W.H. (1987) The fate of the untreated menopause. *Obstetrics and Gynecology Clinics of North America* **14**, 1–11.

van der Putte, S.C.J. (1991) Anogenital 'sweat' glands. Histology and pathology of a gland that may mimic mammary glands. *American Journal of Dermatopathology* **13**, 557–567.

van der Putte, S.C.J. (1993) Ultrastructure of the human anogenital 'sweat' gland. *Anatomical Record* **235**, 583–590.

van der Putte, S.C.J. (1994) Mammary-like glands of the vulva and their disorders. *International Journal of Gynecological Pathology* **13**, 150–160.

van der Putte, S.C.J. & van Group, L.H.M. (1995) Cysts of mammary like glands in the vulva. *International Journal of Gynecological Pathology* **14**, 184–188.

van Niekerk, W.A. (1976) True hermaphroditism. An analytic review with a report of 3 new cases. *American Journal of Obstetrics and Gynecology* **126**, 890–907.

Wakashin, K. (2007) Sanitary napkin contact dermatitis of the vulva: location-dependent differences in skin surface conditions may play a role in negative patch test results. *Journal of Dermatology* **34**, 834–837.

Wallenburg, H.C.S. & Wladimiroff, J.W. (1976) Recurrence of vulvovaginal candidosis during pregnancy. *Obstetrics and Gynecology* **48**, 491–494.

Warkany, J. (1971) *Congenital Malformations*. Year Book Medical Publishers, Chicago.

Wartenberg, H. (1982) Development of the early human ovary and role of the mesonephros in the differentiation of the cortex. *Anatomy and Embryology* **165**, 253–280.

Weiss, J.P., Duckett, J.W. & Snyder, H.M. (1984) Single unilateral vaginal ectopic ureter: is it really a rarity? *Journal of Urology* **132**, 1177–1179.

Wilkins, L. (1960) Masculinisation of female fetus due to use of orally given progestins. *Journal of the American Medical Association* **172**, 1028–1032.

Williams, I.R. & Kupper, T.S. (1996) Immunity at the surface: homeostatic mechanisms of the skin immune system. *Life Sciences* **58**, 1485–1507.

Winkelmann, R.K. (1977) The Merkel cell system and a comparison between it and the neurosecretory or APUD cell system. *Journal of Investigative Dermatology* **69**, 41–46.

Winkelmann, R.K. & Breathnach, A.S. (1973) The Merkel cell. *Journal of Investigative Dermatology* **60**, 2–15.

Woodworth, H., Dockerty, M.B., Wilson, R.B. & Pratt, J.H. (1971) Papillary hidradenoma of the vulva: a clinicopathologic study of 69 cases. *American Journal of Obstetrics and Gynecology* **110**, 501–508.

Yang, C.C., Cold, C.J., Yilmaz, U. & Maravilla, K.R. (2006) Sexually responsive vascular tissue of the vulva. *British Journal of Urology* **97**, 766–772.

Ya-Xian, Z., Suetake, T. & Tagami, H. (1999) Number of cell layers of the stratum corneum in normal skin – relationship to the anatomical location on the body, age, sex and physical parameters. *Archives of Dermatological Research* **291**, 555–559.

Yu, R.C.H., Morris, J.F., Pritchard, J. & Chu, T.C. (1992) Defective alloantigen-presenting capacity of Langerhans cell histiocytosis cells. *Archives of Disease in Childhood* **67**, 1370–1372.

Zah, W., Kalderon, A.E. & Tucci, J.R. (1975) Mixed gonadal dysgenesis. *Acta Endocrinologica. Supplementum* **197**, 1–39.

Zamboni, L. (1971) *Fine Morphology of Mammalian Fertilisation*. Harper & Row, New York.

Chapter 2: Principles of examination, investigation and treatment

F.M. Lewis & S.M. Neill

Cultural and historical considerations

In recent years patients have become much more aware of their own health and better informed about their disease, diagnosis and management. However, attitudes to vulvo-vaginal disease continue to be very much affected by the contemporary social and cultural background. Despite campaigns to educate women about vulval self-examination, encouraging them to talk openly about their symptoms and to seek help early, there is still a certain amount of stigma attached to genital disease. Women are often embarrassed to discuss vulval problems and often fear their symptoms may be due to a sexually transmitted infection. Trotula in the 11th century (Mason-Hohl 1940) said 'since these organs happen to be in a retired location, women on account of modesty and the fragility and delicacy of the state of these parts dare not reveal the difficulties of their sickness to a male doctor'. There is no doubt that women with vulval problems do still often wish to be seen by a female doctor, and those with vulval problems are more likely to be referred to a specialized vulval clinic if seen by a female general practitioner (Cooper & Wojnarowska 2001).

Sociological factors are particularly important in the recognition, acceptance and treatment of sexually transmitted disease; the history of that subject and its interaction with society have been intensively studied (Aral & Holmes 1990, Schwartz & Gillmore 1990, Waugh 1990). The UK is fortunate in its network of clinics for sexually transmitted disease, staffed by specialists in genitourinary medicine and able to deal with the necessary screening and contact tracing. Patients are able to self-refer directly to these clinics and this together with the level of confidentiality provided encourages attendance. These clinics have also become the focus of HIV diagnosis and treatment, and have been useful in the collection of valid statistics about the incidence and trends of sexually transmitted infections.

Cultural practices relating to the vulva are also important. Over the last decade or so, there has been significant publicity and banning of the practice of female genital mutilation, although it is still carried out in Africa. International campaigns aim to eradicate the practice (Kelly & Adams-Hillard 2005) and it is now illegal in many countries. However, 60% of mothers whose children had been subjected to the procedure felt that the practice should be continued for cultural reasons, citing pressure from paternal relatives (Ekenze & Ezegwui 2007). As there is increasing migration of these people to other countries, healthcare workers in the Western world will be seeing these women and need to be aware of the associated cultural issues and all the complications relating to the outlawed practice and their impact on antenatal care (Gordon *et al.* 2007).

Vulval lesions are not well described in the early medical literature, but first appear in the writings of Severinus Pineus in the 16th century and Van den Spieghel in the 17th. The terms used to describe the anatomical structures are often related to their function. The word *vulva* is derived from the Latin word for 'wrapping'. The *vagina* (sheath) and *mons veneris* (hill of Venus) are obvious descriptions. Clitoris, somewhat more obscurely, is usually thought to come from the Greek *kleitoris* meaning 'key' or 'gate-keeper'. Hymen is derived from the Greek *hymen*, meaning membrane. The labia are probably so called in that they are lip like (Latin *labium* – lip) surrounding the vaginal opening.

References to the female genitalia, whether in overt or covert form, are common in art and literature. There are formalized representations on Greek pots and the moulded ceramic 'vulval' plates of Judy Chicago (1996) in her celebration of women down the ages.

Vulval clinics

The International Society for the Study of Vulvo-vaginal Disease (ISSVD) was founded in 1970, originally as the International Society for the Study of Vulvar Disease, and its Fellows must demonstrate a particular interest in vulvo-

Ridley's The Vulva, 3rd edition. Edited by Sallie M. Neill and Fiona M. Lewis. © 2009 Blackwell Publishing, ISBN: 978-1-4051-6813-7.

vaginal conditions. The majority of members are gynaecologists, dermatologists or pathologists, and they come from
many countries. It has addressed problems relating to classification and terminology and, in so doing, has links with
the International Federation of Obstetricians and Gynecologists (FIGO), the World Health Organization (WHO)
and the International Society of Gynecological Pathologists
(ISGP). In addition, several countries now have multidisciplinary groups that meet regularly and also organize postgraduate courses dedicated to teaching about vulval disease.
There is, for example, a British Society for the Study of Vulval Disease, and a European College for the Study of Vulval
Disease was inaugurated in 1996.

A specialized clinic dedicated to vulval and vaginal disorders provides the best setting for the patient to be seen.
The necessary equipment for diagnosis and investigation can
be readily available with access to a team of appropriately
trained ancillary staff. The first vulval clinic was held at
Tulane University School of Medicine, Louisiana, in 1957
(Birch & Collins 1960). Published reports on the clinic offer
an interesting picture of changing therapies and attitudes
(Ridley 1993). Despite an increased number of such clinics,
the workload has risen (Bauer *et al.* 1999, Tan *et al.* 2000).
Ideally, these clinics would be multidisciplinary, which
reduces the need for multiple visits. However, owing to
financial and staffing restrictions, this is not always possible
in practice. In the UK, the majority of vulval clinics are
attended by a dermatologist (British Co-operative Clinical
Group 1999), but links with colleagues in gynaecology,
genitourinary medicine and pathology must be in place.
There are sometimes psychological and psychosexual issues
that need to be addressed and input from psychiatrists and
psychologists may be necessary. This combined approach is
a valuable resource, beneficial in management, teaching and
research. It is recommended that specialists who intend to
run a vulval clinic should have adequate training. A recent
questionnaire survey of fellows of the ISSVD revealed that
29% were self-taught (Murphy 2007), which is far from
ideal.

Patients with vulval problems present to a variety of health
professionals, including gynaecologists, dermatologists, genitourinary physicians, urologists and paediatricians. This can
often lead to confusion and mismanagement with varying
approaches according to the specialist. There are conditions which require the input of different specialists, so it is
important to tailor each patient's treatment. Another area
of confusion will be clinicopathological correlation, so
working closely with the pathologist is essential. In general, dermatologists work closely with pathologists, often
looking at the histological specimens together. This is not
usually the case in other specialties, as the pathologist
often makes the diagnosis without discussing the patient.
It is important that the clinical and histological diagnosis

concur; if there is doubt, repeated biopsies should be taken.
Agreement and understanding of changing classifications
and terminology must occur between clinicians and pathologists to avoid confusion.

The consultation

History

The importance of an accurate and thorough history cannot be overemphasized. Many find it convenient to have a
formal proforma as a basis for history taking, and to then
enlarge upon particular aspects in the light of the individual
patient's problem. A structured form (Fig. 2.1) ensures that
essential information is collected. It is also useful to have
similar baseline data for each patient to be used for future
comparative clinical research.

It is important that the initial interview should take place
in a relaxed and sympathetic atmosphere, as this is the first
encounter with the patient. Building a good rapport with
them at this stage will help them gain confidence in the
consultation. There are some instances when language difficulties will impede good history taking, and an interpreter
or family member may need to help in the history taking.
Unfortunately, this may limit the personal and intimate
information that the patient is willing to give.

There are several areas to be covered in the consultation
(Ridley 1978). A history of the presenting complaint should
include duration and initiating, provoking and alleviating
factors. Previous treatments used and their effects should
be noted, either prescribed or bought 'over the counter'.
A general medical history, including medication taken
and a previous dermatological and gynaecological history,
is essential as the vulval problem may be part of more
widespread disease. When it is deemed relevant, a brief sexual history may be necessary. If the patient is complaining
of pain, an enquiry about other forms of pain syndrome,
such as fibromyalgia or atypical facial pain, may be useful.
Features of the social history, such as smoking, are highly
relevant in conditions such as vulval intraepithelial neoplasia. If a sexually transmitted infection is possible from the
history, a full travel history and assessment by a genitourinary physician would be indicated.

Examination

It follows that the physical examination of such an intimate
area should be conducted with tact and awareness of the
patient's possible discomfort. It is advisable practice to have
a chaperone present (Royal College of Obstetricians and
Gynaecologists 1997), and this is essential when the doctor
carrying out the examination is male. There is evidence
that there are wide variations in policies with regard to the
use of chaperones (Torrance *et al.* 1999), but it is strongly

VULVAL CLINIC   Date:_____

Referral: GP/GU/Derm/Gyn/Urol/Other   Marital status: m/s/d/w

History:

Treatment: Topical_____ Systemic _____

Atopy: Asthma   Hay fever   Eczema

Skin disease: Psoriasis   Sites _____

       Ear piercing Y/N Age: _____ P/Ts (?+ve): _____

Family history: Asthma   Hay fever   Eczema
       Psoriasis

Gynaecological history: Menses_____ Menopause _____ G/P_____ Cx smears_____

Intercourse: Y/N Dyspareunia Y/N Superficial/deep Recovery_____

       Tampons Y/N

Urinary symptoms: _____

GI symptoms: IBS/colitis/Crohn's/oesophageal problems

STD: Y/N Details:_____

Malignancies: _____

Drug history: Allergies:

PMH:

Smoker: Y/N _____/day   Alcohol: _____ U/week

Autoimmune disease:

	Thyroid	IDDM	PA	Vitiligo	Alopecia	Other
Personal						
Family						

Pain: Back/joint   Migraine   Oral
   Facial   Depression
   Dysmenorrhoea PMT

Examination:
Dermatographic: Y/N
Scalp:
Mouth: Tongue   Gingivae   Buccal mucosae
     Soft palate   Hard palate

Eyes   **Nails**
Other

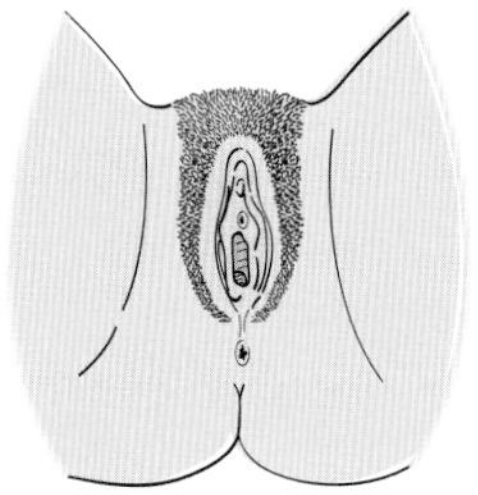

Mons pubis
Labia majora
Labia minora
Clitoris/clitoral hood
I/L sulci
Introitus

Vagina   Perianal
Vestibule   Natal cleft
Perineal body

Diagnosis: _____
Treatment:

Information leaflet: Y/N
Outcome:

Fig. 2.1 Proforma for clinical history and examination.

recommended for examination of the vulva. Even if it is explained that there will be a female chaperone, in certain circumstances a female patient, especially in some religious cultures, will insist on a female doctor. This request should always be respected. Women frequently complain of feeling embarrassed, humiliated or demeaned by a genital examination, but the presence of a chaperone as well as explanation and reassurance will minimize distress.

Further problems with the examination will be posed if the clinic attended is a teaching clinic. It is essential, therefore, before starting the history, to ensure that the patient is content to have more than one doctor and a nurse present. It should not be assumed that the patient is willing to also have an examination in the presence of an observer, so a further request needs to be made before proceeding. Sometimes patients have already experienced some distress in their history giving, which can then be compounded by examining them without their permission. Most patients readily accede, and they will often also agree to the presence of a trainee doctor if the importance of learning is explained.

It is unnecessary to have the patient in the lithotomy position as a full examination of the vulva can be performed with the patient in the dorsal and then (for the perianal area) the left lateral position. The examination must be thorough and methodical, and include a conscious note of all areas of the vulva as well as of the perineum and perianal area. Simple inspection will allow only the mons pubis, the labia majora, the margins of the labia minora, the perineal body and the anus to be seen. Adequate exposure of the vulva requires the separation of the labia majora and minora. The interlabial sulci and inguinal folds need to be inspected carefully. Here again, it is helpful to have on the proforma a list that can be checked, and a diagram to be marked (Fig. 2.1). A good light is essential, as is some form of magnification such as an adjustable magnifying glass on a wall bracket.

The colposcope, giving a magnification of 8–10 times, is not helpful during examination of the vulva. It provides a very small field of examination and shows up little on keratinized skin; moreover, the position that has to be taken up by the patient makes full examination of the whole anogenital area difficult. The use of the colposcope for the investigation of cervical and vaginal lesions cannot be extrapolated to the vulva (Micheletti *et al.* 2008). Colposcopic examination of the vestibule, vagina and cervix may, of course, be indicated at some convenient time for certain patients. There is no place for the routine use of toluidine blue and little for acetic acid, the only point of which at the vulva might be in delineating areas of vulval intraepithelial neoplasia for biopsy. The confusion caused by misplaced emphasis on acetowhite tissue has been considerable, and the light reflection effect produced is essentially non-specific. It has been shown that 30% of women without any vulval symptoms had acetowhite areas outside the vestibule (van Buerden *et al.* 1997).

Examination of the vagina and cervix should be routine in mucocutaneous diseases, vulval intraepithelial neoplasia and vaginal discharge. In some situations, the inguinal lymph glands will need to be palpated. It is always helpful to examine the mouth. Additional information will be gleaned from examination of the mouth, eyes, scalp, nails and other flexural sites, including the umbilicus. This may reveal disease at other sites and give helpful diagnostic clues.

Most children will permit examination of the vulva and perianal area, either lying on the back or, in the case of very small children and babies, on the knee of the mother or other female attendant (Blake 1992). As the labia majora are unformed, visualization is easy, and even the vestibule and hymen are usually readily visible without any need to separate the labia minora. In specific situations, examination under anaesthesia may be required. This may also be the case for adults with painful vaginal adhesions or stenosis.

Findings on examination

It is important when examining the vulva to allow for changes in morphology at different ages and physiological states such as pregnancy. There are also changes which may be variants of normal, and it is important to be aware of these to avoid misdiagnosis and mismanagement.

The vulva in infancy and childhood

During the first few weeks of life, the vulva and vagina are under the influence of maternal hormones received transplacentally (see Chapter 1). The labia minora are relatively prominent in childhood and the hymen is thickened and the orifice difficult to see. Milia, which are blocked eccrine sweat ducts, can be found. The prepubertal introital area is bright red in its normal state, a fact that often gives rise to mistaken suspicion of abnormality. Another important feature in children is the occasional presence of labial adhesions, which can mimic ambiguous genitalia (see Chapter 5). With adhesions, a line of demarcation between the clitoral hood and the labia minora under the clitoris can be seen (Pokorny 1992). The progressive changes encountered between infancy and adolescence have been described by Pokorny (1993).

At puberty, deposition of fat increases the size of the labia majora and the prominence of the mons pubis. As this occurs, the labia minora become more covered and may pigment. The clitoris enlarges and the urethral orifice becomes more evident. Coincidentally, the vestibular glands of Bartholin become active and the hymenal orifice increases in diameter. Periurethral cysts, which spontaneously resolve, may be confused with a microperforate hymen. The development and growth of pubic hair is described in five stages (Tanner 1962). The adult distribution of pubic hair, with the upper limit on the mons pubis and extending to the upper thighs, is usually attained between 12 and 17 years of age.

The vulva in pregnancy

In pregnancy, the vulva may become engorged and varicose veins commonly appear on the labia majora. Hyperpigmentation of the labia majora can be marked.

The vulva in the postmenopausal woman

Although there is a lack of documentation, clinical observation suggests that with increasing age the labia majora apparently diminish in volume, presumably because of a reduction of fat and connective tissue. This is accompanied by a thinning of labial hair due to loss of hair follicles with increasing age and a reduction of pigmentation. Fordyce spots also reduce in number and size. Hormone replacement therapy is now taken by many postmenopausal women; it will tend to restore vaginal and hence introital moistness but will have no effect on the keratinized vulval skin.

Normal variants

In each area of the vulva – the clitoris, labia majora, labia minora, vestibule and hymen – the range of normal appearances is wide, and patients must be given firm reassurance when appropriate. Common benign lesions such as small tags, angiokeratomas and seborrhoeic warts should be confidently diagnosed clinically and require no treatment.

The size of the labia majora varies with age, ethnic origin and parity (Krantz 1977). A degree of asymmetry is common and is usually of no significance, but it has been a presenting sign in neurofibromatosis (Friedrich & Wilkinson 1985). The labia minora can vary significantly in size and may be bifid in their anterior parts in some women. They are often asymmetrical. The edges can be pigmented, and sometimes serrated. The whole of the inner surface of the labia minora can be covered with small sebaceous papules. These are often referred to as Fordyce spots, but the true definition of Fordyce spots is ectopic sebaceous glands, as found on the buccal mucosa. On the vulva, they are not ectopic but at an expected site. They are very prominent in some women but can be seen more clearly if the labia are stretched.

The vestibule is a mucosal surface and it is covered with non-cornifying, stratified epithelium. Its boundaries extend from the hymenal ring to the inner, inferior aspects of the labia minora. In some patients, there may be a distinct line (Hart's line) demarcating the junction of the keratinized

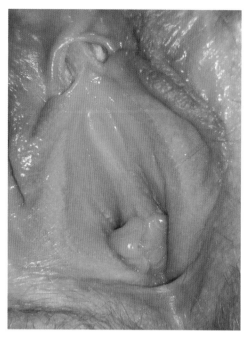

Fig. 2.2 Hart's line demarcating the junction of the keratinized skin of the labia minora with the non-keratinized mucosa of the vestibule.

stratified squamous epithelium of the labium minus and the non-keratinized vestibular mucosa (Fig. 2.2). This was first described by the Edinburgh gynaecologist David Berry Hart in his textbook of gynaecology in 1882 (Hart & Barbour 1882). He wrote 'a line running separates mucous membrane from skin – starting at the base of the inner aspect of the right labium minus, it passes down beside the base of the outer aspect of the hymen, up along the base of the inner aspect of the left labium minus, in beneath the prepuce of the clitoris and down to where it started from'. Routine examination of the vestibule includes the noting of the urethra, the hymen or hymenal ring, and the presence or absence of any minor vestibular gland openings or erythema. Episiotomy scars are generally obvious. Scars from obstetric tears can be seen around the urethra and on the anterior vestibule. They sometimes pigment.

Vestibular papillomatosis is the term used to describe the common finding of a myriad of tiny filamentous projections of the epithelium lining the vestibule and the inner parts of the labia minora (Fig. 2.3). They have had various names; for example, 'vestibular papillae' (Friedrich 1983), 'hirsuties papillaris vulvae' (Altmeyer et al. 1982), vulval squamous papillomatosis (Growdon et al. 1985) and others, including papillomatosis labialis, hirsutoid papillomas of the vulva and pseudocondylomas. It is believed that vestibular papillomatosis is the female equivalent of the tiny symmetrical projections found around the coronal sulcus known as penile pearly papules or hirsutoid papules of the penis

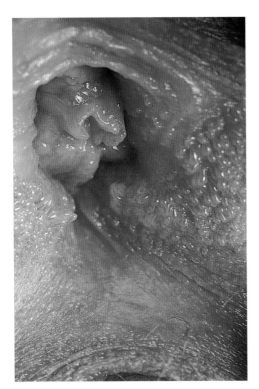

Fig. 2.3 Vestibular papillomatosis. Confluent sheets of tiny filamentous projections of the vestibular epithelium.

(Altmeyer *et al.* 1982). Originally, it was thought that the lesions were induced by the human papillomavirus (HPV), but there is now good evidence to the contrary (Bergeron *et al.* 1990, Moyal-Barracco *et al.* 1990). Clinically, they can be distinguished from viral warts as they are symmetrically distributed in an orderly fashion with each papilla arising from a solitary base and of the same colour as the rest of the vestibular epithelium. The histological features include papillomatosis, acanthosis and occasionally parakeratosis

(Fig. 2.4). The application of 5% acetic acid does not produce acetowhitening confined to the lesions.

Investigations

For the well-trained observer, the diagnosis can often be made on the basis of the history and examination alone. No investigations may be necessary for some patients, e.g. those with vulvodynia (see Chapter 6). For other patients, investigations may be needed to confirm the diagnosis, and these need to be tailored to the clinical features.

Biopsy

Different biopsy techniques have been employed in the diagnosis of vulval disease. Generally, these can be performed under local anaesthesia in the outpatient setting. An adequate explanation of what is involved for the patient should then be followed by the patient's written consent. Standard forms for this are widely available.

The disposable biopsy punch is usually satisfactory for diagnostic, histological samples, and is particularly useful for lesions on the inner aspects of the vulva. These range in size from 2 to 8 mm, but generally the 6 mm size is preferred for an adequate specimen. When the specimen is a biopsy only, care must be taken in interpretation (Crawford *et al.* 1995). This is particularly important for suspected malignant lesions, in which specimens following total excision must be assessed for an accurate tumour depth.

Although the use of a prilocaine/lidocaine cream (EMLA) alone has been reported to allow pain-free punch biopsy of the vulva (Byrne *et al.* 1989), further infiltration with lidocaine 1% or 2% should be used. EMLA certainly reduces the discomfort of the injected local anaesthesia and its absorption can be assisted by adduction of the thighs for 10 minutes or so before infiltrating the lidocaine with a

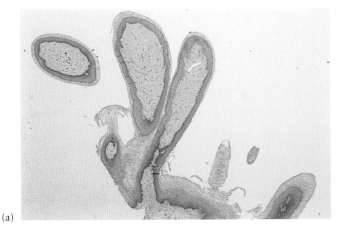

(a)

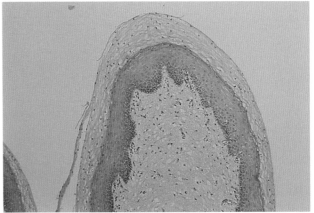

(b)

Fig. 2.4 (a) Histology of vestibular papillomatosis. Low-power magnification showing the papillary projections of the epithelium. (b) Higher power magnification showing normal epithelium with a central core of connective tissue.

fine-needle cartridge syringe or 30-gauge needle. The punched out specimen is removed with sharp scissors. Small biopsies may not require sutures, haemostasis being achieved by pressure or cautery; others may need one or two absorbable sutures, for example with 5.0 Vicryl. Many small lesions such as warts or tags can also be removed in the usual way under local anaesthesia by the hyfrecator, cautery or snipping off.

If EMLA cream is used, it must be taken into account when interpreting the histology. Some histological features such as pale, swollen keratinocytes, basal cell vacuolation and basal layer destruction with subepidermal cleavage are related to the use of this preparation and may lead to misdiagnosis (Cazes et al. 2007). Ultrastructural changes may also be attributable to EMLA and were mistaken for lysosomal storage disease in one series (Vallance et al. 2004).

Specimens for immunofluorescence are, after washing in saline, put into liquid nitrogen or into transport medium. Michel's medium is a useful transport medium with the specimen being stable for 28 days (Vaughan-Jones et al. 1995). Specimens for electron microscopy are put into liquid nitrogen or glutaraldehyde. If an infective cause is suspected, it may be appropriate to send some tissue for bacterial, viral and fungal culture. It is best to discuss these cases with the local laboratory first as requirements for the method of transport may vary.

Cytology

The use of cytological techniques in the diagnosis of vulval disorders is extremely limited. There are conflicting results reported in studies. Histological examination of a tissue sample should always be regarded as the gold standard. However, for a rapid diagnosis of herpes simplex infection, a Tzanck smear is helpful.

Microbiological investigation

Swabs for bacterial and yeast culture, suitable viral transport medium for viral culture and blades for taking scrapings for tinea, Candida and erythrasma will be required. If a sexually transmitted infection is suspected, the patient is best served by referral to a genitourinary medicine clinic for full investigation and screening. In the UK, these clinics are well equipped for investigation and management of these infections together with contact tracing. Serology may be needed to confirm some infectious diseases.

Wood's lamp examination

The Wood's lamp emits ultraviolet rays but includes a filter of Wood's glass to exclude visible light. The changes seen in erythrasma will fluoresce pink under this light, and it can also be useful in the diagnosis of vitiligo as the areas of depigmentation are accentuated.

Patch tests

Patch testing is a measure of delayed type (type IV) hypersensitivity and is used to investigate a suspected allergic contact dermatitis. Small amounts of allergens in suitable concentration are placed on aluminium discs and applied to the back of the patient. These are removed and read at 48 hours, and then read again at 72 hours after application. There are standard series that are used but it is important to extend these for investigation of an anogenital dermatosis to include preservatives and topical steroids, otherwise relevant allergens may be missed.

Patch testing is of no value in the investigation of urticarial (type I) reactions. Prick testing may be required if a semen or latex allergy is suspected. Radioimmunoabsorbent assays can also be helpful in the investigation of type I reactions.

Imaging

It is rare that radiological imaging techniques are needed for the investigation of vulval disorders but they are sometimes required to assess the extent of malignant disease. With the advent of some newer modalities such as computed tomography and magnetic resonance imaging (MRI), imaging of the genital area has improved (Chang 2002). Congenital anomalies such as vaginal atresia and ambiguous genitalia can be evaluated by MRI.

Blood tests

Routine blood tests are of little value unless indicated by the history and examination.

Investigation in children may pose problems and should be carefully planned, often in consultation with colleagues in gynaecology and genitourinary medicine. The unoestrogenized vaginal mucosa can be easily damaged even with cotton-tipped swabs (Pokorny 1993). An alternative is a small 5 mm endoscope with the capacity for irrigation which can be used to examine the vagina in prepubertal children. This can be performed with a topical local anaesthetic in a cooperative child, but is more commonly carried out under general anaesthesia. In a child with a persistent vaginal discharge, or when sexual abuse is suspected, vaginal secretions can be obtained by a 'catheter-within-catheter' technique (Pokorny 1992).

Management

The diagnosis and further management are best discussed in detail with the patient after she has dressed. In some cases, specific areas in the history may need to be checked or explored in more detail and may be volunteered by patients once they are more relaxed. However, there are some instances when it may be appropriate to demonstrate certain things with the aid of a mirror while the patient is still undressed. This can be particularly helpful to explain the correct method and sites of treatment, or to reassure about normal anatomical variants. Digital photography may be useful to monitor changes in vulval pathology over time and also response to treatment. It is recommended that written consent is obtained from the patient for photography, that patient confidentiality is respected and maintained at all times and that laws on data protection are abided by.

For many of the conditions, it will be appropriate to reinforce the verbal explanation and advice given at the time with information leaflets for patients to take away. In the age of the worldwide web, many patients will look up information about their condition on the Internet and it is helpful to give details of trustworthy sites and patient support groups.

Topical treatment in vulval disease

General principles

Many women feel the need to cleanse the vulval area several times a day as they are often worried that a lack of hygiene on their part may have contributed to their vulval symptoms. The transepidermal water loss from the thinner vulval skin is greater than that from forearm skin (Britz & Maibach 1979). It is, therefore, more susceptible to the irritant effects of topical preparations, and the majority of proprietary brands including disposable wipes can cause an irritant dermatitis. Simple washing once daily with tepid water and using an emollient as a soap substitute should be encouraged. Emulsifying ointment is preferred because of the low allergenic potential with this substance. Aqueous cream is an alternative but may sting if the skin is fissured. Soap removes the natural lipids produced by epithelial cells that have an important role in the integrity of the skin barrier.

The majority of topical preparations used for vulval disorders are either creams or ointments. Gels and lotions often sting and are not widely used. An ointment is a water-in-oil emulsion and is a stable compound which rarely requires the addition of preservatives. Ointments form an impermeable layer over the skin that prevents evaporation of water. From the patient's point of view, they are greasy and may not spread so easily. However, they are the preferred vehicle for the delicate vulval skin.

Creams are oil-in-water emulsion preparations. They are less greasy than ointments and spread more easily. Their high water content requires the addition of preservatives to prevent contamination by bacteria and fungi, and to prolong shelf life. These additives can cause an allergic contact dermatitis. It is important to remember that preservatives, stabilizers and other additives are all components of topical

treatment and, if the cutaneous problem flares during treatment, it may be due to an allergic contact dermatitis to one of these agents. Allergy to the steroid molecule itself can rarely occur and is most common with hydrocortisone.

Emollients

In addition to their use as soap substitutes, emollients can also be applied directly if the skin is dry. Barrier preparations, for example zinc and castor oil cream or petroleum jelly, can be useful to protect the skin from the irritant effects of urine. Patients with erosive dermatoses, such as lichen planus, can also benefit from these.

Topical steroids

Topical steroids were first used in 1952 (Sulzberger & Witten 1952). They have revolutionized the treatment of many dermatoses although the mechanism of their anti-inflammatory action is not fully understood. Since the introduction of topical hydrocortisone, many different compounds have been formulated, and they are generally incorporated into a base or vehicle for ease of application. They are ranked in order of potency by their ability to produce vasoconstriction on the skin (McKenzie & Stoughton 1962). In the UK, there are four classes of topical steroid (Table 2.1), whereas in the USA there are seven categories (Table 2.2). The classification of some steroids differs in each system, which may lead to confusion. Sometimes, the topical steroid may be combined with an antimicrobial agent, which may be useful if there is secondary infection, but sometimes the antimicrobial agent can be the cause of a contact allergy. For the non-dermatologist, it is helpful to become familiar with at least one preparation from each category, and to tailor the strength and vehicle to the clinical situation. Generally, ointments are used, but the foam preparations frequently used by gastroenterologists for rectal inflammatory bowel disease can be used for intravaginal application.

If used correctly, topical steroids are safe. Fear of the potential side-effects such as skin atrophy and bruising often preclude their use by anxious patients. Their worries

Table 2.1 UK classification of topical steroids

Class	Potency	Examples
I	Mild	1% hydrocortisone
II	Moderate	Clobetasol butyrate 0.05% Fludroxycortide
III	Potent	Betametasone valerate 0.1% Fluticasone propionate Betamethasone dipropionate 0.05%
IV	Superpotent	Clobetasol propionate 0.05% Diflucortolone valerate 0.3%

Table 2.2 US classification of topical steroids

Class	Potency	Examples
I	Superpotent	Clobetasol propionate 0.05%
		Betamethasone dipropionate 0.05%
II	Potent	Mometasone furoate 0.1%
III	Upper mid-strength	Betamethasone valerate 0.1%
IV	Mid-strength	Fluocinolone acetonide 0.03%
V	Lower mid-strength	Fluticasone propionate
VI	Mild	Fluocinolone acetonide 0.01%
VII	Least potent	1% hydrocortisone

can be further strengthened not only by family and friends but also by healthcare professionals. Many of the product information leaflets included in the packaging state that they should not be used on the genitalia and a thorough explanation on the safe use of topical steroids for vulval disease needs to be given to the patient. The vulva is an area that is naturally occluded and therefore the penetration of the steroid is enhanced. In occluded areas, it has been shown that there is a 'reservoir effect' in which the steroid can stay in the stratum corneum for up to 2 weeks. The topical steroid therefore needs to be applied only once daily (Lagos & Maibach 1998). In children, the use of a cotton-tipped swab can be helpful to apply the treatment to a small area. When deciding about the correct amount to prescribe, a useful measure is the finger tip unit. This is the amount squeezed from a standard tube that covers the distance between the distal interphalangeal joint and the tip of the index finger, and equates to approximately 0.5 g (Long & Findlay 1991). About half this amount is adequate for one application to the vulva.

Other topical treatments

If the vulval dermatosis is weeping and eroded, then soaks can be useful for a short period. The antiseptic potassium permanganate in low dilution (e.g. 1:10000) can be very helpful to dry the area so that topical creams and ointments can then be used. A pad of gauze is soaked in the solution and then applied to the vulva for 10 minutes two or three times a day. It is vital to warn the patient that it will cause brown staining on anything that it comes into contact with, such as all receptacles, clothing, nails and skin. Erosive disease responds quickly and the soaks would not be continued for too long (48 hours is usually sufficient) as the potassium permanganate will cause an irritant dermatitis.

Many of the widely used treatments for psoriasis such as tar and vitamin D derivatives are far too irritant to be used on the vulva and a marked irritant dermatitis can ensue (see Chapter 5).

Imiquimod and topical 5-fluorouracil are used in specific situations to treat vulval intraepithelial neoplasia. These cause a significant inflammatory reaction and need to be applied much less frequently than in extragenital sites. Silver sulphadiazine cream can be used as a soothing rescue if the soreness is particularly severe.

For further details and potential side-effects of topical treatments, see Chapter 5.

References

Altmeyer, P., Chilf, G.-N. & Holzmann, H. (1982) Hirsuties papillaris vulvae (Pseudokondlyome der vulva). *Der Hautarzt* 33, 281–283.

Aral, S.O. & Holmes, K.K. (1990) Epidemiology of sexual behavior and sexually transmitted disease. In: *Sexually Transmitted Diseases*, 2nd edn (eds K.K. Holmes, P.-A. Märdh, P.F. Starling & P.J. Wiesner), pp. 19–36. McGraw Hill, New York.

Bauer, A., Greif, C., Vollandt, R. *et al.* (1999) Vulvar diseases need an interdisciplinary approach. *Dermatology* 199, 223–226.

Bergeron, C., Ferenczy, A., Richart, R.M. & Guralnick, M. (1990) Micropapillomatosis labialis appears unrelated to human papillomavirus. *Obstetrics and Gynaecology* 76, 281–286.

Birch, H.W. & Collins, J.H. (1960) The vulvar clinic. *Southern Medical Journal* 53, 473–477.

Blake, J. (1992) Gynaecologic examination of the teenager and young child. *Obstetrics and Gynecology Clinics of North America* 19, 27–38.

British Co-operative Clinical Group (1999) Genitourinary physicians and vulval clinics: a UK survey. *International Journal of STD and AIDS* 10, 220–223.

Britz, M.B. & Maibach, H.I. (1979) Human labia majora skin: transepidermal water loss in vivo. *Acta Dermato-venereologica. Supplementum* 59, 23–25.

Byrne, M.A., Taylor-Robinson, D., Pryce, D. & Harris, J.R.W. (1989) Topical anaesthesia with lidocaine-prilocaine cream for vulval biopsy. *British Journal of Obstetrics and Gynaecology* 96, 497–499.

Cazes, A., Prost-Squarcioni, C., Bodemer, C. *et al.* (2007) Histologic cutaneous modifications after the use of EMLA cream, a diagnostic pitfall: review of 13 cases. *Archives of Dermatology* 143, 1074–1076.

Chang, S.D. (2002) Imaging of the vagina and vulva. *Radiological Clinics of North America* 40, 637–658.

Chicago, J. (1996) *The Dinner Party*. Penguin Books, Harmondsworth.

Cooper, S.M. & Wojnarowska, F. (2001) The influence of the sex of the general practitioner on referral to a vulval clinic. *Journal of Obstetrics and Gynaecology* 21, 179–180.

Crawford, R.A.F., Todd, P., Fisher, C., Lowe, D.G. & Shepherd, J.H. (1995) Outpatient vulval biopsy: a note of caution. *British Journal of Obstetrics and Gynaecology* 102, 487–489.

Ekenze, S.O. & Ezegwui, H.U. (2007) Genital lesions complicating female genital cutting in infancy: a hospital-based study in South Eastern Nigeria. *Annals of Tropical Paediatrics* 27, 285–290.

Friedrich, E.G. (1983) The vulvar vestibule. *Journal of Reproductive Medicine* 28, 773–777.

Friedrich, E.G. & Wilkinson, E.J. (1985) Vulvar surgery for neurofibromatosis. *Obstetrics and Gynaecology* 65, 135–138.

Gordon, H., Comerasamy, H. & Morris, N.H. (2007) Female genital mutilation. *Journal of Obstetrics and Gynaecology* 27, 416–419.

Growdon, W.A., Fu, Y.S., Lebhertz, T.B. *et al.* (1985) Pruritic vulvar squamous papillomatosis: evidence of human papilloma virus aetiology. *Obstetrics and Gynaecology* **66**, 564–568.

Hart, D.B. & Barbour, A.H. (1882) *Manual of Gynaecology*, p. 6. Maclachlan and Stewart, Edinburgh.

Kelly, E. & Adams-Hillard, P.J. (2005) Female genital mutilation. *Current Opinion in Obstetrics and Gynaecology* **17**, 490–494.

Krantz, K.E. (1977) The anatomy and physiology of the vulva and vagina. In: *Scientific Foundation of Obstetrics and Gynaecology*, 2nd edn (eds E.E. Phillipp, J. Barnes & M. Newton), pp. 65–78. Heinemann, London.

Lagos, B.R. & Maibach, H.I. (1998) Frequency of application of topical steroids: an overview. *British Journal of Dermatology* **139**, 763–766.

Long, C.C. & Findlay, A.Y. (1991) The finger-tip unit – a new practical measure. *Clinical and Experimental Dermatology* **16**, 444–447.

Mason-Hohl, E. (1940) *The Diseases of Women, by Trotula of Salerno*. Ward Ritchie, Los Angeles.

McKenzie, A.W. & Stoughton, R.B. (1962) Method for comparing percutaneous absorption of steroids. *Archives of Dermatology* **86**, 608–610.

Micheletti, L., Bogliatto, F. & Lynch, P.J. (2008) Vulvoscopy. Review of diagnostic approach requiring clarification. *Journal of Reproductive Medicine* **53**, 179–182.

Moyal-Barracco, M., Leibowitch, M. & Orth, G. (1990) Vestibular papillae of the vulva. Lack of evidence for human papillomavirus aetiology. *Archives of Dermatology* **126**, 1594–1598.

Murphy, R. (2007) Training in the diagnosis and management of vulvovaginal diseases. *Journal of Reproductive Medicine* **52**, 87–92.

Pokorny, S.F. (1992) Prepubertal vulvovaginopathies. *Obstetrics and Gynecology Clinics of North America* **19**, 39–68.

Pokorny, S.F. (1993) The genital examination of the infant through adolescence. *Current Opinion in Obstetrics and Gynecology* **5**, 753–757.

Ridley, C.M. (1978) Diagnostic principles and techniques. *Clinical Obstetrics and Gynaecology* **21**, 963–972.

Ridley, C.M. (1993) The 1991 presidential address: International Society for the Study of Vulvovaginal Disease. *Journal of Reproductive Medicine* **38**, 1–4.

Royal College of Obstetricians and Gynaecologists (1997) *Intimate Examinations: a Report of a Working Party*. RCOG, London.

Schwartz, P. & Gillmore, M.R. (1990) Sociological perspectives on human sexuality. In: *Sexually Transmitted Diseases*, 2nd edn (eds K.K. Holmes, P.-A. Märdh, P.F. Starling & P.J. Wiesner), pp. 45–53. McGraw Hill, New York.

Sulzberger, M.B. & Witten, V.H. (1952) The effect of topically applied compound F in selected dermatoses. *Journal of Investigative Dermatology* **19**, 101–102.

Tan, A.L., Jojnes, R., McPherson, G. & Rowan, D. (2000) Audit of a multidisciplinary vulvar clinic in a gynaecologic hospital. *Journal of Reproductive Medicine* **45**, 655–658.

Tanner, J.M. (1962) *Growth at Adolescence*, 2nd edn. Blackwell, Oxford.

Torrance, C.J., Das, R. & Allison, M.C. (1999) Use of chaperones in clinics in genitourinary medicine: survey of consultants. *British Medical Journal* **319**, 159–160.

Vallance, H., Chaba, T., Clarke, L. & Taylor, G. (2004) Pseudo-lysosomal storage disease caused by EMLA cream. *Journal of Inherited and Metabolic Disease* **27**, 507–511.

van Buerden, M., van de Vanger, N., de Craen, A.J. *et al.* (1997) Normal findings in vulvar examination and vulvoscopy. *British Journal of Obstetrics and Gynaecology* **104**, 320–324.

Vaughan-Jones, S., Plamer, I., Bhogal, B.S. *et al.* (1995) Michel's transport medium for immunofluorescence and immunoelectron microscopy in auto-immune bullous diseases. *Journal of Cutaneous Pathology* **22**, 365–370.

Waugh, M.A. (1990) History of clinical developments in sexually transmitted diseases. In: *Sexually Transmitted Diseases*, 2nd edn (eds K.K. Holmes, P.-A. Märdh, P.F. Starling & P.J. Wiesner), pp. 3–16. McGraw-Hill, New York.

Chapter 3: Sexually transmitted diseases of the vulva

N.C. Nwokolo & S.E. Barton

Introduction

The vulva may be the site of a number of sexually transmitted infections. These infections may become manifest at the point of entry of the causative microorganism into the vulval skin, e.g. the primary chancre of syphilis, or following local dissemination as in genital herpes simplex, genital human papillomavirus (HPV) and molluscum contagiosum infections. Pathological processes occurring in the vagina such as candidiasis and trichomoniasis may have a secondary effect on the vulval skin. Sexually transmitted infections (STIs) such as genital herpes and genital warts, as well as non-sexually transmitted conditions such as candidiasis and bacterial vaginosis, may be aggravated by sexual intercourse.

The normal flora of the female genital tract

In adults, the predominant bacterial species within the vagina is *Lactobacillus*, which constitutes over 95% of the normal flora. However, large numbers of other organisms, both anaerobic and aerobic, also colonize the vagina, and alterations in the relative predominance of these organisms may be associated with vaginal symptoms.

Prior to puberty, in the absence of the raised levels of oestrogen associated with the onset of menarche, the vagina is colonized mainly by faecal bacteria and skin commensals and the pH is high (Hammerschlag *et al.* 1978). At the onset of menarche, rising oestrogen levels cause stratification and thickening of the squamous epithelium of the adolescent vagina and vestibule, and a fall in vaginal pH due to the increasing predominance of lactobacilli. Also present in smaller numbers are other species such as *Gardnerella*

vaginalis, Mycoplasma hominis, peptostreptococci and other streptococcal strains and *Bacteroides* species. It is thought that hydrogen peroxide-producing lactobacilli are responsible for maintaining the acidic pH necessary to control the numbers of endogenous bacteria within the vagina (Hawes *et al.* 1996). Following the menopause, oestrogen withdrawal causes a fall in the lactobacilli and a reversion to a premenarchal-like state. Variations in the normal vaginal flora are seen over the course of each menstrual cycle, and external influences also play a part in determining the relative predominance of different organisms (Bartlett *et al.* 1977, Wilks & Tabaqchali 1987, Keane *et al.* 1997).

Screening for sexually transmitted infections

The bulk of screening for STIs in the UK is carried out within genitourinary medicine (GUM) clinics, with limited screening occurring in gynaecology and family planning clinics and general practice.

In GUM, individuals requesting a screen are assessed by a clinician and testing is offered according to symptoms, taking into account the incubation periods of the various infections. A 'full STI screen' generally involves a genital examination during which swabs are taken for chlamydia, gonorrhoea, trichomonas, candidiasis and bacterial vaginosis. Serological testing for syphilis and HIV is also performed. Tests for other infections such as hepatitis B and C and herpes are performed according to clinical need. The advent of nucleic acid amplification testing (NAAT) techniques means that, increasingly, asymptomatic individuals may be offered non-invasive investigations using urine or self-taken vulvovaginal swabs.

Genital examination is performed with the patient either lying supine with knees apart or in the lithotomy position. It is important to have a strong, adjustable light source. Following inspection of the external genitalia for lumps, ulcers and discharge and palpation of the inguinal

Ridley's The Vulva, 3rd edition. Edited by Sallie M. Neill and Fiona M. Lewis. © 2009 Blackwell Publishing, ISBN: 978-1-4051-6813-7.

region for lymphadenopathy, speculum examination is performed.

An appropriately sized, lubricated speculum is inserted into the vagina to expose the cervix. The vaginal walls and cervix are inspected for discharge and lesions. Specimens are collected using a cotton-tipped swab or plastic loop. Vaginal swabs are taken for *Candida*, bacterial vaginosis and trichomoniasis. Specimens for chlamydia and gonorrhoea should be taken from the endocervix. Urethral, rectal and oropharyngeal swabs may also be sent for testing for chlamydia and gonorrhoea depending on clinical circumstances.

In GUM clinics, microscopic examination of vaginal and cervical discharge is performed at the time of examination for candidiasis, bacterial vaginosis, trichomoniasis and gonorrhoea. This allows definitive diagnosis and treatment of these conditions at the initial visit and before formal laboratory results become available. Specimens for microscopy are spread onto a glass slide and allowed to dry for Gram staining (*Candida*, bacterial vaginosis, gonorrhoea) or examined as wet preparations – the specimen is applied to a drop of saline on a glass slide and examined under a coverslip (*Trichomonas*, syphilis using dark-ground microscopy). Specimens for culture are directly inoculated onto appropriate culture media (Sabouraud's medium for *Candida*, New York City or other specific medium for gonorrhoea, and Diamond's or other appropriate medium for *Trichomonas*). When it is not possible to inoculate specimens directly onto culture media, they should be inserted into appropriate transport media. It is important to bear in mind that certain fastidious organisms such as *Neisseria gonorrhoeae* do not survive well in most transport media. Media such as Amies medium with charcoal may prolong the survival of *N. gonorrhoeae*. Specimens for NAAT are generally sent as dry swabs not inoculated into any medium. If in doubt, the local microbiology laboratory should be consulted as to the most appropriate method of transporting specimens.

Infection with protozoa

Trichomoniasis
Trichomonas vaginalis is a motile, flagellated protozoan (Fig. 3.1) which colonizes the lower genital tract of males and females.

Epidemiology
Trichomoniasis is the commonest non-viral sexually transmitted infection with over 170 million adults infected worldwide. In the UK, infection with *T. vaginalis* accounts for approximately 2% of GUM clinic attendances.

It is a significant cause of premature labour and low birth weight and appears to facilitate HIV transmission (Laga *et al.* 1993, Sorvillo & Kernott 1998, Bowden & Garnett 2000).

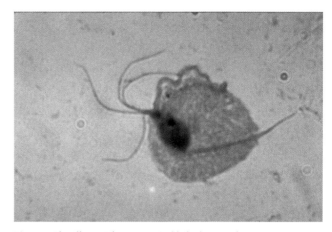

Fig. 3.1 Flagellate trichomonas. Published in Wisdom, A. & Hawkins, D. (1997) *Diagnosis in Color: Sexually Transmitted Diseases*, 2nd edn. Mosby-Wolfe, London; slide 275, p. 159, © Elsevier 1997.

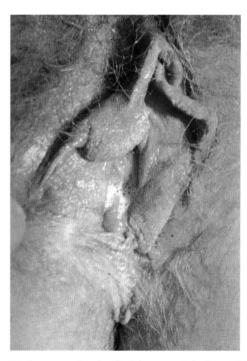

Fig. 3.2 Discharge associated with trichomonas infection. Published in Wisdom, A. & Hawkins, D. (1997) *Diagnosis in Color: Sexually Transmitted Diseases*, 2nd edn. Mosby-Wolfe, London; slide 276, p. 160, © Elsevier 1997.

Clinical features
T. vaginalis has an incubation period of 4–28 days (Hesseltine 1942). Up to 50% of infected women are asymptomatic. Symptoms vary from mild to severe and are mainly due to vulvovaginitis. The discharge is classically frothy, offensive smelling and purulent (Fig. 3.2). Infection of the urethra and paraurethral glands is common. Dysuria may be a feature.

Speculum examination may reveal the classic 'strawberry cervix' seen in about 2% of women (Sherrard 2007), which is due to punctate haemorrhages on the ectocervix.

Diagnosis

The simplest and most commonly used diagnostic test for *T. vaginalis* is microscopy of a wet mount preparation of vaginal fluid in saline. This allows demonstration of the characteristic motile flagellated protozoa and should be performed as soon as possible after the sample is taken as the organisms become less motile over time. Wet mount microscopy has a sensitivity of 60–70% compared with culture in women (Krieger *et al.* 1988, Gelbart *et al.* 1989, Levi *et al.* 1997). Because of the lower sensitivity and specificity of the wet mount preparation compared with culture, ideally vaginal samples should be sent for culture when possible. Newer techniques for the detection of *T. vaginalis* DNA in urine or vaginal secretions use polymerase chain reaction (PCR) technology and in some studies have a greater sensitivity than culture (Madico *et al.* 1998, Caliendo *et al.* 2005). These tests are not yet widely available in the UK.

Treatment

The recommended treatment for trichomoniasis is with oral metronidazole 2 g as a single dose or 400–500 mg twice daily for 5–7 days (Sherrard 2007). Tinidazole 2 g orally as a single dose may also be used. Metronidazole and tinidazole have a cure rate of approximately 95% (Gülmezoglu & Garner 1998). Spontaneous cure occurs in 20–25% (Sherrard 2007). It is important to ensure that the male partners of women with trichomoniasis are treated.

Treatment failure

Lack of response to treatment may be due to poor compliance, failure to treat the male partner, poor absorption, for example because of vomiting, or antimicrobial resistance. Repeating a standard course of treatment will usually result in a response in the first three situations. When resistance is suspected, higher doses or longer courses of metronidazole or tinidazole may be considered, as may the following treatments for which there is only anecdotal evidence: nonoxynol-9 pessaries nightly for 2 weeks and then once weekly for up to 7 months; acetarsol pessaries 2 × 250 mg nightly for 2 weeks; paromomycin sulphate 250 mg pessaries once or twice daily for 2 weeks (Sherrard 2007).

Infection with yeasts

Vulvovaginal candidiasis

Vulvovaginal candidiasis (VVC) is the second most common vaginal infection in the Western hemisphere after bacterial vaginosis (Sobel 1990). *Candida* species are recognized as part of the normal endogenous yeast flora of the vulva and vagina in women of childbearing age, and can be routinely

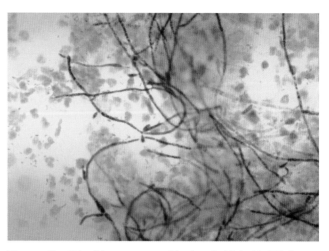

Fig. 3.3 *Candida albicans* spores and hyphae. Published in Wisdom, A. & Hawkins, D. (1997) *Diagnosis in Color: Sexually Transmitted Diseases*, 2nd edn. Mosby-Wolfe, London; slide 251, p. 148, © Elsevier 1997.

isolated in up to 50% of women (Drake & Maibach 1973). Of these, *Candida albicans* is responsible for almost 90% of symptomatic episodes of vulvovaginitis (Sobel 1997). *C. albicans* is an ovoid, budding yeast, which, under the microscope, may be seen as spores or hyphae (elongated filaments resembling a mould mycelium) (Fig. 3.3). Other *Candida* species such as *C. glabrata*, *C. tropicalis*, *C. parapsilosis* and *C. krusei* may also cause symptoms and may be resistant to conventional anti-candidal preparations.

Epidemiology

Approximately 75% of women of reproductive age will experience at least one episode of *Candida* vulvovaginitis in their lifetime (Sobel 1985). However, 10–20% of women with positive vaginal cultures for *Candida* will be asymptomatic (Daniels & Forster 2002).

A number of conditions may be associated with increased colonization of the vagina by *Candida*. These include uncontrolled diabetes mellitus, pregnancy and the use of systemic antibiotics. The association between the oral contraceptive pill and VVC is a matter of debate (Lapan 1970, Spinillo *et al.* 1995, Geiger & Foxman 1996); however, older high-dose oestrogen pills are more likely to cause this problem than the low-dose preparations currently available.

There is little evidence to suggest that modification of carbohydrate intake has any impact on the incidence of VVC in non-diabetic women (Foxman 1990, Weig *et al.* 1999). VVC is rare before menarche and has its highest incidence in the third and fourth decades. Although most women report an increase in the frequency of VVC coincident with the onset of sexual activity, it is not considered to be a sexually transmitted disease. Treatment of the male partners of women with VVC does not prevent infection in women. There are very few data about the prevalence of VVC in

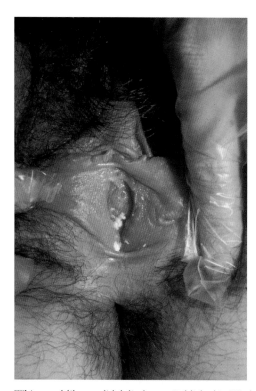

Fig. 3.4 White curd-like candidal discharge. Published in Wisdom, A. & Hawkins, D. (1997) *Diagnosis in Color: Sexually Transmitted Diseases*, 2nd edn. Mosby-Wolfe, London; slide 256, p. 151, © Elsevier 1997.

menopausal and postmenopausal women; however, studies suggest that hormone replacement therapy may be a predisposing factor (Sobel *et al.* 1998).

Clinical features
The cardinal symptom of VVC is pruritus. This may be intense and is usually accompanied by a thick, curd-like discharge (Fig. 3.4). Typically, the discharge is not offensive. Burning, external dysuria and superficial dyspareunia are common. In women with vulvovaginitis, individual symptoms and signs of vaginitis in the absence of laboratory tests are unreliable diagnostic indicators of candidiasis (Anderson *et al.* 2004). Several studies have shown that a subjective diagnosis of *Candida* vulvovaginitis in women with symptoms of pruritus, burning and discharge is inaccurate in 30% of women and leads to inappropriate treatment (Ferris *et al.* 1996, 2002, Linhares *et al.* 2001).

There may be erythema and swelling of the vulva with excoriation and fissuring. A thick cheesy discharge may be seen at the introitus. Speculum examination reveals erythema of the vaginal walls with adherent plaques of white exudate. Erythema may extend outwards and involve the perineum and perianal area.

Diagnosis
Measurement of the pH of vaginal secretions may be

Table 3.1 Treatment schedules for anti-candidal treatments

Drug	Formulation	Dosage regimen
Topical preparations		
Clotrimazole	Pessary	500 mg stat.
Clotrimazole	Pessary	200 mg × 3 nights
Clotrimazole	Pessary	100 mg × 6 nights
Clotrimazole	Vaginal cream (10%)	5 g stat.
Econazole	Pessary	150 mg stat.
Econazole	Pessary	150 mg × 3 nights
Fenticonazole	Pessary	600 mg stat.
Fenticonazole	Pessary	200 mg × 3 nights
Isoconazole	Vaginal tablet	300 mg × 2 stat.
Miconazole	Ovule	1.2 g stat.
Miconazole	Pessary	100 mg × 14 nights
Nystatin	Vaginal cream (100 000 U)	4 g × 14 nights
Nystatin	Pessary (100 000 U)	1–2 × 14 nights
Oral preparations		
Fluconazole	Capsule	150 mg stat.
Itraconazole	Capsule	200 mg b.d. × 1 day

Adapted with permission from www.bashh.org/guidelines/2002/candida_0601.pdf.

helpful in distinguishing VVC from other causes of vulvovaginitis. In VVC the pH is usually normal, whereas in trichomoniasis, for example, the pH is raised. Light microscopy of a Gram-stained vaginal smear demonstrates the presence of yeast blastospores or pseudohyphae in approximately 65–68% of patients with symptomatic VVC (Emmerson *et al.* 1994, Sonnex & Lefort 1999).

When microscopy is negative or unavailable a vaginal swab should be sent for fungal culture using Sabouraud's medium.

Treatment
Treatment should be reserved for symptomatic infection only. In the absence of symptoms, no treatment is required. Several topical and systemic antifungals are available and effective for the treatment of VVC (Table 3.1). There is no difference in the efficacy of single-dose regimens compared with short or longer course regimens (Reef *et al.* 1995). Individuals with severe vulvitis may benefit from the additional application of a low-potency topical steroid preparation.

Recurrent vulvovaginal candidiasis
Recurrent VVC is defined as four or more episodes of microbiologically proven infection in a year. Many women with other recurrent or persistent vulval conditions such as genital herpes, eczema and contact dermatitis are erroneously diagnosed as having recurrent VVC and treated inappropriately with antifungal agents.

The causes of recurrent VVC are unclear but appear more often to be related to abnormal host factors rather than a particularly virulent or resistant organism (Fidel & Sobel

1996). Conditions such as uncontrolled diabetes mellitus or immunosuppression may play a role, but in most cases no underlying cause is found.

Management is usually with an induction course of oral or topical therapy followed by a period of up to 6 months of maintenance therapy. The following maintenance regimens may be considered: fluconazole 100 mg weekly, itraconazole 50–100 mg daily (Reef *et al.* 1995) or clotrimazole 500 mg vaginal pessaries for 6 months (Sobel 1992). It may be necessary to repeat the induction/maintenance treatment courses if symptoms recur. Treatment of the male sex partners of women with recurrent VVC has not been shown to be effective in reducing the number of recurrences (Fong 1992).

Bacterial infections

Bacterial vaginosis

Bacterial vaginosis is the commonest cause of abnormal vaginal discharge in women of childbearing age with a prevalence varying from 5% to 50% (Hay 2006). It generally occurs as a consequence of a disturbance in the vaginal flora resulting in an increase in pH, with overgrowth of *G. vaginalis* and the other anaerobic species described above, together with a reduction in lactobacilli. The characteristic symptom of this condition is an offensive vaginal discharge, due to the production of amines such as putrescine, cadaverine and trimethylamine that give off a characteristic fishy odour (Brand & Galask 1986). Vaginal inflammation is uncommon; hence, the term vaginosis rather than vaginitis. Symptoms may be exacerbated by factors which lead to an increase in vaginal pH such as douching, menstruation and the presence of semen in the vagina. Although bacterial vaginosis occurs more commonly in sexually active women, evidence for its sexual transmission is lacking, and treatment of the sexual partners of women with this condition does not prevent it from recurring (Larsson 1992, Colli *et al.* 1997). Bacterial vaginosis has been associated with pelvic inflammatory disease (Ness *et al.* 2005), post-termination of pregnancy endometritis and late miscarriage (Larsson *et al.* 1992, Hay *et al.* 1994), preterm birth/rupture of membranes and postpartum endometritis (Hay *et al.* 1994).

Diagnosis
The diagnosis may be made by the fulfilment of Amsel's criteria (Amsel *et al.* 1983) or using the Hay–Ison (Ison & Hay 2002) or Nugent (Nugent *et al.* 1991) methods of examination of vaginal discharge.

To fulfil Amsel's criteria, at least three of the following must be present:
1 Thin, white, homogeneous discharge.
2 Clue cells on microscopy of wet mount (clue cells are vaginal epithelial cells covered with multiple Gram-variable

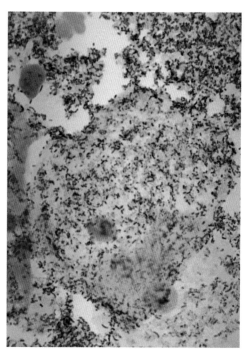

Fig. 3.5 Clue cell. Published in Wisdom, A. & Hawkins, D. (1997) *Diagnosis in Color: Sexually Transmitted Diseases*, 2nd edn. Mosby-Wolfe, London; slide 283, p. 163, © Elsevier 1997.

organisms so that their edges are completely obliterated) (Fig. 3.5).
3 pH of vaginal fluid > 4.5.
4 Release of a fishy odour with 10% potassium hydroxide.

A microscope is not necessary for a diagnosis to be made using Amsel's criteria as long as the other three prerequisites can be demonstrated.

The Hay–Ison method of diagnosis, on microscopy:
• Grade 1 (normal): *Lactobacilli* predominate.
• Grade 2 (intermediate): mixed flora with some *Lactobacilli*, but *Gardnerella* or *Mobiluncus* species also present.
• Grade 3 (bacterial vaginosis): predominantly *Gardnerella* and/or *Mobiluncus* species. *Lactobacilli* are few or absent.

The Nugent score is derived from estimating the relative proportions of different bacteria to produce a score between 0 and 10. A score of < 4 is normal; 4–6 is intermediate; and > 6 indicates bacterial vaginosis. The Hay–Ison and Nugent methods do not lend themselves easily to application outside of a specialist setting. Culture of vaginal fluid may grow *G. vaginalis*; however, this does not give a definitive diagnosis of bacterial vaginosis as this organism may be present as a commensal.

Treatment
Treatment of asymptomatic women is not necessary, although such women if diagnosed incidentally may choose to take treatment. The following treatment regimens are

recommended by the British Association for Sexual Health and HIV (BASHH) (Hay 2006): metronidazole 400–500 mg orally twice daily for 5–7 days; metronidazole 2 g orally as a single dose; metronidazole gel (0.75%) intravaginally once daily for 5 days; clindamycin cream (2%) intravaginally once daily for 7 days; clindamycin 300 mg orally twice daily for 7 days; or tinidazole 2 g orally as a single dose.

Chlamydial infections

Chlamydia trachomatis is an obligate intracellular bacterium with two distinct human biovars that share serological similarities but differ in the clinical syndromes they cause. The trachoma biovar includes the genital tract serovars D, E, F, G, H, I, J and K, which cause genital tract disease, and the trachoma serovars A, B and C, which cause the eye disease trachoma. The LGV biovar contains three strains, L1, L2 and L3, which cause lymphogranuloma venereum. Genital subtypes D–K can cause extragenital disease, including ophthalmia neonatorum and pneumonitis in infants and conjunctivitis in adults.

Genital chlamydia infection

Epidemiology

Genital chlamydia infection, the commonest STI in the UK and USA, has increased in the last decade. This increase is, in part, due to better detection and increased testing. The number of genital chlamydia infections in the UK and USA is highest in women aged 16–19 and in men aged 20–24. A pilot study for the UK National Chlamydia Screening Programme between 1999 and 2000 showed a prevalence of 10.5% in women in the 16–19 age group (UK Department of Health 2004). The burden of disease of genital chlamydial infection is high with its consequences of pelvic inflammatory disease (PID), ectopic pregnancy and tubal infertility, incurring an annual cost to the UK Department of Health of £100 million.

Pathogenesis

Non-LGV serovars of *C. trachomatis* mainly infect squamocolumnar (transitional) and columnar epithelial cells (Schachter 1999); hence, the predilection of this organism for the cervix, urethra, rectum and conjunctiva. Infection is initiated by the attachment of the organism as an infectious, but metabolically inert, form called the elementary body (EB), which then enters the cell via a membrane-bound vesicle called an inclusion body. Differentiation and further replication occur within the inclusion body, following which reorganization takes place, resulting in the formation of further infectious EBs. The EBs are released by cytolysis and go on to infect new cells (Morrison 2003). Infection with *C. trachomatis* is known to be associated with the establishment of persistent low-grade infection that may be present for years (Schachter 1999). However, the mechanisms for this are poorly defined. In cell culture, interferon gamma (IFN-γ) induces the production of non-infectious, atypical organisms which remain viable for over 1 month (Beatty *et al.* 1993). These atypical forms of chlamydia differentiate into infectious EBs when IFN-γ is removed from the cell culture system (Beatty *et al.* 1995).

The clinical effects of chlamydia infection are likely to result from a combination of tissue damage caused by replication of the organism as well as the inflammatory response induced by the organism itself and antigenic material from damaged host cells (Schachter 1999). The inflammatory response to chlamydial organisms is believed to be partly caused by a hypersensitivity induced by chlamydial heat shock proteins (HSPs), constituents of bacteria which share certain antigenic sites with human cells. Women with ectopic pregnancy and tubal infertility have been found to have high levels of antibody to chlamydial HSP-60 (Wagar *et al.* 1990, Toye *et al.* 1993).

Clinical features

The incubation period of *C. trachomatis* is approximately 11 days for men (Schofield 1982); however, there are no studies that give an accurate assessment of the incubation period in women. A review by Korenromp *et al.* (2002) inferred an incubation period of 20 days from a study of women in rural Uganda. Up to 80% of women with genital chlamydia are asymptomatic (Gaydos *et al.* 2004). In women with symptoms, these may include postcoital or intermenstrual bleeding, lower abdominal pain, vaginal discharge or dysuria. Examination may be normal or reveal mucopurulent cervicitis or contact bleeding from the cervix. Women with PID may have adnexal or cervical tenderness.

Complications of genital chlamydia infection

Chlamydial disease may be associated with infection of the Bartholin's glands (Davies *et al.* 1978). Infection may also spread upwards from the cervix into the endometrium and along the fallopian tubes resulting in PID. Seronegative reactive arthritis (sexually associated reactive arthritis; SARA), although rare in women, may occur as a consequence of genital chlamydial infection and may be associated with circinate vulvitis (Thambar *et al.* 1977), a condition clinically similar to circinate balanitis, a psoriasiform eruption on the glans penis seen in men with Reiter's syndrome. Other complications include Fitz-Hugh–Curtis syndrome (chlamydial perihepatitis associated with PID) and adult conjunctivitis.

Diagnosis

The diagnosis of chlamydia should be made using NAAT (Horner & Boag 2006). These demonstrate superior performance to culture and enzyme immunoassay (EIA) (Jespersen *et al.* 2005, Jalal *et al.* 2006), and also lend themselves well

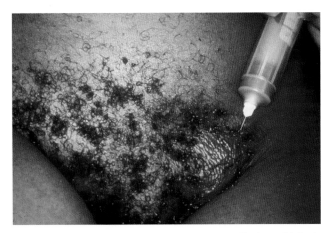

Fig. 3.6 Lymphogranuloma venereum: aspiration of bubo. Published in Wisdom, A. & Hawkins, D. (1997) *Diagnosis in Color: Sexually Transmitted Diseases*, 2nd edn. Mosby-Wolfe, London; slide 49, p. 50, © Elsevier 1997.

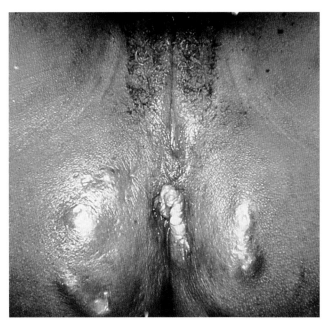

Fig. 3.7 Lymphogranuloma venereum: sinuses.

to non-invasive sampling techniques such as urine testing and vulvovaginal swabs taken by the patient. Suitable samples for chlamydia testing include endocervical, urethral and vulvovaginal swabs as well as first-catch urine samples.

Treatment

Both BASHH and the Centers for Disease Control and Prevention (CDC) recommend a single 1 g dose of azithromycin as the standard treatment for uncomplicated genital chlamydia (Horner & Boag 2006). Alternatives include doxycycline 100 mg twice a day for 7 days, erythromycin 500 mg twice a day for 10–14 days or ofloxacin 200 mg twice a day or 400 mg once a day for 7 days.

Individuals with chlamydia should be screened for other STIs and their partners should be traced and treated.

Lymphogranuloma venereum

Lymphogranuloma venereum (LGV) is uncommon in women outside the developing world, being most common in sub-Saharan Africa, southeast Asia and South America. Since 2003, there has been an ongoing epidemic of this infection in men who have sex with men in the UK and Europe (Health Protection Agency 2008).

LGV is caused by *C. trachomatis* serovars L1, L2 and L3. Unlike genital chlamydial infection, LGV is an invasive, lymphoproliferative disease, characterized by a primary lesion which appears as a small, painless papule, vesicle or ulcer on the vulva and which may go unnoticed (Viravan *et al.* 1996, Mabey & Peeling 2002). This lesion occurs most commonly at the posterior fourchette, but may also occur on the vaginal wall or cervix. The primary stage is followed by a secondary stage, which may occur weeks to months after the primary lesion (Perine & Stamm 1999,

Mabey & Peeling 2002). Only 20–30% of women present with adenopathy (Perine & Stamm 1999). Women may experience proctitis, which is thought to be due to direct inoculation. The secondary phase may be accompanied by systemic symptoms such as fever, myalgia, headaches and weight loss. The tertiary stage of LGV is associated with scarring. Untreated, it can lead to lymphatic obstruction and elephantiasis and stricture and fistula formation in the rectum (Figs 3.6 and 3.7).

Diagnosis

NAAT has increasingly been shown to be useful in identifying men with LGV (Mayaud 2006). Initial evaluation may be undertaken by using NAAT for *C. trachomatis* on appropriate clinical material and sending positive results to a reference laboratory for LGV serological testing, as NAAT does not distinguish non-LGV chlamydia serovars from LGV serovars (Mayaud 2006). However, NAAT has not been well evaluated on clinical samples other than urine, cervical, urethral and rectal swabs. Positive serology at titres > 1:256 strongly supports the diagnosis. Histology may also be helpful.

Treatment

The BASHH guidelines (Mayaud 2006) recommend the following regimens for the treatment of LGV: doxycycline 100 mg twice daily orally for 21 days (or tetracycline 2 g daily or minocycline 300 mg loading dose followed by 200 mg twice daily), or erythromycin 500 mg four times daily orally for 21 days. Investigation for other STIs and contact tracing and treatment are essential for all individuals with LGV (Mayaud 2006).

Gonorrhoea

Neisseria gonorrhoeae is a Gram-negative diplococcus which infects the urethra, cervix, anorectum and pharynx. Involvement of the vagina is unusual because the stratified squamous epithelium of this organ is relatively resistant to infection. In women, genital infection may spread to the surrounding areas including the paraurethral and Bartholin's glands, the fallopian tubes and the endometrium. From the pharynx, infection may disseminate resulting in systemic disease.

Epidemiology

Gonorrhoea is the second most common bacterial STI in the UK. In 2006, there were nearly 20 000 diagnoses of uncomplicated infection. In the UK, rates are highest in 16–19 year old women and 20–24 year old men. Widespread resistance to penicillin and quinolones means that in many countries, including the UK, the only antibiotics that *N. gonorrhoeae* consistently remains sensitive to are the cephalosporins. UK surveillance data show significant levels of *N. gonorrhoeae* resistance to penicillin (11.2%), tetracyclines (44.5%) and ciprofloxacin (14.1%) (Forsyth *et al.* 2000, Fenton *et al.* 2003). Resistance occurs by virtue of plasmid acquisition or as a result of alterations in the amino acid sequence of the gonococcal chromosome.

Clinical features

The incubation period for gonorrhoea is between 2 and 10 days (Wallin 1975, Harrison *et al.* 1979, Platt *et al.* 1983). Approximately 50% of women with gonorrhoea are symptomatic (Bignell 2005). Symptoms may include a vaginal discharge, dysuria, lower abdominal pain and, rarely, intermenstrual bleeding or menorrhagia. Rectal and pharyngeal infections are usually asymptomatic. Examination may be normal or reveal a purulent urethral discharge or mucopurulent cervicitis with or without pelvic tenderness.

Complications

Infection may spread from the urethra to the paraurethral (Skene's) glands and cause oedema of the urethral meatus and sometimes abscess formation. The gonococcus may also infect the Bartholin's glands causing enlargement and, if untreated, abscess formation (Fig. 3.8). Bartholin's abscesses are easily visible and treatment may require surgical intervention. Infection may spread from the cervix into the uterus and thence to the fallopian tubes resulting in salpingitis and PID with the consequent increased risk of tubal infertility, ectopic pregnancy and chronic pelvic pain. Haematogenous spread resulting in disseminated gonorrhoea

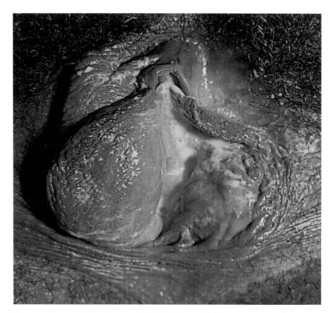

Fig. 3.8 Bartholin's abscess. Published in Wisdom, A. & Hawkins, D. (1997) *Diagnosis in Color: Sexually Transmitted Diseases*, 2nd edn. Mosby-Wolfe, London; slide 213, p. 127, © Elsevier 1997.

is uncommon (Hook & Handsfield 1999, Bignell 2005), but may result in cutaneous lesions, arthralgia or arthritis.

Diagnosis

The Gram-negative diplococci of *N. gonorrhoeae* may be seen on microscopic examination of the cervical or anorectal discharge. In women, the sensitivity of microscopy is between 30% and 50% (Ison 1990, Jephcott 1997, Hook & Handsfield 1999). Culture is 100% specific, but the sensitivity of this technique is variable, depending on collection and transport techniques. In optimal conditions, sensitivity approaches 85–95% (Bignell *et al.* 2006). Samples for culture should be plated directly onto specialized culture media or sent to the laboratory in appropriate transport media. Culture, however, performs suboptimally to the newer DNA detection techniques of NAAT which are being used increasingly in the detection of gonorrhoea (Palladino *et al.* 1999, Akduman *et al.* 2002). NAAT has sensitivities of up to 95% (Van Doornum *et al.* 2001, Van Dyck *et al.* 2001, Knox *et al.* 2002, Moncada *et al.* 2004), but it does not allow for antibiotic sensitivity testing. NAAT technology performs well on urine specimens and self-taken vulvovaginal swabs, allowing testing to be done non-invasively. However, in low-prevalence settings, the positive predictive value may be less than 80% so confirmation by culture is necessary (Van Doornum *et al.* 2001, Katz *et al.* 2004).

Treatment

The treatment of choice is a cephalosporin to which the

majority of organisms are sensitive. The choice of antibiotic used to treat gonorrhoea should be based on local antibiotic sensitivities. The UK BASHH (Bignell 2005) guidelines recommend ceftriaxone 250 mg intramuscularly or cefixime 400 mg orally as a single dose. When the organism is known to be quinolone sensitive, or when the regional prevalence of resistance to a particular antibiotic is less than 5%, alternatives include single doses of the following: ciprofloxacin 500 mg orally or ofloxacin 400 mg. Individuals with gonorrhoea should be screened for other STIs including chlamydia, which may be present in up to 40% of these women. It is mandatory that contact tracing is performed so that sexual partners can receive treatment (Bignell 2005).

Syphilis

This ancient disease is undergoing a resurgence perhaps as a result of an increase in unsafe sex practices, but more importantly because of its association with HIV infection. *Treponema*, subspecies *pallidum*, the causative agent of syphilis, is a spirochaete that causes infection only in humans. Other subspecies of *T. pallidum* are also known to cause human disease; *T. pertenue* is the cause of yaws, a tropical ulcer disease which has largely died out, whereas *T. carateum* causes pinta, a disfiguring condition endemic in South America. The *Treponema* subspecies are morphologically and serologically indistinguishable from one another. The organism cannot be cultured *in vitro*.

Clinical disease with *T. pallidum* is divided into five stages: primary, secondary, early latent, late latent and tertiary. The primary, secondary and early latent stages are associated with high rates of sexual and vertical transmission, while the late latent stage is less infectious although sexual and vertical transmission may still occur. In the tertiary stage, sexual transmission does not occur; however, vertical transmission may occur rarely (Stamm 1999).

Epidemiology

Syphilis remains a common condition worldwide with 12 million cases in 2004 (World Health Organization 2004). Syphilis and its consequences, including congenital syphilis, are associated with significant morbidity and mortality. In the years following the Second World War, rates of syphilis in the Western world declined as a result of more settled conditions and effective antibiotic treatment. Increased rates were again seen in the 1970s and 1980s predominantly in homosexual men, but these tailed off in the early 1990s, coinciding with the safer sex campaigns against HIV. Since the late 1990s, however, rates in men and, to a smaller extent, in women have been on the increase both in the UK and the USA. In England, infectious syphilis rates increased from 0.4/100 000 in 1998 to 8.8/100 000 in 2006. In women, rates increased from 0.2 to 1.3/100 000

over the same time period. The increase is thought to be as a result of localized outbreaks in Bristol, Manchester, Brighton and London over the past few years. A similar picture is seen in the USA where, in the period from 2001 to 2006, there has been an increase in rates in men from 3.0/100 000 to 5.7/100 000. Rates in women increased from 0.8/100 000 in 2004 to 1.0/100 000 in 2006 (CDC 2006a).

Pathogenesis

T. pallidum enters the tissues via small abrasions in mucous membrane or skin. The organism then attaches to local host cells and multiplies, following which it is then carried to the regional lymph nodes. At the site of initial entry, a primary chancre is formed, characterized by perivascular infiltrates of plasma cells, lymphocytes and macrophages together with an obliterative endarteritis. Millions of spirochaetes are present in the primary chancre, which usually appears 2–6 weeks after initial infection. Concurrent with the establishment of the primary lesion, haematogenous dissemination also occurs to distant organs. The resulting treponemal bacteraemia is characterized by the systemic symptoms and signs associated with secondary syphilis. Transplacental transmission to the fetus occurs most commonly in this stage.

The histological changes seen in the primary chancre are also mirrored in the lymph nodes and other organs and explain the spectrum of clinical disease seen in this condition. Cell-mediated and humoral responses are responsible for destroying the majority of organisms; however, some persist, perhaps because the treponemal cell surface presents few targets for the host immune response (Stamm 1999).

The primary and secondary stages are characterized by the development of antibody responses that can be used to assess the progress of disease and response to treatment. Serological responses to syphilis are both specific to *T. pallidum* and non-specific. Non-specific responses are mounted to lipid antigens on the treponemal cell surface and are measured using tests such as the Venereal Disease Reference Laboratory (VDRL) test or the rapid plasma reagin (RPR) test. VDRL and RPR increase in titre from the primary to the secondary stages of disease, fall in latent or treated disease and can be positive in other treponemal and non-treponemal diseases. Specific serological tests detect antibodies to *T. pallidum* only and are positive for life regardless of whether infection is treated or not. Specific tests in current usage include the treponemal enzyme immunosorbent assay (EIA), *T. pallidum* particle agglutination (TPPA) test, *T. pallidum* haemagglutination (TPHA) test and fluorescent treponemal antigen (FTA) test, which may measure immunoglobulin (Ig)G or IgM. The secondary stage can last for several weeks and may be associated with intermittent relapses and remissions. However, it is eventually curtailed by the host immune response. This

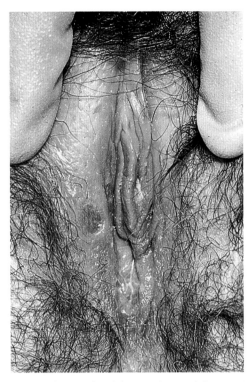

Fig. 3.9 Primary chancre of syphilis on right inner labium majus.

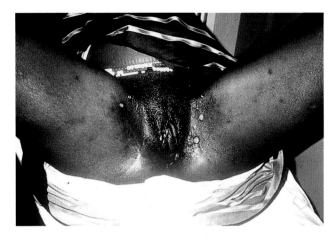

Fig. 3.10 Condyloma lata of secondary syphilis.

stage is followed by complete resolution of clinical symptoms, although specific serological tests remain positive. A period of latency follows the secondary stage in which, although organisms are no longer present in the blood stream, they are still present in many organs. The first 2 years after infection are described as the early latent period (in the USA, this refers to the first year only), during which there is a significant risk of secondary relapse. However, subsequent to this, in the late latent phase, secondary relapse does not occur.

The tertiary stage occurs in about a third of individuals with untreated disease and is characterized by invasion of the tissues of the central nervous system, cardiovascular system, skin, eyes and other organs. It is thought that this is because of declining immune responses (Stamm 1999). This stage usually occurs 3–12 years after infection (French 2007) and is associated with the formation of destructive granulomatous lesions called gummata, which may be found in skin, bones or internal organs. Histologically, a gumma is composed of a granuloma with monocytic and lymphocytic infiltrates and features of an endarteritis. They contain few or no treponemes.

Clinical features

In women, the primary chancre is commonly found on the vulva and starts as a macule, which then becomes papular

and eventually ulcerates (Fig. 3.9). The chancre is usually single and painless, but multiple, painful ulcers may occur. It classically has an indurated clear base without an exudate (Musher 1999). The development of the primary chancre may be accompanied by regional lymph node enlargement. Primary chancres may also occur within the vagina, on the cervix and within the oropharynx, and, as they are painless and often occur in hidden locations, they can go unnoticed. The chancre may persist for up to 6 weeks and is sometimes still present when symptoms of secondary syphilis appear, giving a clue to the diagnosis.

Secondary syphilis is associated with the development of constitutional symptoms including fever, general malaise and a generalized maculopapular rash characteristically involving the palms and soles. The palmar–plantar lesions are bronze coloured and may resemble the psoriasiform lesions of keratoderma blenorrhagica seen in Reiter's syndrome. Occasionally, pustular or vesicular lesions may occur. Oral and genital mucosal involvement can occur with painless superficial 'snail track ulcers' on the palate or larger greyish plaques called mucous patches. These lesions are highly infectious. Condylomata lata are the classical genital lesions seen in secondary syphilis and in women may be present on the vulva and in the perianal area (Fig. 3.10). They are large, wart-like lesions on a broad base and are usually present in warm, moist locations such as the intertriginous areas of the groins and axillae. Other symptoms, including alopecia, uveitis, jaundice, periostitis, glomerulonephritis and meningeal symptoms may also occur as a consequence of systemic vasculitis.

The gummata of tertiary syphilis may rarely occur on the vulva, as squamous lesions or subcutaneous nodules. They sometimes ulcerate and several cases have been described (Matras 1935, Konrad 1936). The differential diagnosis of the vulval lesions of syphilis includes other causes of genital ulceration such as genital herpes, chancroid, lymphogranuloma venereum, pyogenic infections, Behçet's disease and other dermatological ulcerative conditions. Condylomata lata may be difficult to distinguish from genital warts.

Diagnosis
Syphilis may be diagnosed by visualizing treponemes on dark-ground microscopy of fluid from a primary chancre or other infectious syphilitic lesion. Dark-ground microscopy has a sensitivity of between 79% and 97% and a specificity of 77–100% (Hook *et al.* 1985, Romanowski *et al.* 1987, Cummings *et al.* 1996). It is generally not available outside GUM services and, in the majority of cases, the diagnosis is made on serological tests. The treponemal EIA IgM/IgG is the first to become positive about 3 weeks after infection. The TPPA and TPHA tests usually become positive at about 4–6 weeks. The non-specific VDRL and RPR tests are positive at approximately 4 weeks (French 2007). Currently, several point-of-care tests for syphilis are being developed, offering the opportunity for rapid diagnosis (French 2007). Multiplex PCR techniques for the identification of *H. ducreyi* and *T. pallidum* have been developed although they are not in widespread use.

Treatment
Treatment of syphilis depends on the stage of disease. Parenteral penicillin remains the mainstay of treatment with no reports of resistance to this antibiotic. For early disease (primary, secondary and early latent), the UK BASHH guidelines (Goh 2002) recommend procaine penicillin G at a dose of 750 mg intramuscularly (i.m.) for 10 days, or benzathine penicillin 2.4 mU i.m. as a single dose or two doses 1 week apart. Late disease is characterized by slowly multiplying organisms so prolonged treatment with procaine penicillin for 17 days or three doses of benzathine penicillin 1 week apart are recommended (French 2002). The CDC recommends a single dose of benzathine penicillin for early disease and three doses a week apart for late disease (CDC 2006b). Neurosyphilis is treated with prolonged doses of intravenous or intramuscular penicillin (French 2002). In individuals who are allergic to penicillin, desensitization may be performed (CDC 2006b). This may be particularly important in individuals with neurosyphilis and in pregnancy since there are no studies on the efficacy of alternatives to penicillin in the treatment of these conditions. Alternatives to penicillin include doxycycline, erythromycin and azithromycin. Treatment with azithromycin has been associated with treatment failure and resistance (Lukehart *et al.* 2004), so close follow-up of individuals receiving this and other alternatives to penicillin should be undertaken.

Complications of treatment include the Jarisch–Herxheimer reaction, which is an acute inflammatory response to the killing of large numbers of treponemes in what is similar to an endotoxin reaction. About one- to two-thirds of individuals with primary or secondary syphilis will experience fever, chills, arthralgia and headache, which starts approximately 4–6 hours after treatment and subsides within a few hours (Musher 1999). The reaction may be associated with both penicillin and non-penicillin regimens and is not an indication to discontinue treatment. Management is with reassurance and analgesia. Screening for other STIs should be performed, and the sexual contacts of infected individuals should be screened and treated.

Chancroid
Chancroid is an uncommon cause of genital ulceration in the UK and is caused by *Haemophilus ducreyi*, a Gram-negative rod. Infection is prevalent in south-east Asia and Africa, but even in these regions it is declining, possibly as a result of mass syndromic management of STIs. In the 1980s there were several reports of chancroid in the UK in Sheffield, Manchester and Liverpool. The Manchester and Liverpool cases had travelled to endemic areas (Mallard *et al.* 1983, Arya *et al.* 1988).

Clinical features
Chancroid is characterized by the presence of painful genital ulcers and tender inguinal lymphadenopathy. Lesions occur after an incubation period of 3–10 days (Ronald & Albritton 1999, Lewis 2003). In women lesions usually involve the labia, posterior fourchette, perineum and perianal area (Fig. 3.11). Multiple lesions are common and have a ragged edge with a necrotic base containing purulent exudate.

Diagnosis
Diagnosis may be made by culturing material from the base or edge of the ulcer or from pus aspirated from an enlarged

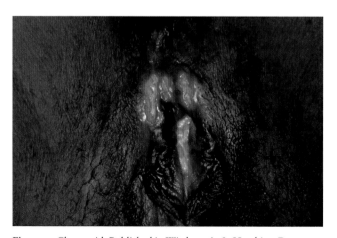

Fig. 3.11 Chancroid. Published in Wisdom, A. & Hawkins, D. (1997) *Diagnosis in Color: Sexually Transmitted Diseases*, 2nd edn. Mosby-Wolfe, London; slide 183, p. 112, © Elsevier 1997.

lymph node. Material should be placed in special culture medium (Lewis 2000). Microscopy has a low sensitivity and is not recommended routinely (Lewis & Ison 2006). Although NAAT has been developed for the simultaneous amplification of DNA targets from *H. ducreyi*, *T. pallidum* and herpes simplex virus (HSV) type 2, it is not yet widely available (Orle *et al.* 1996).

Treatment
The BASHH (Mayaud 2007) recommendations for treatment of chancroid include single doses of each of the following: azithromycin 1 g orally, ceftriaxone 250 mg i.m. or ciprofloxacin 500 mg orally.

Donovanosis
Donovanosis is an ulcerative condition caused by *Klebsiella granulomatis* (formerly *Calymmatobacterium granulomatis*). It is endemic in Papua New Guinea, parts of India, South America and southern Africa and in Australian Aborigines. No cases have been described in the UK in recent years.

Clinical features
In women, symptoms of infection begin with a small papule on the labia, fourchette or elsewhere on the vulva, following which the skin breaks down, forming deep-red, beefy, relatively painless ulcers. Inguinal lymphadenopathy is common. The cervix may be involved, resulting in lesions that mimic a carcinoma, and extragenital lesions may occur in the mouth, larynx, nose and on the chest.

Diagnosis
Diagnosis is made by demonstrating Donovan bodies (pleomorphic, bipolar-staining inclusions in histiocytes) or by culture (Carter *et al.* 1997).

Treatment
Treatment should be for at least 3 weeks or until all lesions are healed (CDC 2006b). Several antibiotic regimens are effective in the treatment of this condition. These include azithromycin 1 g weekly or 500 mg daily; ceftriaxone 1 g daily; doxycycline 100 mg twice daily and co-trimoxazole 960 mg twice daily (Richens 2001, CDC 2006b).

Viral infections

Genital herpes
Epidemiology
HSV types 1 and 2 are typically associated with oropharyngeal and genital infections, respectively. However, although genital herpes infection is most typically associated with the HSV type 2, epidemiological studies have shown that up to 50% of new presentations are caused by HSV type 1 (Ross

et al. 1993, Löwhagen *et al.* 2000, Forward & Lee 2003, Manavi *et al.* 2004). This may be the result of increasing numbers encountering this virus for the first time when they become sexually active and not in childhood as used to be the case, and also because oral sex has become much more commonplace. The strongest risk factor for acquiring genital herpes is a person's lifetime number of sexual partners (Corey & Handsfield 2000). The type 2 virus rarely causes symptomatic oropharyngeal disease, and genital infection remains the most common manifestation of infection with this virus.

The prevalence of HSV2 varies widely from country to country and within different populations in the same country (Smith & Robinson 2002, Weiss 2004). HSV infection is an important cofactor in the transmission of HIV. The majority of people with genital herpes are unaware that they are infected because they either have no symptoms or experience symptoms that neither they nor their physicians recognize as being due to herpes (Fleming *et al.* 1997, Gupta *et al.* 2007).

Pathogenesis
Infection with HSV most frequently occurs following contact of the virus with mucous membrane or abraded skin. Infection is followed by replication in cells of the epidermis and dermis, which may result in vesiculation of the affected tissue. The virus spreads along the lymphatics to the regional lymph nodes and thence to sensory or autonomic nerve root ganglia via local sensory neurones where they lie dormant. Latency may be established after both symptomatic and asymptomatic infection but the mechanisms by which this occurs are incompletely understood (Corey & Wald 1999). The majority of HSV2-infected individuals intermittently reactivate their virus, leading to periods of symptomatic or asymptomatic shedding of virus from skin or mucous membrane. Both host and viral factors influence reactivation. Insertion of HSV2 latency-associated transcripts into an HSV1 virus results in increased viral reactivation in sacral nerve root ganglia (Buchman *et al.* 1979), and those who are immunosuppressed experience more severe and frequent reactivations. Subclinical viral shedding may occur in over 80% of HSV2 infected individuals (Wald *et al.* 2000), and is likely to be the primary mechanism by which transmission occurs.

Clinical features
Initial primary and non-primary episodes Herpes infection may manifest itself clinically for the first time in two different ways: as a first or initial episode non-primary infection or as a true primary infection. First episode non-primary symptoms occur in individuals who have previously been exposed to any type of HSV in the past and in whom antibodies are already present at the time of the initial

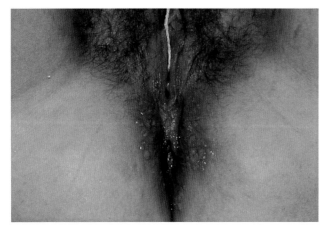

Fig. 3.12 Genital herpes.

symptoms. True primary infection occurs in an HSV sero-negative individual, i.e. one in whom there has been no previous exposure to HSV. Following an incubation period of fewer than 7 days, initial primary genital infection with HSV results. Approximately 20% of individuals develop prodromal symptoms lasting from 2 to 24 hours in which there is localized tingling and/or pain. Following the prodrome, papules appear on the skin, which then become vesicular and may ulcerate. Multiple lesions are usual (Fig. 3.12). Crusting and re-epithelialization follow and healing generally occurs about 3 weeks later without scarring. Viral shedding may continue for up to 16 days in primary infection (Corey 1988). Genital lesions are painful and may involve the vulva, perineum, perianal, urethral and introital regions. There may also be constitutional symptoms including fever, malaise, headache and inguinal lymphadenopathy is common. Sexually acquired HSV can produce extragenital lesions on the buttocks and thighs (Lautenschlanger & Eichmann 2001). Speculum examination in women may reveal cervical ulceration, which occurs in up to 90% of women with first episode infection (Barton et al. 1981, Corey et al. 1983). Individuals with prior exposure to HSV may experience less severe symptoms at the initial episode than those without previous infection. Symptoms of HSV1 are clinically indistinguishable from those of HSV2. Women have more severe symptoms and are more likely to have complications than men (Corey et al. 1983).

Recurrent episodes HSV2 causes, on average, four recurrences a year compared with HSV1, in which individuals tend to experience only one per year. Approximately 90% of people with HSV2 will have at least one recurrence in the 12 month period after infection (Benedetti et al. 1994). Recurrences tend to be milder and less widespread than the initial episode and the period of viral shedding is shorter.

In general, after the first 3 years, recurrences occur less frequently. The time from the initial appearance of vesicles to re-epithelialization is approximately 8 days (Corey & Wald 1999). Individuals with genital herpes may present with atypical symptoms including recurrent itching, fissuring, erythema or linear ulceration (Gupta et al. 2007). Many women with herpes are wrongly diagnosed with recurrent thrush or other vulval conditions (Lautenschlanger & Eichmann 2001).

Complications
Primary genital herpes may be accompanied by both external and internal dysuria in over 80% of women (Corey & Wald 1999). Dysuria may result from irritation caused by urine coming into contact with genital ulcers or autonomic nervous system dysfunction. Autonomic dysfunction may also result in constipation and hyperaesthesia of the perineal and sacral regions. Aseptic meningitis occurs in up to 36% of women (Corey et al. 1983, Corey & Wald 1999, Lautenschlanger & Eichmann 2001).

Herpes in pregnancy
Acquisition of genital HSV in pregnancy may result in spontaneous abortion and preterm delivery (Whitley et al. 1991, Brown et al. 1996) and in the transmission of infection to the neonate during labour. Congenital abnormalities such as chorioretinitis and hydroanencephaly may occur if infection is acquired before the third trimester of pregnancy (Florman et al. 1973, Hutto et al. 1987, Baldwin & Whitley 1989). Neonatal herpes is most frequently seen in infants whose mothers acquire primary infection in the third trimester (Brown et al. 1987) and may have a mortality of up to 80% (Whitley et al. 1991). The majority of infants acquire infection as a result of mucous membrane contact with infected maternal cervicovaginal secretions. In spite of the above, however, in the majority of pregnancies, there is usually very little HSV morbidity except when infection occurs close to the time of delivery (Brown et al. 1997). The prevalence of this condition in the UK is much lower (1.65/100 000 births) than in the USA (20–50/100 000 births) (Whitley 1990, Tookey & Peckham 1996). The reasons for this difference are unclear. Women who have antibodies during pregnancy, having had genital herpes previously, are much less likely to transmit infection to their infants (Brown et al. 1991, 1997). Continuous therapy with aciclovir or valaciclovir from 36 weeks' gestation has been shown to prevent recurrences at term (Scott et al. 1996, 2001, Sheffield et al. 2006). In the absence of recent acquisition of infection or lesions at the time of labour, vaginal delivery may be anticipated. Women presenting with first episode genital herpes at the time of delivery or within 6 weeks of the expected date of delivery should be offered caesarean section (Kinghorn et al. 2007).

Diagnosis

The diagnosis of genital herpes is usually made clinically; however, clinical diagnosis has a sensitivity of less than 40% and results in a false positive diagnosis in up to 20% of individuals (Koutsky *et al.* 1990). For this reason, a clinical diagnosis of genital herpes should be confirmed wherever possible. Viral culture has a specificity of 100% but a sensitivity of only 80% in primary disease and 25–50% in recurrent disease (Corey & Holmes 1983). Swabs from herpetic lesions should be taken as soon as possible after the lesions appear and should be inoculated into specific viral transport media. PCR techniques are up to four times more sensitive and are increasingly being used in the diagnosis of herpes (Gupta *et al.* 2007). Type-specific serology which distinguishes between glycoproteins G1 and G2 of HSV1 and -2, respectively, may be of benefit in ruling out genital HSV2 in an individual in whom culture has failed to provide a diagnosis. However, it does not allow one to distinguish genital symptoms caused by the type 1 virus from those caused by HSV2. Individuals with genital ulceration should always be tested for other causes of ulcers as well as for STIs in general.

Prevention

Condoms have been shown to offer some, but not complete, protection against transmission of genital HSV from seropositive men to their seronegative female partners (Wald *et al.* 2001), but the reverse has not been shown to be the case. The reason for this discrepancy may be that virus is shed from a larger surface area in women than in men, thus potentially exposing men to a higher risk of infection. A study of HSV2 serodiscordant couples in which seropositive partners took daily suppressive valaciclovir reduced transmission by 50% (Corey *et al.* 2004). There were no transmissions in couples who used condoms more than 90% of the time in conjunction with antiviral therapy.

Treatment

Primary herpes Treatment of primary genital herpes with an oral antiviral agent such as aciclovir, valaciclovir or famciclovir reduces both the duration and severity of symptoms. It does not, however, have any influence on the natural history of disease (Mertz *et al.* 1984, Brown *et al.* 2002). Aciclovir has poor bioavailability necessitating frequent dosing. Valaciclovir and famciclovir can be dosed less frequently, but are more expensive (Kinghorn *et al.* 2007).

Treatment should be started within 5 days of the onset of symptoms and as long as new lesions are forming. Even if only a small number of ulcers are seen at the time of presentation, treatment should still be given, as, untreated, progression of symptoms over the first week is common

(Corey & Wald 1999). The following 5 day regimens are commonly recommended: aciclovir 200 mg five times daily; aciclovir 400 mg three times daily; valaciclovir 500 mg twice daily; famciclovir 250 mg three times daily. Treatment may be continued beyond 5 days if new lesions are still forming (Kinghorn *et al.* 2007).

Recurrent herpes Individuals with infrequent recurrences may benefit from taking antiviral treatment with each episode. Oral antivirals reduce the duration of recurrences but should be given early, if possible in the prodromal phase (Nilsen *et al.* 1982, Sacks *et al.* 1996, Spruance *et al.* 1996). Patients should be educated about how to recognize symptoms so as to benefit from early intervention and be able to initiate treatment themselves. The following 5 day regimens are commonly used: aciclovir 200 mg five times daily; aciclovir 400 mg three times daily for 3–5 days; valaciclovir 500 mg twice daily; famciclovir 125 mg twice daily. Shorter courses of treatment have also been shown to be effective (Leone *et al.* 2002, Strand *et al.* 2002, Aoki *et al.* 2006). Studies of individuals with six or more recurrences a year have shown benefit with continuous daily suppressive treatment with one of the three antivirals named above (Kaplowitz *et al.* 1991, Mertz *et al.* 1997, Corey *et al.* 2004). Such individuals suffer fewer or no recurrences. There is good evidence of long-term safety of both aciclovir and valaciclovir (Girard 1996, Reitano *et al.* 1998).

Human papillomavirus infections

These are caused by HPVs, which are small non-enveloped double-stranded DNA viruses that infect the basal epithelial cells of skin and mucous membrane. There are over 100 different subtypes that are responsible for a wide variety of benign and malignant lesions. Types 6 and 11 ('low-risk' types) are the causative agents of anogenital warts (condylomata acuminata) and have little or no potential for malignant transformation, whereas types 16, 18, 31, 33, 45 and 51 ('high-risk' types) have significant potential to cause malignant change and are implicated in the aetiology of cervical and anal cancers. HPV16 and 18 are responsible for the majority of vulval intraepithelial neoplasia (see Chapter 8). HPV16 is the most prevalent of the high-risk types and is seen in at least half of all cases of invasive cervical carcinomas worldwide and some vulval cancers.

Virology

HPVs have an icosahedral capsid enclosing a circular viral genome. The genome has eight open reading frames (ORFs) which code for six early proteins (E1, E2, E4, E5, E6 and E7) and two late proteins (L1 and L2). The E1 and E2 proteins are important for viral replication, and E2 suppresses the expression of E6 and E7, which are important in malignant transformation (Chiang *et al.* 1992, Berg &

Stenlund 1997). E4 codes for proteins that disrupt cytoker-atin networks resulting in the formation of koilocytes, the vacuolated squamous epithelial cells characteristic of HPV infection (Doorbar *et al.* 1991). E5 is involved in cellular transformation and may interact with epidermal growth factor to induce cellular proliferation (Genther *et al.* 2003). E6 and E7 play important roles in cellular transformation via interactions with the p53 tumour suppressor gene, caus-ing downregulation of p53 activity (Hudson *et al.* 1990) as well as accelerated degradation of p53 (Werness *et al.* 1990, Hubbert *et al.* 1992; Zimmermann *et al.* 1999). E7 interacts with retinoblastoma (Rb) gene proteins, increasing degra-dation of these proteins as well as binding to other cellular proteins causing loss of cell cycle control (Munger *et al.* 1989). The L1 and L2 genes encode for the viral capsid proteins and L2 is important in interactions between the virus and host cell. L1 alone or with L2 can self-assemble into virus-like particles (VLPs) when expressed in eukary-otic or prokaryotic expression systems. Although these VLPs lack the virus genome DNA, their morphological and immunological characteristics are very similar to those of naturally occurring HPV and have been the basis for the development of HPV vaccines (Xu *et al.* 2000). Human HPVs do not possess the E3 ORF (Sonnex 1998).

Epidemiology

HPV infection is the commonest viral sexually acquired dis-ease worldwide. It is estimated that 80–85% of individuals will be infected with one or more HPV types during their lifetime (Jenkins *et al.* 1996). The prevalence of HPV infec-tion varies from country to country. In a study of women aged 15–74 without cytological abnormalities, from 11 countries, Clifford *et al.* (2005) demonstrated a prevalence range from 1.4% in Spain to 25.6% in Nigeria. In the UK, there has been a 300% increase in the number of diagnoses of anogenital warts made in GUM clinics over the last 10 years with 83 745 new diagnoses made in 2006. The highest incidence is in young people aged between 16 and 25, and rates of infection decline with age reaching their lowest levels after age 50. Factors associated with an increased risk of acquiring genital warts include number of sexual partners, presence of other sexually transmitted infections, smoking and use of the oral contraceptive pill, although some of this evidence is conflicting (Jamison *et al.* 1995, Franco 1996, Feldman *et al.* 1997, Munk *et al.* 1997; Habel *et al.* 1998, Wen *et al.* 1999). Transmission occurs via direct skin-to-skin contact during sexual activity. Studies show that, although condoms are beneficial for reducing trans-mission and in reducing the duration of symptoms, they do not completely eliminate the risk of transmission. This is likely to be because HPV may be transmitted from infected skin not covered by the condom (Wen *et al.* 1999, Winer *et al.* 2003).

Pathogenesis

In order for infection to occur, HPV is thought to gain access to the basal epithelial cells via abrasions in the skin. Once the virus enters the nucleus its genome becomes epis-omal and early promoter activity begins. Here, low levels of viral DNA synthesis occur and the expression of the viral proteins E6 and E7, important in malignant transforma-tion, is kept in check by the E2 protein, which acts as a sup-pressor of transcription. Infection is initially latent, but, as differentiation proceeds towards the surface, this stimulates late promoter activity leading to the production of late gene products L1 and L2 resulting in viral capsid formation and the production of complete viral particles (Cossart *et al.* 1995). Clinical lesions are thought to represent the clonal expansion of a population of keratinocytes derived from a single HPV-infected basal cell (Sonnex 1998).

Immunology

HPV infection is generally transient, with most infections being cleared within 12–18 months (Hildesheim *et al.* 1994, Ho *et al.* 1998). This suggests that the immune system is important in eradicating disease. The role of humoral im-munity in HPV infection is not clear. An antibody response may be detected approximately 8 months after infection and persists for up to 40 months. Women who develop anti-bodies are more likely to develop persistent infection than women who do not develop antibodies, suggesting that antibodies are not protective and serve only as markers of progression (Carter *et al.* 1996). In immunosuppressed indi-viduals, multiple resistant warts are common, and difficult to treat. These individuals are at increased risk of develop-ing anogenital cancers (Alloub *et al.* 1989, Lowy *et al.* 1994, Matteeli *et al.* 2001).

Clinical features

The incubation period of HPV is from several weeks to up to 18 months; however, the majority of infected indivi-duals will have subclinical disease which will go unnoticed (Sonnex 1998). Infection with genital HPV may manifest as visible warts present on the external genitalia (Fig. 3.13), in the vagina or on the cervix, as premalignant lesions in the form of vulval intraepithelial neoplasia (VIN) (Fig. 3.14), vaginal intraepithelial neoplasia (VAIN) or cervical intraepi-thelial neoplasia (CIN) or as a malignant tumour (Buschke–Lowenstein) (Fig. 3.15). Genital HPV types may also cause lesions at extragenital sites, including the face, oropharynx, conjunctivae and nasal cavity. This section will cover gen-ital warts only.

In women, the commonest site for the development of warts is the vulva; however, involvement of the vagina, cervix and perianal areas is common. Lesions may range from small, flat papules to typical condylomata acumin-ata (Fig. 3.16), which are irregular, fleshy, cauliflower-like

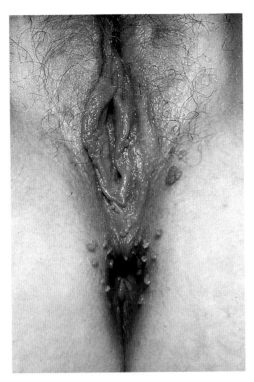

Fig. 3.13 Vulval and perianal papular warts.

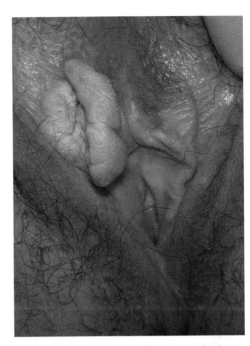

Fig. 3.15 Buschke–Lowenstein tumour arising on a background of lichen sclerosus.

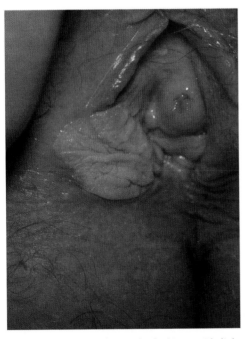

Fig. 3.14 Unifocal verrucous plaque of vulval intraepithelial neoplasia.

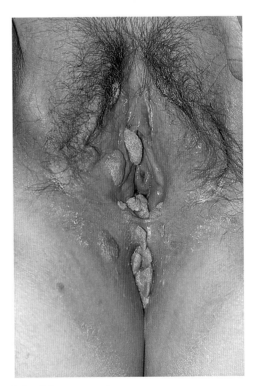

Fig. 3.16 Condylomata acuminata.

lesions that may grow to a very large size if left untreated. Lesions may become extremely large in pregnancy, in the immunosuppressed and in diabetics (Fig. 3.17). Cervical lesions may be subtle and flat, only becoming visible with application of acetic acid, or may appear as more florid condylomata. Visible genital warts are caused by low-risk HPV types 6 and 11 and do not, in general, transform into malignant lesions.

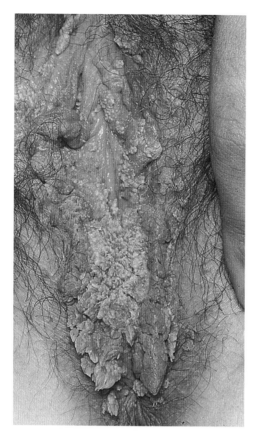

Fig. 3.17 Extensive condylomata acuminata.

Diagnosis

The diagnosis of genital warts is usually made on clinical grounds; however, in cases of doubt (e.g. where a lesion is pigmented or atypical), lesions should be biopsied. Histology reveals a hyperplastic prickle cell layer with elongated dermal papillae and koilocytes which are mature squamous cells with a large clear perinuclear zone (Koutsky & Kiviat 1999). However, a histological report of koilocytosis is not necessarily diagnostic of HPV infection and the clinical picture must be taken into account. There has been a tendency over the last 20 years to attribute many vulval conditions to infection with HPV, with the finding of koilocytes in the histological specimens. Koilocytic atypia has also been found in other vulval inflammatory conditions in the absence of papillomavirus infection (Dennerstein et al. 1994). There is also a problem of the misdiagnosis of koilocytosis in the mucosal epithelium of the vulval vestibule. The heavily glycogenated cells lose their glycogen during processing leaving vacuolated cells resembling koilocytes.

Treatment

The natural history of genital warts is that they may resolve spontaneously, remain unchanged or become florid. Avail-able treatments include 'over-the-counter' self-administered treatment, topical caustics, immunomodulators, physical therapies or surgery. The most appropriate treatment depends on the number, distribution and morphology of warts as well as the patient's choice.

Many of the treatments for warts aim to cause physical destruction of warty tissue, such as cryotherapy with liquid nitrogen, podophyllin, 0.15% podophyllotoxin cream, 0.5% podophyllotoxin solution and trichloroacetic acid. Podophyllotoxin is an antimitotic agent which causes arrest of spindle formation in metaphase, thus preventing cell division. Podophyllin has been associated with severe adverse skin reactions and is inferior to podophyllotoxin; it is therefore no longer recommended for the routine management of anogenital warts (Lassus 1987, Marzukiewicz & Jablonska 1990, Kinghorn et al. 1993, Lacey et al. 2003, Sonnex et al. 2007).

Cryotherapy and podophyllin must be administered by clinicians whereas podophyllotoxin may be self-administered. Imiquimod 5% is a new topical immune modulator inducing interferon and cytokine release, which stimulates both the innate and the cell-mediated immune response. Non-keratinized lesions usually respond well to podophyllotoxin, podophyllin or trichloroacetic acid, while keratinized lesions generally have a better response to cryotherapy or ablative measures such as surgery or electrocautery. Imiquimod is suitable for both keratinized and non-keratinized lesions (Sonnex et al. 2007). Podophyllin and podophyllotoxin are teratogenic and must not be used in pregnancy, but cryotherapy and trichloroacetic acid may be tried. Imiquimod has not yet been licensed for use in pregnancy.

Large lesions may need to be removed by surgical excision. Table 3.2 summarizes commonly used treatments and rates of clearance/recurrence.

Genital warts in children

Genital warts in children always raises the possibility of sexual abuse. Reports of abuse in children with genital warts vary from 0% to 80% (Armstrong & Handley 1997, Moscicki 1998). However, HPV is known to be transmitted by non-sexual means, and a recent epidemiological study from the USA showed that many anogenital HPV infections among preadolescent children are a result of non-sexual horizontal transmission, acquired either perinatally or postnatally (Sinclair et al. 2005). HPV types 3 and 27 are a common cause of hand warts and are found in anogenital warts in 10–20% of children where there is no evidence of sexual abuse (De Villiers 1994, Hammerschlag 1998). HPV subtypes do not appear to show the same high degree of site specificity in children as they do in adults (Armstrong & Handley 1997). It is important to consider the possibility of sexual abuse in all children who present with genital warts.

Table 3.2 Table of treatments, clearance and recurrence rates for anogenital warts

Agent	Self-/physician-administered treatment	Schedule of treatment	Clearance rate after 3 months	Recurrence rate	Notes
Podopyllotoxin	Self	Twice daily applications for 3 consecutive days followed by 4 day break for 4 or 5 cycles	34–77%	10–91%	Avoid in pregnancy
Imiquimod 5%	Self	3 times weekly applications for up to 16 weeks	50–62%	13–19%	Wash off after 6–10 hours. Not approved in pregnancy
Trichloroacetic acid 80–90%	Physician	Weekly applications until resolution	70%	36%	Can be used internally and in pregnancy
Cryotherapy	Physician	Weekly to twice weekly treatments until resolution	63–92%	0–39%	Can be used in pregnancy

Adapted with permission from http://www.bashh.org/guidelines/2007/ NatGuideMgxAGW2007.pdf.

One study showed the positive predictive value of genital warts for sexual abuse was 37% for children aged 2–12 years, and 70% for children over 8 years of age (Sinclair *et al.* 2005). Assessment of children with genital warts must be done in a non-judgemental manner, and should utilize a multidisciplinary team approach. Early involvement of a community paediatric team experienced in child abuse is important.

Human papillomavirus vaccines
Two vaccines against HPV have recently undergone evaluation in large clinical trials. Both vaccines are based on the recombinant expression and self-assembly of the major capsid protein, L1, into VLPs that resemble the outer capsid of the whole virus. The first, Gardasil (Sanofi Pasteur MSD, Maidenhead, UK), a quadrivalent vaccine against HPV types 6, 11, 16 and 18, was shown in the FUTURE I and II studies to reduce the incidence of clinical disease caused by these HPV types including anogenital warts and cervical, vulval and vaginal intraepithelial neoplasia in women between the ages of 15 and 26 (Garland *et al.* 2007). Gardasil was not effective at preventing disease in women already infected with the vaccine HPV types. Gardasil is currently licensed for administration to girls in several countries, including the USA and Australia (Australian Government Department of Health and Ageing 2007, Saslow *et al.* 2007). The United Kingdom Department of Health launched a vaccination programme at the end of 2008 (UK Government News Network 2007) using a second vaccine, Cervarix (GlaxoSmithKline Biologicals, Belgium), a bivalent vaccine against HPV types 16 and18.

Several concerns exist regarding the provision of HPV vaccines, including the anxiety that they will encourage unsafe sexual behaviour and promote premature sexual activity among adolescents. Second, there is as yet no data

about the long-term efficacy of the vaccines, and it remains unclear whether follow-up doses are necessary. Additionally, there are no data about the duration of protection necessary to prevent cancer. It remains to be seen how these issues play out.

Molluscum contagiosum
Epidemiology
Molluscum contagiosum is caused by the molluscum contagiosum virus (MCV), a DNA pox virus, with four distinct subtypes (MCVI, II, III and IV) all of which cause similar disease. MCVI is the commonest cause of childhood molluscum, whereas MCVII more commonly causes infection in adults and is the major cause of infection in HIV-positive individuals. MCVIII and -IV are rare. Infection is prevalent throughout the world, although the true incidence is unknown. A survey of general practices in the UK found an annual incidence of 261/100 000 (Pannell *et al.* 2005), while other authors give a worldwide estimate of between 2% and 8% (Billstein & Mattaliano 1990). In HIV-infected individuals the prevalence ranges from 5% to 18% and disease is more prevalent at lower CD4 counts (Schwartz & Myskowski 1992, Stefanaki *et al.* 2002). Atopic dermatitis, Darier's disease and immunodeficiency may all predispose to infection with MCV. Infection shows a biphasic incidence with peaks in childhood and early adulthood. Transmission of infection is generally by fomites and close physical contact. In adults, it is thought that sexual transmission plays an important role.

Pathogenesis
MCV is a double-stranded DNA virus measuring 200–300 nm in length, making it one of the largest known human viruses. Following infection, the virus establishes itself in the basal layer of the epidermis and multiplies in the

epithelial cell cytoplasm, destroying the cells and forming large inclusion bodies called 'molluscum bodies' containing large numbers of virus particles. The virus is not strongly immunogenic, so reinfection may occur.

Clinical features

After an incubation period of 1 week to 6 months (Low 1946, Brown *et al.* 1981), infection is manifested by the presence of discrete, pearly, umbilicated, papular skin lesions of varying sizes. These most commonly occur on the face, trunk and extremities in children and the lower abdomen, groins and genital region in adults. Immunosuppressed individuals, such as those with HIV infection, may develop extensive, disfiguring lesions, particularly involving the face.

Lesions usually develop over several weeks and may range in diameter from less than 1 mm to over 10 mm. Lesions may be single or multiple and may run into the hundreds in the immunocompromised (Schwartz & Myskowski 1992). They may become inflamed and pustular, healing after the lesions have crusted over. Spontaneous resolution is common but this may take several months.

In women lesions may occur on the lower abdomen, pubis and labia majora and adjacent skin (Fig. 3.18). Lesions do not affect the vagina or cervix. Molluscum contagiosum lesions may be confused with a variety of cutaneous lesions, including genital warts, basal cell carcinoma, cutaneous cryptococcosis, histoplasmosis and keratoacanthoma. A variant of the condition called a 'giant molluscum' may occur, and on the vulva may mimic a large genital wart.

Diagnosis

In the majority of cases, the diagnosis is made on clinical grounds. Where doubt about the diagnosis exists, lesions should be biopsied. Histology is characteristic and demon-strates intraepidermal lobules with central cellular and viral debris (Low 1946, Brown *et al.* 1981). The basal layer is composed of acanthotic prickle cells, and as the cells move towards the surface, virus particles form inclusion bodies which distort the cytoplasm and push the nucleus towards the periphery. The nucleus disappears and the resultant 'molluscum body' can be seen. Intact lesions show little or no inflammatory response while disrupted lesions may demonstrate an intense inflammatory response with the presence of lymphocytes, histiocytes and inflammatory giant cells. MCV cannot be grown in tissue culture.

Treatment

Treatment is mainly for cosmesis as the majority of lesions undergo spontaneous regression. Adults with genital molluscum contagiosum should be offered a screen for sexually transmitted infections. Many different treatment modalities are advocated for the treatment of molluscum contagiosum; however, there is very little evidence for the efficacy of most of these. The first of only two randomized controlled trials (RCTs) of treatment for genital molluscum contagiosum showed a 92% cure rate following treatment with 0.5% podophyllotoxin, compared with 52% in individuals treated with 0.3% podophyllotoxin and 16% in those treated with placebo (Syed *et al.* 1994). A second RCT of treatment for genital molluscum showed that individuals who received 1% imiquimod cream compared with placebo achieved cure rates of 82% and 16%, respectively, after 4 weeks of treatment (Syed *et al.* 1998). Neither of these treatments is licensed either in the UK or by the US Food and Drug Administration for the management of molluscum. Other treatments include cryotherapy, extirpation of the pearly molluscum core manually or with forceps, piercing with an orange stick, diathermy or curettage (Scott 2008a).

Infestations with ectoparasites

Scabies

Scabies is caused by the mite *Sarcoptes scabiei*. Infestation results from close personal, including sexual, contact. Genital infection is common in men with papular lesions on the scrotum and penile shaft but rare on the vulva (Fig. 3.19). The classical signs are usually found on the web spaces of the hands with characteristic burrows (Fig. 3.20). However, crusted or Norwegian scabies (a variant in which extremely large numbers of mites are present causing widespread pruritic, scaly lesions) may be associated with vulval involvement (Bakos *et al.* 2007). Crusted scabies is usually seen in immunocompromised or elderly individuals or in those with physical or mental disability (Billstein 1999). Treatment of non-crusted scabies should be with two applications of permethrin 5% cream or malathion 0.5% aqueous lotion applied to the whole body from the neck

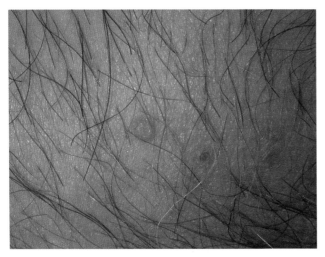

Fig. 3.18 Umbilicated lesion of molluscum contagiosum.

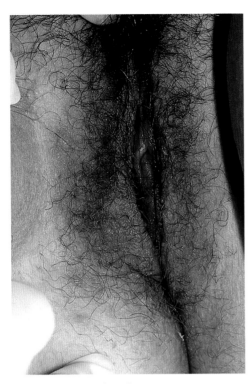

Fig. 3.19 Scabies: lesions on the vulva.

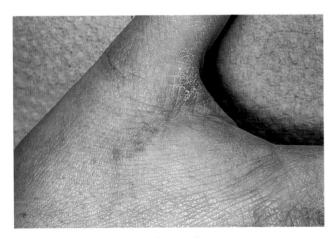

Fig. 3.20 Scabies: lesions in the finger web space.

down and left on for 12 hours; crusted scabies is treated with ivermectin at a dose of 200 μg/kg (Scott 2008b). All members of the family and close contacts should also be treated.

Pubic lice

Phthirus pubis, the 'crab louse' (Fig. 3.21) is sexually transmitted and infests the pubic hair causing itching which may lead to scratching, resulting in erythema and irritation. There may be no symptoms. Examination may reveal blue macules (maculae caeruleae) at feeding sites.

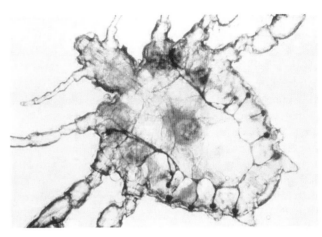

Fig. 3.21 Crab louse.

The pubic louse is also able to attach to the eyelashes, so these should be inspected in those who present with this condition. Infestation is commonly associated with the presence of other STIs and affected individuals should be offered screening. Treatment is with one or two applications of the following:
1 Malathion 0.5%, which should be applied to dry pubic hair and washed out preferably after 12 hours or overnight.
2 Permethrin 1% cream rinse applied to damp pubic hair and washed out after 10 minutes.
3 Phenothrin 0.2% applied to dry hair and washed out after 2 hours.

Infestation of eyelashes can be treated with permethrin 1% lotion, keeping the eyes closed during the 10 minute application, or with a paraffin-based ointment such as simple eye ointment BP applied to the eyelashes twice daily for 8–10 days (Scott 2008c).

HIV infection and vulval disease

The acquisition of HIV infection is more common in women with recurrent vulval HSV infection. Similarly, other conditions that lead to breaks in the vulval and vaginal epithelium, such as syphilis and other ulcerative bacterial conditions (i.e. lymphogranuloma venereum and chancroid), have been associated with higher rates of HIV incidence, particularly in the developing world. Studies are in progress to examine whether improved treatment of vulval ulcerative disease, especially HSV infection, will lead to reduced rates of HIV acquisition. Preliminary data from these studies suggest that prophylactic treatment with aciclovir 400 mg twice daily does not effectively protect against the acquisition of HIV infection (Celum *et al.* 2008).

In a woman with HIV infection, the major risk of developing vulval infections is related to a reduced CD4 count and consequent immune suppression. Significant immune suppression (CD4 counts < 200 cells/ml) is associated with increased rates of vaginal candidiasis, recurrent HSV and bacterial vaginosis. Standard treatment for these infections is sufficient in most patients (BASHH Clinical Guidelines 2006). It is important to exclude resistant HSV in patients with recurrent lesions and a very low CD4 count. After successful treatment of HSV in these cases, it is important to continue with antiviral agents prophylactically.

Longitudinal case-controlled studies of women with HIV have demonstrated that HIV-infected women were at least three times more likely to develop genital warts, although the risk of developing this condition is reduced with higher CD4 counts. Treatment of anogenital warts in immunocompromised individuals can be problematic, although benefits have been reported with immunological therapy (Gilson *et al.* 1999, Saiag *et al.* 2002).

It is likely that women who have acquired HIV infection have also been infected with HPV, particularly HPV16, HPV18, and other high-risk oncogenic subtypes. These are associated with an increased risk of cervical, vulval and anal premalignant and malignant disease.

There has also been an association of HIV infection with abnormal cervical cytology and a higher risk of more rapid progression to severe dysplasia. Currently, there is no evidence that there is a higher rate of VIN or squamous cell carcinoma in HIV-positive women.

Any woman diagnosed with HIV infection should be offered cervical screening at diagnosis, and annually thereafter. It is recommended that at these visits surveillance for vulval or perianal abnormalities is also performed. There is no evidence at present that performing annual colposcopy or anoscopy on HIV-infected women reduces the risk of development of cervical, vulval or anal cancer.

The new vaccines against HPV subtypes given to HIV-positive women who have not previously been infected with HPV may prevent the development of lower genital tract intraepithelial neoplasia (Palefsky 2008). However, it is not clear what effect vaccination after acquisition of infection will have. The plan to vaccinate all young girls should in theory prevent infection, which, in turn, may lead to a reduction in the risk for those who subsequently become HIV infected.

Summary

The vulva can be the primary site of infection in a number of STIs, as well as being secondarily involved as a consequence of a vaginal infection and discharge. Although the vulva is a well-defined anatomical structure for the clinician, many patients are unable to distinguish between the vulva and the vagina when describing their symptoms.

It is therefore important to take an accurate history and perform a thorough examination in all women presenting with lower genital tract symptoms. This information should then lead to appropriate investigations and management of the patient.

Acknowledgement

The authors are grateful to David Hawkins for allowing them to use the original slides that are reproduced in this chapter.

References

Akduman, D., Ehret, J.M., Messina, K. et al. (2002) Evaluation of a strand displacement amplification assay (BD Probetec-SDA) for detection of Neisseria gonorrhoeae in urine specimens. *Journal of Clinical Microbiology* 40, 281–283.

Alloub, M.I., Barr, B.B., McLaren, K.M. et al. (1989) Human papillomavirus infection and cervical intraepithelial neoplasia in women with renal allografts. *British Medical Journal* 298, 153–155.

Amsel, R., Totten, P.A., Spiegel, C.A. et al. (1983) Nonspecific vaginitis: Diagnostic criteria and microbial and epidemiologic associations. *American Journal of Medicine* 74, 14–22.

Anderson, M.R., Klink, K. & Cohrssen, A. (2004) Evaluation of vaginal complaints. *Journal of the American Medical Association* 291, 1368–1379.

Aoki, F.Y., Tyring, S., Diaz-Mitoma, F. et al. (2006) Single-day, patient-initiated famciclovir therapy for recurrent genital herpes: a randomized, double-blind, placebo-controlled trial. *Clinical Infectious Diseases* 42, 8–13.

Armstrong, D.K. & Handley, J.M. (1997) Anogenital warts in prepubertal children: pathogenesis, HPV typing and management. *International Journal of STD & AIDS* 8, 78–81.

Arya, O.P., Cupit, P., Dundon, M.B. et al. (1988) Chancroid in Liverpool. *Genitourinary Medicine* 64, 66.

Australian Government Department of Health and Ageing (2007) The national HPV vaccination program. General Practitioners. Available from: http://www.health.gov.au/internet/standby/publishing.nsf/Content/general-practitioners

Bakos, L., Reusch, M.C., D'Elia, P., Aquino, V. & Bakos, R.M. (2007) Crusted scabies of the vulva. *Journal of the European Academy of Dermatology and Venereology* 21, 682–684.

Baldwin, S. & Whitley, R.J. (1989) Intrauterine herpes simplex virus infection. *Teratology* 39, 1–10.

Bartlett, J.G., Onderdonk, A.B., Drude, E. et al. (1977) Quantitative bacteriology of the vaginal flora. *Journal of Infectious Diseases* 136, 271–277.

Barton, I.G., Kinghorn, G.R., Walker, M.J. et al. (1981) Association of HSV-1 with cervical infection. *Lancet* 2, 1108.

Beatty, W.L., Byrne, G.I. & Morrison, R.P. (1993) Morphologic and antigenic characterization of interferon gamma-mediated persistent Chlamydia trachomatis infection in vitro. *Proceedings of the National Academy of Sciences of the United States of America* 90, 3998–4002.

Beatty, W.L., Morrison, R.P. & Byrne, G.I. (1995) Reactivation of persistent *Chlamydia trachomatis* infection in cell culture. *Infection and Immunity* **63**, 199–205.

Benedetti, J., Corey, L. & Ashley, R. (1994) Recurrence rates in genital herpes after symptomatic first episode infection. *Annals of Internal Medicine* **121**, 847–854.

Berg, M. & Stenlund, A. (1997) Functional interactions between papillomavirus E1 and E2 proteins. *Journal of Virology* **71**, 3853–3863.

Bignell, C. (2005) National guideline on the diagnosis and treatment of gonorrhoea in adults. Available from: http://www.bashh.org/guidelines/2005/gc_final_0805.pdf

Bignell, C., Ison, C.A. & Jungmann, E. (2006) Gonorrhoea. *Sexually Transmitted Infections* **82** (Suppl 4), 6–9.

Billstein, S. (1999) Scabies. In: *Sexually Transmitted Diseases* (eds K.K. Holmes, P.F. Sparling, P.A. Mardh, *et al.*), pp. 645–650. McGraw Hill, New York.

Billstein, S.A. & Mattaliano Jr, V.J. (1990) The 'nuisance' sexually transmitted diseases: molluscum contagiosum, scabies, and crab lice. *The Medical Clinics of North America* **74**, 1487–1505.

Bowden, F.J. & Garnett, G.P. (2000) *Trichomonas vaginalis* epidemiology: parameterising and analysing a model of treatment interventions. *Sexually Transmitted Infections* **76**, 248–256.

Brand, J.M. & Galask, R.P. (1986) Trimethylamine: the substance mainly responsible for the fishy odour often associated with bacterial vaginosis. *Obstetrics and Gynecology* **63**, 682–685.

Brown, S.T., Nalley, J.F. & Kraus, S.J. (1981) Molluscum contagiosum. *Sexually Transmitted Diseases* **8**, 227–234.

Brown, T.J., McCrary, M. & Tyring, S.K. (2002) Antiviral agents: non-antiretroviral [correction of nonantiviral] drugs. *Journal of the American Academy of Dermatology* **47**, 581–599.

Brown, Z.A., Vontver, L.A., Benedetti, J. *et al.* (1987) Effects on infants of a first episode of genital herpes during pregnancy. *New England Journal of Medicine* **317**, 1246–1251.

Brown, Z.A., Benedetti, J., Ashley, R. *et al.* (1991) Neonatal *Herpes simplex* virus infection in relation to asymptomatic maternal infection at the time of labor. *New England Journal of Medicine* **324**, 1247–1252.

Brown, Z.A., Benedetti, J., Selke, S. *et al.* (1996) Asymptomatic maternal shedding of *Herpes simplex* virus at the onset of labor: relationship to preterm labor. *Obstetrics and Gynecology* **87**, 483–488.

Brown, Z.A., Selke, S., Zeh, J. *et al.* (1997) The acquisition of *Herpes simplex* virus during pregnancy. *New England Journal of Medicine* **337**, 509–515.

Buchman, T.G., Roizman, B. & Nahmias, A.J. (1979) Demonstration of exogenous genital reinfection with *Herpes simplex* virus type 2 by restriction endonuclease fingerprinting of viral DNA. *Journal of Infectious Diseases* **140**, 295–304.

Caliendo, A.M., Jordan Green, A.M., Ingersoll, J. *et al.* (2005) Real-time PCR improves detection of *Trichomonas vaginalis* compared with culture using self-collected vaginal swabs. *Infectious Diseases in Obstetrics and Gynecology* **13**, 145–150.

Carter, J.J., Koutsky, L.A., Wipf, G.C. *et al.* (1996) The natural history of human papillomavirus type 16 capsid antibodies among a cohort of university women. *Journal of Infectious Diseases* **174**, 927–936.

Carter, J., Hutton, S., Sriprakash, K.S. *et al.* (1997) Culture of the causative organism of donovanosis (*Calymmatobacterium granulomatis*) in HEp-2 cells. *Journal of Clinical Microbiology* **35**, 2915–2917.

CDC (2006a) Surveillance 2006: national profile. Syphilis. Available from: http://www.cdc.gov/std/stats/syphilis.htm

CDC (2006b) Sexually transmitted diseases. Treatment guidelines. Available from: http://www.cdc.gov/std/treatment/2006/genitalulcers.htm#

Celum C, Wald, A., Hughes, J. *et al.* (2008) HSV-2 suppressive therapy for prevention of HIV acquisition; results of HPTN 039. In: *Proceedings of the Conference on Retroviruses and Opportunistic Infections*, Abstract 32.

Chiang, C.M., Ustav, M., Stenlund, A. *et al.* (1992) Viral E1 and E2 proteins support replication of homologous and heterologous papillomaviral origins. *Proceedings of the National Academy of Sciences of the United States of America* **89**, 5799–5803.

Clifford, G.M., Gallus, S., Herrero, R. *et al.* (2005) Worldwide distribution of human papillomavirus types in cytologically normal women in the International Agency for Research on Cancer HPV prevalence surveys: a pooled analysis. *Lancet* **366**, 991–998.

Colli, E., Landoni, M. & Parazzini, F. (1997) Treatment of male partners and recurrence of bacterial vaginosis: a randomised trial. *Genitourinary Medicine* **73**, 267–270.

Corey, L. (1988) First-episode, recurrent, and asymptomatic *Herpes simplex* infections. *Journal of the American Academy of Dermatology* **18**, 169–172.

Corey, L. & Holmes, K.K. (1983) Genital *Herpes simplex* virus infections: current concepts in diagnosis, therapy, and prevention. *Annals of Internal Medicine* **98**, 973–983.

Corey, L. & Wald, A. (1999) Genital herpes. In: *Sexually Transmitted Diseases* (eds K.K. Holmes, P.F. Sparling, P.A. Mardh, *et al.*), pp. 285–312. McGraw Hill, New York.

Corey, L. & Handsfield, H.H. (2000) Genital herpes and public health: addressing a global problem. *Journal of the American Medical Association* **283**, 791–794.

Corey, L., Adams, H.G., Brown, Z.A. & Holmes, K.K. (1983) Genital *Herpes simplex* virus infections: clinical manifestations, course, and complications. *Annals of Internal Medicine* **98**, 958–72.

Corey, L., Wald, A., Patel, R. *et al.* (2004) Once-daily valacyclovir to reduce the risk of transmission of genital herpes. *New England Journal of Medicine* **350**, 11–20.

Cossart, Y.E., Thompson, C. & Rose, B. (1995) Virology. In: *Genital warts – human papillomavirus infection* (ed. A. Mindel), pp. 1–34. Edward Arnold, London.

Cummings, M.C., Lukehart, S.A., Marra, C. *et al.* (1996) Comparison of methods for the detection of *Treponema pallidum* in lesions of early syphilis. *Sexually Transmitted Diseases* **23**, 366–369.

Daniels, D. & Forster, G. (2002) National guideline on the management of vulvovaginal candidiasis. Available from: http://www.bashh.org/guidelines/2002/candida_0601.pdf

Davies, J.A., Rees, E., Hobson, D. & Karayiannis, P. (1978) Isolation of *Chlamydia trachomatis* from Bartholin's ducts. *The British Journal of Venereal Diseases* **54**, 409–413.

Dennerstein, G.J., Scurry, J.P., Garland, S.M. *et al.* (1994) Human papilloma virus vulvitis: a new disease or an unfortunate mistake? *British Journal of Obstetrics and Gynaecology* **101**: 992–8.

De Villiers, E.M. (1994) Human pathogenic papillomavirus types: an update. *Current Topics in Microbiology and Immunology* **186**, 1–12.

Doorbar, J., Ely, S., Sterling, J. *et al.* (1991) Specific interaction between HPV 16 E1-E4 and cytokeratins results in collapse of the epithelial cell intermediate filament network. *Nature* **352**, 824–827.

Drake, T.E. & Maibach, H.I. (1973) Candida and candidiasis: cultural conditions, epidemiology and pathogenesis. *Postgraduate Medicine* **53**, 83–87.

Emmerson, J., Gunputrao, A., Hawkswell, J. *et al.* (1994) Sampling for vaginal candidiasis: how good is it? *International Journal of STD & AIDS* **5**, 356–358.

Feldman, J.G., Chirgwin, K., Dehovitz, J.A. & Minkoff, H. (1997) The association of smoking and risk of condyloma acuminatum in women. *Obstetrics and Gynecology* **89**, 346–350.

Fenton, K.A., Ison, C.A., Johnson, A.P. *et al.* (2003) Ciprofloxacin resistance in *Neisseria gonorrhoeae* in England and Wales in 2002. *Lancet* **361**, 1867–1869.

Ferris, D.G., Dekle, C. & Litaker, M.S. (1996) Women's use of over-the-counter antifungal medications for gynecologic symptoms. *Journal of Family Practice* **42**, 595–600.

Ferris, D.G., Nyirjesy, P., Sobel, J.D. *et al.* (2002) Over-the-counter antifungal drug misuse associated with patient-diagnosed vulvovaginal candidiasis. *Obstetrics and Gynecology* **99**, 419–425.

Fidel, P.J. & Sobel, J.D. (1996) Immunopathogenesis of recurrent vulvovaginal candidiasis. *Clinical Microbiology Reviews* **9**, 335–348.

Fleming, D., McQuillan, G., Johnson, R. *et al.* (1997) Herpes simplex virus type 2 in the United States 1976–1994. *New England Journal of Medicine* **337**, 1105–1111.

Florman, A.L., Gershon, A.A., Blackett, P.R. & Nahmias, A.J. (1973) Intrauterine infection with *Herpes simplex* virus: Resultant congenital malformations. *Journal of the American Medical Association* **225**, 129–132.

Fong, I.W. (1992) The value of treating the sexual partners of women with recurrent vaginal candidiasis with ketoconazole. *Genitourinary Medicine* **68**, 174–176.

Forsyth, A., Moyes, A. & Young, H. (2000) Increased ciprofloxacin resistance in gonococci isolated in Scotland. *Lancet* **356**, 1984–1985.

Forward, K.R. & Lee, S.H.S. (2003) Predominance of *Herpes simplex* virus type 1 from patients with genital herpes in Nova Scotia. *The Canadian Journal of Infectious Diseases* **14**, 94–96.

Foxman, B. (1990) The epidemiology of vulvovaginal candidiasis: risk factors. *American Journal of Public Health* **80**, 329–331.

Franco, E.L. (1996) Epidemiology of anogenital warts and cancer. *Obstetrics and Gynecology Clinics of North America* **23**, 597–623.

French, P. (2002) UK national guideline for the management of late syphilis. Available from: http://www.bashh.org/guidelines/2002/late$final_b_311202.pdf

French, P. (2007) Syphilis. *British Medical Journal* **334**, 143–147.

Garland, S.M., Hernandez-Avila, M., Wheeler, C.M. *et al.* (2007) Quadrivalent vaccine against human papillomavirus to prevent anogenital diseases. *New England Journal of Medicine* **356**, 1928–1943.

Gaydos, C.A., Theodore, M., Dalesio, N. *et al.* (2004) Comparison of three nucleic acid amplification tests for detection of *Chlamydia trachomatis* in urine specimens. *Journal of Clinical Microbiology* **42**, 3041–3045.

Geiger, A.M. & Foxman, B. (1996) Risk factors for vulvovaginal candidiasis: a case-control study among university students. *Epidemiology* **7**, 182–187.

Gelbart, S., Thomason, J., Osypowski, P. *et al.* (1989) Comparison of Diamond's modified medium and Kupferberg for the detection of *Trichomonas vaginalis*. *Journal of Clinical Microbiology* **27**, 1095–1096.

Genther, S.M., Sterling, S., Duensing, S. *et al.* (2003) Quantitative role of the human papillomavirus type 16 E5 gene during the reproductive stage of the viral life cycle. *Journal of Virology* **77**, 2832–2842.

Gilson, R.J., Shupack, J.L., Freidman-Kien, A. *et al.* (1999) A randomised controlled safety study using imiquimod for the topical treatment of anogenital warts in HIV infected patients. *AIDS* **13**: 2397–2404.

Girard, M. (1996) Safety of acyclovir in general practice: a review of the literature. *Pharmacoepidemiology and Drug Safety* **5**, 325–332.

Goh, B. (2002) UK National guideline on the management of early syphilis. Available from: http://www.bashh.org/guidelines/2002/early$final0502.pdf

Gülmezoglu, A.M. & Garner, P. (1998) Trichomoniasis treatment in women: a systematic review. *Tropical Medicine and International Health* **3**, 553–558.

Gupta, R., Warren, T. & Wald, A. (2007) Genital herpes. *Lancet* **370**, 2127–2137.

Habel, L.A., Van Den Eeden, S.K., Sherman, K.J. *et al.* (1998) Risk factors for incident and recurrent condylomata acuminata among women. A population-based study. *Sexually Transmitted Diseases* **25**, 285–292.

Hammerschlag, M. (1998) Sexually transmitted diseases in sexually abused children: medical and legal implications. *Sexually Transmitted Infections* **74**, 167–174.

Hammerschlag, M.R., Alpert, S., Onderdonk, A.B. *et al.* (1978) Anaerobic microflora of the vagina in children. *American Journal of Obstetrics and Gynecology* **131**, 853–856.

Harrison, W.O., Hooper, R.R., Wiesner, P.J. *et al.* (1979) A trial of minocycline given after exposure to prevent gonorrhea. *New England Journal of Medicine* **300**, 1074–1078.

Hawes, S.E., Hillier, S.L., Benedetti, J. *et al.* (1996) Hydrogen peroxide-producing lactobacilli and acquisition of vaginal infections. *Journal of Infectious Diseases* **174**, 1058–1063.

Hay, P. (2006) National guideline for the management of bacterial vaginosis. Available from: http://www.bashh.org/guidelines/2006/bv_final_0706.pdf

Hay, P.E., Lamont, R.F., Taylor-Robinson, D. *et al.* (1994) Abnormal bacterial colonisation of the genital tract and subsequent preterm delivery and late miscarriage. *British Medical Journal* **308**, 295–298.

Health Protection Agency (2008) Lymphogranuloma venereum. Available from: http://www.hpa.org.uk/infections/topics_az/hiv_and_sti/Stats/STIs/lgv/statistics.hm

Hesseltine, H. (1942) Experimental human vaginal trichomoniasis. *Journal of Infectious Diseases* **71**, 127.

Hildesheim, A., Schiffman, M.H., Gravitt, P.E. *et al.* (1994) Persistence of type-specific human papillomavirus infection among cytologically normal women. *Journal of Infectious Diseases* **169**, 235–240.

Ho, G.Y., Bierman, R., Beardsley, L. *et al.* (1998) Natural history of cervicovaginal papillomavirus infection in young women. *New England Journal of Medicine* **338**, 423–428.

Hook, E.W. & Handsfield, H.H. (1999) Gonococcal infections in the adult. In: *Sexually transmitted diseases* (eds K.K. Holmes, P.F. Sparling, P.A. Mardh, *et al.*), pp. 451–466. McGraw Hill, New York.

Hook, E.W., Roddy, R.E., Lukehart, S.A. *et al.* (1985) Detection of *Treponema pallidum* in lesion exudate with a pathogen specific antibody. *Journal of Clinical Microbiology* **22**, 241–244.

Horner, P.J. & Boag, F. (2006) UK national guideline for the management of genital tract infection with *Chlamydia trachomatis*. Available from: http://www.bashh.org/guidelines

Hubbert, N.L., Sedman, S.A. & Schiller, J.T. (1992) Human papillomavirus type 16 E6 increases the degradation rate of p53 in human keratinocytes. *Journal of Virology* **66**, 6237–6341.

Hudson, J.B., Bedell, M.A., McCance, D.J. & Laimins, L.A. (1990) Immortalization and altered differentiation of human keratinocytes *in vitro* by the E6 and E7 open reading frames of human papillomavirus type 18. *Journal of Virology* **64**, 519–526.

Hutto, C., Arvin, A., Jacobs, R. *et al.* (1987) Intrauterine herpes simplex virus infections. *Journal of Pediatrics* **110**, 97–101.

Ison, C.A. (1990) Laboratory methods in genitourinary medicine: methods of diagnosing gonorrhoea. *Genitourinary Medicine* **66**, 453–459.

Ison, C.A. & Hay, P.E. (2002) Validation of a simplified grading of Gram stained vaginal smears for use in genitourinary medicine clinics. *Sexually Transmitted Infections* **78**, 413–5.

Jalal, H., Stephen, H., Al-Suwaine, A. *et al.* (2006). The superiority of polymerase chain reaction over an amplified enzyme immunoassay for the detection of genital chlamydial infections. *Sexually Transmitted Infections* **82**, 37–40.

Jamison, J.H., Kaplan, D.W., Hamman, R. *et al.* (1995) Spectrum of genital human papillomavirus infection in a female adolescent population. *Sexually Transmitted Diseases* **22**, 236–243.

Jenkins, D., Sherlaw-Johnson, C. & Gallivan, S. (1996) Can papilloma virus testing be used to improve cervical cancer screening? *International Journal of Cancer* **65**, 768–773.

Jephcott, A.E. (1997) Microbiological diagnosis of gonorrhoea. *Genitourinary Medicine* **73**, 245–252.

Jespersen, D.J., Flatten, K.S., Jones, M.F. & Smith, T.F. (2005) Prospective comparison of cell cultures and nucleic acid amplification tests for laboratory diagnosis of Chlamydia trachomatis infections. *Journal of Clinical Microbiology* **43**, 5324–5326.

Kaplowitz, L.G., Baker, D., Gelb, L. *et al.* (1991) Prolonged continuous acyclovir treatment of normal adults with frequently recurring genital *Herpes simplex* virus infection. The Acyclovir Study Group. *Journal of the American Medical Association* **265**, 747–751.

Katz, A.R., Effler, P.V., Ohye, R.G. *et al.* (2004) False-positive gonorrhoea test results with a nucleic acid amplification test: the impact of low prevalence on positive predictive value. *Clinical Infectious Diseases* **38**, 814–819.

Keane, F.E.A., Ison, C.A. & Taylor-Robinson, D. (1997) A longitudinal study of the vaginal flora over a menstrual cycle. *International Journal of STD and AIDS* **8**, 489–494.

Kinghorn, G.R., McMillan, A., Mulcahy, F. *et al.* (1993) An open comparative study of the efficacy of 0.5% podophyllotoxin lotion and 25% podophyllin solution in the treatment of condylomata acuminata in males and females. *International Journal of STD and AIDS* **4**, 194–149.

Kinghorn, G.R., Barton, S., Bickford, J. *et al.* (2007) National guideline for the management of genital herpes. Available from: http://www.bashh.org/guidelines/

Knox, J., Tabrizi, S.N., Miller, P. *et al.* (2002) Evaluation of self-collected samples for *Chlamydia trachomatis, Neisseria gonorrhoeae* and *Trichomonas vaginalis* by polymerase chain reaction among women living in remote areas. *Sexually Transmitted Diseases* **29**, 647–654.

Konrad, K. (1936) Ulceroses Syphilid zwei Jahre nach durchgefuhrer Malariakur. *Zentralblatt fur Hant- und Geschlechtskrankheiten* **53**, 150.

Korenromp, R.L., Sudaryo, M.K., de Vlas, S.J. *et al.* (2002) What proportion of episodes of gonorrhoea and chlamydia becomes symptomatic? *International Journal of STD & AIDS* **13**, 91–101.

Koutsky, L.A. & Kiviat, N.B. (1999) Genital human papillomavirus In: *Sexually Transmitted Diseases* (eds K.K. Holmes, P.F. Sparling, P.A. Mardh, *et al.*), pp. 347–359. McGraw Hill, New York.

Koutsky, L.A., Ashley, R.L., Holmes, K.K. *et al.* (1990) The frequency of unrecognized type 2 *Herpes simplex* virus infection among

women. Implication for the control of genital herpes. *Sexually Transmitted Diseases* **17**, 90–94.

Krieger, J.N., Tam, M.R., Stevens, C.E. *et al.* (1988) Diagnosis of trichomoniasis: comparison of conventional wet mount examination with cytological studies, cultures and monoclonal antibody staining of direct specimens. *Journal of the American Medical Association* **259**, 1223–1227.

Lacey, C.J.N., Goodall, R.L., Tennvall, G.R. *et al.* (2003) Randomised controlled trial and economic evaluation of podophyllotoxin solution, podophyllotoxin cream, and podophyllin in the treatment of genital warts. *Sexually Transmitted Infections* **79**, 270–275.

Laga, M., Manoka, A., Kivuvu, M. *et al.* (1993) Non ulcerative sexually transmitted diseases as risk factors for HIV-1 transmission in women: results from a cohort study. *AIDS* **7**, 95–102.

Lapan, D. (1970) Is the 'pill' a cause of vaginal candidiasis? Culture study. *New York State Journal of Medicine* **70**, 949–951.

Larsson, P.G. (1992) Treatment of bacterial vaginosis. *International Journal of STD & AIDS* **3**, 239–247.

Larsson, P.G., Platz-Christensen, J.J., Thejls, H. *et al.* (1992) Incidence of pelvic inflammatory disease after first-trimester legal abortion in women with bacterial vaginosis after treatment with metronidazole: a double blind, randomized study. *American Journal of Obstetrics and Gynecology* **166**, 100–103.

Lassus, A. (1987) Comparison of podophyllotoxin and podophyllin in treatment of genital warts. *Lancet* **2**, 512–513.

Lautenschlager, S. & Eichmann, A. (2001) The heterogeneous clinical spectrum of genital herpes. *Dermatology* **202**, 211–219.

Leone, P.A., Trottier, S. & Miller, J.M. (2002) Valacyclovir for episodic treatment of genital herpes: a shorter 3-day treatment course compared with 5-day treatment. *Clinical Infectious Diseases* **34**, 958–962.

Levi, M.H., Torres, J., Pina, C. *et al.* (1997) Comparison of the InPouch TV culture system and Diamond's modified medium for detection of *Trichomonas vaginalis. Journal of Clinical Microbiology* **35**, 3308–3310.

Lewis, D.A. (2000) Diagnostic tests for chancroid. *Sexually Transmitted Infections* **76**, 137–141.

Lewis, D.A. (2003) Chancroid: clinical manifestations, diagnosis, and management. *Sexually Transmitted Infections* **79**, 68–71.

Lewis, D.A. & Ison, C.A. (2006) Chancroid. *Sexually Transmitted Infections* **82** (Suppl 4), 19–20.

Linhares, I.M., Witkin, S.S., Miranda, S.D. *et al.* (2001) Differentiation between women with vulvovaginal symptoms who are positive or negative for *Candida* species by culture. *Infectious Diseases in Obstetrics and Gynecology* **9**, 221–225.

Low, R.C. (1946) Molluscum contagiosum. *Edinburgh Medical Journal* **53**, 657.

Löwhagen, G.B., Tunbäck, P., Andersson, K. *et al.* (2000) First episodes of genital herpes in a Swedish STD population: a study of epidemiology and transmission by the use of *Herpes simplex* virus (HSV) typing and specific serology. *Sexually Transmitted Infections* **76**, 179–182.

Lowy, D.R., Kirnbauer, R. & Sciller, J.T. (1994) Genital human papillomavirus infection. *Proceedings of the National Academy of Sciences of the United States of America* **91**, 2436–2440.

Lukehart, S.A., Godornes, C., Molini, B.J. *et al.* (2004) Macrolide resistance in Treponema pallidum in the United States and Ireland. *New England Journal of Medicine* **351**, 154–158.

Mabey, D. & Peeling, R.W. (2002) Lymphogranuloma venereum. *Sexually Transmitted Infections* **78**, 90–92.

Madico, G., Quinn, T.C., Rompalo, A. *et al.* (1998) Diagnosis of

Trichomonas vaginalis infection by PCR using vaginal swab samples. *Journal of Clinical Microbiology* **36**, 3205–3210.

Mallard, R.H., Macauley, M.E., Riordan, R. *et al.* (1983). *Haemophilus ducreyi* infection in Manchester. *Lancet* **2**, 283.

Manavi, K., McMillan, A. & Ogilvie, M. (2004) *Herpes simplex* virus type I remains the principal cause of initial anogenital herpes in Edinburgh, Scotland. *Sexually Transmitted Diseases* **31**, 322–324.

Marzukiewicz, W. & Jablonska, S. (1990) Clinical efficacy of condyline (0.5% podophyllotoxin) solution and cream vs podophyllin in the treatment of external condylomata acuminata. *The Journal of Dermatological Treatment* **1**, 123–126.

Matras, G. (1935) Lues III. Ulcer gummosa. *Zentralbum für Haut und Geshlechtskrankheiten* **51**, 89.

Matteelli, A., Beltrame, A., Graifemberghi, S. *et al.* (2001) Efficacy and tolerability of topical 1% cidofovir cream for the treatment of external anogenital warts in HIV-infected persons. *Sexually Transmitted Diseases* **28**, 343–346.

Mayaud, P. (2006) National guideline for the management of lymphogranuloma venereum (LGV). Available from: http://www.bashh.org/guidelines

Mayaud, P. (2007) National guidelines for the management of chancroid. Available from: http://www.bashh.org/guidelines

Mertz, G.J., Critchlow, C.W., Benedetti, J. *et al.* (1984) Double-blind placebo-controlled trial of oral acyclovir in first-episode genital *Herpes simplex* virus infection. *Journal of the American Medical Association* **252**, 1147–1151.

Mertz, G.J., Loveless, M.O., Levin, M.J. *et al.* (1997) Oral famciclovir for suppression of recurrent genital *Herpes simplex* virus infection in women. A multicenter, double-blind, placebo controlled trial. Collaborative Famciclovir Genital Herpes Research Group. *Archives of Internal Medicine* **157**, 343–349.

Moncada, J., Schachter, J., Hook, E.W. *et al.* (2004) The effect of urine testing in evaluations of the sensitivity of the Gen-Probe Aptima Combo 2 assay on endocervical swabs for *Chlamydia trachomatis* and *Neisseria gonorrhoeae*. *Sexually Transmitted Diseases* **31**, 273–237.

Morrison, R.P. (2003) New insights into a persistent problem – chlamydial infections. *Journal of Clinical Investigations* **111**, 1647–1649.

Moscicki, A. (1998) Genital infections with human papillomavirus (HPV). *The Pediatric Infectious Disease Journal* **17**, 651–652.

Munger, K., Werness, B.A., Dyson, N. *et al.* (1989) Complex formation of human papillomavirus E7 proteins with the retinoblastoma tumor suppressor gene product. *The EMBO Journal* **20**, 4099–4105.

Munk, C., Svare, E.I., Poll, P. *et al.* (1997) History of genital warts in 10 838 women 20 to 29 years of age from the general population. Risk factors and association with Papanicolaou smear history. *Sexually Transmitted Diseases* **24**, 567–572.

Musher, D.M. (1999) Early syphilis In: *Sexually Transmitted Diseases* (eds K.K. Holmes, P.F. Sparling, P.A. Mardh, *et al.*), pp. 479–485. McGraw Hill, New York.

Nandwani, R. on behalf of the Clinical Effectiveness Group of BASHH (2006) UK National Guidelines on the sexual health of people with HIV: sexually transmitted infections. Available from: www.bashh.org. 2006.

Ness, R.B., Hillier, S.L., Kip, K.E. *et al.* (2005) Bacterial vaginosis and risk of pelvic inflammatory disease. *Obstetrics and Gynecology Survey* **60**, 99–100.

Nilsen, A.E., Aasen, T., Halos, A.M. *et al.* (1982) Efficacy of oral acyclovir in the treatment of initial and recurrent genital herpes. *Lancet* **2**, 571–573.

Nugent, R.P., Krohn, M.A. & Hillier, S.L. (1991) Reliability of diagnosing bacterial vaginosis is improved by a standardized method of gram stain interpretation. *Journal of Clinical Microbiology* **29**, 297–301.

Orle, K.A., Gates, C.A., Martin, D.H. *et al.* (1996) Simultaneous PCR detection of *Haemophilus ducreyi*, *Treponema pallidum* and *Herpes simplex* virus types 1 and 2 from genital ulcers. *Journal of Clinical Microbiology* **34**, 49–54.

Palefsky, J. (2008) Human papilloma virus and anal neoplasia. *Current HIV/AIDS report* **5**, 78–85.

Palladino, S., Pearman, J.W., Kay, I.D. *et al.* (1999) Diagnosis of *Chlamydia trachomatis* and *Neisseria gonorrhoeae*, genitourinary infections in males by the Amplicor PCR assay of urines. *Diagnostic Microbiology and Infectious Disease* **33**, 141–146.

Pannell, R.S., Fleming, D.M. & Cross, K.W. (2005) The incidence of molluscum contagiosum, scabies and lichen planus. *Epidemiology and Infection* **133**, 985–991.

Perine, P.L. & Stamm, W.E. (1999) Lymphogranuloma venereum. In: *Sexually Transmitted Diseases* (eds K.K. Holmes, P.F. Sparling, P.A. Mardh, *et al.*), pp. 423–432. McGraw Hill, New York.

Platt, R., Rice, P.A. & McCormack, W.M. (1983) Risk of acquiring gonorrhea and prevalence of abnormal adnexal findings among women recently exposed to gonorrhea. *Journal of the American Medical Association* **250**, 3205–3209.

Reef, S.E., Levine, W.C., McNeil, M.M. *et al.* (1995) Treatment options for vulvovaginal candidiasis. *Clinical Infectious Diseases* **20**, (Suppl 1) 80–90.

Reitano, M., Tyring, S., Lang, W. *et al.* (1998) Valaciclovir for the suppression of recurrent genital herpes simplex virus infection: a large-scale dose range-finding study. International Valaciclovir HSV Study Group. *Journal of Infectious Diseases* **178**, 603–610.

Richens, J. (2001) National guideline for the management of donovanosis (granuloma inguinale). Available from: http://www.bashh.org/guidelines

Romanowski, B., Forsey, E., Prasad, E. *et al.* (1987) Detection of *Treponema pallidum* by fluorescent monoclonal antibody test. *Sexually Transmitted Diseases* **14**, 156–159.

Ronald, A.R. & Albritton, W. (1999) Chancroid and *Haemophilus ducreyi*. In: *Sexually Transmitted Diseases* (eds K.K. Holmes, P.F. Sparling, P.A. Mardh, *et al.*), pp. 515–523. McGraw Hill, New York.

Ross, J.D.C., Smith, I.W. & Elton, R.A. (1993) The epidemiology of *Herpes simplex* types 1 and 2 infection of the genital tract in Edinburgh 1978–1991. *Genitourinary Medicine* **69**, 381–383.

Sacks, S.L., Aoki, F.Y., Diaz-Mitoma, F. *et al.* for the Canadian Famciclovir Study (1996) Patient initiated, twice daily oral famciclovir for early recurrent genital herpes: a randomized, double-blind multicenter trial. *Journal of the American Medical Association* **276**, 44–49.

Saiag, P., Bourgault-Villada, I., Pavlovich, M. & Roudier-Pujol, C. (2002) Efficacy of imiquimod on external anogenital warts in HIV infected patients previously treated by highly active antiretroviral therapy. *AIDS* **16**, 1438–1440.

Saslow, D. Castle, P.E., Cox, J.T., Davey, D.D. *et al.* (2007) American cancer society guideline for human papillomavirus (HPV) vaccine use to prevent cervical cancer and its precursors. *CA: A Cancer Journal for Clinicians* **57**, 7–28.

Schachter, J. (1999) Biology of Chlamydia Trachomatis. In: *Sexually Transmitted Diseases* (eds K.K. Holmes, P.F. Sparling, P.A. Mardh, *et al.*), pp. 391–405. McGraw Hill, New York.

Schofield, C.B.S. (1982) Some factors affecting the incubation period and duration of symptoms of urethritis in men. *The British Journal of Venereal Diseases* **58**, 184–187.

Schwartz, J.J. & Myskowski, P.L. (1992) Molluscum contagiosum in patients with human immunodeficiency virus infection. *Journal of the American Academy of Dermatology* **27**, 583–588.

Scott, G. (2008a) National guideline for the management of molluscum contagiosum. Available from: http://www.bashh.org/guidelines

Scott, G. (2008b) UK National guideline on the management of scabies infestation. Available from: http://www.bashh.org/guidelines

Scott, G. (2008c) UK National guideline on the management of *Phthirus pubis* infestation. Available from: http://www.bashh.org/guidelines

Scott, L.L., Sanchez, P.J., Jackson, G.L. *et al.* (1996) Acyclovir suppression to prevent cesarean delivery after first-episode genital herpes. *Obstetrics and Gynecology* **87**, 69–73.

Scott, L.L., Hollier, L.M., McIntire, D. *et al.* (2001) Acyclovir suppression to prevent clinical recurrences at delivery after first episode genital herpes in pregnancy: an open-label trial. *Infectious Diseases in Obstetrics and Gynecology* **9**, 75–80.

Sheffield, J.S., Hill, J.B., Hollier, L.M. *et al.* (2006) Valacyclovir prophylaxis to prevent recurrent herpes at delivery: a randomized clinical trial. *Obstetrics and Gynecology* **108**, 141–147.

Sherrard, J. (2007) UK National guideline on the management of *Trichomonas vaginalis*. Available from: http://www.bashh.org/guidelines

Sinclair, K.A., Woods, C.R., Kirse, D.J. & Sinal, S.H. (2005) Anogenital and respiratory tract human papillomavirus infections among children: age, gender, and potential transmission through sexual abuse. *Pediatrics* **116**, 815–825.

Smith, J.S. & Robinson, N.J. (2002) Age-specific prevalence of infection with *Herpes simplex* virus Types 2 and 1. *Journal of Infectious Diseases* **186**, S3–S28.

Sobel, J.D. (1985) Epidemiology and pathogenesis of recurrent vulvovaginal candidiasis. *American Journal of Obstetrics and Gynecology* **152**, 924–935.

Sobel, J.D. (1990) Vaginal infections in adult women. *The Medical Clinics of North America* **74**, 1573–1602.

Sobel, J.D. (1992) Treatment of recurrent vulvovaginal candidiasis with maintenance fluconazole. *International Journal of Gynaecology and Obstetrics* **37**, 17–34.

Sobel, J.D. (1997) Vaginitis. *New England Journal of Medicine* **337**, 1896–1903.

Sobel, J.D., Faro, S., Force, R.W., Foxman, B. *et al.* (1998) Vulvovaginal candidiasis: epidemiologic, diagnostic, and therapeutic considerations *American Journal of Obstetrics and Gynecology* **178**, 203–211.

Sonnex, C. (1998) Human papillomavirus infection with particular reference to genital disease. *Journal of Clinical Pathology* **51**, 643–648.

Sonnex, C. & Lefort, W. (1999) Microscopic features of vaginal candidiasis and their relation to symptomatology. *Sexually Transmitted Infections* **75**, 417–419.

Sonnex, C., Birley, H., Fox, P. *et al.* (2007) UK guideline on the management of anogenital warts. Available from: http://www.bashh.org/guidelines

Sorvillo, F. & Kernott, P. (1998) Trichomonas vaginalis and amplification of HIV-1 transmission. *Lancet* **351**, 213–214.

Spinillo, A., Capuzzo, E., Nicola, S. *et al.* (1995) The impact of oral contraception on vulvovaginal candidiasis. *Contraception* **51**, 293–297.

Spruance, S.L., Tyring, S.K., DeGregoria, B. *et al.* and the Valaciclovir study group (1996) A large scale, placebo controlled, dose ranging trial of per oral valaciclovir for episodic treatment of recurrent herpes genitalis. *Archives of Internal Medicine* **156**, 1729–1735.

Stamm, L.V. (1999) Biology of Treponema pallidum. In: *Sexually Transmitted Diseases* (eds K.K. Holmes, P.F. Sparling, P.A. Mardh, *et al.*), pp. 468–472. McGraw Hill, New York.

Stefanaki, C., Stratigos, A.J. & Stratigos, J.D. (2002) Skin manifestations of HIV-1 infection in children. *Clinics in Dermatology* **20**, 74–86.

Strand, A., Patel, R., Wulf, H.C. & Coates, K.M. and the International Valaciclovir HSV Study Group (2002) Aborted genital herpes simplex virus lesions: findings from a randomised controlled trial with valaciclovir. *Sexually Transmitted Infections* **78**, 435–439.

Syed, T.A., Lundin, S. & Ahmad, M. (1994) Topical 0.3% and 0.5% podophyllotoxin cream for self-treatment of molluscum contagiosum in males. A placebo-controlled, double-blind study. *Dermatology* **189**, 65–68.

Syed, T.A., Goswami, J., Abbas, A.O. & Seyed, A.A. (1998) Treatment of molluscum contagiosum in males with an analog of imiquimod 1% in cream: a placebo-controlled, double-blind study. *Journal of Dermatology* **25**, 309–313.

Thambar, I.V., Dunlop, R., Thin, R.N. & Huskisson, E.C. (1977) Circinate vulvitis in Reiter's syndrome. *The British Journal of Venereal Diseases* **53**, 260–262.

Tookey, P. & Peckham, C.S. (1996) Neonatal *Herpes simplex* virus infection in the British Isles. *Paediatric and Perinatal Epidemiology* **10**, 432–442.

Toye, B., Lafirriere, C., Claman, P. *et al.* (1993) Association between antibody to the chlamydial heat shock protein and tubal infertility. *Journal of Infectious Diseases* **168**, 1236–1240.

UK Department of Health (2004) National Chlamydia Screening Programme. Available from: http://www.chlamydiascreening.nhs.uk/ps/assets/pdfs/a-rprt-03_04.pdf

UK Government News Network (2007) HPV vaccine recommended for NHS immunisation programme. Available from: http://www.gnn.gov.uk/environment/fullDetail.asp?ReleaseID=325799&NewsAreaID=2

Van Doornum, G.J., Schouls, L.M., Pijl, A. *et al.* (2001) Comparison between the LCx Probe system and the Cobas Amplicor system for the detection of *Chlamydia trachomatis* and *Neisseria gonorrhoeae* infections in patients attending a clinic for sexually transmitted diseases in Amsterdam, The Netherlands. *Journal of Clinical Microbiology* **39**, 829–835.

Van Dyck, E., Ieven, M., Pattyn, S. *et al.* (2001) Detection of *Chlamydia trachomatis* and *Neisseria gonorrhoeae* by enzyme immunoassay, culture, and three nucleic acid amplification tests. *Journal of Clinical Microbiology* **39**, 1751–1756.

Viravan, C., Dance, D.A.B., Ariyarit, C. *et al.* (1996) A prospective clinical and bacteriologic study of inguinal buboes in Thai men. *Clinical Infectious Diseases* **22**, 233–239.

Wagar, E.A., Schachter, J., Bavoli, P. & Stephens, R.S. (1990) Differential human serologic response to two 60,000 molecular weight *Chlamydia trachomatis* antigens. *Journal of Infectious Diseases* **162**, 922–927.

Wald, A., Zeh, J., Selke, S., Warren, T. *et al.* (2000) Reactivation of genital *Herpes simplex* virus type 2 infection in asymptomatic seropositive persons. *New England Journal of Medicine* **342**, 844–850.

Wald, A., Langenberg, A.G.M. & Link, K. (2001) Effect of condoms on reducing the transmission of *Herpes simplex* virus type 2 from men to women. *Journal of the American Medical Association* **285**, 3100–3106.

Wallin, J. (1975) Gonorrhoea in 1972. A 1-year study of patients attending the VD Unit in Uppsala. *The British Journal of Venereal Diseases* **51**, 41–47.

Weig, M., Werner, E., Frosch, M. & Kasper, H. (1999) Limited effect of refined carbohydrate dietary supplementation on colonization of the gastrointestinal tract of healthy subjects by Candida albicans. *American Journal of Clinical Nutrition* **69**, 1170–1173.

Weiss, H. (2004) Epidemiology of *Herpes simplex virus* type 2 infection in the developing world. *Herpes* **11** (Suppl 1), 24A–35A.

Wen, L.M., Estcourt, C.S., Simpson, J.M. & Mindel, A. (1999) Risk factors for the acquisition of genital warts: are condoms protective? *Sexually Transmitted Infections* **75**, 312–316.

Werness, B.A., Levine, A.J. & Howley, P.M. (1990) Association of human papillomaviruses types 16 and 18 proteins with p53. *Science* **248**, 76–79.

Whitley, R. (1990) *Herpes simplex* virus infections. In: *Infectious diseases of the fetus and newborn infant* (eds J.S. Remmington & J.O. Klein), pp. 282–301. WB Saunders, Philadelphia.

Whitley, R., Arvin, A., Prober, C. *et al.* (1991) Predictors of morbidity and mortality in neonates with *Herpes simplex* virus infections. *New England Journal of Medicine* **324**, 450–454.

Wilks, M. & Tabaqchali, S. (1987) Quantitative bacteriology of the vaginal flora during the menstrual cycle. *Journal of Medical Microbiology* **24**, 241–245.

Winer, R.L., Lee, S.-K., Hughes, J.P. *et al.* (2003) Genital human papillomavirus infection: incidence and risk factors in a cohort of female university students. *American Journal of Epidemiology* **157**, 218–226.

World Health Organization (2004) Disease watch. Syphilis. Available from: http://www.who.int/std_diagnostics/publications/Disease%20watch%20syphilis.pdf

Xu, Y.-F., Zhang, Y.-Q., Xu, X.-M. & Song, G.-X. (2000) Papillomavirus virus-like particles as vehicles for the delivery of epitopes or genes. *Archives of Virology* **151**, 2133–2148.

Zimmermann, H., Degenkolbe, R., Bernard, H.U. & O'Connor, M.J. (1999) The human papillomavirus type 16 E6 oncoprotein can down-regulate p53 activity by targeting the transcriptional coactivator CBP/p300. *Journal of Virology* **73**, 6209–6219.

Chapter 4: Non-sexually transmitted infections of the vulva

F.M. Lewis & S.M. Neill

Sources of infection

The normal flora of the vulva includes diphtherioids (lipophilic and non-lipophilic), micrococci, coagulase-negative staphylococci and lactobacilli. There is a high incidence of *Staphylococcus aureus* on the vulva compared with other sites such as the perianal and forearm skin (Aly *et al.* 1979). The majority of pathogens reach the vulva and vagina through sexual contact, but other infections are not sexually acquired and this chapter deals with these. Infection of the lower genital tract in females is usually exogenous. Some vulval infections, particularly those caused by fungi or pyogenic cocci, may be transferred to the area by the hands. Other modes of transmission are by fomites or through immersion in contaminated water. The proximity of the vulva to the anus allows colonization of the introitus by coliforms (Fair *et al.* 1970), which may then be inoculated into the urethra and bladder by sexual intercourse and cause urinary tract infection. Organisms such as *Candida* species and threadworms may spread to the vulva and vagina from the anus.

Infection with nematodes, tapeworms and flukes

Oxyuriasis (threadworm infection)
Infection with *Enterobius vermicularis* (the threadworm) is common throughout the world, especially in children. The worms live in the bowel, and lay eggs on the perianal and perineal skin at night. These can be shed and ingested or the larvae may hatch and re-enter the gastrointestinal tract. Pruritus ani is the most common symptom, but vulval itching and vulvovaginitis can also occur. Worms are sometimes found in the vagina (Kacker 1973, Chung *et al.* 1997) and there is a report of an egg granuloma affecting the vulva (Sun *et al.* 1991). Other parasitic worms, such as *Ascaris lumbricoides* (roundworm) and *Trichuris trichiura*, have occasionally been found in the vagina (de Mundi *et al.* 1978).

Threadworms are 3–12 mm long, and can be seen on the perianal skin or labia. Eggs can be identified by applying adhesive tape to the perianal skin and examining it microscopically.

General hygiene measures are vital in management. The hands must be washed thoroughly and nails scrubbed before meals and after urination and defaecation. Piperazine is used in children under 2 years of age for 7 days and mebendazole 100 mg as a single dose in older children and adults.

Filariasis
The nematode worms are widely distributed throughout the world. *Wuchereria bancrofti* (found in the tropics), *Brugia malayi* (south-east Asia) and *Brugia timori* (Indonesia) are the species causing infection in humans and are transmitted by mosquitoes carrying infected larvae. These mature in the lymphatic system over a number of years and the subsequent inflammatory reaction gives rise to lymphoedema and, in chronic cases, elephantiasis. Vulval infection is usually due to *W. bancrofti*. Bilateral involvement is usual but the oedema is occasionally greater on one side. Histology of affected lymph nodes is non-specific, but parts of dead worms may be seen. Circulating antigen-specific soluble immune complexes have been shown to be useful in the differential diagnosis of filarial infection and in therapeutic monitoring (Dixit *et al.* 2007).

Diethylcarbamazine is effective treatment but the release of antigen on destruction of the microfilariae can evoke an allergic reaction. Generally, treatment starts with 1 mg/kg/day, increasing over 3 days to 6 mg/kg/day in divided doses, and continued for 3 weeks. Surgical treatment may be needed.

Onchocerciasis
The worm *Onchocerca volvulus* is endemic in the African tropics and in some areas of South America and is transmitted to humans by flies. Cutaneous involvement results in intensely pruritic papules and nodules. If microfilariae are found in the eyes, blindness can result. The vulva is not involved but worms may be seen in vaginal cytology smears. Ivermectin is the treatment of choice.

Ridley's The Vulva, 3rd edition. Edited by Sallie M. Neill and Fiona M. Lewis. © 2009 Blackwell Publishing, ISBN: 978-1-4051-6813-7.

Echinococcosis (hydatid disease)

Echinococcus granularis and *Echinococcus multilocularis* are tapeworms living in the intestines of dogs and other animals. Ova ingested by humans develop into larvae which travel via the bloodstream to distant sites where hydatid cysts develop. Hydatid cysts of the vulva, presenting as painless, subcutaneous swellings, have been reported (Anagnostidis 1935, Ricci 1945, Grassi & Catalano 1957). Treatment is by surgical excision.

Schistosomiasis (bilharzia)

Schistosomiasis is a trematode (fluke) infection endemic in the tropics and subtropics. Three main species affect humans: *Schistosoma mansoni* (Africa, Caribbean, South America), *Schistosoma japonicum* (Far East) and *Schistosoma haematobium* (Africa and Middle East). Eggs from an infected host are passed in faeces or urine and these hatch and release miracidia. These penetrate the body of snails, which act as intermediate hosts. The miracidia develop into cercaria, which are then shed and enter the skin via bathing or wading. From here, they then pass into the bloodstream. Both male and female parasites mature in the portal venous system of the liver and then migrate: *S. mansoni* and *S. japonicum* to the mesenteric vessels and *S. haematobium* to the vesical plexus. Eggs are laid which penetrate blood vessels and, when they reach the surrounding tissues, immunological reactions give rise to dermatitis and infiltrative granulomata.

Vulval lesions occur mainly before puberty (Boulle & Notelovitz 1964, McKee *et al.* 1983) and present as chronic granulomatous infiltrative nodules which may ulcerate (Mawad *et al.* 1992). The labia majora are initially involved, but infection then spreads to the labia minora. The infective lesions can cause vulval hypertrophy (Laven *et al.* 1998) and may mimic condylomata acuminata or malignancies. Scarring and calcification can follow. The delay between infection and the development of the lesions can be up to 3 years (Goldsmith *et al.* 1993).

The diagnosis is made by the presence of ova in urine or faeces. Previously, cytology has been described for the diagnosis of ulcerated lesions (Berry 1971), but now enzyme-linked immunosorbent assays (ELISAs) are available to detect schistosomal immunoglobulins. A wet cervical biopsy crushed between two glass slides was shown to be helpful in diagnosing genital lesions in a series of women with urinary schistosomiasis (Kjetland *et al.* 1996). Histology shows intense inflammatory features with granulomata, numerous eosinophils and pseudoepitheliomatous hyperplasia.

Praziquantel is effective against all human schistosomes. It is given as two or three oral doses of 20 mg/kg over a 24 hour period.

Infection with protozoa

Leishmaniasis

Leishmaniasis is a chronic disease caused by protozoan parasites belonging to the genus *Leishmania*. It is endemic to South America, the Mediterranean and areas of Asia and Africa, and is transmitted by sandflies. Three forms exist: cutaneous, mucocutaneous and visceral (kala-azar). Genital involvement is more common in cutaneous leishmaniasis. The incubation period of cutaneous leishmaniasis can range from 2 weeks to many months (Marsden 1979). The lesions usually start as small papules which enlarge and may ulcerate. Nodular, ulcerative and lupoid forms are described (Feinstein 1978), mainly affecting the face and extremities. After spontaneous recovery from kala-azar, or after successful treatment, patients may develop dermal lesions called leishmanoids. Vulval involvement due to sexual transmission of *Leishmania* from these has been described (Symmers 1960). The vulval lesions need to be distinguished from those of syphilis and donovanosis.

The diagnosis is confirmed by identifying the parasites (known as Leishman–Donovan bodies) in smears or tissue. Specialized media are required for culture. The Montenegro skin test is an intradermal test using leishmanial antigen. It becomes positive in most patients but cannot distinguish between current and past infection. Serological and immunological tests using indirect immunofluorescence and ELISA are now available.

Some lesions may heal spontaneously, but if they are extensive, or caused by an organism which can lead to mucocutaneous destructive disease (particularly *L. braziliensis*), then pentavalent antimony preparations are used. Intralesional or parenteral sodium stilbogluconate (20 mg/kg/day) for 20–28 days is generally given but it is always helpful to take advice from an expert in tropical medicine.

Amoebiasis

Amoebiasis is caused by *Entamoeba histolytica* and primarily affects the gastrointestinal tract. Infection occurs worldwide but is especially common in the tropics and subtropics, where hygiene standards are low (Krogstad *et al.* 1978). Asymptomatic human carriers excrete the cysts and transmission is by the faecal–oral route or via flies, food or water. After ingestion, cysts transform to the pathogenic trophozoites in the bowel, leading to colitis and mucosal ulceration.

The skin is affected in a minority of patients. Cutaneous lesions present as abscesses, which rupture to form painful, irregular, sloughy ulcers or as verrucous plaques. The perineum, vulva (Fig. 4.1) and cervix may be affected, and lymphadenopathy often occurs (Gogoi 1969). Intestinal amoebiasis is usually present, causing diarrhoea and some-

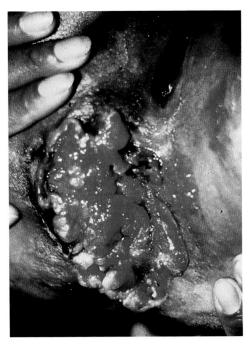

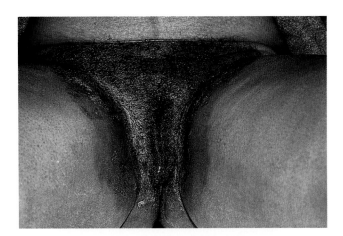

Fig. 4.1 Amoebiasis: large exuberant ulcer with sloughing base.

Fig. 4.2 Tinea cruris: spreading lesions with a scaly edge.

times liver abscesses (El Zawahry & El Komy 1973). The vulva may be involved by direct extension of rectal amoebiasis, but this is regarded as an unusual complication. Sexual transmission can occur via anal intercourse. Only 100 cases of genital disease had been described up until the 1970s (Cohen 1973) and most of these involved the cervix. An isolated case of clitoral amoebiasis has been reported (Majmudar *et al.* 1976).

Genital amoebiasis must be distinguished from other causes of deep ulceration such as donovanosis or lymphogranuloma venereum. The diagnosis is made by identifying motile amoebae in scrapings from the ulcers or from the cervix. Trophozoites or cysts may be found in fresh stool specimens. Histologically, ulceration and necrosis are seen with a mixed inflammatory cell infiltrate in the dermis. *E. histolytica* trophozoites can be identified as eosinophilic structures with prominent nucleoli.

Metronidazole is very effective treatment for cutaneous amoebiasis (Knight 1980), and is used at a dose of 800 mg three times a day for 5 days. For chronic infections in which cysts are present in the faeces, diloxanide furonate 500 mg three times a day for 10 days is given. In resistant cases, intravenous pentamidine is needed.

Mycotic infections

Tinea cruris

Tinea cruris is a fungal infection affecting the groins that is common in men but uncommon in women (Ingram 1955, Blank & Mann 1975). The usual dermatophytic fungi involved are *Trichophyton rubrum*, *Trichophyton mentagrophytes* and *Epidermophyton floccosum*. Heat and humidity are provoking factors, and the condition is most prevalent in people who wear tight, occlusive underwear, particularly during warm weather.

Tinea cruris starts as a small, erythematous scaly patch which may be itchy. The areas slowly extend peripherally with central clearing (Fig 4.2). The groins are chiefly affected, but the infection may spread to the vulva, perineal or perianal areas, either as a continuous rash or as inflamed areas separated by normal skin. If topical steroids have been applied, the appearances may change significantly, and it is then termed tinea incognito. In this form, nodules are often seen and the circumferential scale is usually lost (see Chapter 5). There may well be a focus of infection elsewhere and it is important to examine the rest of the skin and the nails thoroughly. Deep fungal infections of the vulva are very rare, but a trichophytic granuloma of the vulva due to *Microsporum canis* has been reported (Margolis *et al.* 1998). Inflammatory fungal infection of the vulva and mons pubis due to *Trichophyton mentagrophytes* can mimic bacterial infection (Barile *et al.* 2006).

The diagnosis is made by microscopy of scrapings from the edge of the eruption suspended in 10% potassium hydroxide. The main differential diagnoses are flexural psoriasis, erythrasma and cutaneous candidiasis.

Topical terbinafine is the most effective treatment, although imidazole creams are also used. If hair-bearing skin is involved, systemic agents are needed, as the fungus may be deep in the follicle. Terbinafine 250 mg/day or itraconazole 200 mg/day for 2 weeks work well.

Pityriasis versicolor

Pityriasis versicolor (tinea versicolor) is a common superficial fungal infection caused by the lipophilic yeast *Malassezia furfur* (previously termed *Pityrosporum orbiculare*). It is common worldwide but is especially prevalent in warm, humid environments.

Scaly, bran-like macules appear on the trunk and upper limbs. The genital area is often spared but can be involved if the eruption is widespread (Bumgarner & Burke 1949). Affected areas can be hyperpigmented but striking hypopigmentation has been reported to occur in the napkin area of black infants (Jelliffe & Jacobson 1954). It is often the pigmentary change that leads the patient to seek advice, although some may complain of mild pruritus.

The diagnosis is usually made clinically but can be confirmed by the presence of hyphae and spores on microscopy of potassium hydroxide-prepared skin scrapings. Pityriasis versicolor must be distinguished from seborrhoeic dermatitis, pityriasis rosea, erythrasma and secondary syphilis.

Topical clotrimazole applied for 2 weeks is often effective. Selenium sulphide shampoo is commonly used but should not be applied to the vulva as it may be irritant. Widespread disease may require oral treatment and itraconazole 200 mg/day for 7 days is used (Delescluse 1990).

Phycomycosis

Phycomycosis is an invasive fungal infection caused by several different species including *Mucor* and *Basidiobolas*. Infection of the vulva has been described in a diabetic patient (Scott *et al.* 1985) and in a bone marrow recipient (Nomura *et al.* 1997). Both cases resembled necrotizing fasciitis with deep inflammation and ulceration. Amphotericin B and triazoles are effective therapies.

Chromoblastomycosis (chromomycosis)

Chromoblastomycosis is a chronic fungal infection that usually presents as a papule on the foot or leg. Male farm workers are most commonly affected as the pathogenic fungi are found in soil and decaying wood. Vulval involvement is uncommon and was reported in one of five female patients in a series from India (Sharma *et al.* 1999). The organism *Hormodendrum compactum* was isolated from a verrucous lesion on the vulva in one patient (Kakoti & Dey 1957). Itraconazole can be effective but surgery may also be necessary.

Piedra (trichosporis)

Piedra is a superficial infection of the hair shaft where fungal elements adhere to form nodules. There are two forms, black piedra and white piedra, varying in their clinical appearance depending on which part of the hair shaft is infected. The causative organisms are *Piedraia hortae* and *Trichosporon beigelii* and the pubic area is often affected. This is less frequent in women than in men (Kalter *et al.* 1986), but was found in 18% of inguinal specimens from females in an African study (Therizol-Ferly *et al.* 1994). The diagnosis is made by direct microscopy and culture on Saboraud's medium. It must be distinguished from pediculosis, trichomycosis and trichorrhexis nodosa of bacterial origin. Cutting the affected hair and washing with 2% ketoconazole shampoo is an effective treatment. Recurrence is common.

Bacterial infections

Infection with Gram-positive cocci

S. aureus and species of *Streptococcus* are the most common cutaneous pathogens. Primary pyogenic infection is most likely to occur after injury to the skin such as surgery. It can present as folliculitis, furunculosis or as a vulvovaginitis (Lang *et al.* 1958). Secondary bacterial infection can complicate any vulval condition in which the epithelial barrier is compromised. The diagnosis can be confirmed by microscopy and culture of lesional swabs. In acute, severe infections, blood cultures may be indicated to exclude systemic involvement.

Folliculitis and furunculosis

Bacterial folliculitis is an infection of the hair follicle. If the infection is deep and the surrounding tissue becomes involved, a furuncle will result. In the vulval area, shaving, plucking or waxing hair can predispose to folliculitis, and lesions are common on the mons pubis (Fig. 4.3) and outer

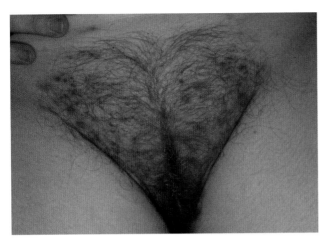

Fig. 4.3 Folliculitis: widespread lesions on the mons pubis.

labia majora. Diabetes mellitus, poor hygiene, immunodeficiency and occlusion of the skin due to obesity can all be aggravating factors. *S. aureus*, carried on the skin and in the nose of 30% of healthy subjects, is the most common cause of both folliculitis and furunculosis.

Superficial disease can be treated with topical antibacterials, such as chlorhexidine or triclosan. Patients with recurrent and persistent lesions may require a prolonged course of oral antibiotics. It is also important to exclude and treat chronic staphylococcal carriage in these patients, who may harbour the organism at other sites such as the groin, axillae and nose.

Impetigo
Impetigo is a superficial bacterial infection which occurs in bullous and non-bullous forms. Staphylococci and streptococci can be causative, whether singly or in combination. The vulva may be involved as part of generalized infection.

Staphylococcal scalded skin syndrome
This syndrome is considered to be one of the staphylococcal toxin-mediated infections in which exfoliative toxins (mainly phage group II types 71 and 55) cleave through the granular layer of the epidermis to form flaccid bullae (Ladhani & Evans 1996). It is most commonly seen in young children but can affect adults, in whom the prognosis is much worse if they are immunosuppressed. After a period of malaise, rapidly spreading erythema is seen with the formation of bullae. These slough after a couple of days to leave moist skin, which then exfoliates. The flexures are classically involved and are often the first areas to be affected.

Histology shows a line of cleavage at the stratum granulosum with the blisters devoid of inflammatory cells. The diagnosis is made clinically as swabs are often negative. ELISAs can identify the toxins. The early phase can resemble

Kawasaki's disease but the rapid progression excludes this. Other differential diagnoses are bullous impetigo and graft-versus-host disease.

Treatment is with penicillinase-resistant penicillins, e.g. flucloxacillin for 7–10 days. Supportive care and expert nursing are important.

Toxic shock syndrome
This is a multisystem disease caused by strains of *S. aureus*, which are able to produce toxic shock syndrome toxin 1. This is isolated from over 90% of cases, and those patients who develop the syndrome have insufficient antibodies against the toxin. In the early 1980s, most cases were seen in young menstruating women in whom the focus of infection was a tampon (Shands *et al.* 1980). Now, cases related to tampon use are rare and it is seen mainly in patients after surgical procedures. There is a sudden onset of high fever with systemic symptoms, and, in some cases, a rapid progression to septic shock. A diffuse macular rash is seen with erythema of the mucous membranes. The nidus of infection must be removed and treatment is supportive with high-dose penicillinase-resistant antibiotics.

Cellulitis
On the vulva, *Streptococcus pyogenes* is the most common cause of cellulitis. Spreading inflammation is seen, which may extend deeply. Systemic features are often present. Cellulitis may complicate lymphoedema of the vulva and recurrent infection can itself lead to further lymphatic damage. Treatment is with oral or parenteral penicillin or erythromycin.

Bartholin's gland abscess
Acute infection of the Bartholin's duct leading to abscess formation may be caused by *S. aureus*, *Neisseria gonorrhoeae*, *Pseudomonas aeruginosa*, *Escherichia coli* and *Streptococcus faecalis*. Painful swelling occurs on the affected labium majus and patients are often systemically unwell. Initial treatment is with antibiotics, but this may be followed by marsupialization or incision and drainage. Patients over 40 or those with treatment-resistant lesions must be biopsied to exclude malignancy. Streptococcal toxic shock-like syndrome can follow a Bartholin's gland abscess (Shearin *et al.* 1989).

Corynebacterial infection

Erythrasma
This is a localized, superficial infection caused by *Corynebacterium minutissimum*. The organism is part of the normal skin flora, but its growth is helped by the moist and occluded environment found in the axillae, groins, natal cleft and between the toes. It is more common in adults than

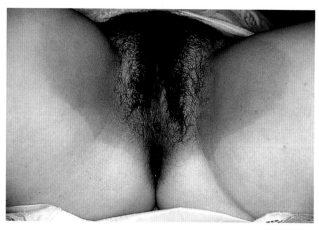

Fig. 4.4 Erythrasma.

in children and predisposing factors include diabetes (Somerville *et al.* 1970), obesity and immunosuppression. Well-defined, brownish, scaly patches appear in the affected areas (Fig. 4.4). The differential diagnosis is from tinea cruris, intertrigo and seborrhoeic dermatitis. Under Wood's light, erythrasma may, but not invariably, show coral-pink fluorescence (Mattox *et al.* 1993), caused by the presence of a porphyrin. It is possible to culture *C. minutissimum* in special media from skin scrapings. Topical azoles such as clotrimazole or miconazole are usually effective treatments. For extensive disease oral erythromycin 250 mg four times a day for 2 weeks is useful. However, recurrence is common.

Trichomycosis (nodosa)

Trichomycosis is caused by at least three species of corynebacteria (Freeman *et al.* 1969). Small nodules of different colours – yellow, red or black (White & Smith 1979) – are firmly attached to the hairs of the axillae or pubic area. Occasionally, sweat may appear red and stain clothing. The bacteria may inflict some damage to the shafts of the hairs (Orfanos *et al.* 1971), and can produce a cement-like substance (Shelley & Miller 1984). Trichomycosis must be differentiated from piedra and pediculosis pubis. The diagnosis is made by microscopy and culture of affected hairs, which fluoresce under examination with Wood's light. It is treated by clipping off or shaving the affected hairs and applying an antibacterial preparation such as clindamycin lotion.

Cutaneous diphtheria

Diphtheria, caused by *Corynebacterium diphtheriae*, classically causes inflammation and tonsillar membranes associated with severe toxaemia. In developed countries it is now a rare disease owing to immunization programmes. Cutaneous infection is common in the tropics and deep ulcers with adherent slough can result. Vulval infection has been described in adults (Parks 1941, Machnicki 1953), and in children (Hunt 1954). Treatment is with diphtheria antitoxin and penicillin.

Mycobacterial infections

Tuberculosis (*Mycobacterium tuberculosis*)

The lung is the most common site of tuberculosis but other organs may be infected, either directly or by spread from distant areas. Tuberculosis of the female genital tract is not uncommon, particularly in developing countries. However, large studies have shown that vulval tuberculosis is rare in comparison with infection of the upper genital tract (Nogales-Ortiz *et al.* 1979, Agarwal & Gupta 1993). It may occur as a primary exogenous infection through contact with sputum or secretions from a sexual partner with pulmonary or urogenital tuberculosis (Bjornstad 1947), by distal spread from the upper genital tract or by haematogenous spread from tuberculosis elsewhere. An association between tuberculosis and HIV infection is well known, and genitourinary tuberculosis is more common in HIV-positive patients.

In primary infection, the initial lesion is an inconspicuous brown-red papule, but this is often missed so that the clinical picture is dominated by inguinal or femoral adenitis. The primary tuberculous lesion usually heals after a few months, but the enlarged glands may persist and break down. In other forms of vulval tuberculosis, nodules appear which develop into ulcers with soft, ragged edges or indurated fungating masses. These can be mistaken for one of the ulcerating sexually transmitted infections (Sardana *et al.* 2001). In the chronic stage, fibrosis leads to scarring and sinus formation. Involvement of regional lymph nodes may lead to caseation and scarring, or to vulval lymphoedema (Ashworth 1974). Infection of Bartholin's glands, usually unilateral, presents as a painless, hard vulval swelling, or as a cold abscess (Schaefer 1959). Erosive perineal and vulval lesions were described as part of generalized papulonecrotic tuberculid in a child (Ramdial *et al.* 1998).

Tuberculous lesions of the vulva must be distinguished from lymphogranuloma venereum, donovanosis and carcinoma. Histology of biopsy material may show tubercles and caseation, and tubercle bacilli may be demonstrated by microscopy of pus or tissue sections stained by a Ziehl–Nielsen technique. Suspected tuberculous material may be cultured to differentiate the organism from opportunist mycobacteria. Treatment is with antituberculous chemotherapy, and expert advice should be sought especially if there is evidence of resistant strains.

Leprosy (*Mycobacterium leprae*)

There is a spectrum of clinical types of leprosy depending on the host's ability to develop specific cell-mediated immunity

(Ridley & Joplin 1966). The female genital tract may be infected by haematogenous spread with involvement of the ovaries, cervix, uterus and fallopian tubes (Bonar & Rabson 1957). Direct infection of the vulva can also occur (Grabstold & Swan 1952).

Other bacterial infections

Actinomycosis

Actinomycosis is a rare disease caused by *Actinomyces israelii* and *Actinomyces gerencseriae*. These are anaerobic or microphilic Gram-positive, non-acid-fast bacilli which tend to form fungus-like colonies in tissue. They are regularly found in the mouths of healthy adults, and sporadically in the gastrointestinal and genital tracts. They cause a chronic granulomatous infection with abscess formation and draining sinuses, through which the characteristic sulphur granules emerge. Genital tract infection is rare but usually arises from extension of bowel disease (Wagman 1975). Colonization of intrauterine contraceptive devices within the cervical canal may occur and is usually asymptomatic. Invasive actinomycotic infections associated with these devices have been described, involving the cervix, uterus and adnexae (Lomax *et al.* 1976, Purdie *et al.* 1977). Three cases of actinomycosis affecting the vulva alone have been described previously (Daniel & Mavrodin 1954). Penicillin is the treatment of choice, but prolonged high doses may be required. Tetracyclines, erythromycin and clindamycin are alternatives.

Mycoplasma infection

Mycoplasmas are the smallest free-living organisms. *Mycoplasma hominis* and *Ureaplasma urealyticum* are found in the genital tract and colonization is related to sexual activity (McCormack *et al.* 1972). Although *M. hominis* was first isolated from a Bartholin's gland abscess (Dienes & Edsall 1937), it is not a major cause of the disease (Lee *et al.* 1977). *M. hominis* is often found in cultures from patients with bacterial vaginosis, but its role in the disease is uncertain. This organism and *M. genitalium* are implicated in pelvic inflammatory disease and in postpartum and post-abortion fever (Taylor-Robinson 1995). *U. urealyticum* can cause urethritis in men, but is not known to cause any disease of the lower urogenital tract in women.

Mixed infections

Necrotizing fasciitis (synergistic gangrene)

This is a rapidly spreading necrosis of subcutaneous fat and fascia. It is imperative to make an early diagnosis as it is life threatening with a mortality rate of 20–40%. Although invasive streptococci group A account for about 10% of cases, the majority are polymicrobial (Cabrera *et al.* 2002)

with mixed anaerobes including Bacteroides species (Rea & Wyrick 1970). The earliest sign is an erythematous or violaceous discoloration of the skin, with subcutaneous induration and oedema and marked tenderness. Later, blisters and subcutaneous necrosis develop, and gas formation may be detected clinically or radiologically (Fisher *et al.* 1979). Generally, the disease is less common in women than in men, but the vulva is a site of predilection. Factors that predispose to the disease, or worsen the prognosis, are diabetes mellitus, corticosteroid therapy, debilitating diseases and irradiation for malignancy. Cases have been described after pelvic surgery (Borkawf 1973), in episiotomy sites (Shy & Eschenbach 1981, Sutton *et al.* 1985), as a complication of vulval squamous cell carcinoma (Adelson *et al.* 1991) or vulval abscesses (Roberts & Hester 1972) and in a patient receiving chemotherapy for acute myelogenous leukaemia (Hoffman & Turnquist 1989).

It is important to distinguish necrotizing fasciitis from extensive pyoderma gangrenosum (Hutchinson *et al.* 1976), as the treatment for this is with high-dose steroids – radically different from the immediate surgical debridement and high-dose antibiotic therapy necessary to increase the chances of survival in necrotizing fasciitis. Early treatment is vital as, in one series of 29 patients, 15 patients had a delay of more than 48 hours between presentation and treatment, and 11 of these died (Stephenson *et al.* 1992).

Infection with viruses

Varicella and zoster

Varicella and zoster are caused by herpesvirus varicellae (varicella zoster virus). Varicella (chickenpox) is the primary infection and the virus then persists in the sensory root ganglion cells. Zoster (shingles) occurs when the virus is reactivated. This is most likely to occur in the elderly and in those with impaired cell-mediated immunity (e.g. Hodgkin's lymphoma, HIV infection or immunosuppressive therapy). Histology shows ballooning of the cytoplasm, eosinophilic inclusions and multinucleate giant cells.

The incubation period of varicella causing chickenpox is 14–20 days. Widespread papules then appear which become vesicular and eventually crust over. Some may be haemorrhagic. There is associated fever and malaise. Mucosal surfaces can be involved, including the vulva. The lesions heal over a period of 2 weeks but may scar.

In zoster, pain is often in the prodrome and may be the presenting feature. Red papules, which evolve into vesicles and pustules, then appear in a dermatomal distribution, usually unilateral. Transient lymphadenopathy often accompanies the lesions. Lumbosacral nerves are involved in 15% of cases and, if the S3 dermatome is affected, vulval lesions will occur (Fig. 4.5). Vaginal lesions have also been

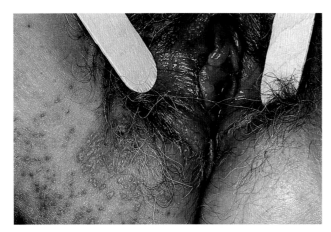

Fig. 4.5 Vulval herpes zoster: the third sacral nerve root is involved.

recorded (Janson 1959) and acute retention of urine can result from involvement of S2 (Waugh 1974). Up to 30% of patients over 40 can develop postherpetic neuralgia with allodynia a predominant symptom. It is the initiating event in some patients with vulvodynia.

Diagnosis is usually straightforward but may be confirmed by electron microscopy of vesicle fluid or by tissue culture. An immediate test is the Tzanck smear, which will show multinucleated giant cells. Generally, varicella in children does not require treatment, but in adults, in whom the disease may be more severe, aciclovir 800 mg five times per day for 7 days is the drug of choice. Alternatives are the more expensive valaciclovir 1 g/day or famciclovir 500–750 mg three times daily for 7 days. Famciclovir started within 72 hours of the onset of symptoms can reduce the duration of postherpetic neuralgia (Tyring et al. 1995). The addition of oral steroids may be helpful to diminish postherpetic neuralgia (Tyring 2007). Severe infection in the immunocompromised may require high-dose intravenous antiviral therapy.

Herpes simplex

Genital infection with herpes simplex is usually sexually acquired and, although the majority are type II infection, type I can also occur (see Chapter 3). Atypical herpes simplex infection may be seen in those who are immunosuppressed. Lesions resembling a verrucous carcinoma were seen in a pregnant patient with common variable immunodeficiency (Beasley et al. 1997). The infection failed to respond to aciclovir but did resolve with intravenous foscarnet.

Epstein–Barr virus

Epstein–Barr virus (EBV) is another human herpes virus which selectively infects B lymphocytes. It causes infectious mononucleosis but primary infection may be asymptomatic. It has also been associated with several B-cell

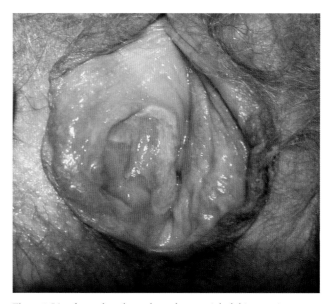

Fig. 4.6 Lipschutz ulcer: large deep ulcer on right labium majus.

lymphoproliferative disorders and nasopharyngeal carcinoma. No link has been found with vulval neoplasia (Cheung et al. 1993).

Acute painful ulcers in young non-sexually active women were described by Lipschutz in 1913. These are now considered to be a toxic reaction to infection and have been described in association with EBV infection, typhoid and paratyphoid fever. In some cases, EBV has been isolated from the ulcers (Portnoy et al. 1984, Halvorsen et al. 2006), and in one case the lesion mimicked a lymphoma (Eghbali et al. 1989). Lipschutz-type ulcers occur mainly in teenagers (Lampert et al. 1996, Barnes et al. 2007) and start as a haemorrhagic blister that rapidly enlarges and ulcerates. The base of the ulcers is covered by a thick slough (Fig. 4.6). They are usually located on the inferior, posterior aspect of the vulva. On occasions two ulcers may occur in apposition ('kissing' lesions). They are often painful and distressing to the patient until the correct diagnosis is made, as initially there is always the suspicion that this has been a sexually acquired problem. Resolution is slow but eventually healing occurs spontaneously usually without scarring. Smaller, shallower ulcers can be treated with a potent topical corticosteroid and potassium permanganate soaks. Large deep ulcers may require the addition of a short 2 week course of oral prednisolone.

Orf

Orf is caused by a parapoxvirus and is widespread in sheep and lambs. Human lesions occur after direct inoculation and lesions are most common on the hands of farmers and meat handlers. Small red papules appear, which enlarge to form haemorrhagic pustules. A case of vulval orf in a child who lived on a farm has been described (James 1968).

Cytomegalovirus

Primary infection with, or reactivation of, latent cytomegalovirus is recognized in immunosuppressed patients. Infection of the cervix has been reported (Brown *et al.* 1988), but a woman with AIDS developed disseminated cytomegalovirus infection of the whole genital tract (Friedmann *et al.* 1991). Cytomegalovirus was detected in the epithelium and macrophages of the vulva, vagina and cervix.

Other infections

The vulva has been rarely involved in some other infective processes, either directly or as a secondary phenomenon.

Pseudocellulitic plaques of the buttocks and vulva were an unusual clinical presentation in a patient with primary parvovirus B19 infection (Delbrel *et al.* 2003). More recently, reports of a 'bathing trunk' eruption with genital involvement have been seen in a child (Buttler *et al.* 2006) and in an adult (Kramkimel *et al.* 2008) (Fig. 4.7a,b).

In one case, *Borrelia burgdorferi* was demonstrated by polymerase chain reaction in vulval lesions (Orelli *et al.* 1998). The patient presented with swelling and soreness of the right labium majus. Histology revealed follicular lymphocytic hyperplasia, consistent with pseudolymphoma. The lesions healed completely after 3 weeks of doxycycline treatment.

A coagulopathy secondary to Rickettsial infection led to a post-traumatic vulval haematoma in one patient (Dietrich *et al.* 2005).

Although smallpox is now eradicated, there are reports of accidental vaccinia of the vulva with the virus being transmitted from recently vaccinated individuals (Haim 1976, Kanra *et al.* 1980). If smallpox vaccination becomes necessary, then this may be seen more frequently.

Vulval infection in children

The normal bacterial environment of the vulva differs in the child as there is an absence of lactobacilli and a more alkaline pH. Diphtherioids and *Staphylococcus epidermidis* are prevalent (Heller *et al.* 1969). This can make the genital tract more prone to bacterial infection, but may protect it from candidiasis. Another factor is that the distance between the anus and perineum is shorter, and poor hygiene habits such as back to front wiping after defaecation can lead to introduction of organisms from the bowel to the vulva. The inner aspect of the vulva is relatively exposed in the child as the fat pads of the labia majora and mons pubis have not developed, and organisms can readily spread.

Infection in children can occur via several routes. Transplacental (e.g. congenital syphilis) and perinatal transmission in the birth canal (e.g. herpes simplex, streptococcal infections and lower genital tract warts) is important in neonates and infants. In older children, poor hygiene can spread threadworms and bacteria on towels and flannels, by direct contact. Sexual abuse is not normally a cause of the usual bacterial infections, unless the infection is one such as syphilis or gonorrhoea.

Vulvovaginitis

Inflammation of the vulval (vulvitis) and vaginal (vaginitis) epithelia can occur separately, but it is rare for the vulva not to be involved in vaginal infection as the associated discharge affects the vulva. The main symptoms are itching, soreness and dysuria (Koumantakis *et al.* 1997). When the primary problem is a vaginitis, the child may present with few symptoms, the parents being more concerned by the discharge. A useful sign suggesting a heavy discharge is a degree of pigmented erythema and scaly rim on the inner dependent parts of the labia majora (Pokorny 1992).

(a)

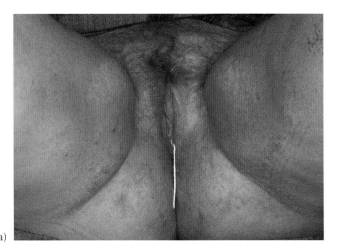

(b)

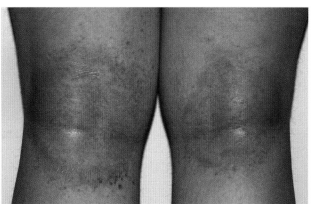

Fig. 4.7 (a) Bathing trunk eruption secondary to parvovirus B19 infection. (b) Flexural lesions may occur at other sites.

Physical findings include a discharge and erythema. In severe cases, erosions can develop. The diagnosis is made by culture of lesional swabs. Investigation should include high vaginal swabs, which must be taken with due regard to the unoestrogenized mucosa (see Chapter 2). The exclusion of foreign bodies, vaginal tumours and lower genital tract abnormalities will usually call for the help of an appropriately trained specialist, and possibly an examination under anaesthesia.

Potential pathogens are *Haemophilus influenzae,* and groups A and B beta-haemolytic streptococci. Although uncommon, *Shigella* species can produce an acute vaginitis in children (Gryngarten *et al.* 1994). *Trichomonas vaginalis* vulvovaginitis may occur in children through sexual contact, but female infants born to women with trichomoniasis can acquire the infection during delivery, although the risk is low (Bramley 1976). The organisms disappear from the vagina in about 6 weeks, when the influence of maternal oestrogens has waned. It has been suggested that trichomonads may be a rare cause of neonatal pneumonia (McLaren *et al.* 1983). In the 1800s, epidemics of gonococcal vulvovaginitis occurred in institutions owing to poor hygiene (Holt 1905), but this cause is now rare (Farrell *et al.* 1981). In prepubertal girls, infection with *N. gonorrhoeae* is likely to be due to sexual contact.

When the child presents with intense vulval or perianal pruritus, threadworm (*Enterobius vermicularis*) infection is the most likely cause. Poor local hygiene, with resulting faecal contamination, is often a predisposing factor.

A persistent, malodorous, purulent or blood-stained discharge raises the possibility of a retained foreign body (Pokorny 1994, Farrington 1997). This form can be particularly difficult to differentiate from child sexual abuse, since the history may be unreliable and the hymen disrupted, with recurrent bleeding, in both cases. These symptoms may also occur when a foreign body has been spontaneously extruded, leaving hymenal changes and a granular reddening of the vaginal wall which, if the diagnosis is firm, can be effectively treated with an oestrogen cream applied to the vulva for up to 2 weeks (Pokorny 1992).

Resolution of vulvitis may be followed by the appearance of adhesions of the clitoral hood (Pokorny 1992).

Congenital syphilis

With the increased incidence of syphilis, the features of congenital syphilis are important to recognize (Chakraborty & Luck 2008). Transmission to the fetus is usually via the placenta, but can occur during delivery if there are external genital lesions. As the time from primary infection in the mother to pregnancy increases, the risk to the baby reduces. In mothers with untreated infection, there is a higher incid-

ence of low birth weight and intrauterine death. One of the early manifestations of congenital syphilis is persistent rhinitis, and this may be accompanied by non-tender lymphadenopathy and hepatosplenomegaly. Bullous, papular and papulosquamous lesions appear on the vulva as part of the characteristic dermatosis. Mucous patches and moist erosions also occur. Vulval condylomata lata develop later, typically towards the end of the first year of life. Other features may be present owing to gumma formation in other organs including bone and cardiovascular and nervous systems.

Any exposed infant should be thoroughly investigated for active infection. Parenteral penicillin G is the treatment of choice.

Herpes simplex

Infection by either herpes simplex virus (HSV) 1 or 2 can occur in children. Perinatal infection is dealt with in Chapter 3. Genital herpes in older children has the same clinical features as in adults (Fig. 4.8) except that cervical infection does not occur. Children can transmit HSV to the vulva from infection in their own mouths (Nahmias *et al.* 1968), and occasionally a mother's herpetic whitlow may be responsible. Sexual transmission of HSV to abused children is well known (Gardner & Jones 1984).

Perianal streptococcal dermatitis (cellulitis)

This is caused by group A beta-haemolytic streptococci (Amren *et al.* 1966) and presents as demarcated erythema around the anal canal and spreading out onto the buttocks (Fig. 4.9). It is most commonly seen in children (Krol 1990),

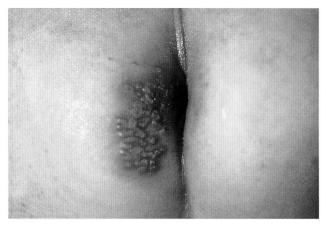

Fig. 4.8 Genital herpes in a child.

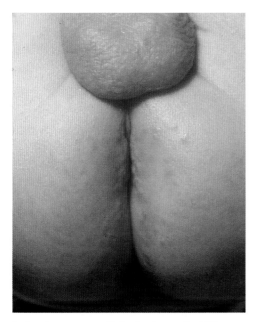

Fig. 4.9 Perianal streptococcal infection in a male child.

but occasionally occurs in adults (Neri *et al.* 1996). It is often associated with pain and secondary constipation. The diagnosis is confirmed by swabs and penicillin is the treatment of choice (Marks & Maksimak 1998, Herbst 2003).

Toxin-mediated perineal erythema

Rapidly desquamating perineal erythema mediated by superantigens to staphylococci and streptococci can occur in young adults but has also been reported in children (Patrizi *et al.* 2008). It must be differentiated from the perineal eruption seen in Kawasaki's disease (see Chapter 5).

References

Adelson, M.D., Miranda, F.R. & Strumpf, K.B. (1991) Necrotising fasciitis: a complication of squamous cell carcinoma of the vulva. *Gynaecology Oncology* **42**, 98–102.

Agarwal, J. & Gupta, K.J. (1993) Female genital tuberculosis-a retrospective clinico-pathologic study of 501 cases. *Indian Journal of Pathology and Microbiology* **36**, 389–397.

Aly, R., Britz, M. & Maibach, H.I. (1979) Quantitative microbiology of human vulva. *British Journal of Dermatology* **101**, 445–448.

Amren, D.E., Anderson, A.S. & Wanamaker, C.W. (1966) Perianal cellulitis associated with group A streptococci. *American Journal of Disease in Childhood* **112**, 546.

Anagnostidis, N. (1935) Kyste hydatique de la grande lèvre de la vulve et mécanisme de sa production. *Gynécologie et Obstétrique* **32**, 356–358.

Ashworth, F.L. (1974) Tuberculous lymphoedema. *British Medical Journal* **4**, 167–169.

Barile, F., Filotico, R., Cassano, N. & Vena, G.A. (2006) Pubic and vulvar inflammatory tinea due to *Trichophyton mentagrophytes*. *International Journal of Dermatology* **45**, 1375–1377.

Barnes, C.J., Alio, A.B., Cunningham, B.B. *et al.* (2007) Epstein–Barr virus associated genital ulcers: an under recognized disorder. *Paediatric Dermatology* **24**, 130–134.

Beasley, K.L., Cooley, G.E., Kao, G.F. *et al.* (1997) Herpes simplex vegetans: atypical genital herpes infection in a patient with common variable immunodeficiency. *Journal of the American Academy of Dermatology* **37**, 860–863.

Berry, A. (1971) Evidence of gynaecological bilharziasis in cytologic material. A morphological study for cytologists in particular. *Acta Cytologica* **15**, 482–486.

Bjornstad, R. (1947) Tuberculous primary infection of genitalia: two cases of venereal genital tuberculosis. *Acta Dermato-venereologica* **27**, 106–109.

Blank, F. & Mann, S.J. (1975) *Trichophyton rubrum* infections according to age, anatomical distribution and sex. *British Journal of Dermatology* **92**, 171–174.

Bonar, B.E. & Rabson, A.S. (1957) Gynaecological aspects of leprosy. *Obstetrics and Gynecology* **9**, 33–38.

Borkawf, H.I. (1973) Bacterial gangrene associated with pelvic surgery. *Clinical Obstetrics and Gynecology* **16**, 40–45.

Boulle, A. & Notelovitz, M. (1964) Bilharzia of the female genital tract. *South African Journal of Obstetrics and Gynaecology* **18**, 48–50.

Bramley, M. (1976) Study of female babies of women entering confinement with vaginal trichomoniasis. *British Journal of Venereal Diseases* **52**, 58–62.

Brown, S., Senekjian, E.K. & Montag, A.G. (1988) Cytomegalovirus infection of the uterine cervix in a patient with acquired immunodeficiency syndrome. *Obstetrics and Gynecology* **71**, 489–491.

Bumgarner, F.E. & Burke, R.C. (1949) Pityriasis versicolor. Atypical clinical and mycological variants. *Archives of Dermatology* **59**, 192–194.

Buttler, G.J., Mendelsohn, S. & Franks, A. (2006) Parvovirus B19 infection presenting as 'bathing trunk' erythema with pustules. *Australasian Journal of Dermatology* **47**, 286–268.

Cabrera, H., Skoczdopole, L., Marini, M. *et al.* (2002) Necrotizing gangrene of the genitalia and perineum. *International Journal of Dermatology* **41**, 847–851.

Chakraborty, R. & Luck, S. (2008) Syphilis is on the increase: the implications for child health. *Archives of Disease in Childhood* **93**, 105–109.

Cheung, A.N.Y., Khoo, V.S., Kwong, K.Y. *et al.* (1993) Epstein–Barr virus in carcinoma of the vulva. *Journal of Clinical Pathology* **46**, 849–851.

Chung, D.I., Kong, H.H., Yn, H.S. *et al.* (1997) Live *Enterobius vermicularis* in the posterior fornix of the vagina in a Korean woman. *Korean Journal of Parasitology* **35**, 67–69.

Cohen, C. (1973) Three cases of amoebiasis of the cervix uteri. *Journal of Obstetrics and Gynaecology of the British Commonwealth* **80**, 476–480.

Daniel, C. & Mavrodin, A. (1954) L'actinomycose génitale de la femme. *Revue Française de Gynécologie et d'Obstétrique* **29**, 1–11.

Delbrel, X., Sibaud, V., Cogrel, O. *et al.* (2003) Pseudo-cellulitis plaques and Koplick spot: a particular form of parvovirus B19 primo-infection. *La Revue de Medecine Interne* **24**, 317–319.

Delescluse, J. (1990) Itraconazole in tinea versicolor: a review. *Journal of the American Academy of Dermatology* 23, 551–554.

de Mundi Zamorano, A., del Alano, C.M., de Blas, L.L. & Alvarez san Cristobal, A. (1978) Egg of *Trichiuris trichiuria* in a vaginal smear. *Acta Cytologica* 22, 119–120.

Dienes, L. & Edsall, G. (1937) Observations on the L-organisms of Kleinberger. *Proceedings of the Society for Experimental Biology and Medicine* 36, 740–745.

Dietrich, J., Perlman, S. & Hertweck, S.P. (2005) Post-traumatic vulvar haematoma secondary to coagulopathy caused by Rickettsial infection. *Journal of Paediatric and Adolescent Gynaecology* 18, 175–177.

Dixit, V., Gupta, A.K., Bisen, P.S. *et al.* (2007) Serum immune complexes as diagnostic and therapeutic markers in lymphatic filariasis. *Journal of Clinical Laboratory Annals* 21, 114–118.

Eghbali, H., Lacut, J.Y. & Hoernie, B. (1989) Genital infectious mononucleosis mimicking high grade non-Hodgkin's lymphoma. *Médecine et Maladies Infectieuses* 19, 83–86.

El Zawahry, M. & El Komy, M. (1973) Amoebiasis cutis. *International Journal of Dermatology* 12, 305–310.

Fair, W.R., Timothy, M.M., Miller, M.A. *et al.* (1970) Bacteriologic and hormonal observations of the urethra and vaginal vestibule in normal premenopausal women. *Journal of Urology* 104, 426–431.

Farrell, M.K., Billmire, M.E., Sharroy, J.A. *et al.* (1981) Prepubertal gonorrhoea: a multidisciplinary approach. *Pediatrics* 67, 151–153.

Farrington, P.F. (1997) Paediatric vulvo-vaginitis. *Clinical Obstetrics and Gynaecology* 40, 135–140.

Feinstein, R.J. (1978) Cutaneous leishmaniasis. *Dermatology* 1, 45–50.

Fisher, J.R., Conway, M.J. & Takeshita, R.T. (1979) Necrotising fasciitis. Importance of roentgenographic studies for soft-tissue gas. *Journal of the American Medical Association* 241, 803–807.

Freeman, R.G., McBride, M.E. & Knox, J.M. (1969) Pathogenesis of trichomycosis axillaris. *Archives of Dermatology* 100, 90–99.

Friedmann, W., Schäfer, A., Kretschmer, R. *et al.* (1991) Disseminated cytomegalovirus infection of the female genital tract. *Gynaecology and Obstetrics Investigation* 31, 56–57.

Gardner, M. & Jones, J.G. (1984) Genital herpes acquired from the sexual abuse of children. *Journal of Pediatrics* 104, 243–244.

Gogoi, M.P. (1969) Amoebiasis of the female genital tract. *American Journal of Obstetrics and Gynaecology* 105, 1281–1286.

Goldsmith, P.C., Leslie, T.A., Sams, V. *et al.* (1993) Lesions of schistosomiasis mimicking warts on the vulva. *British Medical Journal* 307, 556–557.

Grabstold, H. & Swan, L. (1952) Genitourinary lesions in leprosy, with special reference to atrophy of the testis. *Journal of the American Medical Association* 149, 1287–1291.

Grassi, G. & Catalano, G. (1957) Case of echinococcal cyst of the labium majus. *Policlinica; sezione practica* 64, 1383–1384.

Gryngarten, M.G., Turco, M.L., Escobar, M.E. *et al.* (1994) Shigella vulvo-vaginitis in prepubertal girls. *Adolescent Paediatric Gynaecology* 7, 86–89.

Haim, S. (1976) Accidental vaccinia of the vulva. *Cutis* 17, 308–309.

Halvorsen, J.A., Brevig, T., Aas, T. *et al.* (2006) Genital ulcers as initial manifestation of Epstein-Barr virus infection: two new cases and review of the literature. *Acta Dermato-venereologica* 86, 439–442.

Heller, R.H., Joseph, L.M. & Davis, H.J. (1969) Vulvovaginitis in the pre-menarchal child. *Journal of Paediatrics* 74, 370–377.

Herbst, R. (2003) Perineal streptococcal dermatitis/disease: recognition and management. *American Journal of Clinical Dermatology* 4, 555–560.

Hoffman, M.S. & Turnquist, D. (1989) Necrotising fasciitis of the vulva during chemotherapy. *Obstetrics and Gynecology* 74, 483–484.

Holt, L.E. (1905) Gonococcus infections in children, with especial reference to their prevalence in institutions and means of prevention. *New York Medical Journal* 81, 521–526, 589–592.

Hunt, E. (1954) Ulcers of the vulva. In: *Diseases Affecting the Vulva*, 4th edn, p. 122. Henry Kimpton, London.

Hutchinson, P.E., Summerly, R. & Lawson, R.S. (1976) Progressive postoperative gangrene: a reminder. *British Journal of Dermatology* 194, 89–95.

Ingram, J.T. (1955) Tinea of the vulva. *British Medical Journal* 2, 1500.

James, J.R.E. (1968) Orf in man. *British Medical Journal* 3, 804–806.

Janson, P. (1959) Seltere Zoster verlaufeformen. *Zeitschrift für Haut und Geschlechtskrankheiten* 26, 292.

Jelliffe, D.B. & Jacobson, F.W. (1954) The clinical picture of tinea versicolor in negro infants. *Journal of Tropical Medicine and Hygiene* 57, 290–292.

Kacker, T.P. (1973) Vulvovaginitis in an adult with threadworms in the vagina. *British Journal of Venereal Diseases* 49, 314–315.

Kakoti, L.M. & Dey, N.C. (1957) Chromoblastomycosis in India. *Journal of the Indian Medical Association* 28, 351.

Kalter, D.C., Tschen, J.A., Cernoch, P.K. *et al.* (1986) Genital white piedra: epidemiology, microbiology and therapy. *Journal of the American Academy of Dermatology* 14, 982–993.

Kanra, G., Sezer, V.M., Secmeer, G. & Oran, O. (1980) Accidental vaccinia vulva vaginitis. *Cutis* 26, 267–268.

Kjetland, E.F., Poggensee, G., Helling-Giese, G. *et al.* (1996) Female genital schistosomiasis due to Schistosoma haematobium. Clinical and parasitological findings in women in rural Malawi. *Acta Tropical* 62, 239–255.

Knight, R. (1980) The chemotherapy of amoebiasis. *Journal of Antimicrobial Chemotherapy* 6, 577–593.

Koumantakis, E.E., Hassan, E.A., Deligeoroogiou, E.K. & Creatsas, G.K. (1997) Vulvovaginitis during childhood and adolescence. *Journal of Pediatric and Adolescent Gynaecology* 10, 39–43.

Kramkimel, N., Leclerc-Mercier, S., Rozenberg, F. *et al.* (2008) An adult presenting with a bathing-trunk eruption associated with primary infection to human parvovirus B19. *British Journal of Dermatology* 158, 407.

Krogstad, D.J., Spencer, H.C. & Healy, G.R. (1978) Current concepts in parasitology: amoebiasis. *New England Journal of Medicine* 298, 262–265.

Krol, A.L. (1990) Perianal streptococcal dermatitis. *Paediatric Dermatology* 7, 97–100.

Ladhani, S. & Evans, R. (1996) Staphylococcal scalded skin syndrome. *Archives of Disease in Childhood* 78, 85–88.

Lampert, A., Assier-Bonnet, H., Chevallier, B. *et al.* (1996) Lipschutz's genital ulceration: a manifestation of Epstein-Barr primary infection. *British Journal of Dermatology* 135, 663–665.

Lang, W.R., Israel, S.L. & Fritz, M.A. (1958) Staphylococcal vulvovaginitis: a report of two cases following antibiotic therapy. *Obstetrics and Gynecology* 11, 352–354.

Laven, J.S., Vleugels, M.P., Dofferhoff, A.S. & Bloembergen, P. (1998) Schistosomiasis haematobium as a cause of vulvar hypertrophy. *European Journal of Obstetrics, Gynecology and Reproductive Biology* 79, 213–216.

Lee, Y.H., Rankin, J.S., Albert, S. *et al.* (1977) Microbiological investigation of Bartholin's gland abscesses and cysts. *American Journal of Obstetrics and Gynaecology* 129, 150–153.

Lipschutz, B. (1913) Über eine eigenartige Geschwürsform des weiblichen Genitales (ulcus vulvae acutum). *Archives of Dermatological Research* 114, 363–396.

Lomax, C.W., Harbert, G.M. & Thornton, W.N. (1976) Actinomycosis of the female genital tract. *Obstetrics and Gynecology* 48, 341–346.

Machnicki, S. (1953) Diphtheria of the vulva and vagina. *Zeitschrift für Haut- und Geschlechtskrankheiten* 86, 386.

Majmudar, B., Chaiken, M.C. & Lee, K.U. (1976) Amoebiasis of clitoris mimicking carcinoma. *Journal of the American Medical Association* 236, 1145–1146.

Margolis, D.J., Weinberg, J.M., Tangoren, I.A. *et al.* (1998) Trichophytic granuloma of the vulva. *Dermatology* 197, 69–70.

Marks, V.J. & Maksimak, M. (1998) Perianal streptococcal cellulitis. *Journal of the American Academy of Dermatology* 18: 587–588.

Marsden, P.D. (1979) Current concepts in parasitology: leishmaniasis. *New England Journal of Medicine* 300, 350–355.

Mattox, T.F., Rutgers, J., Yoshimori, R.N. *et al.* (1993) Non-fluorescent erythrasma of the vulva. *Obstetrics and Gynecology* 81, 862–864.

Mawad, N.M., Hassanein, O.M., Mahmoud, O.M. & Taylor, M.G. (1992) Schistosomal vulval granuloma in a 12 year old Sudanese girl. *Transactions of the Royal Society of Tropical Medicine and Hygiene* 86, 644.

McCormack, W.M., Almeida, P.C., Bailey, P.E. *et al.* (1972) Sexual activity and vaginal colonisation with genital mycoplasmas. *Journal of the American Medical Association* 221, 1375–1377.

McKee, P.H., Wright, E. & Hutt, M.S.R. (1983) Vulval schistosomiasis. *Clinical and Experimental Dermatology* 8, 189–194.

McLaren, L.C., Davis, L.E., Healy, G.R. *et al.* (1983) Isolation of *Trichomonas vaginalis* from the respiratory tract of infants with respiratory disease. *Pediatrics* 71, 888–890.

Nahmias, A.J., Dowdle, W.R., Naib, Z.M. *et al.* (1968) Genital infection with herpes simplex viruses 1 and 2 in children. *Paediatrics* 42, 659–666.

Neri, L., Bardazzi, F., Marzaduri, S. & Patrizi, A. (1996) Perianal streptococcal dermatitis in adults. *British Journal of Dermatology* 135, 796–798.

Nogales-Ortiz, F., Tarancon, I. & Nogales, F.F. (1979) The pathology of female genital tuberculosis. A 31 year study of 1436 cases. *Obstetrics and Gynecology* 53, 422–428.

Nomura, J., Ruskin, J., Sahebi, F. *et al.* (1997) Mucomycosis of the vulva in a transplant recipient. *Bone Marrow Transplant* 8, 859–860.

Orelli, S., Schnarwyler, B., Maurer, R. *et al.* (1998) Vulväres Pseudolymphom: Nachweis der Infektion mit *Borrelia burgdorferi* mittels Polymerasekettenreaktion. *Gynäkol Geburtshilfliche Rundsch* 38, 143–145.

Orfanos, C.E., Schloesser, E. & Mahrie, G. (1971) Hair destroying growth of *Corynebacterium tenuis* in the so-called trichomycosis axillaris. *Archives of Dermatology* 103, 632–636.

Parks, J. (1941) Diphtheritic vaginitis in the adult. *American Journal of Obstetrics and Gynecology* 41, 714–718.

Patrizi, A., Raone, B., Savoia, F. *et al.* (2008) Recurrent toxin-mediated perineal erythema: eleven paediatric cases. *Archives of Dermatology* 144, 239–243.

Pokorny, S.F. (1992) Prepubertal vulvovaginopathies. *Obstetric and Gynecology Clinics of North America* 19, 39–58.

Pokorny, S.F. (1994) Long term intravaginal presence of foreign bodies in children. A preliminary study. *Journal of Reproductive Medicine* 39, 931–935.

Portnoy, J., Ahronheim, G.A., Ghibu, F. *et al.* (1984) Recovery of Epstein–Barr virus from genital ulcers. *New England Journal of Medicine* 311, 966–968.

Purdie, D.W., Carty, M.J. & McLeod, T.I. (1977) Tubo-ovarian actinomycosis and the IUCD. *British Medical Journal* 2, 1392.

Ramdial, P.K., Mosam, A., Mallett, R. *et al.* (1998) Papulonecrotic tuberculid in a 2 year old girl: with emphasis on extent of disease and presence of leucocytoclastic vasculitis. *Paediatric Dermatology* 15, 450–455.

Rea, W.J. & Wyrick, W.J. (1970) Necrotising fasciitis. *Annals of Surgery* 172, 957–963.

Ricci, J. (1945) *One Hundred Years of Gynecology, 1800–1900*, p. 470. Blakiston, Philadelphia.

Ridley, D.S. & Jopling, W.H. (1966) Classification of leprosy according to immunity. A five group system. *International Journal of Leprosy and other Mycobacterial Disease* 34, 255–273.

Roberts, D.B. & Hester, L.L. (1972) Progressive synergistic bacterial gangrene arising from abscesses of the vulva and Bartholin's gland. *American Journal of Obstetrics and Gynecology* 114, 285–290.

Sardana, K., Koranne, R.V., Sharma, R.C. *et al.* (2001) Tuberculosis of the vulva masquerading as a sexually transmitted disease. *Journal of Dermatology* 28, 505–507.

Schaefer, G. (1959) Diagnosis and treatment of female genital tuberculosis. *Clinical Obstetrics and Gynecology* 2, 530–535.

Scott, R.A., Gallis, H.A. & Livengood, C.H. (1985) Phycomycosis of the vulva. *American Journal of Obstetrics and Gynecology* 153, 675–676.

Shands, K.N., Schmid, G.P., Dan, B.B. *et al.* (1980) Toxic-shock syndrome in menstruating women: association with tampon use and *Staphylococcus aureus* and clinical features in 52 cases. *New England Journal of Medicine* 303, 1436–1442.

Sharma, N.L., Sharma, R., Grover, P.S. *et al.* (1999) Chromoblastomycosis in India. *International Journal of Dermatology* 38, 846–851.

Shearin, R.S., Boehlke, J., Karanth, S. *et al.* (1989) Toxic shock-like syndrome associated with Bartholin's gland abscess: a case report. *American Journal of Obstetrics and Gynaecology* 160, 1073–1074.

Shelley, W.B. & Miller, M.A. (1984) Electron microscopy, histochemistry and microbiology of bacterial adhesion in trichomycosis axillaris. *Journal of the American Academy of Dermatology* 10, 1005–1014.

Shy, K.K. & Eschenbach, D.A. (1981) Fatal perineal cellulitis from an episiotomy site. *Obstetrics and Gynecology* 54, 292–298.

Somerville, D.A., Seville, R.H., Cunningham, R.C. *et al.* (1970) Erythrasma in a hospital for the mentally subnormal. *British Journal of Dermatology* 82, 355–358.

Stephenson, H., Dotters, D.J., Katz, V. & Droegmueller, W. (1992) Necrotising fasciitis of the vulva. *American Journal of Obstetrics and Gynecology* 166, 1324–1327.

Sun, T., Schwartz, N.S., Sewell, C. *et al.* (1991) Enterobius egg granuloma of the vulva and peritoneum: review of the literature. *American Journal of Tropical Medicine and Hygiene* 45, 249–253.

Sutton, G.P., Smitz, L.R., Clark, D.H. & Bennett, J.E. (1985) Group B streptococcal necrotising fasciitis arising in an episiotomy. *Obstetrics and Gynecology* 66, 733–736.

Symmers, W.S. (1960) Leishmaniasis acquired by contagion. A case of marital infection in Britain. *Lancet* 1, 1276.

Taylor-Robinson, D. (1995) The history and role of *Mycoplasma genitalum* in sexually transmitted diseases. *Genitourinary Medicine* 71, 1–8.

Theirzol-Ferly, M., Kombila, M., Gomez de Diaz, M. *et al.* (1994) White piedra and Trichosporon species in equatorial Africa. I. History and clinical aspects: an analysis of 449 superficial inguinal specimens. *Mycoses* 37, 249–253.

Tyring, S.K. (2007) Management of herpes zoster and post-herpetic neuralgia. *Journal of the American Academy of Dermatology* 57, 136–142.

Tyring, S., Barbarash, R.A., Nahlik, J.E. *et al.* (1995) Famciclovir for the treatment of acute herpes zoster: effects on acute disease and post-herpetic neuralgia. *Annals of Internal Medicine* 123, 89–96.

Wagman, H. (1975) Genital actinomycosis. *Proceedings of the Royal Society of Medicine* 68, 228–230.

Waugh, M.A. (1974) Herpes zoster of the anogenital area affecting urination and defaecation. *British Journal of Dermatology* 90, 235–238.

White, S.W. & Smith, J. (1979) Trichomycosis pubis. *Archives of Dermatology* 115, 444–445.

Chapter 5: Non-infective cutaneous conditions of the vulva

S.M. Neill & F.M. Lewis

Introduction

In this chapter the cutaneous conditions that have a predilection for the vulva and those which are common at this site as part of more generalized dermatological disease will be discussed.

It is recognized that some conditions tend to be clinically and histologically less distinct when they occur in the vulval area. Clinically, this is particularly the case for lesions occurring on keratinized surfaces where the typical morphological features of the dermatoses are altered. The dampness and frictional forces exerted at a flexural site lead to maceration. Secondary bacterial or candidal overgrowth and irritant contact dermatitis from the topical treatments or incontinence can also complicate the clinical picture. A dermatosis that would be white and scaly on a non-flexural site becomes macerated, soggy and covered in keratinous debris.

Histologically, difficulties arise with interpretation on mucosal surfaces, e.g. with long-standing lichen planus.

Finally, it should be remembered that neoplastic conditions can resemble benign dermatoses (Fig. 5.1) and it is important to always biopsy early on any dermatitis or lesion that is not responding to treatment.

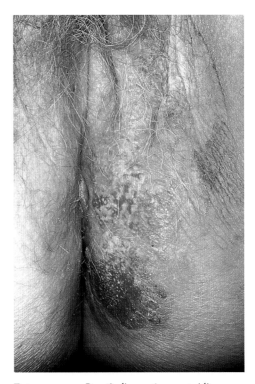

Fig. 5.1 Extramammary Paget's disease: 'eczematoid' appearance.

History

Classification of non-infective, non-neoplastic lesions

The reason various classifications were introduced for vulval skin diseases was because gynaecologists were the main physicians dealing with vulval disease. They had no formal training in dermatology and struggled to try to identify the different dermatoses which, as already mentioned, were atypical and would have also proven difficult

Ridley's The Vulva, 3rd edition. Edited by Sallie M. Neill and Fiona M. Lewis. © 2009 Blackwell Publishing, ISBN: 978-1-4051-6813-7.

for dermatologists themselves. A brief summary of the previous classifications is mentioned not only for historical information but also to help understand and interpret the past literature.

The first descriptions of vulval disease towards the end of the 19th century were confusing, as was exemplified by the various terms allocated to lichen sclerosus (see below). The dermatological and gynaecological literature developed separately and many different names were given to identical conditions. Jeffcoate and Woodcock (1961) preferred to sweep away the former plethora of terms and to substitute the all-embracing concept of a 'dystrophy'. This in turn led to the classification adopted by the fledgling International Society for the Study of Vulval Disease (ISSVD) in 1976

(Friedrich 1976), featuring lichen sclerosus and dystrophy, the latter of mixed and hypertrophic types, with and without atypia. Later, atypia was taken up into the new concept of intraepithelial neoplasia, which was given its own separate classification. The classifications were later directed primarily at the epithelial dermatological disorders. Nonmalignant conditions were classified as lichen sclerosus, other dermatoses and squamous cell hyperplasia in 1987 (Ridley *et al.* 1989). This again was not a helpful classification because the term squamous hyperplasia is a histological description and not a clinical diagnosis. The ISSVD has recently proposed a further classification based on histological patterns found on biopsy (Lynch *et al.* 2007). However, as dermatologists are well aware, it is a combination of the clinical picture and the histological findings that eventually lead to the correct diagnosis, and this can be very challenging in vulval disease. The authors feel that a separate classification is not necessary for vulval disease especially as there are no separate classifications for infections, malignancies or dermatological conditions at other flexural sites of the body. It is important not to concentrate all one's dermatological knowledge to one site; the condition may affect the vulval skin, but it might also be just one manifestation of a disease that can affect other skin sites and internal organs.

Symptoms

A variety of symptoms can result from a vulval dermatosis. A number of conditions may be asymptomatic and it is the clinical appearance that draws the patient's attention to the problem and in turn then to seek help. Itching, or pruritus, is the commonest complaint. It is best defined as a sensation that leads to a desire to scratch. Lesions tend to be more pruritic at this site than elsewhere. This may be attributable in part to the local environment, and in part to psychological and psychosexual factors. The mechanism of itch is not well understood, but it is probably mediated by free unmyelinated nerve endings, distinct from those mediating pain, near the dermal–epidermal junction. Encephalins (opioids), in conjunction with histamine released from mast cells, and perhaps prostaglandin E and neuropeptides, are also likely to be involved. The sensation is greatly influenced by psychological factors and by warmth. Rarely, intense pruritus arises on normal skin. Itching and rubbing are frequently followed by the thickening of lichenification, to which the genital area appears to be especially susceptible. This change was at one time termed neurodermatitis, referring to the role of the nerve fibres rather than to a psychological origin, and the term may have influenced the practice of treatments such as alcohol injections and denervation procedures. The term is now best avoided.

The inflammatory element in many vulval dermatoses and the presence of erosion understandably often give rise to soreness. However, symptoms consisting predominantly of pain, burning and soreness, with no visible signs, or persisting after adequate treatment and resolution of a dermatitis, are likely to be in the category of a sensory abnormality, usually vulval vestibulodynia or dysaesthetic vulvodynia (see Chapter 6). Itch can also be centrally mediated.

Genetic disorders

Epidermolysis bullosa

This term is applied to a genetically determined group of conditions, inherited by way of either dominant or recessive genes. They are characterized by increased fragility of the skin and mucosae, with a tendency to form bullae, which may arise spontaneously or in response to mild trauma. The appearances and pathogenesis are heterogeneous; the different types are now classified according to the pathogenetic mechanisms involved. The forms that involve the genital area are the junctional type, in which the splitting occurs in the lamina lucida of the basement membrane, and the dystrophic type, in which the splitting takes place below the lamina densa (Petersen *et al.* 1996). The early onset, often with a family history, together with the presence of lesions elsewhere, will usually make the diagnosis of epidermolysis bullosa straightforward.

Extensive erosions and ulceration which heal with scarring can affect the anogenital area (Fig. 5.2). One patient is reported who had anal scarring leading to constipation and bladder compression, narrowing of the vestibule and partial fusion of the labia (Shackleford *et al.* 1982). Vaginal adhesions have also been described (Steinkampf *et al.* 1987).

Genetic counselling and prenatal diagnosis may be offered where appropriate. Many patients have been helped by the support group the Dystrophic Epidermolysis Bullosa Research Association (DEBRA). Expert nursing support and education with special attention to the avoidance of the trauma of friction and pressure is required. These patients need a multidisciplinary approach to their management.

Darier's disease (keratosis follicularis)

This acantholytic disorder of keratinization is inherited by way of an autosomal dominant gene. It is caused by mutations in the *ATP2A2* gene which encodes the sarco- and endoplasmic reticulum ATPase type 2. These mutations result in abnormal keratinocyte adhesion with loss of desmosomes and breakdown of desmosome–keratin intermediate filament attachment. Not all patients will give a family history, however, and reasons for this include nonrecognition of mild early disease, non-paternity and new mutations.

The lesions tend to develop in childhood or adolescence and to worsen gradually, with fluctuations but no remissions.

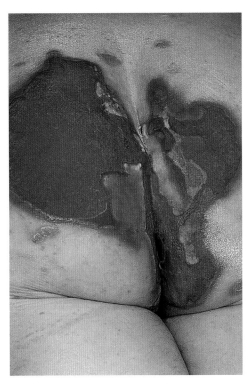

Fig. 5.2 Epidermolysis bullosa, junctional type: anogenital ulceration.

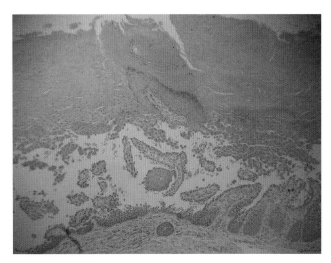

Fig. 5.3 Histology of benign familial chronic pemphigus showing acantholysis.

The primary lesions consist of horny papules. All aspects of the vulva, as well as skin and mucosal surfaces elsewhere, are often involved. Oral lesions are well recognized but vaginal lesions do not appear to have been recorded. Maceration and secondary bacterial infection is common, leading to malodorous masses, which are common in the genital area. The lesions are also susceptible to viral infection, of which the herpes simplex virus is the commonest. Lesions are aggravated by heat and warmth, and also by oral lithium carbonate.

Histologically there is dyskeratosis with the formation of corps ronds and grains, clefts within the epidermis and focal areas of acantholysis in the suprabasal layer (Fig. 5.3).

The differential diagnosis is mainly from benign familial chronic pemphigus (Hailey–Hailey disease), which can show considerable overlap with Darier's disease both clinically and histologically. The morphology of extragenital lesions will usually be helpful, particularly those of nail changes, since, although both may show white bands, Darier's alone has red bands with a split or notch. Horny papules and palmar pits are typical of Darier's disease.

Bland emollients, corticosteroids and antibacterial agents are of limited value. The apparent resemblance to the lesions of vitamin A deficiency (of which there is no evidence) led to the trial of retinoids. Topical retinoic acid may help a little, but is irritant. Oral acitretin is of great benefit,

although less so in flexural lesions; but unfortunately this therapy is limited by its teratogenicity and side-effects. Isotretinoin is another option that may be more useful in women of childbearing age as the time after stopping therapy to safe conception is much shorter than that recommended with acitretin. Radiotherapy, dermabrasion, laser treatment, photodynamic therapy and topical 5-fluorouracil have been employed, with varying success.

Benign familial chronic pemphigus (Hailey–Hailey disease)

This rare dermatosis is inherited through an autosomal dominant gene. Not all patients will give a positive family history; lack of recognition of mild lesions, and the relatively late onset, may be the reason rather than a mutation. The disease is caused by mutations in the calcium pump gene *ATP2C1*, which leads to a defect in keratinocyte adhesion.

Lesions usually appear between the second and fourth decades, and affect the genital area as well as flexures elsewhere. Vaginal involvement has been reported (Václavínková & Neumann 1982, Brandrup *et al.* 1990). In general, the condition fluctuates and tends to improve with time. The appearance is typically of moist, red plaques with fissuring and erosions (Fig. 5.4), but pustules and vesicles may also be seen. The lesions are sore and itchy and may be exacerbated by heat, friction, pregnancy and contact allergy (Ponyai *et al.* 1999). Secondary infection, with herpes simplex, bacteria or *Candida*, can aggravate the problem. Squamous cell carcinoma (SCC) has been described on a background of Hailey–Hailey disease (Ochiai *et al.* 1999, Cockayne *et al.* 2000), but oncogenic human papillomavirus infection was a factor in both cases.

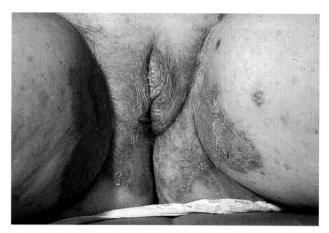

Fig. 5.4 Benign familial chronic pemphigus: moist, scaly, fissured erythema.

Histology shows suprabasal splitting and extensive intra-epidermal acantholysis, the latter giving rise to the description of a 'dilapidated brick wall'. Occasionally, there are a few corps ronds or grains high up in the epidermis. Immunofluorescence is negative.

The differential diagnosis is mainly from Darier's disease, the difference relying on the specific histological and clinical features. Sometimes, the appearance is mistaken for macerated eczema or psoriasis but, when there is resistance to treatment, a biopsy should be performed. Occasionally, anogenital lesions may be mistaken for warts.

Treatment includes avoidance of friction, bland emollients and mild antibacterial washes, together with a topical corticosteroid. The potency of the topical steroid needed depends on the severity of disease and may require a combined preparation with an antibacterial or antifungal agent. Topical tacrolimus has been reported to be of benefit (Sand & Thomsen 2003). Long-term antibiotics by mouth, and occasionally courses of oral steroids, can be useful. Good results have been reported with oral ciclosporin (Berth-Jones *et al.* 1995), and more recently a patient with perineal disease improved with the use of alefacept (Hurd *et al.* 2008). Grenz rays have been shown to help and a variety of drugs and surgical procedures have yielded variable success (Burge 1992). Photodynamic therapy (Ruiz-Rodriguez *et al.* 2002) and laser (Kruppa *et al.* 2000, Collet Villette *et al.* 2005) have been used with some success. Recent interest has been shown in the use of botulinum toxin for axillary Hailey–Hailey disease (Lapiere *et al.* 2000) but its use has not been reported in vulval disease.

Cases have been reported in which the lesions were apparently confined to the vulva but, in the light of more recent cases, these were probably examples of acantholytic dermatosis (see below).

Variants of Darier's disease or Hailey–Hailey disease

Unilateral linear acantholytic lesions with features suggestive of Darier's disease or of benign familial chronic pemphigus have been described. They are probably best regarded as special forms of epidermal naevi. There is one report involving the anogenital area in a child starting at the age of 3 months whose mother and maternal grandmother had anogenital vesicular lesions, raising the possibility of a forme fruste of benign familial chronic pemphigus (Vakilzadeh & Kolde 1985). There may also be a distinct variant, genital acanthloytic dyskeratosis (see below).

Netherton's syndrome (ichthyosis linearis circumflexa)

This rare condition is determined by an autosomal recessive gene. Ichthyosis linearis circumflexa is associated with trichorrhexis invaginata or other abnormalities of the hair shaft. The skin is red and scaly and the changes are marked in the flexures. Kübler *et al.* (1987) have reported a patient with a vulval carcinoma superimposed on the warty tissue.

Dyskeratosis congenita

This rare condition, commoner in males and usually inherited through an X-linked recessive gene, is characterized by cutaneous atrophy and pigmentation with a nail dystrophy. Leukoplakia of the oral cavity may be accompanied by similar changes in the eye and urogenital mucosa. Carcinomas are frequent, affecting the skin, mucosae and other organs, and one female patient described by Sorrow and Hitch (1963) had a carcinoma of the cervix and vagina.

Epidermolytic hyperkeratosis (bullous congenital ichthyosiform erythroderma)

This genodermatosis is caused by mutations in the genes encoding keratins 1 and 10. It presents at birth with erythroderma, blistering and erosions but with time severe hyperkeratosis develops. Hyperkeratotic lesions involving the vulva and vagina have been described (Quinn & Young 1997, Swann *et al.* 2003).

White sponge naevus

White hyperkeratotic lesions of the oral mucosa, often inherited as an autosomal dominant condition, are seen. In some cases, genital lesions have also been present (Dégos & Ebrard 1958). Vulval lesions have been described (Buchholz *et al.* 1985, Nichols *et al.* 1990). White plaques are seen on the tongue and inner aspects of the vulva (Figs 5.5 and 5.6).

Histology of the white plaques shows acanthosis, individual cell keratinization and large vacuolated cells.

If symptoms are present, treatment with topical tetracycline has been helpful in oral lesions, and so is worth trying for the genital area (McDonagh *et al.* 1990, Lim & Ng 1992).

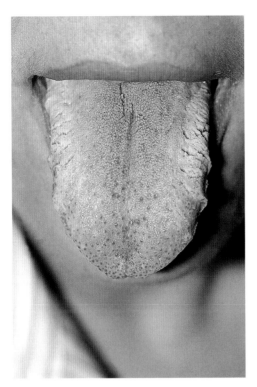

Fig. 5.5 White sponge naevus: white plaques on the tongue.

Goltz syndrome (focal dermal hypoplasia)

In this rare genetic disorder, linear abnormalities of pigmentation, atrophy and telangiectasia are often present at birth. Fat herniation then develops in the streaks. Raspberry-like papillomas can appear at any site but there is a predilection for the perineal and perianal skin.

Pseudoxanthoma elasticum

This condition may be inherited by way of autosomal recessive or dominant genes and over 90 different nonsense and missense mutations have been identified. The elastic tissue, ground substance and collagen are abnormal and the main hazard is the serious risk of systemic vascular lesions including those of the retina. Although there are potential risks in pregnancy, Viljoen *et al.* (1987) found only a small increase in the number of spontaneous abortions, but a tendency to develop marked striae. Cases involving the vulva and vagina have been reported (Szymanski & Caro 1955, Goodman *et al.* 1963).

The lesions are yellowish papules, which may become confluent, often with purpura and telangiectasia. Lesions typically affect the neck and axillae and have a 'plucked chicken' appearance. Angioid streaks are visible on the retina.

Histologically, the main feature is the presence of dystrophic elastic fibres showing deposition of calcium. No treatment is possible apart from limited surgical removal if indicated.

Ehlers–Danlos syndrome

Ehlers–Danlos syndrome (EDS) is now known to comprise at least 10 types, all characterized by different abnormalities of the connective tissue. In type IV, inherited as an autosomal dominant condition, the skin is transparent and fragile, with minor hyperelasticity. Arterial and bowel rupture may be fatal. The fault lies in the production of type III collagen. Rudd *et al.* (1983) studied 20 women in four families with EDS type IV. Ten had been pregnant with a total of 20 pregnancies and five patients had died as a result. Complications and fatalities had arisen from rupture of bowel, large vessels or uterus, lacerations of the vagina and postpartum haemorrhage. Twelve of the liveborn babies had EDS IV and two died during delivery; two pregnancies were aborted. Lurie *et al.* (1998) have reviewed further cases of EDS IV and discussed management. This appears to be the main type of EDS in which there are risks in pregnancy.

There is one report of postcoital laceration and bruising of the vulva in a patient with presumed EDS (Tucker & Yell 1999).

Neurofibromatosis

The neurofibromatoses occur in various forms; of these, type 2 rarely manifests cutaneous signs. The others, of which

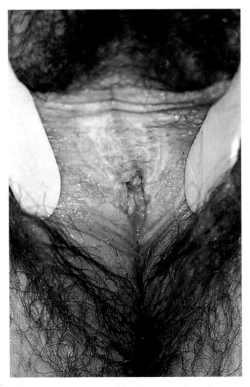

Fig. 5.6 White sponge naevus: white plaques at the vulva.

type 1 (von Recklinghausen's disease) is the commonest, are characterized by tumours, discussed in Chapter 9, and by so-called freckling which, while usually in the axillae, has been reported in the vulval area (Crowe 1964).

Cowden's disease (multiple hamartoma syndrome)

This is a hamartomatous condition involving ectodermal, mesodermal and endodermal tissues. It is an autosomal dominant condition caused by a mutation in the *PTEN* tumour suppressor gene. The skin may show acral, facial and oral mucosal lesions. The vulva may be affected by the acral type, namely keratotic papillomas, sometimes showing a follicular origin (Burnett *et al.* 1975, Brownstein *et al.* 1979), or by other lesions, e.g. an apocrine cystadenoma (Salem & Steck 1983). Excision of any troublesome lesion is indicated.

Dowling–Degos disease (reticular pigmented anomaly of the flexures)

This is probably inherited as an autosomal dominant condition and is characterized by reticulate pigmentation in the flexures which can involve the vulva (O'Goshi *et al.* 2001) (Fig. 5.7). It tends to present in the third or fourth decade and comedone-like lesions on the neck and pitted scarring can also be seen. There is one case in which the genital area was the only site involved (Milde *et al.* 1992).

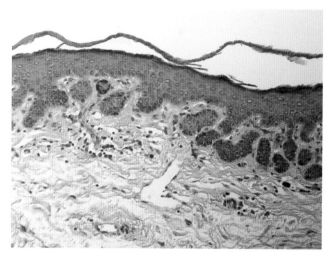

Fig. 5.8 Histology of Dowling–Degos syndrome: the epidermis has numerous thin, branching downgrowths with melanin concentrated at their tips.

The histology is diagnostic with irregular elongation of branched rete ridges with a concentration of melanin at the tips. The melanocyte count is normal (Fig. 5.8).

Galli–Galli disease is a variant of Dowling–Degos disease with acantholysis as an additional feature (Gilchrist *et al.* 2008). The flexural pigmentation is similar but erythematous papules are seen on the trunk and proximal limbs.

Conditions associated with systemic disease

Necrolytic migratory erythema (glucagonoma syndrome)

This distinctive eruption mainly affects the lower abdomen, genital area, thighs and buttocks. It is associated with glucose intolerance and hyperglucagonaemia secondary to α-cell tumours of the pancreas. However, a similar picture has been reported in patients with cirrhosis and diabetes but without a glucagonoma or glucagonaemia. The cause of the rash is unknown but theories include deficiencies of amino acids and essential fatty acids and elevation of epidermal arachidonic acid caused by a raised plasma glucagon.

It usually affects middle-aged females. Patients present with generalized malaise, weight loss, stomatitis, glossitis and often diabetes. The lesions are erythematous and bullous, extending and then healing at the edges to form a serpiginous pattern (Fig. 5.9). The clinical picture is fairly typical but pustular psoriasis, bullous dermatoses and acrodermatitis enteropathica must be considered.

The histology shows epidermal necrolysis and a mild lymphocytic dermal infiltrate.

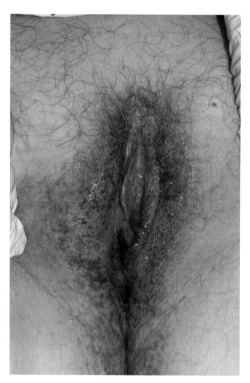

Fig. 5.7 Dowling–Degos syndrome: speckled and confluent pigmentation.

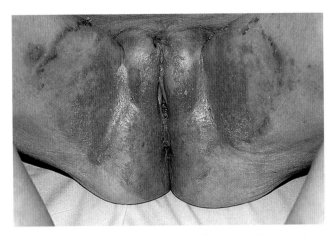

Fig. 5.9 Glucagonoma syndrome: scaly and moist serpiginous rash.

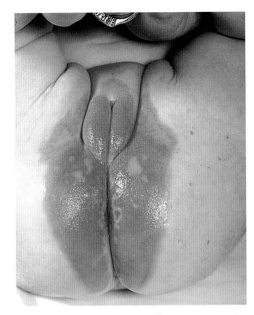

Fig. 5.10 Acrodermatitis enteropathica: fiery erythema of the anogenital area.

Surgical removal of the tumour usually leads to rapid improvement. Secondary deposits may be present at the time of diagnosis and require treatment. Hepatic artery embolization and therapy with octreotide acetate, a synthetic octapeptide analogue of somatostatin, have been shown to be helpful.

Acrodermatitis enteropathica

This condition is related to zinc deficiency. It may be inherited in an autosomal recessive manner, with presentation in infancy, or acquired. The acquired form may be secondary to total parenteral nutrition, Crohn's disease, jejuno-ileal bypass surgery, alcoholism, prematurity, penicillamine given for cystinuria or Wilson's disease, or chelating agents given for iron overload in thalassaemia. Adults may have the acquired type, or have relapses of the genetic type, as in the patient of Verburg et al. (1974) who developed lesions in pregnancy having been previously well controlled on zinc therapy.

The lesions are red, eroded and vesicopustular; they affect not only the genital area (Fig. 5.10) but also other parts, particularly the face (Fig. 5.11). The scalp hair becomes fine and sparse with loss of hair. The course is chronic in the absence of treatment.

The histology is non-specific so the diagnosis is made on the clinical features and confirmed by low serum zinc. However, falsely low values may be found in hypoalbuminaemia. It must be distinguished from candidiasis and seborrhoeic dermatitis. A rare differential diagnosis is Netherton's syndrome. The genital lesions may be similar (Greene & Muller 1985) but there are additional features of ichthyosis, atopy and hair abnormalities.

Oral elemental zinc is the accepted treatment and zinc levels should be monitored regularly. A similar picture to acrodermatitis enteropathica can be seen in pellagra.

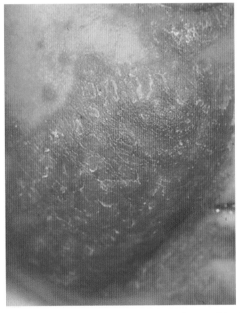

Fig. 5.11 Acrodermatitis enteropathica: fiery erythema of the face.

Inflammatory bowel disease

Ulcerative colitis and Crohn's disease are the two major forms of inflammatory bowel disease and, although they share common symptoms and signs, they are separate entities with different medical and surgical treatments. There are occasions when the distinction of one from the other is not always possible.

Ulcerative colitis

Anogenital lesions are much rarer than in Crohn's disease. Verbov (1973) found only one definite example out of 40 patients and Galbraith *et al.* (2005) describes a perianal ulcer in one child in a series of nine paediatric cases. A pustular vegetative eruption in the groins clinically suggestive of pemphigus has been described. The histology showed only scant acantholysis, and immunofluorescence was negative and the entity was named pemphigus vegetans, Hallopeau type or pyodermite végétante. Genital lesions are rare but there are some reports of Behçet's syndrome occurring in patients with ulcerative colitis (Kobashigawa *et al.* 2004).

Crohn's disease

Anogenital lesions are common and can occur in up to 30% of patients. Crohn's disease affects the whole of the intestinal wall with a tendency to form fistulous tracts. Adjacent structures are frequently involved so gynaecological disease is not uncommon (Fellers *et al.* 2001). Vaginal delivery and episiotomy may be followed by lesions of Crohn's.

Lesions that occur where there is no contiguous bowel disease or at sites clearly away from the anogenital skin are referred to as metastatic (Fig. 5.12) and often occur in the flexures.

Lesions of Crohn's disease, whether contiguous with affected bowel or metastatic, may precede or follow the recognition of bowel disease, often by many years, and even after resolution or removal of the affected intestine. Children and adolescents as well as adults may be affected. The patients present with oedema, often very marked and sometimes with lymphangiectases, firm swelling, oedematous perianal tags and ulcers, fissures, sinuses and fistulae (Figs 5.13 and 5.14). 'Knife cut' fissures are characteristic in the interlabial sulci (Fig. 5.15). The oedema and swelling may occur without gastrointestinal involvement (Martin & Holdstock 1997) and may be unilateral. Symptoms are often severe and may include dyspareunia. The course is chronic and neoplastic changes may occur. Bowen's disease was reported in one case (Prezyna & Kalyanaraman 1977), and vulval carcinoma has been described although it is rare (Greenstein *et al.* 1985). The mechanism for malignant change is unclear but may result from the long-standing inflammatory process, from a defect in immune status or from the effect of the immunosuppressive drugs used in treatment.

Histology may show non-caseating granulomas or only oedema.

The clinical features are variable. Histology may be non-specific, making diagnosis difficult, particularly in the absence of bowel disease. The main differential diagnosis is

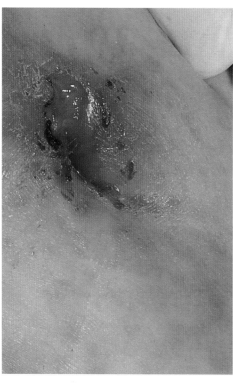

Fig. 5.12 Crohn's disease: metastatic umbilical lesion.

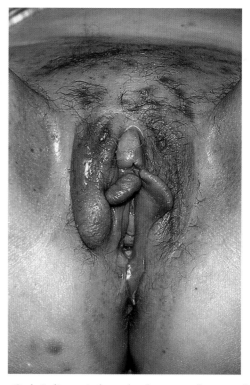

Fig. 5.13 Crohn's disease: indurated oedema, tags, fissures and sinuses.

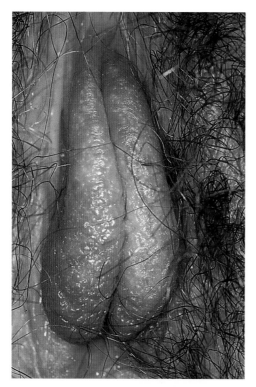

Fig. 5.14 Crohn's disease: oedema of the labia minora.

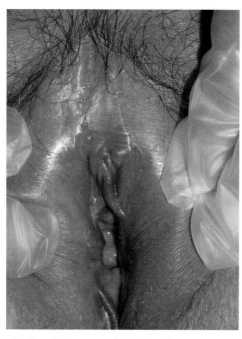

Fig. 5.15 'Knife cut' fissures seen in Crohn's disease.

hidradenitis suppurativa. The presence of bridged scars and comedones in the latter condition is helpful, but the two conditions may coexist (Burrows & Russell-Jones 1992). Other diagnoses to consider include pyoderma gangrenosum, Behçet's syndrome and a chronic atypical infection.

The management of genital Crohn's, particularly if there is active intestinal disease, should involve a multidisciplinary team and will include careful investigation to exclude fistulous tracts. The lesions respond to some extent to medical treatment of the bowel condition. These measures include oral steroids, antibiotics, especially metronidazole, and immunosuppressive drugs such as azathioprine and ciclosporin. Infliximab is used in recalcitrant cases and for fistulous disease. There is one report of infliximab use followed by methotrexate for maintenance to treat pyostomatitis vegetans in association with Crohn's (Bens et al. 2003). The second-generation biologicals may prove successful in the future.

Topical treatment, in the form of potent corticosteroids may prove useful for superficial ulceration and lymphoedema. Topical tacrolimus can also be effective. Nutritional deficiencies, including zinc, are often present and should be corrected. Limited surgery to tags and sinuses is worth considering, and the carbon dioxide laser is effective in treating lymphangiectases. Removal of adjacent diseased bowel can help, but healing may be poor. Vulvectomy (Kao et al. 1975) or excision and grafting (Reyman et al. 1986) have been considered in desperate cases. Care should be taken during vaginal delivery to avoid excessive trauma.

Acute febrile neutrophilic dermatosis (Sweet's syndrome)

Sweet (1979) reviewed a group of patients whom he had earlier reported as having this condition of unknown aetiology. They had fever, painful, erythematous, raised plaques on the skin and neutrophilia; the condition occurred mainly in middle-aged women. Vulval involvement has been reported (Lindskov 1984, Keefe et al. 1988). There have been reports of its association with Behçet's syndrome (Lee & Barnetson 1996) and myeloproliferative disorders. There may be an association or overlap with pyoderma gangrenosum (Lebbe et al. 1992) and both conditions have occurred together in myeloproliferative disease and may be part of a continuum (Caughman et al. 1983, Kuroda et al. 1995).

Histologically, there is leukocytoclasis and a severe inflammatory process, which, although predominantly neutrophilic, may in some instances be lymphocytic or mixed.

The response to oral prednisolone or dapsone is usually good.

Pyoderma gangrenosum

The aetiology of this rare condition is undetermined, but there is a strong association with rheumatoid arthritis and ulcerative colitis, and sometimes Crohn's disease as well as with myeloproliferative disorders. Its indolent ulcerative lesions have been reported at the vulva (McCalmont et al. 1991, Lebbe et al. 1992), although the diagnosis is often difficult to make with certainty. There are reports of herpes simplex complicating pyoderma gangrenosum (Tai & Kelly 2005).

There are multiple punched out, pepperpot-like, small ulcers, or a single large ulcer, set in an area of induration. The edges tend to be violaceous, overhanging and oedematous. The initial lesion may be a single pustule which rapidly enlarges and ulcerates.

The histology is usually inflammatory but non-specific, although there may be evidence of a vasculitis.

The differential diagnosis is mainly from infective ulceration or neoplasia, but the rapidity of onset and progression makes the latter less likely. The correct diagnosis is vital since treatment is not surgical, but medical.

Topical steroids and tacrolimus may be effective. Oral prednisolone or ciclosporin are the two most successful systemic agents (Vidal *et al.* 2004). Azathioprine, dapsone or minocycline may be effective in a limited number of cases. There is one case report of a patient with resistant vulval pyoderma gangrenosum responding to intravenous immunoglobulin (Cummins *et al.* 2007).

Amyloidosis

Lesions are typically glassy or waxy, showing purpura and telangiectasia (Fig. 5.16). Nodular lesions have been described. Vulval examples are rare but Northcutt & Vanover (1985) describe a woman aged 53 with nodular lesions that were reddish, ulcerated and suggestive of malignancy. The lesions recurred 6 years after excision but the patient remained well with no evidence of systemic disease. Histology showed dermal amyloid material of immunoglobulin light chain origin.

Cases of vulval amyloid in association with myeloma have been described (Taylor *et al.* 1991, Buezo *et al.* 1996). Lichen amyloidosis affecting the vulva has also been reported (Gorodeski *et al.* 1988).

Histology shows amyloid as amorphous masses. Staining is positive with Congo red and there is green birefringence with polarized light. The typical straight filaments of immunoglobulin light chain amyloid are seen on electron microscopy. It surrounds vessel walls, accounting for the purpura noted clinically.

The patient should be evaluated for any evidence of systemic disease, as treatment will depend on this. Localized deposits can be treated by surgical excision or laser.

Sarcoidosis

Cutaneous lesions of sarcoidosis may occur alone or in association with systemic disease. The cutaneous lesions have a varied morphology and may be plaques, macular, papular (Fig. 5.17), nodular, annular and rarely ulcerative. Genital lesions are uncommon, but have been described by

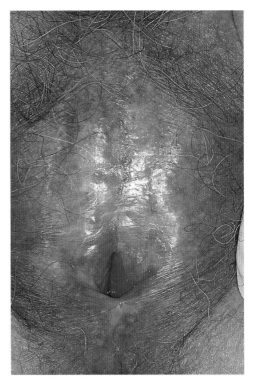

Fig. 5.16 Vulval amyloidosis: atrophy and loss of architecture.

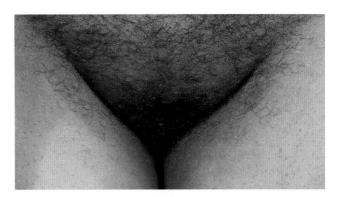

Fig. 5.17 Papular lesions of sarcoid on mons pubis with mild acanthosis nigricans in genitocrural folds.

de Oliveira Neto (1972). Neill *et al.* (1984) reported an example of flexural genital lesions. The lesions were extensive, painless, shallow ulcers affecting the submammary and perianal area and the labia majora; histology was compatible with sarcoidosis. Tatnall *et al.* (1985) reported on a patient with papular lesions of the vulva and perianal areas. The patient had a raised serum angiotensin-converting enzyme, a positive Kveim test and pulmonary lesions; the histology was that of sarcoidosis. There have been five cases of vulval sarcoid reported in the literature to date (Decavalas *et al.* 2007). The fifth case in this last report was a painful lesion arising in an episiotomy scar.

Histology shows epithelioid cells aggregated into discrete non-caseating granulomas with multinucleate giant cells, sometimes cuffed with lymphoid cells.

Topical, intralesional or oral steroids are first-line treatment. Extensive disease may require methotrexate.

Other granulomatous conditions

Some of the reported cases with granulomatous histology may still have been cases of Crohn's disease, with the cutaneous lesions preceding the onset of bowel disease. However, some cases have been categorized as variants of the Melkersson–Rosenthal syndrome (Wagenberg & Downham 1981, Hackel *et al.* 1991). A patient with systemic lupus erythematosus and granulomatous vulval lesions of unknown aetiology developed a SCC at the age of 31. There was also evidence of infection with human papillomavirus types 6 and 11 (Samaratunga *et al.* 1991).

Langerhans cell histiocytosis

Langerhans cell histiocytosis (LCH), previously known as histiocytosis X, may affect the vulva as a solitary manifestation or as part of a widely disseminated disease process. It is probably best regarded as a disorder of immune regulation (Axiotis *et al.* 1991) and occurs in forms which are benign and localized (eosinophilic granuloma), chronic and progressive (Hand–Schuller–Christian) and acute with systemic illness (Letterer–Siwe).

Vulval lesions can occur from 8 months to 85 years (Axiotis *et al.* 1991). In infants, the typical presentation is of yellowish, often purpuric, papules in the napkin area and elsewhere. In adults, the lesions are papular or nodular, sometimes ulcerated.

The characteristic histology is an upper dermal infiltrate of large histiocytic cells which abut onto the dermoepidermal junction. The cells have distinctive bean-shaped nuclei. There is often a lymphocytic infiltrate deeper in the dermis with eosinophils. The Langerhans cells stain positively for S100 protein and electron microscopy reveals the characteristic Birbeck granules.

The differential diagnosis is wide, including neoplasia and dermatoses; definitive diagnosis depends on the specific histology.

Treatment is that of the underlying disease process, and includes excision where feasible, radiotherapy, steroids, vinblastine, vincristine and other chemotherapeutic agents, thalidomide and PUVA (psoralen and UVA treatment) (Axiotis *et al.* 1991, Mottl *et al.* 2007).

Malacoplakia

This condition results from an inadequate or atypical inflammatory response to *Escherichia coli* and other common bacterial pathogens.

It is due to macrophage dysfunction, which results in an inadequate histiocytic response. Primary or acquired immunodeficiency has been noted in nearly 40% of patients (Kogulan *et al.* 2001). It was first described in the bladder, but genital tract involvement is well recognized and was reviewed by Chen and Hendricks (1985). A recent review of the published literature revealed that 40% occurred in the genital area (Kohl & Hans 2008) and typically papules, nodules, ulcers and draining sinuses may be found. Vaginal involvement frequently presents with bleeding.

The clinical differential diagnosis includes Crohn's disease, other granulomatous conditions and malignancy.

The histological appearance is typical and includes sheets of macrophages with an eosinophilic foamy cytoplasm (von Hansemann cells) and characteristic intracytoplasmic 'targetoid' inclusions (Michaelis–Gutmann bodies). The inclusion bodies can be demonstrated with Perls' iron, Prussian blue and periodic acid–Schiff stains. A Gram stain may also reveal intracellular and extracellular bacteria.

Chen and Hendriks (1985) found treatment with cholinergic agonists, which raise the level of cyclic guanosine monophosphate in mononuclear cells, helpful. Long-term antibiotics and surgery are required. Van Furth *et al.* (1992) reported good results with ciprofloxacin, which penetrates well into macrophages, in a patient with malacoplakia of the bladder.

Ligneous disease

This rare condition is usually manifested as a membranous or pseudomembranous conjunctivitis but can affect other tissues, including the lower genital tract. Ocular involvement usually precedes genital lesions (Rubin *et al.* 1989) but there are a few exceptions (Scurry *et al.* 1993a, Schuster & Seregard 2003). Recently, it has been shown that ligneous conjunctivitis is caused by type 1 plasminogen deficiency, a form of inherited hypoplasminogenaemia. A case of this association and extensive ligneous involvement of the female genital tract has been reported (Lotan *et al.* 2007).

The clinical appearance is of firm and sometimes necrotic plaques and nodules, which recur and spread after local biopsy or destructive procedures, and local factors such as trauma seem to be a trigger.

There is a subepidermal hyaline deposit, which is amorphous and eosinophilic and contains albumin, fibrin and immunoglobulin, together with a variable mixed cellular component and sometimes areas of granulation tissue (Fig. 5.18). The epidermis may be ulcerated or hyperplastic. Stains for amyloid are negative.

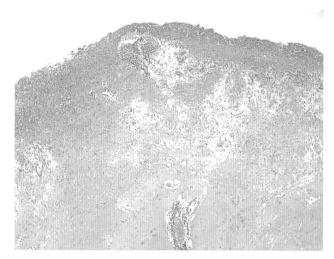

Fig. 5.18 Ligneous disease: deep amorphous hyaline material (courtesy of J. Scurry).

Most of the literature on treatment of ligneous disease is confined to the management of ocular disease. Successful therapy has included surgical excision followed by topical heparin and corticosteroids. There are reports of improvement with oral contraceptives as they can raise plasminogen levels (Teresa-Sartori *et al.* 2003). Replacement therapy with intravenous plasminogen has shown significant improvement of ligneous conjunctivitis but because of the short half-life of the protein daily treatment is required (Schott *et al.* 1998). It is also very important to keep mucosal trauma, including surgical intervention and biopsies, to a minimum.

Lupus erythematosus

In a series of 121 patients with lupus erythematosus (LE), both male and female, Burge *et al.* (1989) found that 21% of those with systemic disease and 24% of those with chronic cutaneous disease had mucosal involvement (nose, eyes, mouth). No specific genital lesions were found in 48 female patients with systemic LE, although one had vaginal lesions possibly secondary to Sjögren's syndrome. Vulval lesions were, however, found in two out of 42 women with chronic cutaneous LE. Of these two, one had erythema with ulceration and later scarring near the introitus; the other had erythema and white reticulate vulval lesions, with lichen planus-like lesions in the mouth. The histology of LE and lichen planus can be similar and it is possible that the features in this second case were due to lichen planus. The two conditions can co-exist.

Vulval involvement in LE is rare but discoid LE has been reported (Bilenchi 2004) and there is one case report of a patient with systemic LE who developed a plaque of cutaneous lupus on the left labium majus (Jolly & Patel 2006).

Sjögren's syndrome

Sjögren's syndrome is characterized by dryness of mucous membranes as a result of reduced glandular function secondary to lymphocytic infiltration. Many patients produce autoantibodies, particularly anti-SS-A (Ro) and SS-B (La). Most cases are associated with other autoimmune diseases, especially rheumatoid arthritis, systemic sclerosis and LE. The predominant symptoms are xerostomia and dry eyes.

Although anogenital symptoms are not uncommon in affected patients, the true incidence of vulval or vaginal involvement is unknown. Bloch *et al.* (1965) described 62 cases and commented that vaginal dryness was present in 20 of the 59 women (11 of them premenopausal). Patients complained of burning and dyspareunia and the mucosa was noted to be red but a biopsy in one patient was non-specific. In a case–control study of 36 women with 43 controls, 61% of the patients with Sjögren's syndrome described dyspareunia and 55% vaginal dryness, compared with 39% and 33% of controls respectively (Marchesoni *et al.* 1995). In a study of patients presenting with dyspareunia who also complained of musculoskeletal symptoms, four of the 11 were found to have primary Sjögren's syndrome with positive antibodies and salivary gland histology (Mulherin *et al.* 1997). It was noted that the vaginal symptoms seemed to predate the ocular and oral symptoms by many months. It is unclear which anogenital glands may be involved in causing these symptoms as the vagina contains no glandular structures, with moisture being mainly the result of transudation.

There are individual case reports of vaginal atresia (Ricard-Rothiot *et al.* 1979) and vulval amyloidosis (Konishi *et al.* 2007) occurring in association with Sjögren's syndrome. However, some patients have both Sjögren's syndrome and lichen planus.

No specific treatment is available and drugs given for associated disease appear to be of little help. Symptomatic treatment with lubricating agents is indicated.

Dermatomyositis

There is one case report of vulval involvement in dermatomyositis (Lavery *et al.* 1985). Dermatomyositis may be associated with an underlying malignancy and there is one case report of its occurrence in a patient with cervical carcinoma (Celebi *et al.* 2001). A reticulosarcoma of the vulva occurred in a patient with dermatomyositis who was on azathioprine, and it was felt that the immunosuppressive treatment was a factor in the malignancy (Wishart 1973).

Behçet's syndrome

This syndrome was originally defined in 1937 as a triad of oral and genital ulceration and ocular lesions (uveitis). It is now recognized as a multisystem disease that may sometimes be diagnosed only after a period of observation of an evolving clinical picture. In 1990 diagnostic criteria were outlined by an International Study Group for Behçet's syndrome. The diagnosis is made when a patient has recurrent oral ulceration in combination with at least two of the following: recurrent genital ulceration, eye lesions, cutaneous lesions or a positive pathergy test (sterile pustules following trauma such as a needle prick). Cutaneous lesions include pyodermatous plaques, erythema nodosum and folliculitis.

The causative agent may be viral, and the pathogenesis of the lesions is probably an autoimmune vascular response. An association with human leukocyte antigen (HLA)-B51 has been described but immunogenetic factors may vary in different parts of the world. The important differential diagnosis is from recurrent aphthous disease, but scarring would be unusual. Aphthous ulceration is also associated with as strong family history, and there will be no pathergy.

The onset is usually in adult life before the age of 50 years. The oral ulcers are indistinguishable from recurrent aphthous ulcers. The vulval ulcers are recurrent, painful and often on the labia minora (Fig. 5.19). They eventually heal, often with scarring. Vaginal ulcers have been reported (Morgan *et al.* 1988) in an atypical case.

Histologically, the appearances may be non-specific or show thrombosed arterioles or other manifestations of arteriolar or venous disease.

Management may be difficult and should involve a multidisciplinary approach. The oral and genital ulceration can be the most symptomatic for the patient, but the retinal disease can lead to blindness and neurological complications to severe disability. Many drugs are employed, with varying success, e.g. colchicine, steroids, dapsone, levamisole, thalidomide and immunosuppressive drugs. Colchicine and aspirin are used to prevent acute exacerbations, corticosteroids for ocular and neurological involvement and anti-coagulants for thrombotic disease. When the genital ulcers are mild, topical corticosteroids are helpful. Thalidomide is effective for mucosal ulcers, although difficult to obtain. Alli *et al.* (1997) report good results, from intralesional recombinant human granulocyte/macrophage colony-stimulating factor (rhGM-CSF) for a large genital ulcer. In severe disease, the biological agents may be useful (Estrach *et al.* 2002).

Recurrent aphthous ulceration

Mild recurrent aphthous ulceration affecting the mouth is common, but some patients have the major form, with more severe scarring lesions (Fig. 5.20), and it may then be associated with recurrent vulval ulceration. The onset is usually in childhood or adolescence and there are no features of systemic disease. There may be a family history. The major differential diagnoses for the vulval ulcers are herpes simplex, Stevens–Johnson syndrome and Behçet's syndrome.

The aetiology is uncertain. There may be cross-reactions between bacterial antigens and the mucosa and some significant HLA links have been reported.

The vulval ulcers are sharply defined, of varying sizes, with a yellowish base and a red halo (Fig. 5.21). The histology is non-specific.

Multiple topical and systemic therapies have been used. Topical corticosteroids, applied in an adhesive base, and tetracyclines are useful for vulval ulcers. Topical local anaesthetic agents, such as 5% lidocaine ointment, may also have a role.

Other non-infective ulcers

Other ulcers, particularly those described in the older literature, are difficult to categorize and may not be distinct

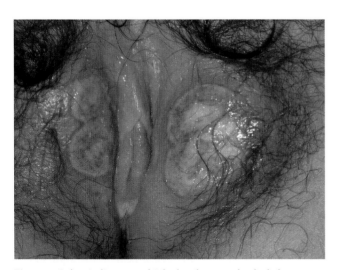

Fig. 5.19 Behçet's disease: multiple slough-covered vulval ulcers.

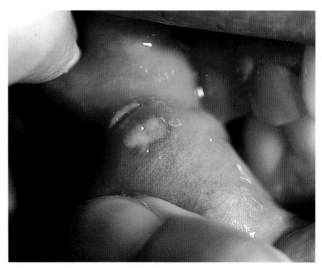

Fig. 5.20 Major aphthous ulcer of the mouth.

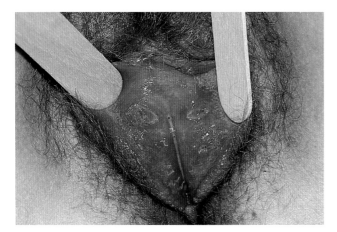

Fig. 5.21 Major aphthous ulcers of the vulva.

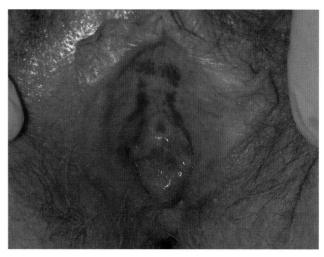

Fig. 5.22 Residual rust-red pigmentation of haemosiderin deposition on the vulval vestibule after lichen planus.

entities. Sutton's ulcers (Sutton 1935) were described, originally in 1913, as recurrent, solitary or few, deep and painful, more often occurring in the mouth than at the vulva; they may well have been identical to major aphthous ulcers.

Lipschutz (1913) described ulcers of sudden onset with fever and pain in young girls. These are now known to be associated with infection (see Chapter 4). They have also been reported in patients with pityriasis lichenoides (Burke *et al.* 1969).

Boyce and Valpey (1971) reported an outbreak of painful ulcers in the wives of servicemen returning from Asia who were themselves symptom free. Muram and Gold (1993) have reported vulval ulcers, not caused by infection or by leukaemic infiltration, in girls with myelocytic leukaemia, and the authors postulated a multifactorial aetiology.

Pigmentary disorders

There is considerable variation in the normal pigmentation of the keratinized vulval skin depending on ethnicity, age and hormonal status. These appearances are usually even and diffuse and do not pose problems with diagnosis.

Pigmentation due to haemosiderin deposition can also occur and tends to have a reddish-brown tinge, rather than the brownish- or bluish-black colour found with melanin. It occurs as a result of extravasation of blood and is a feature of lichen sclerosus, Zoon's vulvitis, caruncles and prolapsed tissue of cervical, vaginal, rectal or urethral origin (Fig. 5.22).

However, in some cases the pigmentation presents a greater diagnostic challenge. It may be patchy, extensive or asymmetrical and such lesions should always be biopsied and then subjected to good clinicopathological correlation. Benign lesions such as seborrhoeic keratoses may mimic

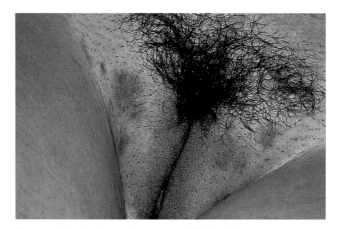

Fig. 5.23 Macular hyperpigmentation of lichen planus.

vulval malignant melanoma clinically, and the diagnosis is made on histological grounds.

Hyperpigmentation

Post-inflammatory pigmentation
This frequently follows lichen planus (Fig. 5.23), in which the pigmentation may be persistent. It can also occur after lichen sclerosus or a fixed drug eruption. When it is clear that there has been a preceding inflammatory dermatosis, the diagnosis of post-inflammatory hyperpigmentation is straightforward, but if there is any doubt, or atypical features, a biopsy should be performed. Histologically, there is pigmentary incontinence, with pigmented macrophages in the upper dermis.

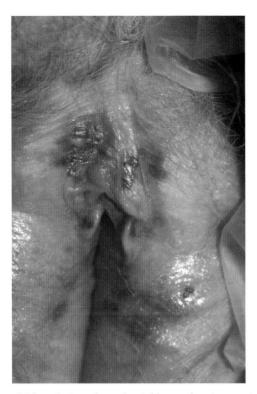

Fig. 5.24 Melanosis: irregular and variable macular pigmentation.

Melanosis

In some cases of vulval pigmentation, histology will reveal only basal hypermelanosis, often with an increased number of melanocytes and some pigmentary incontinence but no melanocytic proliferation. Clinically, these lesions can be very irregular in distribution and colour, often mimicking melanoma (Fig. 5.24). There has been debate about suitable terminology for these lesions. Many use the term vulval melanosis but idiopathic lenticular mucocutaneous pigmentation has been suggested (Gerbig & Hunziker 1996). In a review of 10 reported cases in men and seven in women (Barnhill *et al.* 1990), the term genital lentiginosis was used when there was evidence of melanocytic hyperplasia (sometimes requiring special stains for demonstration), and the term melanosis was reserved for those cases when it was absent.

There is debate about whether these lesions are at risk of malignant change. If the analogy with apparently similar (though solitary) oral lesions is used, these lesions are unlikely to become malignant. However, follow-up is recommended and photographs or diagrams are important aids. Lesions that have changed in any way should be biopsied.

Laugier–Hunziker syndrome is an acquired disorder characterized by benign macular pigmentation of the oral and genital mucosa and longitudinal melanonychia occurs in 50–60% of cases. The dermatoscopic features have been studied in this condition and parallel linear streaks of pigment are seen in the vulval lesions (Gencoglan 2007). There is one case in which a patient developed genital pigmentation as part of Laugier–Hunziker syndrome 1 year after commencing levodopa (Vega Gutierrez 2003). Two years later, she developed Addison's disease with an increase in the melanosis.

Lentigines

Lentigines may be sporadic, or part of a syndrome. Pigmented macules on the vulva have been described as part of the LAMB syndrome (lentigines, atrial myxoma, mucocutaneous myxomas, blue naevi) (Reed *et al.* 1986, Rhodes *et al.* 1986). In the Carney complex (cutaneous and atrial myxomas, mucocutaneous pigmentation, endocrine abnormalities and schwannomas), facial pigmentation is usual, but multiple blue/black macules on the vulva were the presenting feature in one case (Pandolfini *et al.* 2001). These also occur in Dowling–Degos disease (see p. 90). Any lentiginous change must be biopsied to exclude atypical lentiginosis, which is a precursor of melanoma.

Vaginal pigmentation

Melanocytes are found in the vagina in only 3% of women, but pigmented macules, melanosis and malignant melanoma are all recognized. Any pigmented vaginal lesion should be biopsied. Cervical melanosis is also recognized (Deppisch 1983).

Acanthosis nigricans

All forms of this disease, including pseudoacanthosis nigricans seen in obese patients, are now thought to be related to insulin resistance. In one study, acanthosis nigricans was a frequent finding in hirsute, hyperandrogenic women and was invariably found on the vulva (Grasinger *et al.* 1993). In children, it is benign and may be hereditary. In adults, some cases may be linked with malignancy, usually an adenocarcinoma. Very rarely, the condition is drug induced; nicotinic acid (Tromovitch *et al.* 1964) and triazinate (Greenspan *et al.* 1985) have been incriminated.

The lesions chiefly affect the neck, the mucosae and the flexures, and the genital area is a site of predilection (Fig. 5.17). They are dark, at first velvety and then warty, and all aspects of the vulva may be involved. If the acanthosis nigricans is a cutaneous manifestation of underlying malignancy, the onset is usually rapid and may be accompanied by tripe palms and lip involvement.

The histology shows hyperkeratosis and papillomatosis, some acanthosis and pigmentation. Horny inclusions are sometimes present.

Treatment is aimed at the underlying disease process. Hyperinsulinaemia must be corrected and weight loss may be helpful. Keratolytics, retinoids, dermabrasion and laser treatment have all been tried.

Confluent and reticulated papillomatosis (Gougerot–Carteaud syndrome)

This is an uncommon condition in which reticulate and pigmented papules usually affect the neck and upper trunk. Cases have been reported in the mons pubis region (Hallel-Halevy *et al.* 1993). It often responds well to minocycline.

Miscellaneous causes of pigmentation

Trichomycosis and chromhidrosis may lead to some discoloration of the skin. A proprietary laxative, Dorbanex, was reduced in the bowel to dithranol and was responsible for staining of skin in contact with faeces as well as reddish-brown discoloration of urine and vaginal secretions (Barth *et al.* 1984). Related compounds may cause similar effects.

Vulval and vaginal pigmentation has been described secondary to the ingestion of bismuth (Weiner 1940) and quinacrine (Lutterloh & Shellenberger 1946).

Hypopigmentation

Post-inflammatory hypopigmentation

Hypopigmentation is a common sequel of inflammation, especially obvious in darker skin (Fig. 5.25). Post-inflammatory hypopigmentation is usually incomplete and ill defined.

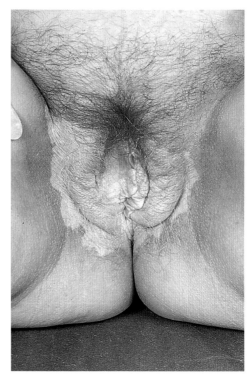

Fig. 5.26 Vitiligo: total loss of pigment in a symmetrical pattern.

Vitiligo

Vitiligo is of uncertain aetiology but autoimmune and neurohumoral mechanisms have been suggested. There is complete depigmentation of an area of skin that is in all other respects normal. The patch is well defined and the condition is usually symmetrical (Fig. 5.26). In hairy areas, the hair may or may not retain its colour.

Histology shows reduced numbers or a complete absence of melanocytes. Those that are present are apparently normal but non-functional. There is a mild lymphocytic infiltrate.

The two main differential diagnoses of vitiligo are the pale thickening of lichenification and lichen sclerosus. Distinguishing it from lichen simplex and lichen sclerosus is usually straightforward as there is no epidermal change in vitiligo. However, diagnostic difficulties arise when it occurs together with lichen sclerosus.

There is no effective treatment; measures that might be tried elsewhere would be inappropriate at this site.

Disorders of skin appendages

Disorders of sebaceous glands

Sebaceous glands may be clinically apparent on the labia majora and minora, either as yellowish specks known as Fordyce spots and analogous to the oral lesions, or as

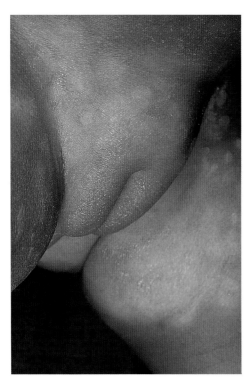

Fig. 5.25 Post-inflammatory hypopigmentation in a child with a psoriasiform napkin rash.

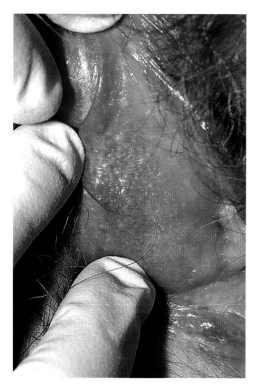

Fig. 5.27 Fordyce spots: aggregated yellow specks on the inner labium minus.

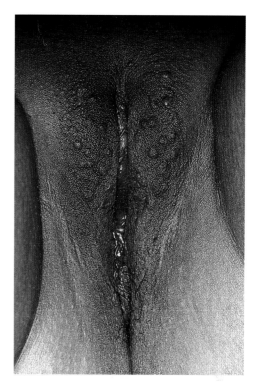

Fig. 5.28 Syringomas: multiple skin-coloured papules.

aggregated sheets (Fig. 5.27). On the labia minora, they end where Hart's line marks the boundary of the vestibule. Secretion from the glands may accumulate between the labia, and patients who complain of soreness or a subjective sensation of swelling in this area often have unusually profuse glands. Blockage of the sebaceous gland may lead to the formation of painful papules or pustules in the childbearing years. Patients describe a flare of their symptoms usually in the 10 days prior to the onset of their menses.

Rocamora *et al.* (1986) have described a case in which sebaceous lobules surrounding a duct formed soft polypoid lesions. They were thought to represent sebaceous gland hyperplasia.

Treatment is not usually indicated, but, if they give rise to symptoms, cautery or hyfrecation is effective for non-inflamed lesions. Inflamed lesions can be treated with a mild topical corticosteroid. The occasional use of a topical retinoid can be tried but the patient must be warned that its use is contraindicated in pregnancy, and probably best avoided in those trying to conceive.

Disorders of sweat glands

Eccrine miliaria

Occlusion of the sweat gland orifices, under conditions of heat and humidity, leads to the appearance of papulovesicles. They are encountered mainly in infants. The obstruction may result in a subcorneal vesicle or in vesiculation proximal to a deeper obstruction at the dermoepidermal junction. The problem is self-limiting.

Syringomas

These benign adenomas of the eccrine sweat ducts appear as skin-coloured papules at the vulva, with or without lesions elsewhere (Fig. 5.28).

Apocrine miliaria

These are poorly documented, but probably not uncommon, appearing as transient painful papules often with a cyclical (menstrual) pattern. Grimmer (1968) reported them in an elderly woman.

Chromhidrosis

This refers to the secretion of coloured sweat, usually arising in apocrine glands. The colour varies from black or brown to yellow or green. The vulva is not a common site, but Joosse *et al.* (1964) reported lesions there. Areas of pigmentation under the skin were found to be a lipofuscin, probably a normal tissue constituent; however, the granules were larger than normal and more numerous. Surgical treatment, sometimes considered elsewhere, is unlikely to be feasible in the genital area.

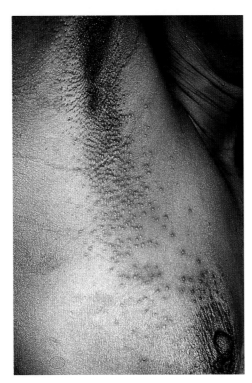

Fig. 5.29 Fox–Fordyce disease: skin-coloured papules in and around a flexure.

Fox–Fordyce disease

This rare eruption of unknown aetiology is characterized by closely packed, skin-coloured papules, which are very itchy and which affect the axillae, breasts and anogenital area (Fig. 5.29). They develop after puberty and become more itchy at menstruation, improving in pregnancy and after the menopause.

The ducts of the apocrine glands are obstructed by keratin plugs, leading to retention of sweat. There may be surrounding inflammation. Complete obstruction of a duct can result in rupture of a retention vesicle.

The contraceptive pill may improve the symptoms by suppressing ovulation. Topical corticosteroids are of limited value. Phototherapy or topical retinoids to exfoliate the surface have been tried. Pimecrolimus has been reported to be of help (Pock *et al.* 2006). Surgical measures may be used as a last resort.

Disorders of hair

Pilonidal sinuses

The classical site for these lesions is the sacrococcygeal area, but rare occurrences on the vulva have been reported (Radman & Bhagavan 1972). They arise as a reaction to an ingrowing hair. The lesion is painful and may present as an abscess requiring incision and drainage. The definitive treatment is excision. The histological features show a sinus tract lined by granulation tissue with fragments of hair.

Pseudofolliculitis pubis is a similar reaction to ingrowing hairs on the mons pubis. It is analogous to that seen in the beard area (sycosis barbae). It may be precipitated by shaving or waxing. Avoidance of traumatic depilation, and, in some severe cases, permanent removal of the hair by laser or electrolysis, may be required.

Hidradenitis suppurativa
Aetiology

This inflammatory neutrophilic folliculitis has in the past been considered to involve mainly the apocrine glands. Yu and Cook (1990), however, considered that the basic pathogenesis is in the follicular epithelium rather than in the apocrine gland, a view supported by Boer and Weltevreden (1996), who found that the earliest event is a spongiform infundibular folliculitis. Although it appears that the apocrine gland is not the primary target in the disease it still may play an aetiological role as the distribution of the disease is limited to the areas where apocrine glands are present. The shearing force in flexural zones has been forwarded as a factor but this does not explain buttock lesions. The disease has been compared to acne, but there is no increased secretion of sebum; however, it is possible that there is an apocrine glandular secretion that might be a triggering factor.

Although numerous bacteria are found in association with hidradenitis suppurativa (Oprica & Nord 2006) they are not considered to be causative. *Streptococcus milleri* is frequently found in the lesions and there is some response to antibiotic agents. A study of 42 women showed a significant incidence of clinical and biochemical endocrine abnormalities, suggesting that an alteration of androgen metabolism might be involved (Mortimer *et al.* 1986a). The patients had irregular periods, premenstrual exacerbation of their disease, acne and hirsutes, a higher concentration of free testosterone and a higher free androgen index than did normal control subjects. However, hidradenitis suppurativa is often worse in overweight patients; Barth *et al.* (1996) found that these findings are no longer significant when the results are controlled for body weight, and concluded that there is no evidence of hyperandrogenism. The skin's innate and adaptive immune responses may be at fault. Antimicrobial peptides are produced after injury or microbial insult and these can act as immune effectors stimulating cytokine and chemokine production (Bardan *et al.* 2004). It is possible that these cutaneous responses are abnormal in hidradenitis suppurativa.

Clinical features

It is rare before puberty and tends to involute after the menopause, although cases occasionally do still occur after

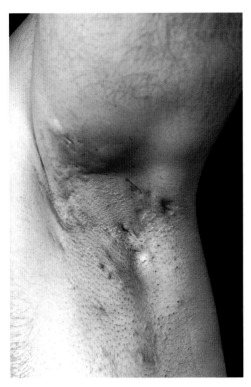

Fig. 5.30 Hidradenitis suppurativa: comedones and bridged scars in a flexure.

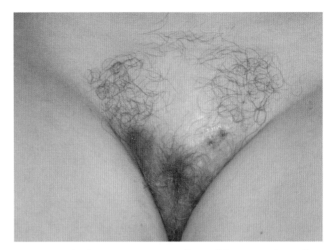

Fig. 5.31 Hidradenitis suppurativa: oedema of the mons pubis with inflamed sinus tract and bridged comedone on the right.

this time (Barth *et al.* 1996). Anogenital lesions are common, being found in the genitocrural folds, mons pubis, labia majora, perianal skin and buttocks. The axillae and breasts may also be affected. A pilonidal sinus may also be present. Afro-Caribbean patients are reportedly affected more often than Caucasians. Tender nodules form, soften and may lead to abscesses; spontaneous discharge is uncommon. Widespread sinuses, induration and scarring develop and there may be fistulae that open into the anus. An important characteristic and diagnostic feature is the presence of bridged scars and comedonal plugs (Figs 5.30 and 5.31).

Histology
The main histological changes include folliculitis and ductal occlusion. There is secondary involvement of the apocrine and eccrine glands (Jemec & Hansen 1996). Sinus tracts lined by keratinized epithelium are formed and are seen more often if there is evidence of occlusion of the duct. There is often distension of apocrine glands and accumulations of polymorphs, which tend to migrate to adjacent tissue. The gland may become necrotic, with an infiltrate of lymphocytes, plasma cells and macrophages. Ultimately, the changes lead to abscesses, fibrosis, foreign body reactions and sometimes pseudoepitheliomatous hyperplasia.

Complications
In addition to scarring, SCC has been reported in long-standing disease (Short *et al.* 2005), and one case of squamous cell carcinoma with hidradenitis was associated with a paraneoplastic neuropathy (Rosenzweig *et al.* 2005). Verrucous carcinomas have also been described (Cosman *et al.* 2000), and one case of clear cell acanthoma (Zedek *et al.* 2007).Other complications in severe disease include anaemia, arthropathy, urethral fistula and amyloidosis (Montes-Romero *et al.* 2008).

Differential diagnosis
The differential diagnosis is in the early stages from a simple folliculitis, and later from deep infections and, in particular, from Crohn's disease, which it may closely resemble and with which it may sometimes coexist.

Management
General measures should include weight reduction and cessation of smoking. Mild disease can be managed initially with antiseptic washes and topical antibiotic lotions. Moderate to severe disease requires long-term oral antibiotics and often surgical intervention (Slade *et al.* 2003). The first-line treatment is an oral tetracycline for 12 weeks initially. In a retrospective trial, 10 weeks of a combination of clindamycin and rifampicin proved to be effective in that eight out of 14 patients went into remission (Mendonça & Griffiths 2006).

The new biological agents may prove to be helpful, but the results are variable and serious side-effects a problem (Moschella 2007). The synthetic retinoids etretinate and isotretinoin have been used but teratogenicity and side-effects limit their use.

Antiandrogen therapy was found helpful in a double-blind cross-over study (Mortimer *et al.* 1986b), and finasteride, a selective inhibitor of type II 5α-reductase, has been used (Joseph *et al.* 2005). Ciclosporin has also been reported as being effective (Buckley & Rogers 1995). Severe recalcitrant disease that fails to respond to medical therapies results in extreme destruction and debility, and here the best approach is surgical (Slade *et al.* 2003). Small areas may be excised with primary closure, but sometimes grafting or healing by secondary intention is required. There may, however, be recurrence in spite of these surgical measures. The carbon dioxide laser is helpful for small areas (Finley & Ratz 1996).

Alopecia areata

Alopecia areata is a common condition in the aetiology of which genetic, autoimmune and other immune factors are probably involved.

Genital hair is lost in alopecia totalis. Patchy loss may be seen in milder examples of the disease. The patches are often centrally placed, round, non-inflamed and asymptomatic. Histology shows follicles that are smaller and higher in the dermis than usual, and in the early stages there is a lymphocytic infiltrate around the hair bulb. Treatment of alopecia areata in general is unsatisfactory and not usually indicated at this site. In the majority of patients the hairs will regrow spontaneously.

Drug reactions

The adverse cutaneous effects of some drugs, both topical and systemic, on the vulval skin can be predicted; the virilization seen with topical testosterone being one such example. In other cases, reactions may be idiosyncratic. The vulva may also be involved in some generalized drug reactions such as Stevens–Johnson syndrome and toxic epidermal necrolysis.

Vulval involvement in systemic drug reactions

Fixed drug eruption

A fixed drug eruption (FDE) characteristically occurs at the same site or sites each time the causative drug is ingested. Its mechanism remains essentially unexplained.

In a study of the site specificity of fixed drug eruptions, the genital mucosa was the most frequently affected area (Ozkaya-Bayazit 2003), but the problem is significantly more common in males. In a study of 29 patients with FDE involving the genital area, only two cases occurred in women, one affecting the vagina and the second affecting the vulva (Sehgal & Gangwan 1986). A series of 13 women presenting with chronic vulvitis, presumed to be the manifestation of FDE, has been reported (Fischer 2007). The main drugs implicated were non-steroidal anti-inflammatory

preparations and COX-2 inhibitors. Other cases affecting the vulva have been reported with dapsone (Sinha 1982) and trimethoprim (Hughes *et al.* 1987). Seminal fluid as a cause of a fixed drug eruption, involving other areas in addition to the vulva and vagina, was described by Best *et al.* (1988). Co-trimoxazole excreted in vaginal fluid has been reported to cause a FDE on the penis (Gruber *et al.* 1997).

Vulval involvement usually presents as acute swelling that may go on to blister and erode; there may also be more typical extragenital lesions at the same time (Fig. 5.32a,b). The characteristic lesion is an erythematous patch, which may become oedematous and sometimes bullous hours after the drug is ingested. This then subsides to leave pigmentation, which can persist for a very long time. There may be a single lesion or multiple lesions. The clinical differential diagnosis is from herpes simplex and from other causes of an acute blister or plaque, and in the quiescent stage from melanocytic lesions and pigmented intraepithelial neoplasia.

Histological examination shows epidermal necrosis with dermal inflammation. The late changes are those of melanin deposition in the epidermis and in dermal melanophages.

The history is all important in making this diagnosis, and it is essential to specifically enquire about over-the-counter medication. A challenge test can be diagnostic and discontinuation of the offending drug is curative.

Stevens–Johnson syndrome

This is the severe form of erythema multiforme with mucosal involvement being the cardinal feature. Cutaneous lesions are not always present. The condition can occur spontaneously but attacks can be precipitated by herpes simplex infection or drugs, most commonly sulphonamides, tetracyclines and penicillins.

The onset is acute and often accompanied by systemic symptoms. In the genital area, painful, shallow ulcers and flaccid bullae on all aspects of the labia and the surrounding skin are seen (Fig. 5.33). Vaginal stenosis (Graham-Brown *et al.* 1981) and vulvovaginal adenosis (Emberger *et al.* 2006) have been described as sequelae (see below).

The histology shows a perivascular infiltrate and extravasation of red cells, oedema and varying degrees of epidermal necrosis, particularly of the basal layer. Subepidermal bullae may form.

The diagnosis is usually easily made but it can be difficult to differentiate from the early phases of toxic epidermal necrolysis. If the typical cutaneous lesions of erythema multiforme are present, this will be helpful.

In those cases where the syndrome is precipitated by recurrent herpesvirus attacks, long-term aciclovir is beneficial as a preventive measure. Good nursing is essential, and in severe cases the patient should be under the care of a burns unit. Treatment is mainly supportive as for toxic epidermal necrolysis as the role of steroids and other disease-modifying

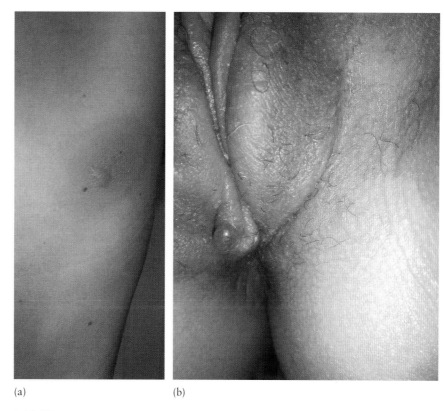

Fig. 5.32 (a) Typical lesion of fixed drug eruption on the arm and (b) associated vulval oedema and blister.

(a)   (b)

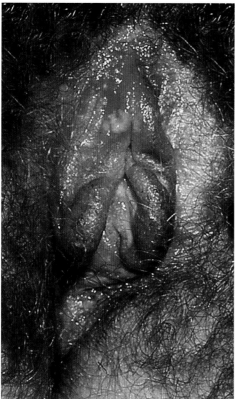

Fig. 5.33 Stevens–Johnson syndrome: multiple vulval ulcers and erosions.

treatments is not established. Bonafe *et al.* (1990) found treatment with the laser helpful in dealing with adhesions; surgical procedures may also be employed (Chapter 10).

Toxic epidermal necrolysis

This is a severe illness which still carries a significant mortality. Idiopathic cases may occur, but there is often a drug that is responsible, commonly a phenazone or a sulphonamide.

The onset is acute with systemic illness and exquisitely painful lesions rapidly causing denudation of the epidermis. The vulval area is often involved, which can lead to vulvo-vaginal scarring (Meneux *et al.* 1997). The soreness and erythema may start in the vulval area.

Histology shows necrosis of the whole epidermis with a subepidermal bulla and basal cell destruction.

Expert nursing is essential and admission to a burns unit is often indicated. Any suspected drug must be withdrawn. Treatment is mainly supportive. The role of steroids and immunoglobulin is still controversial.

Ulcerative lesions

Nicorandil, a vasodilator used in the treatment of angina, is well known to cause oral and perianal ulceration. Vulval involvement has also been reported (Claeys *et al.* 2006).

Genital ulceration with foscarnet has been described in HIV-positive women (Lacey *et al.* 1992, Caumes *et al.*

1993); the ulcers healed when the drug was withdrawn, and did not recur when it was restarted and the area washed after micturition, as recommended by the manufacturer. It is likely that the effect is an irritant one, related to high levels in the urine.

Miscellaneous

Retinoids can cause vulvitis and vaginitis as part of their intensely drying effect on mucous membranes (Thomson 1986). One study has also shown a higher rate of vulvo-vaginal candidiasis in patients taking the oral retinoid acitretin, and it was felt that this was an effect of the drug (Sturkenboom *et al.* 1995).

A vaginitis possibly related to oral lithium was reported by Srebrnik *et al.* (1991).

Occasionally, drugs are implicated in precipitating bullous disease and cases of anogenital cicatricial pemphigoid have been reported secondary to clonidine (van Joost *et al.* 1980) and penicillamine (Shuttleworth *et al.* 1985).

Clitoral priapism lasting up to 3 days has been described after trazodone (Pescatori *et al.* 1993), citalopram (Berk & Acton 1997), nefazodone (Brodie-Meijer *et al.* 1999) and olanzipine (Bucur & Mahmood 2004). Treatment includes discontinuation of the causative drug and administration of adrenergic agonists.

The serotonin reuptake inhibitors fluoxetine (Michael & Mayer 2000) and paroxetine (Michael & Andrews 2002) have been associated with vaginal anaesthesia.

Adverse effects of topical treatments

Topical steroids

These drugs are extremely useful in the management of vulval dermatoses and, if used correctly, are very safe. However, if a potent steroid is applied incorrectly to the keratinized skin in an occluded area for prolonged periods, atrophy, telangiectasia and eventually striae can develop (Fig. 5.34). Some of the change may be reversible if the treatment responsible is stopped.

A papular, erythematous eruption is sometimes seen on the thighs, buttocks and inguinal folds. This has many features in common with peri-oral dermatitis – a rosacea-like condition seen primarily on the peri-oral skin of young females who have been applying topical steroids. The treatment is to withdraw the topical steroid and oral tetracyclines may be needed concomitantly.

If a fungal infection is mistaken for an eczematous process and a topical steroid applied, the scaling is lost and is replaced by papules and nodules without the usual features of tinea cruris (Fig. 5.35). This picture is then termed tinea incognito and may require systemic antifungals for treatment.

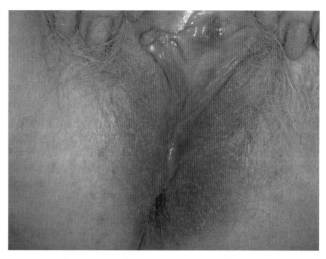

Fig. 5.34 Telangiectasia after excessive overuse of potent topical steroid to treat lichen sclerosus.

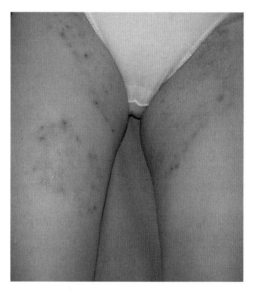

Fig. 5.35 Tinea incognito.

Irritant dermatitis

Many topical agents used to treat skin at other sites are too irritant to use in the vulval area. An irritant dermatitis can follow which may be severe and eroded. This particularly applies to preparations used to treat psoriasis such as tar and vitamin D analogues (Fig. 5.36).

Allergic contact dermatitis

Allergic contact dermatitis is discussed later.

Miscellaneous topical drug effects on the vulva

Dextropropoxyphene suppositories have led to ulceration of the anus, rectum and vagina (Laplanche *et al.* 1984,

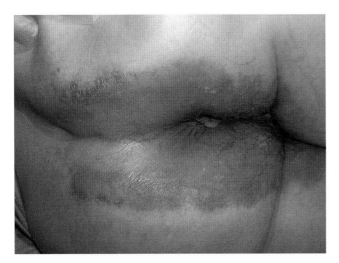

Fig. 5.36 Severe irritant dermatitis after applying calcipotriol to flexural area.

Fenzy & Bogomoletz 1986). Anorectal ulceration has been described with the abuse of ergotamine tartrate suppositories in four patients (Eigler *et al.* 1986).

Donlan and Scutero (1975) attributed a rash accompanied by an eosinophilic pneumonia to a vaginal cream containing a sulphonamide, allantoin and aminacrine.

When an aperient containing anthraquinone was in use (Dorbanex) the urine, skin and vaginal secretions became brownish in colour (Barth *et al.* 1984).

Bullous (blistering) diseases

Blistering may be a feature of epidermolysis bullosa, benign familial chronic pemphigus (Hailey–Hailey disease) and Darier's disease, all of which are discussed above. Those conditions that rarely, if ever, affect the vulva, such as porphyria, dermatitis herpetiformis, pemphigoid gestationis and pemphigus foliaceus, will not be included here.

Immunobullous disorders

These disorders affect skin and mucosae and anogenital involvement is common in several types. Marren *et al.* (1993), for example, in a large series of female patients with immunobullous disease found that such lesions occurred in over 50% of their adult patients with bullous or cicatricial pemphigoid; in the patients with linear immunoglobulin (Ig)A disease they were found in 80% of the children and almost 50% of the adults.

Aetiology and classification

The pathogenesis of the immunobullous disorders lies in the development of antibodies that react against normal epidermal and basement membrane zone tissue. The target antigens are those molecules promoting adhesion between the cells and of the cells to the underlying dermis, hence the development of a blister. Immunofluorescence (IMF) of non-lesional skin and sometimes of other sites is an all-important technique in investigation. Indirect IMF, using the patient's serum, can also be useful.

Bullous pemphigoid

Bullous pemphigoid (BP) mainly affects the elderly, but cases have been described in children (see below). It is characterized by IgG autoantibodies against the hemidesmosomal antigens BP230 and BP180 at the basement membrane.

The bullae are tense, although rupture with the formation of erosions is common, and they often arise from an erythematous base. Both keratinized and non-keratinized skin may be involved (Fig. 5.37).

Histology shows subepidermal bullae, and direct IMF shows IgG at the basement membrane zone (Fig. 5.38). The antigen is located in the basal epidermal cells. Indirect IMF shows a circulating IgG antibody.

Epidermolysis bullosa acquisita

Epidermolysis bullosa acquisita (EBA) is a rare condition in which clinical and histological findings, including those

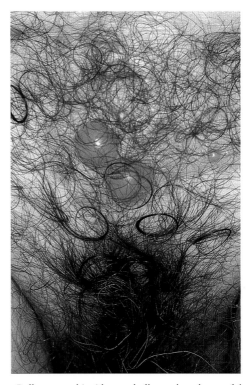

Fig. 5.37 Bullous pemphigoid: tense bullae and erythema of the pubic area.

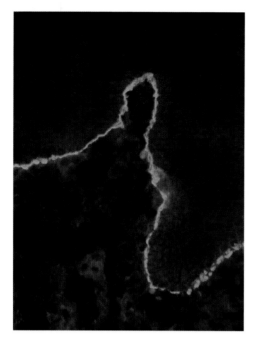

Fig. 5.38 Direct immunofluorescence in bullous pemphigoid: linear band of immunoglobulin G seen at the basement membrane (courtesy of B. Bhogal).

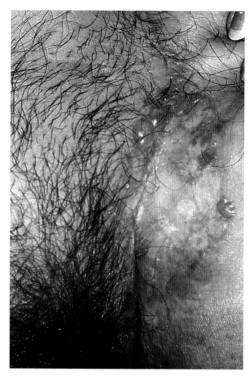

Fig. 5.39 Cicatricial pemphigoid: tense bullae with scarring in the genitocrural area.

of IMF, are similar to those of BP. With salt-split skin preparations, however, the antibody binds to the floor of the blister, i.e. to dermal components. Most patients have IgG autoantibodies targeting the non-collagenous domain of type VII collagen in the anchoring fibrils but a small group demonstrate antibodies to the collagenous domain or have IgA antibodies. Park *et al.* (1997) reported an example in a 6 year old girl with genital involvement. In Marren's study of 140 patients with blistering disorders, one of the two adults and one of the three children with EBA had vulval lesions (Marren *et al.* 1993).

Cicatricial pemphigoid

In cicatricial pemphigoid (CP) the histological findings are identical to those of BP, as are those of IMF when they are positive. The diagnosis is primarily a clinical one, although Setterfield *et al.* (1996a) have demonstrated that the DQB1*0301 allele is found in a significant majority of patients with CP. However, evolution from BP to CP has been described (Banfield *et al.* 1997). It can affect adults and children. Cases that may have been drug induced have also been reported (see above).

The findings at the vulva range from a scarcely discernible obliteration of sulci to a gross distortion of the labia and introitus. Scarring is a prominent feature (Fig. 5.39) and can mimic that of lichen sclerosus. The vagina is often involved, as are also the eyes, mouth and larynx (Fig. 5.40).

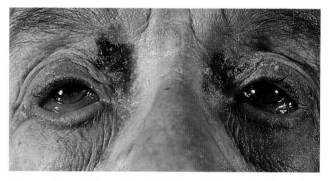

Fig. 5.40 Cicatricial pemphigoid: bullae on the face and obliteration of the conjunctival sulci.

Linear IgA disease of children (chronic bullous disease of childhood) and of adults

These conditions present with tense bullae. In children, in whom the vulval and perianal areas are sites of predilection, the blisters are often described as having a clustered appearance (Fig. 5.41). The condition sometimes, but not always, remits at puberty. At all ages scarring may ensue.

The histology is of a subepidermal bulla, and on IMF there is a linear band of IgA at the basement membrane zone. In children particularly, circulating IgA antibody may be found.

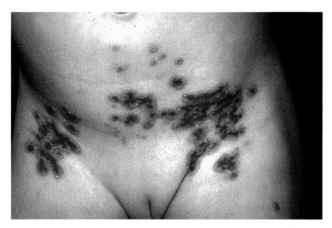

Fig. 5.41 Linear immunoglobulin A disease in a child: clustered bullae of the lower abdomen and groin.

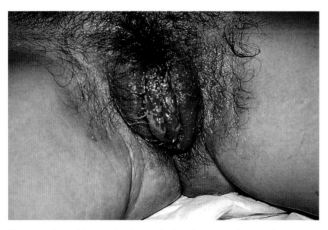

Fig. 5.42 Pemphigus vulgaris: marked oedema, erosions and ulceration.

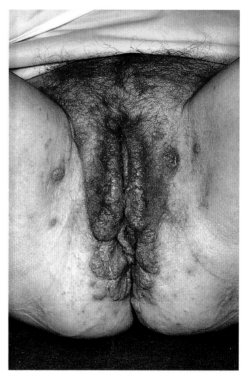

Fig. 5.43 Pemphigus vulgaris, vegetans type: confluent bullous masses.

Pemphigus vulgaris

Pemphigus vulgaris is a rare disease of skin and mucosae often affecting the vulva, with IgG autoantibodies directed against the cell surface of keratinocytes. In general, the condition begins in middle life, but has been described in children. Familial cases may occur. An atypical form of the disease with vulval involvement was associated with angiofollicular lymph node hyperplasia (Castleman's syndrome) in a case reported by Coulson *et al.* (1986). A patient with vulval intraepithelial neoplasia (VIN) treated with imiquimod developed pemphigus on the vulva after treatment (Campagne *et al.* 2003).

The bullae are painful, flaccid and easily eroded (Fig. 5.42). In pemphigus vegetans, a more benign and chronic variant, heaped up masses are a feature (Fig. 5.43). The vagina, and also the cervix (Lonsdale & Gibbs 1998), may be affected. There is one case in which pemphigus vulgaris was confined to the vagina with the presenting feature

being a chronic vaginal discharge (Batta *et al.* 1999). In a follow-up study of 34 patients with pemphigus involving the vulva or vagina, no sequelae were seen long term (Malik & Ahmed 2005).

Histology shows suprabasal acantholysis, and hence intraepidermal bullae. In pemphigus vegetans, downward proliferation of epithelial strands is associated with papillomatosis, acanthosis, hyperkeratosis and eosinophilic infiltration of the dermis. Direct IMF shows deposition of the IgG antibody in the intercellular spaces (Fig. 5.44) and indirect IMF demonstrates circulating IgG antibodies.

Differential diagnosis of the immunobullous disorders

Apart from the exclusion of herpes simplex virus infections, in which the lesions are usually acute, the main difficulty is in distinguishing these conditions from each other, and from lichen planus and lichen sclerosus. The distinction from lichen planus and lichen sclerosus may present difficulties since bullae are readily eroded and may therefore not be visible as such, and the histology may not always be diagnostic. The distinction can be particularly difficult with CP, in which IMF findings may be negative. Repeat biopsies, IMF testing and careful observation over a period of time will often be required. The appearance of more easily recognized lesions at other sites can often give support to a provisional diagnosis.

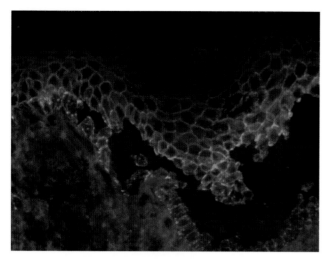

Fig. 5.44 Direct immunofluorescence in pemphigus: immunoglobulin G seen on the surface of keratinocytes (courtesy of B. Bhogal).

Management of immunobullous disorders

The general principles of using bland emollients, soaks of potassium permanganate for open areas, appropriate agents for secondary infection and potent topical corticosteroids for eroded and blistered areas will apply. However, many patients will require systemic therapy and should always be under the supervision of a dermatologist, in cooperation as necessary with the gynaecologist and the ophthalmologist. Corticosteroids are generally used initially but other immunosuppressive agents may be needed including dapsone, azathioprine, mycophenolate and ciclosporin.

Inflammatory dermatoses

Intertrigo

This non-specific inflammation of the flexures, brought about by heat, sweating, obesity and friction, is common in the groins, genitocrural folds and natal cleft. It is further aggravated by diabetes, incontinence and immobility. The ill-defined erythema is often malodorous and secondarily infected with mixed bacteria and *Candida*. In the case of *Candida*, small, outlying, scaly satellite lesions are often present and the main lesions tend to have a macerated edge. This infection is not necessarily associated with a *Candida* vulvovaginitis. The histology shows non-specific changes. It must be distinguished from flexural psoriasis, in which the border is sharper, from seborrhoeic dermatitis and from erythrasma, which is brownish with well-defined edges and shows a coral-pink fluorescence under Wood's light.

The management is to treat predisposing factors and topical barriers such as zinc oxide or Metanium ointments

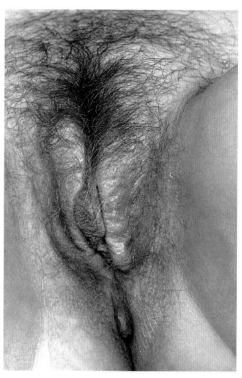

Fig. 5.45 Psoriasis: well-defined erythema of the labia majora and perianal area.

are useful. Mild topical corticosteroids combined with antibacterial or antifungal agents, for example miconazole/hydrocortisone, can be extremely helpful.

Psoriasis

The pattern of psoriasis most commonly affecting the vulva is flexural psoriasis. Psoriasis is genetically determined, but various trigger factors will provoke it in susceptible individuals. Friction and occlusion may initiate or perpetuate flexural lesions. The differential diagnosis includes intertrigo, seborrhoeic dermatitis and eczema. In all these conditions, the margins are less well defined. The presence of more typical disease elsewhere is often helpful.

The silvery scaling of psoriasis seen elsewhere is lost in flexural areas, but the erythema and sharp outline tend to remain (Fig. 5.45). Fissuring in the natal cleft is common. The mons pubis and labia majora are frequently involved and, here, the appearance is scalier (Fig. 5.46). Psoriasis is not a scarring dermatosis, but some patients with psoriasis appear to have loss of the labia minora (Albert *et al.* 2004). However, it is impossible to be certain in these cases that there was not previous lichen sclerosus or lichen planus. In the clinics, many of the patients with lichen sclerosus either have psoriasis themselves or have a first-degree relative with this condition (Simpkin & Oakley 2007, Eberz *et al.* 2008).

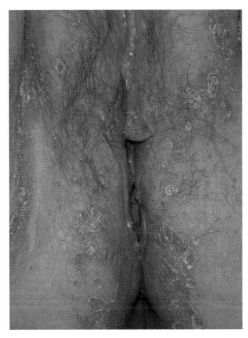

Fig. 5.46 Psoriasis: beefy red, well-defined erythema on the inner aspects with more characteristic scaly lesions on outer aspects.

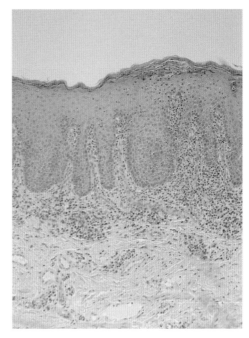

Fig. 5.47 Psoriasis histology: hyperkeratosis and parakeratosis overlying an acanthotic epidermis and loss of the granular layer. Polymorphs are seen within the epidermis.

Psoriasis does not generally affect mucosal surfaces, except in the rare pustular form and in the lesions of Reiter's disease. However, some patients who have definite psoriasis elsewhere, and perhaps perianal lesions, complain of itching of the inner aspects of the vulva. In a series of 93 women with psoriasis, 44% complained of vulval symptoms but lesions were only seen in 23.7% (Zamirska *et al.* 2008). Sometimes all there is to see is a mild erythema in the interlabial sulci and a build-up of keratinous debris. It is interesting that there is an association between psoriasis and complications of pregnancy, such as recurrent abortions, hypertension and caesarean deliveries (Ben-David *et al.* 2008). The authors postulate that this may be due to the autoimmune factors involved in psoriasis.

The typical histology should show parakeratosis, acanthosis with elongation of the rete ridges and a reduced or absent granular layer, often with collections of neutrophils in the epidermis (Fig. 5.47). There may also be papillary oedema and perivascular dermal inflammation. Unfortunately, flexural psoriasis does not always exhibit these characteristic histological features.

Seborrhoeic dermatitis

This common condition has eczematous and psoriasiform features and is probably caused by the yeast *Pityrosporum ovale*. Lesions occur most commonly on the scalp, nasolabial folds and forehead, ears and chest. The genitocrural area and natal cleft may also be involved with ill-defined,

orange–pink and slightly scaly lesions (Fig. 5.48). Secondary infection sometimes occurs.

The histology is non-specific or psoriasiform. The rash is often difficult or impossible to distinguish from psoriasis; lesions vary, resembling first one and then the other, and treatment and management are as for psoriasis.

Management of psoriasis and seborrhoeic dermatitis

Bland emollients, for example emulsifying ointment or aqueous cream, together with a moderately potent topical corticosteroid are usually effective. Occasionally, a more potent preparation may be needed initially, particularly for lesions on the inner aspects of the vulva. Milder preparations are used for maintenance. Tar, dithranol and calcipotriol, although good for psoriasis in other areas, are irritant in the genital area and should be avoided. Tacrolimus or pimecrolimus, calcineurin inhibitors, may be effective treatment but are poorly tolerated on the vulval skin. In severe psoriasis, systemic agents may be needed, but they are not as effective when treating flexural disease.

Reiter's disease

The condition is defined as a non-suppurative polyarthritis of more than 1 month's duration following an enteric or more commonly a lower genital tract infection. Urethritis and/or cervicitis are common, as is conjunctivitis. Subjects with the HLA-B27 are particularly susceptible. Patients

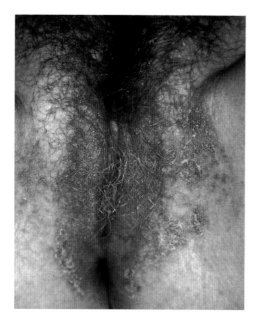

Fig. 5.48 Impetiginized seborrhoeic eczema (courtesy of Shireen Velangi).

often have a psoriasiform rash on the feet and hands, which presents as a pattern that is clinically indistinct from psoriasis. In men, a circinate balanitis is common. The equivalent vulvitis is very rare (Haake & Altmeyer 1988). One patient had striking lesions originally thought to be of mucocutaneous candidosis (Edwards & Hansen 1992). Scaling and crusting involved the keratinized skin of the genital area, she had a vaginal discharge and white papules on the cervix and, later, white papules that became eroded and affected the whole of the vulva including the mucosal aspects.

The histology is that of pustular psoriasis, with hyperkeratosis, parakeratosis, an absent granular layer and prominent polymorph microabscesses in the epidermis.

The differential diagnosis is usually from candidosis, and from psoriasis with which it may constitute a spectrum. However, two rare conditions may sometimes have to be considered: IgA pemphigus and subcorneal pustulosis (see below).

If a chlamydial infection is suspected as the initiating feature, the sexual partner should be screened and a course of a tetracycline given. Mild lesions can be controlled with topical corticosteroids. Long-term treatment may be complex, requiring systemic agents such as methotrexate and retinoids. Supervision by a dermatologist and a rheumatologist will be necessary. Psoriasis and Reiter's disease are both significantly more severe and difficult to control in individuals who are HIV positive.

IgA pemphigus (intraepidermal IgA pustulosis)

This condition is characterized by widespread pustules and may affect the genital area. It appears to be essentially a neutrophilic disorder. Histologically, there is acantholysis and an intraepidermal or subcorneal pustule, with intercellular IgA deposition on IMF. IgA paraproteinaemia may also be found.

Subcorneal pustulosis (Sneddon–Wilkinson disease)

This condition of unknown aetiology is characterized by waves of superficial pustules in a circinate pattern. It may affect the vulva. Its aetiology is unknown. Histologically, the pustules are subcorneal and filled with neutrophils. IMF is negative.

The clinical differential diagnosis of both these conditions includes pemphigus, pustular psoriasis and Reiter's disease. Histology and IMF findings are helpful. The pustules in subcorneal pustulosis are more superficial and acantholysis is seen in IgA pemphigus. Both conditions respond well to dapsone.

Eczema

Eczema is characterized by epidermal spongiosis, with or without acanthosis, and a dermal perivascular lymphohistiocytic infiltrate. It appears in a wide variety of clinical patterns, at the genital area as elsewhere. Eczema and dermatitis are synonymous terms, except when the word 'dermatitis' has been incorporated in the name of some particular disease, e.g. acrodermatitis enteropathica or dermatitis herpetiformis. The skin may become thickened from scratching and there may be erosions, excoriations and fissuring (Fig. 5.49).

Atopic eczema

Patients rarely complain of vulval involvement even when there is severe and widespread eczema elsewhere. However, in patients complaining of itching, with an atopic background and perhaps a few signs elsewhere, minimal erythema, which is often found between the labia, perianally and in the natal cleft is probably a manifestation of eczema. It responds to appropriate treatment.

Irritant and allergic eczematous reactions

These can be difficult to distinguish, and indeed may coexist. The clinical features are diffuse erythema, often with flexural maceration secondarily infected with bacteria and *Candida*. In a severe allergic contact dermatitis, oedema and even blistering may occur. Subsequent lichenification will render the area thick and pale.

The differential diagnosis will include a *Candida* vulvovaginitis, in which there is usually a vaginal discharge, and psoriasis or seborrhoeic dermatitis, in which the distinction may be more difficult, much depending on the history, the presence of lesions elsewhere and the unfolding of events.

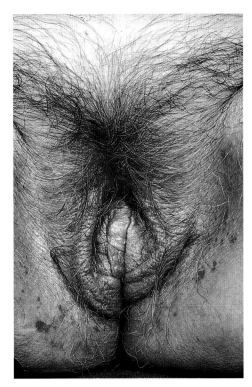

Fig. 5.49 Severe lichenified eczema with excoriations, labial oedema and maceration.

Histology of both types of reactions shows spongiosis, sometimes acanthosis and parakeratosis, and some dermal inflammatory infiltrate.

Irritant reactions

Irritant reactions are those in which there is a direct effect on the tissues, without any allergic mechanism. Elsner *et al.* (1990) have noted the particular susceptibility of the vulval skin in this respect. A wide variety of topical treatments can be responsible, e.g. tar, podophyllin. Dequalinium has caused genital necrosis in both sexes (Tilsley & Wilkinson 1965). Cosmetic preparations such as deodorant sprays and wet wipes can also be irritant. Bubble baths are potentially irritant if the concentration is high. Rycroft and Penney (1983) incriminated bromination of swimming pools.

Some women describe symptoms of vulval irritation during the menstrual period. However, studies have shown that the labia majora are less sensitive to irritation induced by the menses itself than other skin sites (Farage *et al.* 2000). Mechanical friction from sanitary protection is another factor and sanitary pads are now designed to reduce mechanical irritation (Farage *et al.* 2004).

Allergic reactions (allergic contact dermatitis)

In a true allergic reaction, there is a specific immunological reaction involving the skin immune system to specific aller-gens. Figures for the incidence of contact dermatitis in the anogenital area are somewhat variable. Marren *et al.* (1992) found clinically relevant allergies in 39 out of 135 patients (35%) who had been referred for patch testing because response to treatment was slow or the diagnosis uncertain. The patients had a variety of underlying conditions, the largest groups being lichen sclerosus, eczema and those in whom the diagnosis was uncertain. Lewis *et al.* (1994a) reported results in 69 patients referred for testing, in which 40 (58%) had positive results considered relevant. Goldsmith *et al.* (1997), however, carried out a retrospective survey on 201 patients who had been referred for testing over a period of 14 years. Of these, 103 had involvement of the vulva, 42 of the perianal area and 56 involvement of both sites. Those with vulval lesions alone had positive relevant findings in 19%, those with perianal disease alone in 33%, but those in whom both areas were involved there were positive relevant findings in 43%. A recent prospective study of 43 patients with vulval pruritus showed 44% to have relevant patch test reactions (Haverhoek *et al.* 2008). In all studies, the relevant positive reactions were mainly to medicaments, local anaesthetics, corticosteroids and scented products. It seems, therefore, that patients with vulval lesions *per se* do not have frequent sensitivity reactions, but that these problems are commoner in those with perianal involvement or, particularly, with involvement of both areas. The explanation might be related to the greater extent of skin involvement, or could reflect differences in reactivity of the two sites. It is important that extended patch testing is done for patients with a suspected allergic contact dermatitis of the vulva as many of the relevant allergens are outside the standard test series, and will be missed with basic testing.

Many individual cases have been reported. Vaginal preparations (Corazza *et al.* 1992) and an intrauterine device (Romaguera & Grimalt 1981) have been responsible. Perfumes and disinfectants (Sterry & Schmoll 1985) or other additives (Williams *et al.* 2007) in sanitary pads can cause allergic dermatitis. Reactions to contraceptives are well recognized (Bircher *et al.* 1993). The antifungal agent nifuratel was responsible for another case of connubial contact dermatitis (di Prima *et al.* 1990). Lewis *et al.* (1994b) described a cello player with an unusual relevant allergy, to colophony, found in the resin used on the instrument. Seminal fluid may, rarely, produce a type IV reaction rather than the commoner immediate type I (Kint *et al.* 1994).

Management

In all cases of eczema, any known or suspected causative agent should be withdrawn. In the acute stage, bathing with potassium permanganate 1 in 10 000 is soothing. This can be carried out by sitting in a plastic bowl or small bath (the solution causes staining) or by the application of gauze or other soft material that has been soaked in the liquid. Bland emollients such as emulsifying ointment or aqueous cream are used for washing and as moisturizers. Topical corticosteroids, often requiring the addition of an antibacterial or antifungal agent (e.g. miconazole/hydrocortisone, or fusidic acid/betamethasone valerate, or a combination of clobetasol butyrate, oxytetracycline and nystatin), according to severity, are valuable. When the condition has settled, patch testing is indicated if an allergy is suspected.

Lichen simplex and lichenification

'Lichen' is a term used in describing many lesions that have an appearance of closely set papules as their main characteristic; hence, lichen simplex, lichen planus, lichen sclerosus. They have some resemblance to the mossy surface of lichen on a tree. However, the terms 'lichenoid', as in many drug rashes, and 'lichenoides', as in an entity such as pityriasis lichenoides chronica, stem from lichen planus only and imply resemblance to the distinctive features of lichen planus, rather than to those of lichen simplex and lichenification. In lichen planus and lichen sclerosus, genuine closely set papules are indeed to be found, but in lichen simplex and lichenification the appearance is that of thickening overall. The normal skin markings are magnified as a result and this gives the impression of multiple papules.

The terms lichen simplex and lichenification refer to a thickening of the skin, manifested histologically mainly as acanthosis and hyperkeratosis, which is the response to prolonged itching and subsequent rubbing. Some individuals are particularly likely to show this reaction. In lichen simplex, the change occurs on skin that was clinically normal, whereas in lichenification the change is superimposed on some underlying dermatosis, e.g. eczema or psoriasis. Once lichenification occurs, an 'itch–scratch–itch' cycle is set up which may go on for many years.

The clinical features are those of thickened, slightly scaly, pale or earthy-coloured skin with accentuated markings and a diffuse outline. There may be erosions and fissuring. Excoriations as a result of scratching may be seen and the lichenification may be more marked on the side opposite the dominant hand (Fig. 5.50).

The histology shows hyperkeratosis, parakeratosis, acanthosis, a prominent granular layer, lengthened rete ridges and a variable chronic inflammatory infiltrate (Fig. 5.51). There is lamellar thickening of the papillary dermis and sometimes perineural fibrosis. All the epidermal components are hyperplastic, and the labelling index is increased. There may be some evidence of an underlying dermatological condition. The phenomenon called multinucleated atypia of the vulva by McLachlin *et al.* (1994), who reported 12 cases, has been ascribed to a non-specific change found not uncommonly in lichenified skin (le Boit 1996).

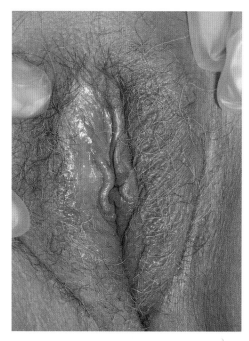

Fig. 5.50 Lichen simplex showing thickening and increased pigmentation involving the left labium majus.

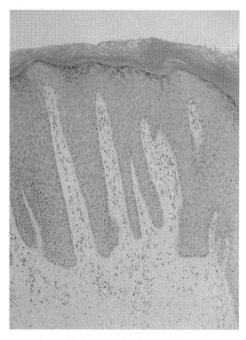

Fig. 5.51 Histology of lichen simplex showing hyperkeratosis, acanthosis and elongation of the rete ridges.

The treatment is essentially that of eczema, but the potent topical corticosteroids, for example betamethasone valerate 0.1% or even clobetasol propionate 0.05%, are often needed initially to break the cycle of itching and rubbing. A mildly anxiolytic antihistamine such as hydroxyzine at night is helpful. The symptoms of pruritus often respond fairly quickly to a topical steroid but, unless the lichenification resolves, the itch–scratch cycle will remain and the symptoms will recur. A graduated reduction in the frequency of application of the topical steroid is helpful.

Lichen sclerosus

History of terminology

A number of terms have been used in the past to describe vulval disease that was characterized by pallor, atrophy and appeared to be associated with malignant change. In all probability, the majority of these were examples of lichen sclerosus and some lichen planus. Lichen sclerosus is a condition defined clinically by Hallopeau (1887, 1889) and histologically by Darier (1892). The disease was initially considered to be a variant of lichen planus (lichen plan sclereux).

The first description of atrophic change on the vulva was referred to as 'ichthyosis'. Schwimmer (1878) introduced the term 'leukoplakia', which was used to imply potentially malignant change in white patches of mucosal or muco-cutaneous tissues. Later, Breisky (1885) described vulval 'kraurosis', which was translated by Shelley and Crissey (1953) as

> ... the labia are apparently missing, in that they are plastered to the mucous surface of the labia majora, so that the edges alone remain indicated by narrow furrows. From the mons veneris to the urethral orifice the integument is drawn tight over the clitoris ... The general effect of this extensive shrivelling is a striking smallness and inflexibility of the vestibular portion of the vulva ... which may indeed ... offer abnormal resistance ... in coitus ... The skin ... appears whitish and dry ... while the adjacent skin parts involved are shiny and dry, pale reddish grey, covered also with faded whitish spots, and show ectatic vascular branching here and there.

Perrin (1901) pointed out the essential identity of kraurosis and 'leukoplasia vulvo-orale' (leukoplakia) but Berkeley and Bonney (1909) and Bonney (1938) argued that the two conditions were distinct and should be subdivided into 'kraurosis', characterized by benign inflammatory changes of the vestibule and introitus, and 'leukoplakic vulvitis', characterized by white areas which had a malignant potential. The account by Berkeley and Bonney of leukoplakic vulvitis described vulval and perianal lesions and some on the thighs, appearing red, later white, cracked, smooth and atrophic; histologically, there was at first a thickened epidermis, with a dermal infiltrate, a subepidermal homogeneous zone and a loss of elastic tissue, culminating in a thin epidermis and dermal sclerosis with no inflammatory cells. The term leukoplakia was used here to refer to changes in keratinized skin. Kraurosis, on the other hand, was described as being confined to the introitus, vestibule, urethral orifice and sometimes the clitoris. The tissue was red, shiny, later 'pale yellow and glistening'. There was vaginal stenosis, with disappearance of the labia minora and clitoris. Histologically, there was striking atrophy, much inflammation and no subepidermal homogeneous zone. Interestingly Jayle (1906) reported that atrophy of the vulval tissue could occur without leukoplakia. It was likely that these were cases of lichen planus.

The incidence of malignancy in kraurosis or leukoplakic vulvitis recorded in the papers of Berkeley and Bonney (in all, 19 cases in 10 years) was not stated but, in every case of carcinoma encountered by the authors (58 in 10 years), leukoplakic vulvitis was present. It was correlated with 'maximum hypertrophy of the interpapillar epithelial processes'. Ormsby and Mitchell (1922) clearly recognized that vulval kraurosis was indistinguishable from lichen sclerosus in a patient with vulval and extragenital lesions; yet this was not recognized by others for a considerable time. In the USA, Taussig (1929) also contributed to the debate; he described a leukoplakic vulvitis, which began as a hypertrophic condition but ended as an atrophic one, with an inflammatory infiltrate and a subepidermal 'collagenous' zone. He used the term kraurosis for the end stage of this leukoplakic vulvitis. X-ray therapy was one of the favoured treatments of leukoplakic vulvitis in the early days, which may have been a factor in the incidence of malignancy. Otherwise, it was treated with wide excision because of the risk of recurrence. Surgical removal of kraurosis was also advocated.

Wallace (1971) summarized a series of accounts by himself and Whimster, trying to simplify the terminology surrounding kraurosis, leukoplakic vulvitis and leukoplakia, with regard to their relationship to lichen sclerosus. They proposed that cases indisputably showing typical lichen sclerosus, clinically and histologically, should be noted as such, that the terms kraurosis and leukoplakic vulvitis should be dropped, and that when the appearance originally described by Breisky as kraurosis was seen without clear evidence of lichen sclerosus it should be termed 'primary atrophy'. Primary atrophy therefore consisted of cases with no clinical evidence of extragenital lichen sclerosus, no perianal lichen sclerosus and no recognizable vulval lichen sclerosus papules, but there was still some potential for malignant change. The histological changes accompanying primary atrophy as described by Wallace and Whimster were an atrophic epidermis, reduced elastic tissue, hyalinized collagen and some inflammatory cells – changes that would all be compatible with lichen sclerosus – but, for some reason, they decided to categorize it separately. Furthermore, they wished to retain the term leukoplakia as a histological entity, characterized by marked dermal hyalinization, sometimes a dermal infiltrate, and a hyperkeratotic epidermis with lengthened, irregular and forked rete pegs with or without cellular atypia. It was distinguishable from lichenification by its lesser degree of acanthosis, spongiosis and parakeratosis, as well by the irregularity of the epidermal downgrowths and the marked hyalinization. They noted the presence of leukoplakia adjacent to 20 squamous carcinomas, and regarded it as premalignant. In retrospect, it seems as if they were describing something very similar to the 'maximum hypertrophy of the interpapillar epithelial processes' of Berkeley and Bonney. They differed from Taussig in viewing this change as a sequel to rather than as a precursor of atrophy, and, although the leukoplakia was usually found arising on lichen sclerosus or on primary atrophy, they believed that occasionally it developed on a vulva that was apparently otherwise normal or that showed just lichenification.

It was at this stage that Jeffcoate and Woodcock (1961) tried to simplify the situation; beginning with an analysis of all putative causes of vulval malignancy (and noting with perspicacity the possibility of a 'field change') they then went on to consider leukoplakia and leukoplakic vulvitis. They commented that the clinician expected the pathologist to give the diagnosis of leukoplakia, whereas the pathologist felt that it was a clinical diagnosis and would have no part in it. The authors analysed too the confusion noted above between the writings of Berkeley and Bonney and those of Taussig, and then turned to lichen sclerosus. Here, they saw that between lichen sclerosus and clinical leukoplakia and kraurosis there was no essential difference. Their conclusion was that the same end point might come from different aetiological factors, and that 'the vulval and perianal regions are subject to chronic skin changes, the particular characteristics of which are probably conditioned by environment rather than causes' and '. . . irrespective of their appearances, all these intractable skin changes, for which a specific cause is not clear, are best given clinically an all-embracing and non-committal title such as "chronic epithelial dystrophy"'.

From this concept stemmed the 1976 ISSVD classification of non-malignant epithelial disorders as lichen sclerosus, hypertrophic and mixed dystrophy (Friedrich 1976). Abolition of the terms lichen sclerosus et atrophicus, leukoplakia, neurodermatitis, leukokeratosis, Bowen's disease, erythroplasia of Queyrat, carcinoma simplex, leukoplakic vulvitis, hypoplastic vulvitis and kraurosis vulvae was recommended. The decision to refer to lichen sclerosus rather than to lichen sclerosus et atrophicus was not controversial. This was the case too as regards the other deletions, with the exception of Bowen's disease, which was to be retained only as Bowenoid papulosis, for a specific clinical picture.

Correlation with the current position

It is now accepted that kraurosis, leukoplakic vulvitis and primary atrophy are essentially cases of lichen sclerosus or lichen planus. Leukoplakia was one of the terms recommended for abolition in 1976, which undoubtedly was a sensible decision as many gynaecologists were inclined to carry out unnecessary surgery because of the premalignant associations with the term. Nevertheless, the histological appearance described by Wallace and Whimster as leukoplakia is recognized today as lichen sclerosus with epithelial hyperplasia and the malignant potential is unknown, but if it is accompanied by differentiated vulval intraepithelia neoplasia (atypia confined to the lower epidermis) it is probably the precursor of malignancy. This aspect is discussed below (see Lichen sclerosus and malignancy).

Aetiology

Familial incidence is well recognized and it may affect both sexes, for example father and daughter, and has been noted in identical and non-identical twins. The link with autoimmune disease is also established with about 21% of patients having an autoimmune disease, 22% a family history and 44% one or more circulating autoantibodies. Those with other autoimmune disease do not differ significantly in clinical respects from those without (Meyrick Thomas et al. 1988). Until recently, the HLA findings, which one would expect to be distinctive in some way, were inconclusive. Marren et al. (1995) and Powell et al. (2000), in their studies of class II antigens, of which DR and DQ are known to be linked with other autoimmune conditions, found a significant association of patients compared with controls with DQ7, and with DR7, DQ8 or DQ9, singly or together. There was also a suggestion that A2 might exert a protective role in that it tended to be absent in patients who had extensive extragenital lesions, and that linkage of DR4 with DQ8 was commoner in those without marked structural change of the anogenital area. An immunohistochemical study of the alterations in the epidermis, dermis and infiltrate supported an autoimmune aetiology (Farrell et al. 1999). Circulating IgG autoantibodies to the glycoprotein extracellular matrix protein 1 (ECM1) have been demonstrated in the sera of about 75% of female patients with lichen sclerosus (Chan et al. 2004).

The pathogenesis remains uncertain. Lavery (1984), noting that some cases were associated with achlorhydria, speculated on interactions between urogastrone (epidermal growth factor) and somatostatin. Friedrich and Kalra (1984), believing that testosterone topically was effective, found lower levels of dihydrotestosterone in patients with lichen sclerosus and suggested that the enzyme 5α-reductase might be involved.

An infective agent has been sought. Cantwell (1984) described pleomorphic, variably acid-fast bacilli in lichen sclerosus and in the closely related morphoea. Others have suggested that the spirochaete *Borrelia burgdorferi* is involved (Schempp et al. 1993), although findings have been conflicting (Abele & Anders 1990, Raguin et al. 1992).

However, a study (Farrell *et al.* 1997) using vulval tissue has shown no spirochaetal forms, and coccoid bodies that were seen appeared to be mast cells rather than bacilli.

Studies of cell kinetics (Oikarinen *et al.* 1991) showed that active regeneration and synthesis of collagen, as well as concomitant loss of connective tissue, took place. A study of epidermal differentiation using keratin markers showed that keratins 6 and 16, associated with increased cell turnover, were expressed suprabasally, and keratins 1 and 10, markers of cornifying epithelium, persisted in spite of the apparent atrophy of the epidermis. Soini *et al.* (1994) have shown, in a study of proliferating cell nuclear antigen, that vulval skin affected by lichen sclerosus has a wide range of proliferative capacity and that high levels are associated with overexpression of wild-type *p53*. Tan *et al.* (1994) also showed an altered *p53* expression and epidermal cell proliferation in vulval lichen sclerosus, compared with normal vulval skin and with extragenital lichen sclerosus. Newton *et al.* (1987), using flow cytometry, found both aneuploidy and a hyperproliferative pattern in some cases. Carli *et al.* (1991) found an increase of CD1a+ Langerhans cells at all stages of the disease, supporting the concept of an abnormality of the skin immunological system, and the study of Marren *et al.* (1997a), demonstrating a lack of correlation between duration of symptoms and histological appearances, suggests a continuing inflammatory process in which activated Langerhans cells may be involved.

Clinical features

Lichen sclerosus is found at all ages, in all parts of the body and in both sexes, but there is a predilection for the anogenital skin. There are two peak incidences in females – one in the premenarche and the second in the menopause. It may present at a very young age, e.g. at 1 year. The main symptom is severe itch and, if there are erosions or fissures, pain. Some patients experience dyspareunia and sexually active women report that they refrain from intercourse because of the problem. Constipation is a common presentation in children with perianal lichen sclerosus as the disease in the anal canal tends to fissure, causing painful defaecation. About 11% of women with anogenital lichen sclerosus have extragenital lesions, but this is seen rarely in children. The primary lesion is an ivory–white papule, flat, polygonal and often with a central plug or dell. The papules are scattered or confluent in plaques (Fig. 5.52). Bullae, purpura, marked atrophy and pallor are frequent features. The lesions occur anywhere, including nails (Ramrakha-Jones *et al.* 2001), scalp (Foulds 1980) and eyelid (Fig. 5.53). The Köbner phenomenon is often seen and the disease appears at the sites of pressure under straps or belts and in scars of various types, including burns (Meffert & Grimwood 1994) and surgical scars (Pass 1984). It has also been reported at a vaccination site (Anderton & Abele 1976), in skin previously

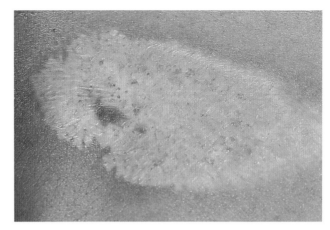

Fig. 5.52 Lichen sclerosus: large plaque on the back, showing confluent crinkly atrophy with some 'delling'.

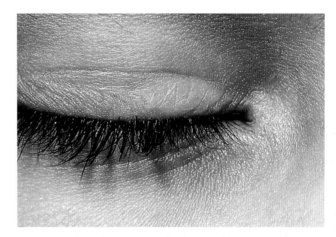

Fig. 5.53 Lichen sclerosus: smooth, white, crinkly plaque of the eyelid.

treated with radiotherapy (Yates *et al.* 1985) and on a congenital haemangioma (Ostlere *et al.* 1996). Weigand (1993), prompted by finding histological features identical to those of lichen sclerosus in some large skin tags, has suggested that occlusion and pressure may be factors in the development of lichen sclerosus. Whimster (1973) noted that lichen sclerosus developed in a split-skin graft transferred to the vulva from the thigh, whereas vulval lichen sclerosus skin reverted to normal when transferred to the thigh. Lichen sclerosus may develop or recur not only in skin grafts (Foulds 1980) but also in a myocutaneous graft (di Paola *et al.* 1982).

Children often have more ecchymosis, haemorrhagic changes and frank bleeding owing to their physical activity in play, for example riding bikes, and again this may be due to the Köbner phenomenon (Figs 5.54 and 5.55). These changes may mimic sexual abuse, which can lead to false

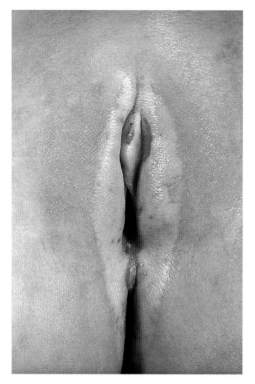

Fig. 5.54 Lichen sclerosus in a child: shiny, smooth pallor with a haemorrhagic blister.

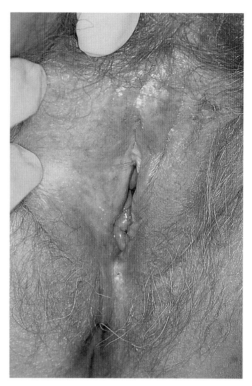

Fig. 5.56 Lichen sclerosus: pallor and atrophy, with loss of labia minora.

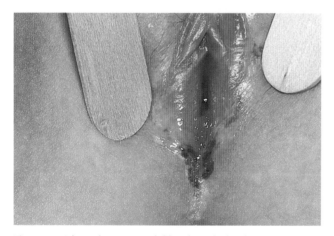

Fig. 5.55 Lichen sclerosus in a child with marked ecchymosis and no labia minora.

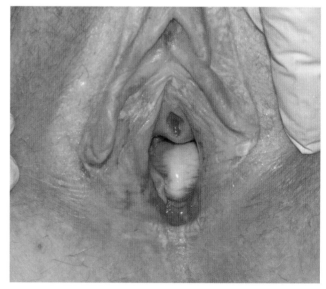

Fig. 5.57 Lichen sclerosus affecting prolapsed mucosa.

accusations for the family and a delay in the correct diagnosis and treatment. However, it is also possible that the abuse could precipitate lichen sclerosus as a Köbner phenomenon in a predisposed child (Warrington & de San Lazaro 1996).

In adults, the lesions may appear on the perineum, inner labia majora, labia minora and clitoris. There may be extension into the genitocrural folds. There is scarring with loss of the labia minora, sealing of the clitoral hood and

burying of the clitoris (Fig. 5.56). The introitus is not usually narrowed as lichen sclerosus does not appear to affect mucosal epithelia. Vaginal disease does not occur unless there is a marked prolapse (Fig. 5.57). Presumably, the prolapsed tissue in a response to trauma becomes cornified and then develops the lichen sclerosus. A few patients

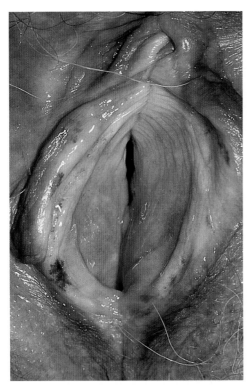

Fig. 5.58 Lichen sclerosus: waxy pallor and ecchymosis on inner aspect of labia minora.

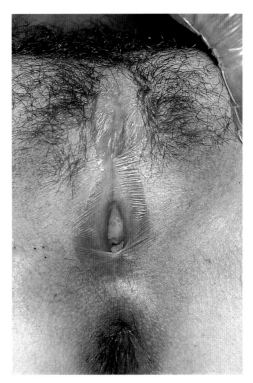

Fig. 5.60 Lichen sclerosus: loss of architecture and midline fusion.

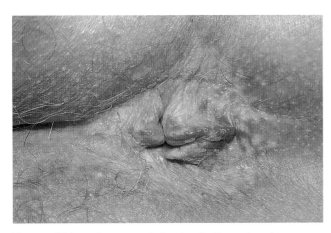

Fig. 5.59 Lichen sclerosus: typical perianal pallor and erosions.

with marked disease have little if any scarring, despite the changes of waxy pallor and ecchymosis (Fig. 5.58). There is often a figure-of-eight configuration when the vulva and perianal area are both affected and very occasionally there is extension into the natal cleft (Fig. 5.59) and buttocks. Perianal involvement occurs in about 30% of cases and is commoner in children. Anterior and posterior fusion in the midline is seen in some patients, and may proceed to leave

only a posteriorly situated narrowed opening (Fig. 5.60). However, the signs may be minimal and limited to tiny white patches and papules (Fig. 5.61), or confined to the clitoral area with pallor and minimal adhesion of the clitoral hood. Milia may also occur transiently (Leppard & Sneddon 1975).

The frequency of oral lesions is small, and Brown *et al.* (1997), in reporting two cases, discusses the problem of accurate diagnosis without histological confirmation. However, cases with confirmatory histology have been reported on the lip (Kelly *et al.* 2006) and tongue (Chaudhry *et al.* 2006).

Histology

The epidermis may be thin and flat but is sometimes hyperkeratotic with some acanthosis and elongated rete pegs. The typical feature is hyalinization of the dermis, bordered inferiorly by an aggregation, usually band-like, of chronic inflammatory cells (Fig. 5.62). The elastin fibres are reduced in the area of sclerosis and extravasated red cells are commonly seen. IMF may show fibrin deposition at the epidermal junction. Marren *et al.* (1997b) have reported distortions of the basement membrane zone, which may be a cause or an effect of the disease. An in-depth study of the histology, with a system of grading, was carried out by Hewitt (1986). There is no correlation of duration of disease and the histological changes (Marren *et al.* 1997a).

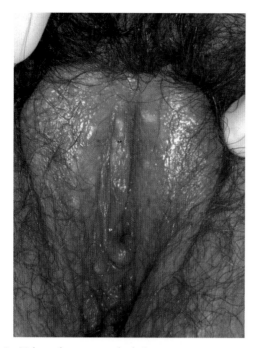

Fig. 5.61 Lichen sclerosus: papular lesions.

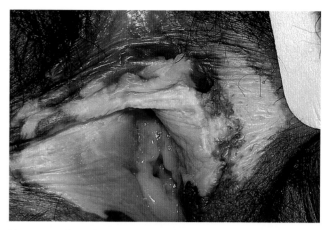

Fig. 5.63 Lichen sclerosus, associated with vitiligo.

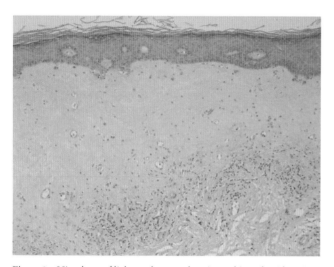

Fig. 5.62 Histology of lichen sclerosus showing a thinned epidermis, subepidermal hyalinization and inflammatory infiltrate underneath.

Differential diagnosis

Vitiligo in terms of pallor and distribution closely resembles lichen sclerosus but there will be no textural changes in the skin. However, lichen sclerosus and vitiligo can occur together and the lichen sclerosus may be overlooked as the changes may be very subtle (Fig. 5.63). Scarring bullous disorders will also enter the differential diagnosis, particularly mucous membrane pemphigoid, and both IMF and histological examinations are needed. Vaginal, ocular or oral lesions are helpful if present, and may be confirmatory evidence of this disease or lichen planus.

The main difficulty is usually to differentiate extragenital lesions of lichen sclerosus from morphoea, and genital ones from lichen planus. The three conditions appear to be closely related; there is, for example, a close resemblance to each in the various stages of graft-versus-host disease (GVHD). Connelly and Winkelmann (1985) reported cases in which they were all combined. The confusion histologically and clinically is usually seen with the superficial variant of morphoea. Classical morphoea tends to be firmer, with a violaceous halo, and resolves to leave brownish areas. Shono *et al.* (1991) showed some differences in the lectin staining patterns between the two, and Hacker (1994) found single-stranded DNA antibodies in many examples of morphoea but in none of (vulval) lichen sclerosus. Patterson and Ackerman (1984) concluded that the conditions were distinct, favouring as criteria for the diagnosis of lichen sclerosus a vacuolar change at the dermal–epidermal junction and a lichenoid lymphocytic infiltrate beneath the papillary dermis, whereas in (extragenital) morphoea the subcutis and reticular dermis show sclerosis and inflammatory infiltration.

Lichen planus may clinically be very similar to lichen sclerosus and there is a histological overlap as areas of lichenoid change are seen in lichen sclerosus. The presence of oral lesions is not evidence enough to confirm that the vulval problem is lichen planus as vulval lichen sclerosus can be associated with oral lichen planus (Marren *et al.* 1994). However, vaginal involvement is supportive of a diagnosis of erosive lichen planus. Lichen planus may be underdiagnosed since those patients with vulval signs compatible with lichen sclerosus may not undergo vaginal examination. The histology can be difficult to interpret, with minimal hyalinization or interface dermatitis to differentiate the two; IMF is helpful if it shows the cytoid bodies associated with lichen planus. Carli *et al.* (1997) have described higher expression of fibrogenic cytokines in lichen sclerosus than in lichen planus, which may prove useful as a distinguishing feature. In some cases, however, differentiation may be impossible, the clinical and histological features seeming to vary within the clinical course, and it may well be that the two conditions are part of a spectrum rather than two distinct entities.

Management and course

The treatment for both children and adults is a potent topical corticosteroid ointment in conjunction with the use of a soap substitute (Neill *et al.* 2002). Irritants such as bubble baths and highly perfumed soaps should be avoided. The regimen currently recommended is 0.5% clobetasol propionate ointment (Dermovate) once a day for the first month, alternate days treatment for the second month and twice a week for the third month. This treatment seems to work for the majority of patients, but there are no randomized controlled trials comparing different potencies of steroids or frequency of application. The patient is then reviewed and, if the response has been good, it is then recommended that the ointment is used as and when required. This treatment stops the itch rapidly, settles the inflammation and therefore reduces scarring. It is safe as the amount used is small and a 30 g tube will last the adult patient at least 3 months and the children often a year. Using a less potent steroid successfully in children has been recorded (Fischer & Rogers 1997). In many cases the appearance virtually returns to normal, but the pallor of scarring remains and the architectural loss will not be reversed. The residual permanent pallor as a result of scarring sometimes makes it difficult at future examinations to know whether the disease is active or burnt out. A lack of textural change or ecchymosis helps clinically but a biopsy is often required. Rarely, an allergy or intolerance to the topical medication may develop and an ointment rather than the cream formulation is better as less preservatives are incorporated in the former. Patch testing will demonstrate whether there is an allergy to the steroid or one of the excipients of the ointment. A potent topical steroid can reactivate human papillomavirus or herpes simplex.

The course in children is usually improvement of signs and symptoms with treatment and most seem to have little problem after the menarche. In some the symptoms disappear for a number of years but recurrences do occur in the reproductive years. In the series described by Wallace (1971) of 32 patients presenting as young adults, 19 had had symptoms as children, although in a larger series of 350 patients (Meyrick Thomas *et al.* 1996) only 11 had been similarly affected.

Lichen sclerosus seems to occur independent of whether or not the patient is taking hormone replacement therapy, and the patient may be assured that such therapy will have no effect on the disease process. There is no role for the use of oestrogen or testosterone creams in lichen sclerosus. Testosterone has been shown to be no better than petrolatum in treating lichen sclerosus (Sideri *et al.* 1994) and does not maintain the improvement brought about by clobetasol propionate (Cattaneo *et al.* 1996). Since a retinoid has been shown to reduce connective tissue degeneration in lichen sclerosus (Niinimäki *et al.* 1989), these agents are worth considering in difficult cases. Oral retinoids may have a limited role in hyperkeratotic and hypertrophic lichen sclerosus that is unresponsive to topical corticosteroids but they are not helpful in atrophic lichen sclerosus. Topical retinoids, on the other hand, are helpful in hyperkeratotic lichen sclerosus. Virgili *et al.* (1995) have used them in combination with a topical corticosteroid. Laser treatment has been employed but does not seem likely to prove beneficial (Kartamaa & Reitamo 1997). Recently, the topical calcineurin inhibitors tacrolimus (Virgili *et al.* 2007) and pimecrolimus (Nissi *et al.* 2007) have been recommended for the treatment of lichen sclerosus. The use of these agents should be limited to those rare cases of lichen sclerosus that have failed to respond to an ultrapotent topical steroid and the use of these agents should be for a short course to bring the disease under control. They should not be used as maintenance therapy when treating a condition that has a risk of malignant transformation until the long-term risk of these immunosuppressants is known. Ciclosporin (Bulbul Baskan *et al.* 2007) and UVA1 (Beattie *et al.* 2006) have also been used for recalcitrant lichen sclerosus.

Surgery is indicated only to correct problems related to scarring and in the cases of preneoplastic or neoplastic change. Removal of lichen sclerosus surgically does not reduce the risk of SCC (Meyrick Thomas *et al.* 1996).

Pregnancy and delivery are unlikely to be significantly affected by lichen sclerosus. If dyspareunia persists with resolution of the lichen sclerosus it is important to ensure that there is no mechanical problem such as narrowing of the introitus. If there was significant anterior or posterior sealing this could be corrected with surgery (see Chapter 10), but it is important to use the potent topical corticosteroid in the immediate postoperative period to avoid koebnerization and resealing. Dilators may also be needed. If there is dyspareunia in the absence of an anatomical abnormality then secondary vulvodynia may be the problem and this will respond to the addition of 5% lidocaine ointment topically. The other consideration in these cases is whether there are psychosexual factors at play and, if that is the case, then referral to a psychosexual therapist would be indicated. Patients' concepts of sexual and obstetric disabilities were reviewed by Dalziel (1995).

Follow-up visits are often dictated by the resources available. In the UK, financial and staffing constraints dictate that follow-up is restricted to those patients who have disease that is poorly controlled or in those who have already had a malignancy or preneoplastic change (Jones *et al.* 2008). These patients will need to be reviewed three or four times a year. Patients discharged to their primary care physician who need regular topical steroids should be seen at least once a year by their doctor, but this does not always happen in practice (Balasubramaniam & Lewis 2007).

An information sheet with treatment instructions as well as advice on follow-up is useful for the patient's reference.

Lichen sclerosus and malignancy

SCC is a rare but real complication of lichen sclerosus. A few cases in adolescent girls have been reported (Roman *et al.* 1991), but in the main it occurs in older age groups (Fig. 5.64). In clinical reports, the incidence of SCC in lichen sclerosus is of the order of 4–6% (Wallace 1971, Meyrick Thomas *et al.* 1996). This series, as others that have been reported, included patients who had presented with their carcinomas, not having been diagnosed with lichen sclerosus previously.

When pathological specimens of SCC are examined, however, the incidence is much higher (Leibowitch *et al.* 1990, Walkden *et al.* 1997). The variation in figures reflects the thoroughness of examination of vulvectomy specimens and the criteria used to diagnose lichen sclerosus. In recent

years, it has become gradually accepted that there are two aetiological patterns of incidence in vulval SCC. One applies to mainly younger women, and is often associated with the oncogenic types of human papillomavirus, and the other is relevant in older women, in whom many of the lesions are associated with lichen sclerosus (Crum 1992). Ageing, mutations, the human papillomavirus and lichen sclerosus may all interact in the older group (Crum *et al.* 1997).

A related aspect is that of the histological precursor of malignancy. In the younger age group SCC appears to be a development of undifferentiated VIN, often multifocal; in those of the older group without lichen sclerosus, it tends rather to arise from a solitary plaque on an otherwise normal vulva. However, in the case of the patient with lichen sclerosus with a SCC, if VIN is found it is more frequently the differentiated type of VIN and epithelial hyperplasia is usually a prominent feature (Leibowitch *et al.* 1990, Carli *et al.* 1995). The association of this type of VIN with SCC in lichen sclerosus was well described by Abell (1965). The epithelial hyperplasia may mask or replace histological evidence of lichen sclerosus in the vicinity of the tumour and so contributes towards a falsely low estimate of the incidence of lichen sclerosus in SCC. This epithelial hyperplasia is distinct from lichen simplex or lichenification and more akin to the 'leukoplakia' described by Wallace and Whimster. The clinical presentation is of an erythematous, ulcerated or hyperkeratotic papule, plaque or nodule (Fig. 5.64). The carcinoma tends to arise on the clitoris or labia minora, sites of predilection for lichen sclerosus. It is striking how often a patient presents with an SCC on lichen sclerosus that has been undiagnosed, and usually untreated, and which may be entirely asymptomatic. It will be interesting to see whether effective treatment of lichen sclerosus with a potent topical steroid will prevent the development of SCC in the future.

Prospective surveys of women known to have lichen sclerosus would furnish valuable information, such as that of Carli *et al.* (1995), who made a longitudinal cohort study of 211 patients. The number of invasive SCCs significantly exceeded that in an age-matched group; the cumulative risk was 14.8% compared with 0.06% in the general population. Meanwhile, it would seem reasonable to conclude that there is indeed an increased risk of malignancy and, therefore, that advice to the patients, and their supervision, should be very careful. It is difficult, however, to discover those women with asymptomatic disease or those who do not seek medical help – a group whose initial presentation is with the vulval carcinoma.

Malignant melanoma in children has been reported in lichen sclerosus (Rosamilia *et al.* 2006), but it must be noted that junctional and compound naevi may be mistaken for malignant melanoma when they are superimposed on lichen

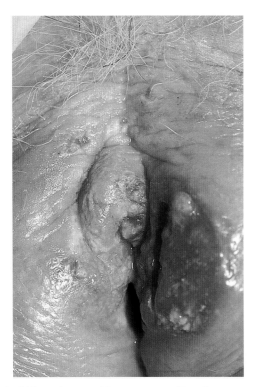

Fig. 5.64 Lichen sclerosus with a squamous cell carcinoma.

sclerosus in children and adolescents (Ackerman 1988). Basal cell carcinomas on a background of lichen sclerosus have also been reported (Meyrick Thomas *et al.* 1985) and many of the cases of verrucous carcinomas are seen in patients with lichen sclerosus (Brisigotti *et al.* 1989).

Lichen planus

Lichen planus is an inflammatory disorder with manifestations on the skin, genital and oral mucous membranes. The characteristic lesions are violaceous, flat papules, which, on keratinized skin, often show white streaks over their surface known as Wickham's striae. Similar papular lesions may be found on the mucosal surfaces, but there are also erosive and hypertrophic variants at these sites. The incidence of genital disease is unknown but, in one study of patients attending a vulval clinic, the prevalence of vulval lichen planus was 3.7% (Micheletti *et al.* 2000).

Aetiology

The pathogenesis is unknown but it is probably an immunological response by T cells activated by, as yet, unidentified antigens. Weak circulating basement membrane zone antibodies have been shown to be present in 61% of patients with erosive lichen planus of the vulva (Cooper *et al.* 2005). Lichen planus-like eruptions can be produced by drugs and are seen in GVHD. Lichenoid reactions can occur on the buccal mucosa adjacent to amalgam restorations and patients often have positive patch test reactions to relevant allergens, their disease improving when the allergen is withdrawn. However, no similar antigens have been shown for genital disease. There has been interest in the role of the hepatitis C virus as a trigger antigen in lichen planus. There does seem to be a significant association between hepatitis C infection and lichen planus in southern Europe and Japan, but not in northern Europe (Carrozzo & Pellicano 2008). Screening for those with vulval lichen planus in this latter population is therefore unnecessary. Familial cases are well recognized, as is an association with autoimmune conditions. HLA findings are conflicting, but there may be an association with HLA-DR1 (Valsecchi *et al.* 1988). There may be different HLA associations with different clinical patterns of disease (Setterfield *et al.* 2006).

Clinical features

The anogenital lesions of lichen planus may be divided into three main groups according to their clinical presentation – classical, hypertrophic and erosive – although there is sometimes overlap. In all cases, it is important to examine the rest of the skin, including the nails, scalp and mouth and conjunctivae. In addition, oesophageal lesions should be sought if the patient has erosive lichen planus and symptoms of dysphagia or pain.

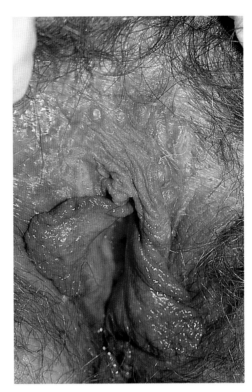

Fig. 5.65 Lichen planus: papules and areas of pallor on the anterior part of the vulva.

In the classical form, typical papules will be found on the keratinized anogenital skin (Fig. 5.65), with or without striae on the inner aspects of the vulva (Fig. 5.66). Hyperpigmentation frequently follows their resolution, particularly in the dark-skinned subject (Fig. 5.23). This type of lichen planus may be asymptomatic, and vulval involvement, as part of a generalized eruption, is likely to be underdiagnosed since the area may not routinely be examined. Vulval lesions were found in 19 of 37 women with cutaneous lichen planus, with four of the 19 having had no symptoms (Lewis *et al.* 1996). In a study of women with oral lichen planus, 57% also had vulval involvement (Belfiore *et al.* 2006). Half of these patients were asymptomatic. Vaginal lesions have not been systematically studied in those with classical lichen planus, but probably do not occur. A case of the rare variant lichen planus pemphigoides involving the vulva was reported in a 10 year old child, an unusual age since lichen planus is rarely seen in childhood (Hernando *et al.* 1992). There are some patients who present with very little inflammatory change but significant pigmentation occurring almost exclusively in the flexural zones.

Hypertrophic lesions are relatively rare and can be difficult to diagnose. They particularly affect the perineum and perianal area, presenting as thickened warty plaques

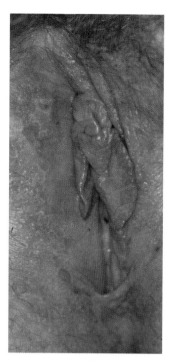

Fig. 5.66 Reticulated network of white striae of lichen planus.

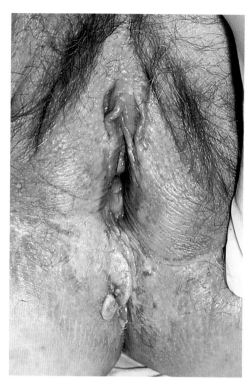

Fig. 5.67 Lichen planus: hypertrophic lesions of the perineum and perianal area.

which may become ulcerated, infected and painful. Because of these features, they can mimic malignancy (Fig. 5.67). They do not appear to be accompanied by vaginal lesions.

Erosive disease is the commonest form of lichen planus to affect the genital area with lesions involving the inner aspects of the vulva and the vagina. There may be accompanying cutaneous lesions, but this is not always the case. A distinctive pattern of erosive disease also involving the gingival mucosa was described as the vulvovaginal–gingival (VVG) syndrome by Pelisse *et al.* (1982). Some use the term plurimucosal lichen planus (Bermejo *et al.* 1990). It has been shown that there is a significant association of the VVG syndrome with the HLA-DQB1*0201 allele when compared with the immunogenetics of other clinical patterns of lichen planus (Setterfield *et al.* 1996b, 2006). It seems, therefore, that patients with vulvovaginal–oral lesions represent a distinct genetic subset.

The vulval lesions are chronic and painful and involve the inner aspects of the labia minora and the vestibule. Striae are sometimes visible at the margins of the lesions. In many patients, the lesions appear as frank erosions or erythematous patches, on a vulva that is otherwise normal in appearance. In others, atrophic changes may be marked, with fusion and scarring of the clitoris and labia minora, leading to a significant loss of the normal architecture (Fig. 5.68). This picture is often indistinguishable from lichen sclerosus clinically or histologically.

The vaginal lesions in erosive lichen planus are important as failure to recognize these early and start treatment can lead to scarring and complete stenosis. The lesions consist

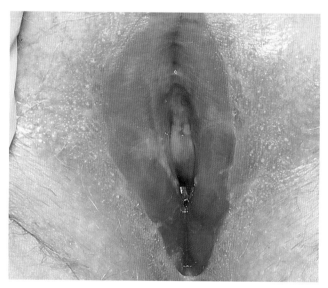

Fig. 5.68 Vulvovaginal–gingival syndrome of lichen planus. Extensive erosive disease, with a white lacy network at the periphery and loss of architecture.

of friable telangiectatic areas with patchy erythema, which are responsible for the common symptoms of postcoital bleeding, dyspareunia and a variable discharge, which is often serosanguinous. With ongoing inflammation, synechiae develop, and in severe cases vaginal stenosis will follow. The vagina may be shortened to such an extent that it barely

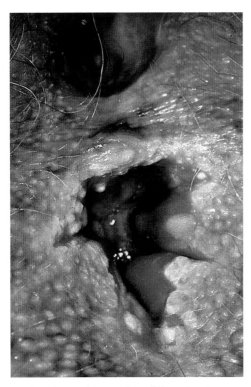

Fig. 5.69 Lichen planus: close-up view of the perianal area.

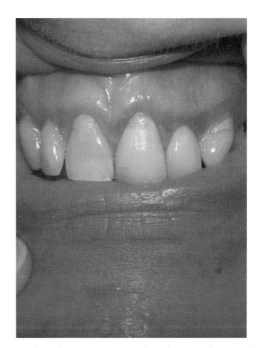

Fig. 5.71 Lichen planus: gingivitis in the vulvovaginal–gingival syndrome.

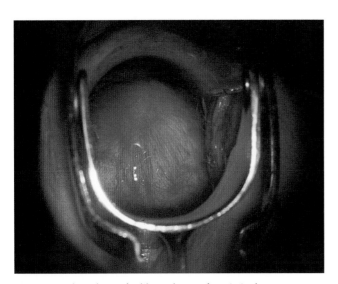

Fig. 5.70 Lichen planus: friable erythema of cervix in the vulvovaginal–gingival syndrome.

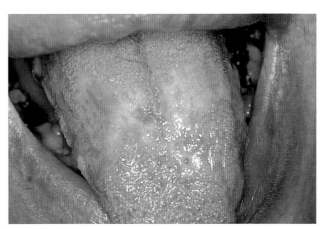

Fig. 5.72 Lichen planus: white plaques on the tongue.

admits the tip of a finger. It is likely that earlier reports of 'desquamative vaginitis' were, in fact, examples of erosive lichen planus. A number of patients have involvement of the anal margin (Fig. 5.69) and the cervix may also be involved (Eisen 1994, Pelisse 1996) (Fig. 5.70).

The gingivitis, which mainly affects the buccal surface, may be mild or severe, and is primarily erosive (Fig. 5.71), although reticulate lesions may also be seen (Eisen 1994).

Buccal lesions may occur and the tongue is often affected, with whitish or bald patches on the dorsal and lateral borders (Fig. 5.72).

A patient was reported with conjunctival lesions (Moyal-Barracco *et al.* 1993). The vulvovaginal–gingival syndrome may also be associated with lacrymal duct stenosis (Fig. 5.73) as well as oesophageal and external auditory canal disease (Setterfield *et al.* 2006).

Course and potential for malignancy

The papulosquamous lesions tend to clear completely, but the postinflammatory hyperpigmentation may linger for many months. In the erosive and hypertrophic forms, the course is chronic with perhaps some fluctuations but few

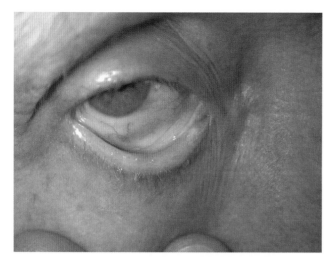

Fig. 5.73 Loss of punctum of lacrymal duct due to scarring lichen planus.

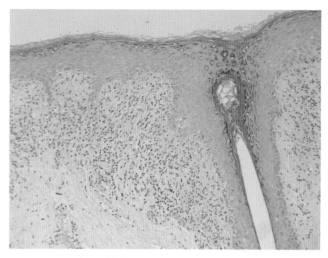

Fig. 5.74 Histology of lichen planus showing a prominent granular layer, saw tooth pattern of the rete ridges and a band-like infiltrate along the dermoepidermal junction.

remissions. Once atrophy has occurred, this will be permanent. One study reports a good prognosis in erosive lichen planus with three-quarters of patients having an improvement in their symptoms (Cooper & Wojnarowska 2006), but this has not been supported by other studies as most patients experience ongoing symptoms (Setterfield *et al.* 2006).

The potential for malignancy in oral lichen planus is generally accepted, and in genital lesions there also appears to be an increased risk of malignancy, although its degree is uncertain. With the possible exception of one case (Crotty *et al.* 1980) there have been no reported malignancies in the vulvovaginal–gingival syndrome. In other forms, SCC (Lewis & Harrington 1994) and SCC *in situ* (Franck & Young 1995) have been reported. Studies of patients with established vulval malignancy have demonstrated associated lichen planus (Zaki *et al.* 1997, Derrick *et al.* 2000) in the surrounding epithelium.

VIN is a precursor of invasive malignancy and the histological changes may be subtle. Patients may present with patches of glassy erythema on a background of lichen planus and clinicopathological correlation is vital in order to make the diagnosis. These patients need close follow-up.

Histology
The histology of lichen planus shows hyperkeratosis in areas of keratinized skin, acanthosis that is typically irregular with a saw-tooth appearance, an increased granular layer and basal cell liquefaction (Fig. 5.74). The hyperkeratosis and acanthosis are especially marked in the hypertrophic form. Sometimes there are apoptotic eosinophilic basal and prickle cells, the so-called colloid bodies. There is a band-like dermal infiltrate mainly composed of T cells and closely

apposed to the dermis; in chronic hypertrophic lesions this feature is less evident. Immunofluorescence reveals shaggy staining of the basement membrane zone for fibrinogen and IgM, cytoid bodies and sometimes granular IgG or IgA.

In the erosive form of the disease, characteristic histological epidermal changes are not always seen, and are evident in only about 70% of patients.

Differential diagnosis
The differential diagnosis of vulval lichen planus is mainly of the immunobullous diseases, especially those associated with scarring, and lichen sclerosus. If vaginal lesions are present, this excludes lichen sclerosus. Without vaginal lesions, the differentiation from lichen sclerosus can be difficult to make unless there is unequivocal histological evidence of subepidermal hyalinization to confirm lichen sclerosus, or interface changes and cytoid bodies to offer convincing evidence of lichen planus. The presence of definite lichen planus elsewhere by no means allows in itself a confident diagnosis of vulval lichen planus, since overlap with lichen sclerosus is well recognized (Marren *et al.* 1994). IMF findings to support cicatricial pemphigoid are helpful, but often negative in that condition, the diagnosis of which is mainly clinical. Lichenoid drug eruptions may occasionally have to be considered (van Voorst Vader *et al.* 1988), as may Zoon's vulvitis (see later).

Hypertrophic lichen planus can also present diagnostic difficulty, particularly when exacerbated by infection. With solitary or sparse lesions, malignancy is often suspected. With more diffuse lesions, lichen sclerosus with secondary lichenification, lichen simplex or protuberant viral warts may be considered.

Management

The mainstays of topical therapy are potent topical corticosteroids, together with bland emollients and barrier creams. The most potent topical steroid is usually required, i.e. clobetasone propionate 0.05%, in a carefully monitored regimen (as described above). The preferred vehicle is the ointment, which is well tolerated. Preparations in an adhesive base, as used in the mouth, are on the whole not tolerated well at the vulva. When there is an element of secondary infection, combinations of a corticosteroid with an antibacterial or antifungal agent is helpful. In the vulvovaginal–gingival syndrome, topical ciclosporin and retinoic acid have been used but with little success, although Eisen (1994) found that both ciclosporin and retinoic acid were more helpful when combined with a corticosteroid than when used alone. The new calcineurin inhibitors have been reported to be of benefit but this is not sustained. Tacrolimus has been used with effect in vulval lichen planus (Byrd et al. 2004) and there is one series reporting the use of pimecrolimus (Lonsdale-Eccles & Velangi 2005). Caution must be used as there are reports of SCC developing in patients with lichen sclerosus treated with tacrolimus (Ormerod 2005), and concern has been expressed about the use of these agents in a condition that is known to undergo malignant change in some patients. These preparations should, therefore, be used for short periods in those who are unresponsive to topical steroids.

Delivery of corticosteroids to the vagina is not easy. A proprietary preparation containing hydrocortisone (Colifoam), introduced with an applicator, is useful. Prednisolone suppositories may be used in more severe cases. Synechiae can be treated in a more conventional way by dilators in conjunction with corticosteroids, and this approach should always follow surgical attempts to remove adhesions or reduce stenosis. Isolated surgical procedures will not help and will invariably lead to further scarring of the vagina. In a small series of five patients, improvement was seen after treatment with topical steroids, tacrolimus ointment, methotrexate and surgical dilatation (Kortekangas-Savolainen & Kiilholma 2007). Regular sexual intercourse will help to preserve patency, but is often impractical because of dyspareunia.

The patient who does not respond adequately to topical measures can be challenging. There is no consensus and little evidence base for the use of systemic agents. Oral steroids are used, for example prednisolone 40 mg/day, tapered off over a few weeks; courses can be repeated as necessary for severe flares. In the vulvovaginal–gingival syndrome there is general agreement that azathioprine, dapsone, griseofulvin, chloroquine and minocycline, all tried empirically, are of little or no benefit; oral ciclosporin may be considered. Retinoids can be very helpful in hypertrophic cases. The new biological agents have been used in oral and cutaneous disease. Efaluzimab (Heffernan et al. 2007)

and basiliximab (Rebora et al. 2002) have been effective but their use has not been evaluated in vulval disease. All these potentially toxic therapies need careful monitoring and are best supervised by a dermatologist.

Zoon's vulvitis

Zoon first described lesions of glazed erythema localized to the glans penis and prepuce that were characterized by a plasma-rich inflammatory infiltrate in the dermis with no epidermal atypia. Later he went on to describe the condition affecting vulval skin (Zoon 1955), as did Garnier (1954). The condition appears to be noted more in men, as in a series of 19 cases reported by Souteyrand et al. (1981) only one was a woman. It is likely that plasma cell vulvitis (PCV; vulvitis circumscripta plasmacellularis) is not a single disease entity but represents a reaction pattern to another inflammatory condition. It is often the histological pattern seen when biopsies are taken from the vestibular mucosal epithelium in long-standing lichen planus or the postinflammatory erythema seen after lichen planus or other inflammatory conditions affecting the vulval vestibule. A plasma cell-rich infiltrate in a vestibular biopsy may be a misleading finding because plasma cells are commonly found in inflammatory conditions of the vestibule as it is a mucosal epithelium. There is therefore some doubt whether PCV is a distinct clinicopathological entity, and many of the reports of vestibular Zoon's may well be cases of lichen planus Scurry et al. (1993b).

Clinical features

Clinically the lesions in the male are striking, with glistening red areas, often speckled and haemorrhagic, affecting the glans and prepuce; in the female they are similar but perhaps less well defined and are found in the vestibule and labia minora, whereas the typical site in men is the glans and prepuce. The glans clitoris is rarely affected. The patients may be asymptomatic but some complain of itching but more commonly a burning sensation, dyspareunia, dysuria, pink-tinged vaginal discharge and occasional bleeding when the area is wiped.

Histology

The essential features are epidermal thinning, absent horny and granular layers and distinctive lozenge-shaped keratinocytes with widened intercellular spaces (Fig. 5.75). There is a dense inflammatory infiltrate in the dermis composed largely of plasma cells, with dilated blood vessels and surrounding haemosiderin deposition. Russell bodies and dermal–epidermal splitting have also been described. Some reports have tended to stress the plasma cells and the haemosiderin rather than the epidermal changes, although the latter were noted by Kavanagh et al. (1993) and Scurry et al. (1993b).

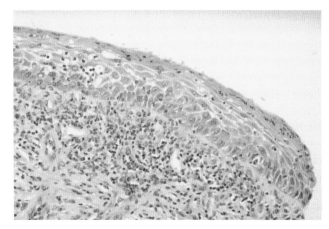

Fig. 5.75 Histology of Zoon's-like inflammation showing marked spongiosis of the epidermis and lozenge-shaped keratinocytes.

Diagnosis

As already discussed there remains some doubt as to whether or not Zoon's vulvitis is a definite entity, the diagnosis tending to be attached rather too easily to any purpuric lesion in which plasma cells and haemosiderin are histologically found. An overlap with lichen aureus in women has also been described (Li *et al.* 2003). Purpuric telangiectatic and lichenoid balanitis share features with the pigmented persistent dermatoses and Jonquières & de Lutsky (1980) reported Zoon's vulvitis with clinical lesions that had the same histology as this entity. The term chronic vulval purpura was used by Kato *et al.* (1990) and may provide a more useful descriptive term (Li *et al.* 2003). These changes may all represent a mucosal reaction to a chronic erosive process such as lichen planus, pemphigus and pemphigoid. The differential diagnosis would also include a fixed drug eruption.

Management

A trial of topical corticosteroids can help some patients as can topical flamazine or clindamycin. However, using a barrier preparation such as Vaseline petroleum jelly is useful for the dysuria and topical 5% lidocaine may alleviate the burning sensation. Topical tacrolimus has not proven to be effective in vulval Zoon's (Virgili *et al.* 2008). Five cases were treated successfully with topical misoprostol (Gunter & Golitz 2005). Morioko *et al.* (1988) reported good results in an atypical case with intralesional interferon α.

Plasma cell orificial mucositis (plasmocytosis circumorificialis)

An entity similar to Zoon's balanitis was described involving the lips, but also occasionally the vulva (Aiba & Tagami 1989). There was a dense infiltrate of plasma cells but apparently no haemosiderin deposition. Although the authors grouped their cases with those reported as Zoon's balanitis

or vulvitis, it seems possible, on clinical and histological grounds, that the condition is distinct.

Angiolymphoid hyperplasia with eosinophilia

This angiomatous inflammatory condition, whose relationship to Kimura's disease is disputed, presents as erythematous intradermal or subcutaneous nodules, and only very rarely affects the vulva or perianal area (Scurry *et al.* 1995). Surgical removal may be effective and oral retinoids can also be helpful (Marcoux *et al.* 1991).

Lesions related to blood and lymphatic vessels

Varicose veins

Vulval varicosities may be seen in 4% of women (Bell *et al.* 2007) (Fig. 5.76). They are common in pregnancy, when increased pelvic blood flow is relevant, but hormonal factors may also be involved, as the veins often enlarge in the first trimester. After delivery, some lesions thrombose spontaneously, but if they do not do so, and when there are no varicosities of the leg, further investigation by venography and computed tomography scan is indicated.

Vulval and perivulval varicose veins are usually accompanied by varicosities in the leg veins. They may be the consequence of chronic pelvic congestion, portal hypertension or obstructive pelvic lesions. Ovarian vein incompetence can lead to varicosities in the vulva and legs (Hobbs 2005).

Management

When the vulval varices are a problem, elevation of the foot of the bed during sleep and supporting garments are helpful. Active treatment includes ligation or sclerosant injections and the use of a pelvic support.

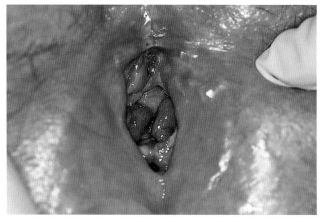

Fig. 5.76 Varicosities: engorged veins in the vestibular area, in a patient who also had lichen sclerosus.

Oedema

Most cases of vulval oedema are due to leakage through, or increased pressure in, capillaries. There are numerous causes for this but the lax tissue of the vulva readily accumulates fluid. Rarely, a direct passive transfer effect can also result in vulval oedema in patients undergoing peritoneal dialysis, in which the channel can be a small hernia or a defect of the peritoneal fascia (Cooper *et al.* 1983, Kopecky *et al.* 1985). Acute, but self-limiting unilateral vulval oedema has also been described after instillation of adhesion barrier solution at laparoscopy (Pados *et al.* 2005). No classification for the types of oedema exists but a useful method is to differentiate acute and chronic causes.

Acute vulval oedema

A degree of oedema is often seen in patients with acute inflammatory conditions such as candidiasis or eczema. This settles with treatment of the primary problem. Urticaria or angio-oedema, including hereditary angio-oedema, may affect the vulva. Dermographism has been suspected of being involved in vulval problems (Lambiris & Greaves 1997) and pressure urticaria is also a possible cause.

Type 1 allergic reactions to latex in condoms and to surgical gloves are increasingly recognized, and are of great concern since potentially fatal reactions may occur if the patient is unaware of the problem and is examined by someone wearing latex-containing gloves. Reactions have been reported during delivery. A further cause of this type of acute oedema is allergy to seminal fluid. This is undoubtedly an entity, but is rare. A careful history is vital – the symptoms start a few minutes after intercourse but do not occur if condoms are used. The important differential diagnosis is vestibulodynia and many women who come suspecting that this is the problem have this condition (see Chapter 6). The mechanisms involved in seminal fluid allergy were reviewed fully by Jones (1991) and Kint *et al.* (1994), the latter authors reporting a case in which type I allergy to seminal plasma was, unusually, possibly combined with a type IV reaction to it. The responsible agent is thought to be a glycoprotein. The patients are usually atopic. The reaction can start at the first intercourse, or begin later. There has been speculation that the occurrence at the first intercourse could be accounted for by intrauterine exposure to the relevant prostatic protein antigen from a male twin, the presence of whom may not always have been known; an alternative explanation is cross-sensitization. The signs may be local or may spread to other areas and even lead to anaphylaxis. Abstinence or the use of a condom is effective management. Desensitization has variable results but may be successful (Lee Wong *et al.* 2008) and intravaginal cromoglycate prior to intercourse may be helpful. Successful conception may be achieved by artificial insemination using the partner's seminal fluid which has been processed to remove allergenic components (Ferré-Ybarz *et al.* 2006).

Vulval oedema has been reported in the ovarian hyperstimulation syndrome, a rare complication following ovulation in cases of infertility (Luxman *et al.* 1996). The mechanism was thought to be fluid retention, decreased oncotic and increased hydrostatic pressure. Gross vulval oedema has been described in pre-eclampsia (Rainford 1970). Prepartum oedema is reported in a woman with a twin pregnancy who was receiving tocolytic drugs to inhibit early labour (Trice *et al.* 1996). The authors postulated a combination of factors, involving glucocorticoids, terbutaline and magnesium sulphate, and noted that β-mimetic drugs such as terbutaline are recognized to cause pulmonary oedema and have been found in association with vulval oedema. Postpartum oedema has been reported following the use of a birthing chair (Davenport & Richardson 1986), and fatal cases have been reported by Ewing *et al.* (1979) in which patients died of vascular collapse and may have had an infective origin.

Chronic vulval oedema

Chronic vulval lymphoedema can follow repeated episodes of acute oedema in which there is lymphatic damage. Primary lymphoedema, secondary to congenital lymphatic hypoplasia, can sometimes be improved by surgery, and may be investigated by lymphangiography. Large amounts of fluid may be discharged locally. An immune deficit was associated, perhaps because of loss of lymphatic fluid into the gut, in the case of severe lymphoedema involving the genital area reported by Shelley and Wood (1981).

Secondary lymphoedema may follow chronic inflammatory disease such as hidradenitis suppurativa or Crohn's disease, infections such as filariasis, obstruction by malignant deposits, surgery (especially if associated with lymphadenectomy) and radiotherapy given, for example, for carcinoma of the cervix or endometrium. The vulva becomes indurated and often verrucose; small lymphatic vesicles (lymphangiectases) may develop (Fig. 5.77). Such vesicles, however, may also appear without overt clinical evidence of lymphoedema (Ambrojo *et al.* 1990), and indeed sometimes in the absence of any underlying cause. They may give rise to diagnostic difficulties, being mistaken for warts or other infections.

The histology of lymphangiectases shows dilated lymphatic vessels lined by a single layer of endothelial cells (Fig. 5.78) and can be difficult to distinguish from that of lymphangiomata circumscripta. It may be indeed that all lymphangiectases, whether arising spontaneously or induced by lymphatic blockage, should be regarded under the heading of lymphangioma circumscriptum.

Chronic lymphoedema, usually unilateral (Fig. 5.79), has been described in women who have undertaken intensive cycling and has been termed bicyclist's vulva (Baeyens

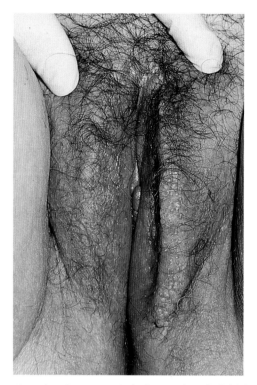

Fig. 5.77 Lymphangiectases: vesicular lesions along the left labium majus giving it a verrucous appearance.

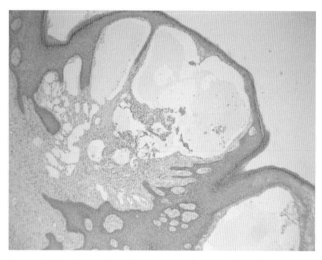

Fig. 5.78 Histology of lymphangiectases showing dilated lymphatic vessels lined by a single layer of endothelial cells.

et al. 2002). Lymphoscintigraphy in three cases showed abnormalities which were thought to be due to repeated compression of the inguinal lymphatic vessels.

Management
The skills of a dedicated lymphoedema service nurse can be of great help. Massage, skin care and advice on support

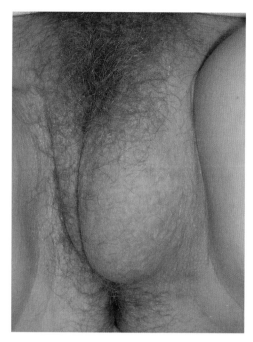

Fig. 5.79 Cyclist's vulva: unilateral lymphoedema left labium majus.

garments are important and some are benefited by referral to a patient support group. Lymphangiectases respond to treatment with the carbon dioxide laser (Landthaler *et al.* 1990). Lymphaticovenular anastomosis has been reported as a successful treatment in one case of acquired lymphangioma circumscriptum (Montegi *et al.* 2007).

In both types of lymphoedema, the affected tissue is subject to recurrent streptococcal infections, which in turn increase the obstruction and predispose to further attacks. The patient described by Buckley and Barnes (1996), who appeared to have the former type, developed extensive vesiculation following repeated attacks. The cellulitis is associated with pain, fever and malaise. It is treated with phenoxymethyl penicillin plus flucloxacillin, or by co-amoxiclav, or by erythromycin if the subject is allergic to penicillin. Phenoxymethyl penicillin or erythromycin can also be given over long periods with benefit to prevent attacks.

In both types of lymphoedema, moreover, a lymphangiosarcoma or angiosarcoma may occasionally develop (Huey *et al.* 1985).

Miscellaneous conditions

Genital papular acantholytic dyskeratosis
Duray *et al.* (1983) described three examples of the nodular lesions on the vulva with the histological changes of acantholysis. The lesions did not recur after excision. Chorzelski *et al.* (1984) then reported a patient whose papular vulval lesions were suggestive of Darier's disease, and essentially

similar case reports followed (Bell *et al.* 2001). A case with disseminated lesions has been described (Ciupinska *et al.* 1998). The histological changes are similar to those seen in Darier's disease or Hailey–Hailey disease, but there is no family history and it is now considered a distinct clinical entity. Time may show that it is a forme fruste of either Darier's or Hailey–Hailey disease.

Acquired dyskeratotic leukoplakia

Under this title, James and Lupton (1988) described a woman of 38 who developed white plaques of the palate, lips and gums, followed by similar lesions on the labia minora. There was no family history and the status of the condition remains uncertain. The histology showed clusters of dyskeratotic cells in the epidermis but sparing the basal layer, and did not appear to fit in with that of any known entity.

Treatment with oral steroids and retinoids, and with the laser, was ineffective.

Vulvovaginal adenosis

Vulvovaginal adenosis is defined by the presence of metaplastic cervical or endometrial epithelium in the vagina or vulva. It may arise from the remnants of embryonic paramesonephric epithelium. Kranl *et al.* (1998) have described vaginal adenosis occurring spontaneously and it is found coincidentally in up to 10% of women. It has also been suggested that prolonged oral contraceptive use may lead to its development. Adenosis in the upper vagina is well recognized as a result of *in utero* exposure to diethyl stilboestrol taken by the mother in pregnancy. It may also occur after trauma, for example treatment with 5-fluorouracil (Goodman *et al.* 1991), or following laser therapy (Sedlacek *et al.* 1990). Vulval and lower vaginal adenosis is rarer and appears usually to arise following severe erosive inflammatory disease such as Stevens–Johnson syndrome (Bonafe *et al.* 1990), toxic epidermal necrolysis (Adornato 2000), lichen planus (Singer *et al.* 1994), pemphigus and as a complication of laser therapy.

Vaginal adenosis may be associated with the development of vaginal adenocarcinoma (Yaghsezian *et al.* 1992).

The pathogenesis is unknown but one explanation is the unmasking of the remnant tissue of Mullerian (paramesonephric) origin.

The adenosis is red and friable, and the main differential diagnosis is from endometriosis.

Graft-versus-host disease

The first reports of genital involvement in GVHD were made in the 1990s. Erythema and erosions can occur and may be seen in up to 49% of patients 2 years after transplant (Zantomio *et al.* 2006). The main risk factor appeared to be the stem cell source – a higher risk of GVHD was seen with peripheral blood progenitor cells than with marrow transplantation. Early recognition is important. Many patients will respond to superpotent topical steroids (Stratton *et al.* 2007) and ciclosporin has also been used topically (Spiryda *et al.* 2003).

Traumatic lesions

Obstetric trauma may lead to serious haematomas, but a variety of other injuries are reported. The patient of Rege and Shukla (1993) presented with a genital ulcer that proved to be connected by a sinus to a dislocated and osteomyelitic symphysis pubis. Injury may lead in due course to abscesses, keloids, cysts, neuromas, calculi, areas of endometriosis or granulation tissue. Most of these are easily managed surgically.

Non-obstetric injuries can occur by a number of mechanisms. In one series of 17 patients, straddle injuries from sexual assault or falls were the commonest cause (Habek & Kulas 2007). Intracoital injury leading to rupture of the posterior fornix, and injuries by foreign objects were also seen. Vulval haematomas have been reported after snowboarding injuries (Kanai *et al.* 2001) and goring (Okur *et al.* 2005). Up to 30% of those with traumatic injuries will have coexisting urological injury which must be investigated appropriately (Goldman *et al.* 1998).

Genital and perineal burns are more common in children but have been described in adults from hot liquids (Roberts *et al.* 2007) and also secondary to a suicide attempt involving fireworks (Weiler-Mithoff *et al.* 1996).

Genital self-mutilation is less common in females than in males, but may present with unexplained vaginal bleeding (Alao *et al.* 1999). Artefactual damage may present in a number of different ways. One case of recurrent vaginal ulceration was treated with infibulation (McQueen 1974).

Vulval disease in children

Many dermatological disorders can affect children but there are some specific conditions that are seen much more commonly in the paediatric group. Congenital abnormalities have been described in Chapter 1 and infections in Chapters 3 and 4.

Of those presenting with vulval symptoms, the majority have an inflammatory dermatosis, with eczematous conditions being most common. In one series, 33% were found to have a dermatitis, 17% psoriasis and 18% lichen sclerosus (Fischer & Rogers 2000). In another series of paediatric patients, few cases of psoriasis was found (Powell 2006).

Labial adhesions

Some agglutination of the labia minora is common in infancy. It is thought to be related to the hypo-oestrogenized state of

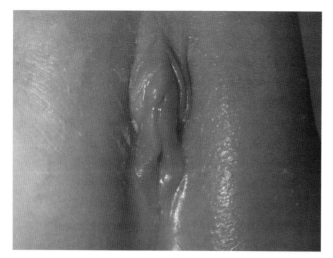

Fig. 5.80 Labial adhesions: midline fusion, leaving a small posteriorly placed opening.

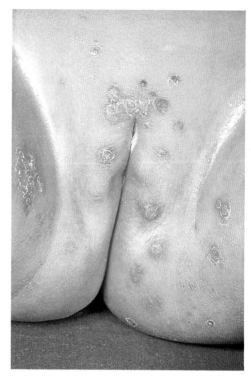

Fig. 5.81 Napkin rash: papules and small nodules.

the vulva in childhood, in combination with mild inflammation (Fig. 5.80). They were found in 1.8% of children attending a general paediatric clinic with a peak incidence of 3.3% between the ages of 13 and 23 months (Leung *et al.* 1993). They are unusual in infants less than 2 months of age because of the persistent influence of maternal oestrogens, but, in this age group, congenital abnormalities or an imperforate hymen are important differential diagnoses. A useful distinguishing sign is a line of demarcation between the clitoral hood and the labia minora seen in labial adhesions (Pokorny 1992). In the older child, lichen sclerosus as a potential cause for agglutination must be excluded and adhesions have been reported after calcinosis cutis (Bernardo *et al.* 1999), although this is very rare.

About 80% of labial adhesions will resolve spontaneously within 1 year but treatment is advised if there are problems with micturition. These may present as pooling of urine behind the fused labia minora, or, if fusion is more extensive and almost complete, only a tiny pin-hole meatus may be left anteriorly leading to difficulty starting the stream. Generally, topical oestrogens are applied once daily and can be effective in around 90% of case series reported (Tebruegge *et al.* 2007). Side-effects of this therapy include vulval pigmentation and breast enlargement but these are mild and resolve after cessation of treatment. Occasionally, digital separation is required, and the use of topical oestrogens after this treatment can prevent recurrence (Soyer 2007). The continued use of emollients is also encouraged. Surgical separation should be reserved for those who are resistant to topical treatment or for those who develop urinary retention.

Napkin rashes

In infancy the napkin area is the site of a variety of eczematous rashes. Irritant dermatitis is the most common but psoriasis and seborrhoeic dermatitis can also occur. It can be very hard to differentiate these entities.

Primary irritant napkin dermatitis

An irritant napkin dermatitis is one of the commonest cutaneous problems seen in infancy. The frequency and severity of napkin dermatitis has reduced in the developed world, probably owing to improvements in napkin materials used. However, there is not yet enough evidence from randomized controlled trials to support or refute the use of disposable napkins in order to prevent napkin dermatitis. Contact with faeces is the most important irritant factor but urine, friction, excessive hydration and chemical irritation from topically applied preparations are also involved. Infection is a secondary event and *Candida albicans* may be an exacerbating factor.

Confluent erythema is seen, particularly over the convexities of the buttocks, labia majora and mons pubis. Papular lesions can develop and a particularly severe form of irritant dermatitis is known as Jacquet's erosive dermatitis (see below) (Fig. 5.81). This tends to occur in older children in whom erosive and ulcerated lesions are seen.

Allergic contact dermatitis

This is rare in children and is not likely to occur in young babies. It has been reported to dyes (Alberta *et al.* 2005) and

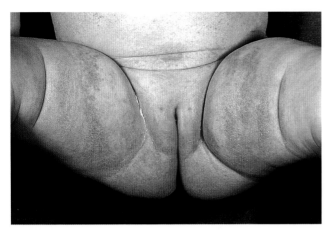

Fig. 5.82 Napkin rash: patchy erythema sparing the flexures.

also to the rubber components of disposable napkins (Roul *et al.* 1998). The holster distribution of this latter type has led to the term 'lucky Luke' dermatitis.

Psoriasiform napkin rash

This form shows erythematous patches with clearly defined margins, but the typical silvery scales seen in psoriasis at other sites are generally lost owing to the moist environment in the genital area (Fig. 5.82). Most of these children do not have the psoriatic diathesis or the HLA patterns seen in psoriasis. However, some do seem to be more likely to develop it later. In one series of 18 patients, two developed psoriasis and two atopic eczema (Rasmussen *et al.* 1986). It is also possible that psoriasis can koebnerize after an irritant napkin dermatitis.

Seborrhoeic dermatitis

Seborrhoeic dermatitis tends to develop before 3 months of age. Salmon-coloured plaques, usually extending out to the inguinal folds, are seen. There may be a greasy scale on the surface and similar scaling on the scalp is frequently seen. It tends to clear after a few months.

Differential diagnosis of napkin rashes

Langerhans cell histiocytosis is an important differential diagnosis of a resistant napkin eruption. The potentially fatal form, Letterer–Siwe disease, usually occurs in the first year of life and may present with a rash resembling eczema in the napkin area. Acrodermatitis enteropathica is another condition to bear in mind if response to treatment is poor. There may be typical lesions elsewhere. Infections such as congenital syphilis, a primary *Candida* infection or herpes simplex are unlikely to present diagnostic difficulty.

Management of napkin rashes

The management of an irritant napkin dermatitis is to increase the frequency of napkin changing and to avoid the use of occlusive pants. Emollients should be used as soap substitutes and then a barrier cream applied. Weak topical steroids (no more potent than hydrocortisone) will help, particularly if a combined preparation with an antibacterial or antifungal is used. The use of potent topical steroids is strongly discouraged as wasting (Johns & Bower 1970) and systemic absorption can occur because of the occlusion in the area.

Perianal dermatitis of the newborn

This is a rare condition, and arises in the first week or so of life as an erythematous, often oedematous, patch round the anus. It clears with simple measures in a few weeks and is thought to be an inflammatory response to faecal irritants. It may or may not be associated with a napkin rash.

Pseudoverrucous papules and nodules

These lesions were first described in patients with urostomies and five children with urinary incontinence were reported to have similar lesions (Goldberg *et al.* 1992) (Fig. 5.81). Histology showed psoriasiform features and it is likely to be due to irritant factors as it improved when they were removed. Other authors believe that these lesions, Jacquet's erosive dermatitis and infantile granuloma gluteale represent variants in a spectrum of a common condition (Robson *et al.* 2006).

Infantile gluteal granuloma

This was described in 1971 by Tappeiner and Pfleger and tends to be commoner in males. Proposed aetiological factors include occlusion, the use of topical corticosteroids and candidal infection. A similar entity has been described in two adults in association with the use of topical benzocaine (Robson *et al.* 2006). The typical lesions are oval, livid nodules affecting the whole napkin area, and they may arise on a background of irritant napkin rash, sometimes as it is improving. They can mimic molluscum contagiosum infection. They regress after a few weeks but may leave scars. Histology shows dermal oedema, a dense granulomatous infiltrate of plasma cells and lymphocytes, together with fibrinoid necrosis and deposition of haemosiderin. Similar cases have been reported in incontinent elderly women, in whom corticosteroids were not a factor (Maekawa *et al.* 1978). Treatment is withdrawal of topical steroids if relevant and any occlusive factors must be minimized.

Kawasaki's disease

Kawasaki's disease is an acute multisystem disorder of unknown aetiology, with serious complications such as coronary artery aneurysms. In a series of 58 patients, 67% presented with a scaly, erythematous perineal eruption and this may be an early sign of the disease (Friter & Lucky 1988).

Bullous disease in children

Blistering disorders in children are uncommon. In one series of 130 children with vulval problems, only two cases of BP were seen (Fischer & Rogers 2000). They are important to recognize as both BP (Levine *et al.* 1992) and cicatricial pemphigoid (Hoque *et al.* 2006) have been mistaken for childhood sexual abuse. Bullous dermatosis of childhood is described earlier.

Bullous pemphigoid

It is known that BP in children is a true variant of the adult form of the disease (Nagano *et al.* 1994). A review found 50 cases of childhood BP in the literature that had been confirmed by direct and indirect immunofluorescence (Fisler *et al.* 2003). Many cases affect the vulva alone and are non-scarring, responding well to oral or topical steroids. They propose that localized vulval pemphigoid should be regarded as a subtype of the disease.

Cicatricial pemphigoid

This is known to affect the vulva in children and has been reported as confined to the vulva in one case (Hoque *et al.* 2006).

Traumatic lesions in children

The majority of accidental injuries in children are falls in a straddle position often involving bicycle riding. The labia minora are most commonly involved as the soft tissue is compressed against the pubic symphysis and rami – hence they are often linear (West *et al.* 1989). Hymenal injuries are rarely the result of unintentional injury and, if seen, the possibility of sexual abuse must be investigated.

Genital and perineal burns generally occur in the context of more widespread injury and are rarely isolated. The majority are due to hot liquids but flame injury, contact and electrical burns are seen (Angel *et al.* 2002).

Hair tourniquet syndromes have been reported in children involving the labia minora (Bacon & Burgis 2005) and clitoris (Alverson 2007), with one case resulting in strangulation and autoamputation of the clitoris (Kuo *et al.* 2002).

Sexual abuse in children

Some vulval dermatoses can mimic child sexual abuse, e.g. the ecchymosis seen in lichen sclerosus and the erosion and ulceration in mucous membrane pemphigoid. It is possible for sexual abuse to occur together with skin disease and the two are not mutually exclusive. Any suspicion of sexual abuse must be followed through and the child referred to an expert in the field. Clear pathways of referral must be in place for best practice (Adams *et al.* 2007, Royal College of Paediatrics and Child Health 2008).

The most important evidence is considered to be a clear statement from the child. Physical signs alone are rarely sufficient for the diagnosis. Forensic evidence is helpful if it yields positive findings such as the presence of seminal fluid in the vagina or evidence of gonorrhoea or syphilis in the absence of perinatal transmission. However, the presence of genital warts alone is not diagnostic as they are well recognized to occur in non-sexually abused children. Abuse does not necessarily result in abnormal physical signs, and these must be interpreted with care and in the light of other evidence. However, there are often signs and indeed injuries which, if present, must be noted in assessment. A scar or laceration of the hymen, or of the anal mucosa extending onto the perineal skin, is highly suggestive of abuse. Under the influence of maternal hormones, the vulva may appear swollen in the neonate, and there may be a vaginal discharge; the hymen may be thickened and pinkish white in colour up to the age of 4 years. A horizontal hymenal diameter of more than 1 cm is not diagnostic of abuse, nor is anal dilatation thought to be a reliable sign of anal abuse in the absence of other evidence. The utmost care in history taking and examination is essential, and therefore referral to those who have specific training in this area is mandatory.

References

Abele, D.C. & Anders, K.H. (1990) The many faces and phases of borreliosis II. *Journal of the American Academy of Dermatology* **23**, 401–410.

Abell, M.R. (1965) Intraepithelial carcinoma of epidermis and squamous mucosa of vulva and perineum. *Surgical Clinics of North America* **46**, 1179–1198.

Ackerman, A.B. (1988) Melanocytic proliferation that simulates malignant melanoma histopathologically. In: *Pathology and Recognition and Malignant Melanoma* (eds M.C. Mihm, G.F. Murphy & N. Kaufman), pp. 166–167. Williams & Wilkins, Baltimore.

Adams, J.A., Kaplan, R.A., Starling, S.P. *et al.* (2007) Guidelines for medical care of children who may have been sexually abused. *Journal of Pediatric and Adolescent Gynaecology* **20**, 163–72.

Adornato, M.C. (2000) Toxic epidermal necrolysis associated with quinidine administration. *New York State Dental Journal* **66**, 38–40.

Aiba, S. & Tagami, H. (1989) Immunoglobulin-producing cells in plasma cell orificial mucositis. *Journal of Cutaneous Pathology* **16**, 207–210.

Alao, A.O., Yolles, J.C. & Huslander, W. (1999) Female genital self-mutilation. *Psychiatric Services* **50**, 971.

Albert, S., Neill, S., Derrick, E.K. & Calonje, E. (2004) Psoriasis associated with vulval scarring. *Clinical and Experimental Dermatology* **29**, 354–356.

Alberta, L., Sweeney, S.M. & Wiss, K. (2005) Diaper dye dermatitis. *Paediatrics* **116**, 450–452.

Alli, N., Karakayali, G., Kahraman, I. & Artüz, F. (1997) Local intralesional therapy with rh GM-CSF for a large genital ulcer in Behçet's disease. *British Journal of Dermatology* **136**, 639–640.

Alverson, B. (2007) A genital hair tourniquet in a 9 year old girl. *Paediatric Emergency Care* **23**, 169–170.

Ambrojo, P., Cogolludo, E.F., Aguilar, A., Sánchez Yus, E. & Sánchez de Paz, F. (1990) Cutaneous lymphangiectases after therapy for carcinoma of the cervix – a case with unusual clinical and histological features. *Clinical and Experimental Dermatology* 15, 57–59.

Anderton, R.L. & Abele, D.C. (1976) Lichen sclerosus et atrophicus in a vaccination site. *Archives of Dermatology* 112, 1787.

Angel, C., Shu, T., French, D. *et al.* (2002) Genital and perineal burns in children: 10 years of experience at a major burn centre. *Journal of Paediatric Surgery* 37, 99–103.

Axiotis, C.A., Merino, M.J. & Duray, P.H. (1991) Langerhans cell histiocytosis of the female genital tract. *Cancer* 67, 1650–1660.

Bacon, J.L. & Burgis, J.T. (2005) Hair thread tourniquet syndrome in adolescents: a presentation and review of the literature. *Journal of Paediatric and Adolescent Gynaecology* 18, 155–156.

Baeyens, L., Vermeesch, E. & Bourgeois, P. (2002) Bicyclist's vulva: observational study. *British Medical Journal* 325, 138.

Balasubramaniam, P. & Lewis, F.M. (2007) Long term follow up of patients with lichen sclerosus: does it really happen? *Journal of Obstetrics and Gynaecology* 27, 282.

Banfield, C.C., Papadavid, E., Frith, P., Allen, J. & Wojnarowska, F.T. (1997) Bullous pemphigoid evolving into cicatricial pemphigoid? *Clinical and Experimental Dermatology* 22, 30–33.

Bardan, A., Nizet, V. & Gallo, R.L. (2004) Antimicrobial peptides and the skin. *Expert Opinion in Biological Therapy* 4, 53–59.

Barnhill, R.L., Albert, L.S., Shama, S.K. *et al.* (1990) Genital lentiginosis: a clinical and histopathologic study. *Journal of the American Academy of Dermatology* 22, 453–460.

Barth, J.H., Reshad, H., Darley, C.R. & Gibson, J.R. (1984) A cutaneous complication of Dorbanex therapy. *Clinical and Experimental Dermatology* 9, 95–96.

Barth, J.H., Layton, A.M. & Cunliffe, W.J. (1996) Endocrine factors in pre- and post-menopausal women with hidradenitis suppurativa. *British Journal of Dermatology* 134, 1057–1059.

Batta, K., Munday, P.E. & Tatnall, F.M. (1999) Pemphigus vulgaris localised to the vagina presenting as a chronic vaginal discharge. *British Journal of Dermatology* 140, 945–947.

Beattie, P.E., Dawe, R.S., Ferguson, J. & Ibbotson, S.H. (2006) UVA1 phototherapy for genital lichen sclerosus. *Clinical and Experimental Dermatology* 31, 343–347.

Belfiore, P., Di Fede, O., Cabibi, D. *et al.* (2006) Prevalence of vulval lichen planus in a cohort of women with oral lichen planus: an interdisciplinary study. *British Journal of Dermatology* 155, 994–998.

Bell, H.K., Farrar, C.W. & Curley, R.K. (2001) Papular acantholytic dyskeratosis of the vulva. *Clinical and Experimental Dermatology* 26, 386–388.

Bell, D., Kane, P.B., Liang, S. *et al.* (2007) Vulvar varices: an uncommon entity in surgical pathology. *International Journal of Gynaecological Pathology* 26, 99–101.

Ben-David, B., Sheiner, E., Hallak, M. & Levy, S. (2008) Pregnancy outcome in women with psoriasis. *Journal of Reproductive Medicine* 53, 183–187.

Bens, G., Laharie, D., Beylot-Barry, M. *et al.* (2003) Successful treatment with infliximab and methotrexate of pyostomatitis vegetans associated with Crohn's disease. *British Journal of Dermatology* 149, 181–184.

Berk, M. & Acton, M. (1997) Citalopram associated clitoral priapism: a case series. *International Clinical Psychopharmacology* 12, 121–122.

Berkeley, C. & Bonney, V. (1909) Leukoplakic vulvitis and its relation to kraurosis vulvae and to carcinoma vulvae. *Proceedings of the Royal Society of Medicine* 3, 29–31.

Bermejo, A., Bermejo, M.D., Román, P., Botella, R. & Bagán, J.V. (1990) Lichen planus with simultaneous involvement of the oral cavity and genitalia. *Oral Surgery, Oral Medicine and Oral Pathology* 69, 209–216.

Bernardo, B.D., Huettuer, P.C., Merrit, D.F. *et al.* (1999) Idiopathic calcinosis cutis presenting as labial adhesions in children: report of two cases with literature review. *Journal of Paediatric and Adolescent Gynaecology* 12, 157–160.

Berth-Jones, J., Smith, S.G. & Graham-Brown, R.A.C. (1995) Benign familial chronic pemphigus (Hailey–Hailey disease) responds to cyclosporin. *Clinical and Experimental Dermatology* 20, 70–72.

Best, C.L., Walters, C. & Adelman, D.C. (1988) Fixed cutaneous eruptions to seminal-plasma challenge: a case report. *Fertility and Sterility* 50, 532–534.

Bilenchi, R. (2004) Discoid lupus erythematosus of the vulva. *Lupus* 13, 815–816.

Bircher, A.J., Hirsbrunner, P. & Langauer, S. (1993) Allergic contact dermatitis of the genitals from additives in condoms. *Contact Dermatitis* 28, 125–126.

Bloch, K.J., Buchanan, W.W., Wohl, M.J. & Bunim, J.J. (1965) Sjögren's syndrome. *Medicine* 44, 187–231.

Boer, J. & Weltevreden, E.F. (1996) Hidradenitis suppurativa or acne inversa. A clinicopathological study of early lesions. *British Journal of Dermatology* 135, 721–725.

Bonafe, J.L., Thibaut, I. & Hoff, J. (1990) Introital adenosis associated with Stevens–Johnson syndrome. *Clinical and Experimental Dermatology* 15, 356–357.

Bonney, V. (1938) Leukoplakic vulvitis and the conditions likely to be confused with it. *Proceedings of the Royal Society of Medicine* 31, 1057–1060.

Boyce, D.C. & Valpey, J.M. (1971) Acute ulcerative vulvitis of obscure etiology. *Obstetrics and Gynecology* 38, 440–443.

Brandrup, F., Petri, J. & Aegidius, J. (1990) Acantholytic lesions in the vagina. *British Journal of Dermatology* 123, 691–692.

Breisky, D. (1885) Über Kraurosis Vulvae. *Zeitschrift für Heilkunde* 6, 69–80.

Brisigotti, M., Moreno, A., Murcia, C., Matías-Giuiu, X. & Prat, J. (1989) Verrucous carcinoma of the vulva. A clinicopathologic and immunohistochemical study of 5 cases. *International Journal of Gynecological Pathology* 8, 1–7.

Brodie-Meijer, C.C., Diemont, W.L. & Buijs, P.J. (1999) Nefazodone-induced clitoral priapism. *International Journal of Psychopharmacology* 14, 257–258.

Brown, A.R., Dunlap, C.L., Bussard, D.A. *et al.* (1997) Lichen sclerosus of the oral cavity: a report of two cases. *Oral Surgery, Oral Medicine, Oral Pathology, Oral Radiology and Endodontics* 84, 165–170.

Brownstein, M.H., Mehregan, A.R., Bikowski, B., Lupulescu, A. & Patterson, J.C. (1979) The dermatopathology of Cowden's syndrome. *British Journal of Dermatology* 100, 667–673.

Buchholz, F., Schubert, C. & Lehmann-Willenbrock, E. (1985) White sponge nevus of the vulva. *International Journal of Gynaecology and Obstetrics* 23, 505–507.

Buckley, D.A. & Barnes, L. (1996) Vulvar lymphangiectasia due to recurrent cellulitis. *Clinical and Experimental Dermatology* 21, 215–216.

Buckley, D.A. & Rogers, S. (1995) Cyclosporin-responsive hidradenitis suppurativa. *Journal of the Royal Society of Medicine* 88, 289–290.

Bucur, M. & Mahmood, T. (2004) Olanzipine induced clitoral priapism. *Journal of Clinical Psychopharmacology* 24, 572–573.

Buezo, G.F., Peçnas, P.F., Firaga, J., Alegre, A. & Aragües, M. (1996) Condyloma-like lesions as the presenting sign of multiple myeloma associated amyloidosis. *British Journal of Dermatology* **135**, 665–666.

Bulbul Baskan, E., Turan, H., Tunali, S., Toker, S.C. & Saricaoglu, H. (2007) Open-label trial of cyclosporine for vulvar lichen sclerosus. *Journal of the American Academy of Dermatology* **57**; 276–278.

Burge, S.M. (1992) Hailey–Hailey disease: the clinical features, response to treatment and prognosis. *British Journal of Dermatology* **126**, 275–282.

Burge, S.M., Frith, P.A., Juniper, R.P. & Wojnarowska, F.W. (1989) Mucosal involvement in systemic and chronic cutaneous lupus erythematosus. *British Journal of Dermatology* **121**, 727–741.

Burke, D.A., Adams, R.M. & Arundell, F.D. (1969) Febrile ulceronecrotic Mucha–Habermann's disease. *Archives of Dermatology* **100**, 200–206.

Burnett, J.W., Goldner, R. & Calton, G.J. (1975) Cowden's disease: report of 2 additional cases. *British Journal of Dermatology* **93**, 329–336.

Burrows, N.P. & Russell-Jones, R. (1992) Crohn's disease in association with hidradenitis suppurativa. *British Journal of Dermatology* **126**, 523–529.

Byrd, J.A., Davis, M. & Rogers, R.S. (2004) Recalcitrant symptomatic vulvar lichen planus. Response to topical tacrolimus. *Archives of Dermatology* **140**, 715–720.

Campagne, G., Roca, M. & Martinez, A. (2003) Successful treatment of a high-grade intraepithelial neoplasia with imiquimod, with vulvar pemphigus as a side effect. *European Journal of Obstetrics and Gynaecology and Reproductive Biology* **109**, 224–227.

Cantwell, A.R. (1984) Histologic observations of pleomorphic, variably acid-fast bacteria in scleroderma, morphoea, and lichen sclerosus et atrophicus. *International Journal of Dermatology* **23**, 45–52.

Carli, P., Cattaneo, A., Pimpinelli, N. *et al.* (1991) Immunohistochemical evidence of skin immune system involvement in vulvar lichen sclerosus and atrophicus. *Dermatologica* **182**, 18–22.

Carli, P., Cattaneo, A., de Magnis, A. *et al.* (1995) Squamous cell carcinoma arising in lichen sclerosus: a longitudinal cohort study. *European Journal of Cancer Prevention* **4**, 491–495.

Carli, P., Moretti, S., Spallanzani, A., Berti, E. & Cattaneo, A. (1997) Fibrogenic cytokines in vulvar lichen sclerosus. An immunohistochemical study. *Journal of Reproductive Medicine* **42**, 161–165.

Carrozzo, M. & Pellicano, R. (2008) Lichen planus and hepatitis C virus infection: an updated critical review. *Minerva Gastroenterology and Dietology* **54**, 65–74.

Cattaneo, A., Carli, P., de Marco, A. *et al.* (1996) Testosterone maintenance therapy. *Journal of Reproductive Medicine* **41**, 99–102.

Caughman, W., Stern, R. & Haines, H. (1983) Neutrophilic dermatoses of myeloproliferative disorders. *Journal of the American Academy of Dermatology* **9**, 751–758.

Caumes, E., Gatineau, M., Bricaire, F. *et al.* (1993) Foscarnet-induced vulvar erosion. *Journal of the American Academy of Dermatology* **28**, 799 (letter).

Celebi, S., Gül, A., Kamali, S. *et al.* (2001) Amyopathic dermatomyositis associated with cervical carcinoma. *Clinical Rheumatology* **20**, 438–440.

Chan, I., Oyama, N., Neill, S.M. *et al.* (2004) Characterization of IgG autoantibodies to extracellular matrix protein 1 in lichen sclerosus. *Clinical and Experimental Dermatology* **29**, 499–504.

Chaudhry, S.I., Morgan, P.R. & Neill, S.M. (2006) An unusual tongue. *Clinical and Experimental Dermatology* **31**, 831–832.

Chen, K.T.K. & Hendricks, E.J. (1985) Malakoplakia of the female genital tract. *Obstetrics and Gynecology* **65**, S84–S87.

Chorzelski, T.P., Kudejko, J. & Jablonska, S. (1984) Is papular acantholytic dyskeratosis of the vulva a new entity? *American Journal of Dermatopathology* **6**, 557–560.

Ciupinska, M., Kalbarczyk, K. & Jablonska, S. (1998) Disseminated papular acantholytic dyskeratosis. *Journal of the European Academy of Dermatology and Venereology* **11**, 55–58.

Claeys, A., Weber-Muller, F., Trechot, P. *et al.* (2006) Cutaneous, perivulvar and perianal ulcerations induced by nicorandil. *British Journal of Dermatology* **155**, 494–496.

Cockayne, S.E., Rassl, D.M. & Thomas, S.E. (2000) Squamous cell carcinoma arising in Hailey-Hailey disease of the vulva. *British Journal of Dermatology* **142**, 540–542.

Collet Villette, A.-M., Richard, M.A., Fouquet, F. *et al.* (2005) Treatment of Hailey-Hailey disease with carbon dioxide laser. *Annals of Dermatology and Venereology* **132**, 637–640.

Connelly, M.G. & Winkelmann, R.K. (1985) Coexistence of lichen sclerosus, morphea and lichen planus. Report of 4 cases and review of the literature. *Journal of the American Academy of Dermatology* **12**, 844–851.

Cooper, S.M. & Wojnarowska, F. (2006) Influence of treatment of erosive lichen planus of the vulva on its prognosis. *Archives of Dermatology* **142**, 289–294.

Cooper, J.C., Nicholls, A.J., Simms, J.M. *et al.* (1983) Genital oedema in patients treated by continuous ambulatory peritoneal dialysis. *British Medical Journal* **286**, 1923–1924.

Cooper, S.M., Dean, D., Allen, J. *et al.* (2005) Erosive lichen planus of the vulva: weak circulating basement membrane zone antibodies are present. *Clinical and Experimental Dermatology* **30**, 551–556.

Corazza, M., Virgili, A. & Mantovani, L. (1992) Vulvar contact dermatitis from nifuratel. *Contact Dermatitis* **27**, 273–274.

Cosman, B.C., O'Grady, T.C. & Pekarske, S. (2000) Verrucous carcinoma arising in hidradenitis suppurativa. *International Journal of Colorectal Disease* **15**, 342–346.

Coulson, I.H., Cook, M.G., Bruton, J. & Penfold, C. (1986) Atypical pemphigus vulgaris associated with angiofollicular lymph node hyperplasia (Castleman's disease). *Clinical and Experimental Dermatology* **11**, 656–663.

Crotty, C.P., Su, W.P.D. & Winkelmann, R.K. (1980) Ulcerative lichen planus. Follow up of surgical excision and grafting. *Archives of Dermatology* **116**, 1252–1256.

Crowe, F.W. (1964) Axillary freckling as a diagnostic aid in neurofibromatosis. *Annals of Internal Medicine* **61**, 1142–1143.

Crum, C.P. (1992) Carcinoma of the vulva: epidemiology and pathogenesis. *Obstetrics and Gynecology* **79**, 448–458.

Crum, C.P., McLachlin, C.M., Tate, J.E. & Mutter, G.L. (1997) Pathobiology of vulvar squamous neoplasia. *Current Opinion in Obstetrics and Gynecology* **9**, 63–69.

Cummins, D.L., Anhalt, G.J., Monahan, T. & Meyerle, J.H. (2007) Treatment of pyoderma gangrenosum with intravenous immunoglobulin. *British Journal of Dermatology* **157**, 1235–1239.

Dalziel, K.L. (1995) Effect of lichen sclerosus on sexual function and parturition. *Journal of Reproductive Medicine* **40**, 351–354.

Darier, J. (1892) Lichen plan scléreux. *Annales de Dermatologie et de Syphiligraphie* **3**, 833–837.

Davenport, D.M. & Richardson, D.A. (1986) Labial adhesions secondary to postpartum vulvar edema. Report of 2 cases. *Journal of Reproductive Medicine* **31**, 523–527.

Decavalas, G., Adonakis, G., Androutsopoulos, G., Gkermpesi, M.

& Kourounis, G. (2007) Sarcoidosis of the vulva: a case report. *Archives of Gynecology and Obstetrics* **275**, 203–205.

Dégos, R. & Ebrard, G. (1958) Leukokératose papillomateuse bucco-génitale. *Bulletin de la Société Française de Dermatologie et Syphiligraphie* **65**, 242.

de Oliveira Neto, M.P. (1972) Sarcoidose com lesoes da vulva. *Revista Brasileira de Medicina* **29**, 134–139.

Deppisch, L.M. (1983) Cervical melanosis. *Obstetrics and Gynecology* **62**, 525–526.

Derrick, E.K., Ridley, C.M., Kobza-Black, A. *et al.* (2000) A clinical study of 23 cases of female anogenital carcinoma. *British Journal of Dermatology* **143**, 1217–1223.

di Paola, G.R., Rueda-Leverone, N.G. & Becardi, M.G. (1982) Lichen sclerosus of the vulva recurrent after myocutaneous graft: a case report. *Journal of Reproductive Medicine* **27**, 666–668.

di Prima, T.M., de Pasquale, R. & Nigro, M.A. (1990) Connubial contact dermatitis from nifuratel. *Contact Dermatitis* **22**, 117–118.

Donlan, C.J. & Scutero, J.V. (1975) Transient eosinophilic pneumonia secondary to the use of a vaginal cream. *Chest* **67**, 232–233.

Duray, P.H., Merino, M.J. & Axiotis, C. (1983) Warty dyskeratoma of the vulva. *International Journal of Gynecological Pathology* **2**, 286–293.

Eberz, B., Berghold, A. & Regauer, S. (2008) High prevalence of concomitant anogenital lichen sclerosus and extra-genital psoriasis in adult women. *Obstetrics and Gynecology* **111**, 1143–1147.

Edwards, L. & Hansen, R. (1992) Reiter's syndrome of the vulva. The psoriasis spectrum. *Archives of Dermatology* **128**, 811–814.

Eigler, F.W., Schaarschmidt, K., Gross, E. & Richter, H.J. (1986) Anorectal ulcers as a complication of migraine therapy. *Journal of the Royal Society of Medicine* **79**, 424–426.

Eisen, D. (1994) The vulvovaginal–gingival syndrome of lichen planus. *Archives of Dermatology* **130**, 1379–1382.

Elsner, P., Wilhelm, D. & Maibach, H.I. (1990) Multiple parameter assessment of vulvar irritant contact dermatitis. *Contact Dermatitis* **23**, 20–26.

Emberger, M., Lanschnetzer, C.M., Laimer, M. *et al.* (2006) Vaginal adenosis induced by Stevens-Johnson syndrome. *Journal of the European Academy of Dermato-Venereology* **20**, 896–898.

Estrach, C., Mpofu, S. & Moots, R.J. (2002) Behçet's syndrome: response to infliximab after failure of etanercept. *Rheumatology* **41**, 1213–1214.

Ewing, T.L., Smale, L.E. & Elliott, F.A. (1979) Maternal deaths associated with postpartum vulvar edema. *American Journal of Obstetrics and Gynecology* **134**, 173–179.

Farage, M., Warren, R. & Wang-Weigand, S. (2000) The vulva is relatively insensitive to menses-induced irritation. *Cutaneous and Ocular Toxicology* **24**, 243–246.

Farage, M.A., Meyer, S.J. & Walter, D. (2004) Development of a sensitive test method to evaluate mechanical irritation potential of mucosal skin. *Skin Research Technology* **10**, 85.

Farrell, A.M., Millard, P.R., Schomberg, K.H. & Wojnarowksa, F. (1997) An infective aetiology for lichen sclerosus: myth or reality? *British Journal of Dermatology* **137** (Suppl 50), 25.

Farrell, A.M., Marren, P., Dean, D. & Wojnarowska, F. (1999) Lichen sclerosus: evidence that immunological changes occur at all levels of the skin. *British Journal of Dermatology* **140**, 1087–1092.

Fellers, E.D., Ribaudo, S. & Jackson, N.D. (2001) Gynecologic aspects of Crohn's Disease. *American Family Physician* **64**, 1725–1728.

Fenzy, A. & Bogomoletz, W.V. (1986) Anorectal ulceration due to abuse of dextropropoxyphene and paracetamol suppositories. *Journal of the Royal Society of Medicine* **80**, 62 (letter).

Ferré-Ybarz, L., Basagana, M., Coroleu, B., Bartolome, B. & Cistero-Bahima, A. (2006) Human seminal plasma allergy and successful pregnancy. *Journal of Investigative Allergy and Clinical Immunology* **16**, 314–316.

Finley, E.M. & Ratz, J.L. (1996) Treatment of hidradenitis suppurativa with carbon dioxide laser excision and secondary intention healing. *Journal of the American Academy of Dermatology* **34**, 465–469.

Fischer, G. (2007) Vulvar fixed drug eruption: a report of 13 cases. *Journal of Reproductive Medicine* **52**, 81–86.

Fischer, G. & Rogers, M. (1997) Treatment of childhood vulvar lichen sclerosus with a potent topical corticosteroid. *Pediatric Dermatology* **14**, 235–238.

Fischer, G.O. & Rogers, M. (2000) Vulvar disease in children: a clinical audit of 130 cases. *Paediatric Dermatology* **17**, 1–6.

Fisler, R.E., Saeb, M., Liang, M.G. *et al.* (2003) Childhood bullous pemphigoid: a clinico-pathological study and review of the literature. *American Journal of Dermatopathology* **25**, 183–189.

Foulds, I.S. (1980) Lichen sclerosus et atrophicus of the scalp. *British Journal of Dermatology* **103**, 197–200.

Franck, J.M. & Young, A.W. (1995) Squamous cell carcinoma in-situ arising within lichen planus of the vulva. *Dermatologic Surgery* **21**, 890–894.

Friedrich, E.G. (1976) New nomenclature for vulvar disease. Report of the committee on terminology. *Obstetrics and Gynecology* **47**, 122–124.

Friedrich, E.G. & Kalra, P.S. (1984) Serum levels of sex hormones in vulvar lichen sclerosus and the effect of topical testosterone. *New England Journal of Medicine* **310**, 488–491.

Friter, B.S. & Lucky, A.W. (1988) The perineal eruption of Kawasaki's syndrome. *Archives of Dermatology* **124**, 1805–1810.

Galbraith, S.S., Drolet, B.A., Kugathasan, S. *et al.* (2005) Asymptomatic inflammatory bowel disease presenting with mucocutaneous findings. *Pediatrics* **116**, 439–444.

Garnier, G. (1954) Vulvite érythémateuse circonscrite bénigne à type érythroplasique. *Bulletin de la Société Française de Dermatologie et de Syphilographie* **61**, 102–103.

Gencoglan, G. (2007) Dermoscopic findings in Laugier-Hunziker. *Archives of Dermatology* **143**, 631–633.

Gerbig, A.W. & Hunziker, T. (1996) Idiopathic lenticular mucocutaneous pigmentation or Laugier–Hunziker syndrome with atypical features. *Archives of Dermatology* **32**, 844–845.

Gilchrist, H., Jackson, S., Morse, L. & Nesbitt, L.T. (2008) Galli-Galli disease: a case report and review of the literature. *Journal of the American Academy of Dermatology* **58**, 299–302.

Goldberg, N.S., Esterley, N.B., Rothman, K.F. *et al.* (1992) Perianal pseudoverrucous papules and nodules in children. *Archives of Dermatology* **128**, 240–242.

Goldman, H.B., Idom, C.B. & Dmochowski, R.R. (1998) Traumatic injuries of the female external genitalia and their association with urological injuries. *Journal of Urology* **159**, 956–959.

Goldsmith, P.C., Rycroft, R.J.G., White, I.R. *et al.* (1997) Contact sensitivity in women patients with anogenital dermatoses. *Contact Dermatitis* **36**, 174–175.

Goodman, A., Zukerberg, L.R., Nikrui, N. & Scully, R.E. (1991) Vaginal adenosis and clear cell carcinoma after 5-fluorouracil treatment for condyloma. *Cancer* **68**, 1628–1632.

Goodman, R.M., Smith, E.W., Paton, D. *et al.* (1963) Pseudoxanthoma elasticum: a clinical and histological study. *Medicine* **42**, 297–334.

Gorodeski, I.G., Cordoba, M., Shapira, A. & Bahary, C.M. (1988) Primary localized cutaneous lichen amyloidosis of the vulva. *International Journal of Dermatology* **27**, 259–260.

Graham-Brown, R.A.C., Cochrane, G.W., Swinhoe, J.R., Sarkany, I. & Epsztejn, L.J. (1981) Vaginal stenosis due to bullous erythema multiforme (Stevens–Johnson syndrome). *British Journal of Obstetrics and Gynaecology* 88, 1156–1157.

Grasinger, C.C., Wild, R.A. & Parker, I.J. (1993) Vulvar acanthosis nigricans: a marker for insulin resistance in hirsute women. *Fertility and Sterility* 59, 583–586.

Greene, S.L. & Muller, S.A. (1985) Netherton's syndrome. Report of a case and review of the literature. *Journal of the American Academy of Dermatology* 13, 329–337.

Greenspan, A.H., Shupack, J.L., Foo, S.H. & Wise, A.C. (1985) Acanthosis nigricans like eruption hyperpigmentation secondary to triazinate therapy. *Archives of Dermatology* 121, 232–235.

Greenstein, A.J., Gennuso, R., Sachar, D.B. *et al.* (1985) Extraintestinal cancers in inflammatory bowel disease. *Cancer* 56, 2914–2921.

Grimmer, H. (1968) Apokrine miliaria der Vulva (subcorneale Schweissdrüsen-retention). *Zeitschrift für Haut und Geslechts-Krankheit* 43, 123–132.

Gruber, F., Stasić, A., Lenković, M. & Brajac, I. (1997) Postcoital fixed drug eruption in a man sensitive to trimethoprim–sulpha-methoxazole. *Clinical and Experimental Dermatology* 22, 144–145.

Gunter, J. & Golitz, L. (2005) Topical misoprostol therapy for plasma cell vulvitis: a case series. *Journal of Lower Genital Tract Disease* 9, 176–180.

Haake, N. & Altmeyer, P. (1988) Vulvovaginitis circinata bei Morbus Reiter. *Hautarzt* 39, 748–749.

Habek, D. & Kulas, T. (2007) Non-obstetric vulvovaginal injuries: mechanism and outcome. *Archives of Gynecology and Obstetrics* 275, 93–97.

Hackel, H., Hartmann, A.A. & Burg, G. (1991) Vulvitis granulomatosa and anoperineitis granulomatosa. *Dermatologica* 182, 128–131.

Hacker, S.M. (1994) Absence of anti-single stranded DNA antibodies in vulvar lichen sclerosus and atrophicus. *Archives of Dermatology* 130, 1454–1455.

Hallel-Halevy, D., Grunwald, M.H. & Halevy, S. (1993) Confluent and reticulate papillomatosis (Gougerot-Carteaud) of the pubic region. *Acta Dermato-venereologica* 73, 155.

Hallopeau, H. (1887) Leçons cliniques sur les maladies cutanées et syphilitiques. *L'Union Médicale* 43, 742–747.

Hallopeau, H. (1889) Lichen plan scléreux. *Annales de Dermatologie et de Syphiligraphie* (2nd series) 10, 447–449.

Haverhoek, E., Reid, C., Gordon, L. *et al.* (2008) Prospective study of patch tests in patients with vulval pruritus. *Australasian Journal of Dermatology* 49, 80–85.

Heffernan, M.P., Smith, D.I., Bentley, D. *et al.* (2007) A single-center, open-label, prospective pilot study of subcutaneous efaluziamb for oral erosive lichen planus. *Journal of Drugs in Dermatology* 6, 310–314.

Hernando, L.B., Sebastian, F.V., Sanchez, J.H., Romero, P.O. & Diez, L.I. (1992) Lichen planus pemphigoides in a 10 year old girl. *Journal of the American Academy of Dermatology* 26, 124–125.

Hewitt, J. (1986) Histologic criteria for lichen sclerosus of the vulva. *Journal of Reproductive Medicine* 31, 781–787.

Hobbs, J.T. (2005) Varicose veins arising from the pelvis due to ovarian vein incompetence. *International Journal of Clinical Practice* 59, 1195–1203.

Hoque, S.R., Patel, M. & Farrell, A.M. (2006) Childhood cicatricial pemphigoid confined to the vulva. *Clinical and Experimental Dermatology* 31, 63–64.

Huey, G.R., Stehman, F.B., Roth, L.M. & Ehrlich, C.E. (1985) Lymphangioma of the edematous thigh after radiation therapy for carcinoma of the vulva. *Gynecologic Oncology* 20, 394–401.

Hughes, B.R., Holt, P.J.A. & Marks, R. (1987) Trimethoprim associated fixed drug eruption. *British Journal of Dermatology* 116, 241–242.

Hurd, D.S., Johnston, C. & Bevins, A. (2008) A case report of Hailey-Hailey disease treated with alefacept (Amevive). *British Journal of Dermatology* 158, 399–401.

James, W.D. & Lupton, G.P. (1988) Acquired dyskeratotic leukoplakia. *Archives of Dermatology* 124, 117–120.

Jayle, F. (1906) Le kraurosis vulvae. *Revue de Gynécologie et de Chirurgie Abdominale* 10, 633–668.

Jeffcoate, T.N.A. & Woodcock, A.S. (1961) Premalignant conditions of the vulva, with particular reference to chronic epithelial dystrophies. *British Medical Journal* 2, 127–134.

Jemec, G.B.E. & Hansen, U. (1996) Histology of hidradenitis suppurativa. *Journal of the American Academy of Dermatology* 34, 994–999.

Johns, A.M. & Bower, B.D. (1970) Wasting of napkin area after repeated use of fluorinated steroid. *British Medical Journal* 1, 347–348.

Jolly, M. & Patel, P. (2006) Looking beyond the ordinary: genital lupus. *Arthritis and Rheumatism* 55, 821–822.

Jones, W.R. (1991) Allergy to coitus. *Australian and New Zealand Journal of Obstetrics and Gynaecology* 31, 137–141.

Jones, R.W., Scurry, J., Neill, S. & MacLean, A.B. (2008) Guidelines for the follow-up of women with vulvar lichen sclerosus in specialist clinics. *American Journal of Obstetrics and Gynecology* 198, 496.

Jonquières, E.D.L. & de Lutsky, F.K. (1980) Balanites et vulvites pseudo-érythroplasiques chroniques. Aspects histopathologiques. *Annales de Dermatologie et de Vénéréologie* 107, 173–180.

Joosse, L.A., Koudstaal, J. & Oswald, F.H. (1964) Chromidrosis vulvae. *Tijdschrift voor Verloskunde und Gynecologie* 64, 179–187.

Joseph, M.A., Jayaseelan, E., Ganapathi, B. *et al.* (2005) Hidradenitis suppurativa treated with finasteride. *Journal of Dermatological Treatment* 16, 75–78.

Kanai, M., Osada, R., Maruyama, K. *et al.* (2001) Warning from Nagano: increase of vulvar hematoma and /or lacerated injury from snowboarding. *Journal of Trauma* 50, 328–331.

Kao, M.S., Paulson, J.D. & Askin, F.B. (1975) Crohn's disease of the vulva. *Obstetrics and Gynecology* 46, 329–333.

Kartamaa, M. & Reitamo, S. (1997) Treatment of lichen sclerosus with carbon dioxide laser vaporization. *British Journal of Dermatology* 136, 356–359.

Kato, T., Kuramoto, Y., Tadaki, T., Hashimoto, K. & Tagami, H. (1990) Chronic vulvar purpura. *Dermatologica* 180, 174–176.

Kavanagh, G.M., Burton, P.A. & Kennedy, C.T.C. (1993) Vulvitis chronica plasmacellularis (Zoon's vulvitis). *British Journal of Dermatology* 129, 92–93.

Keefe, M., Wakeel, R.A. & Kerr, R.E.I. (1988) Sweet's syndrome, plantar pustulosis and vulval pustules. *Clinical and Experimental Dermatology* 13, 344–346.

Kelly, S.C., Helm, K.F. & Zaenglein, A.L. (2006) Lichen sclerosus of the lip. *Pediatric Dermatology* 23, 500–502.

Kint, B., Degreef, H. & Dooms-Goossens, A. (1994) Combined allergy to human seminal plasma and latex: case report and review of the literature. *Contact Dermatitis* 30, 7–11.

Kobashigawa, T., Okamoto, H., Kato, J. *et al.* (2004) Ulcerative colitis followed by the development of Behçet's disease. *Internal Medicine* 43, 243–247.

Kogulan, P.K., Smith, M., Seidman, J. *et al.* (2001) Malakoplakia involving the abdominal wall, urinary bladder, vagina, and vulva: case report and discussion of malakoplakia-associated bacteria. *International Journal Gynecological Pathology* **20**, 403–406.

Kohl, S.K. & Hans, C.P. (2008) Cutaneous malakoplakia. *Archives of Pathology & Laboratory Medicine* **132**, 113–117.

Konishi, A., Fukuoka, M. & Nishimura, Y. (2007) Primary localised cutaneous amyloidosis with unusual clinical features in a patient with Sjögren's syndrome. *Journal of Dermatology* **34**, 394–396.

Kopecky, R.T., Funk, M.M. & Kreitzer, P.R. (1985) Localized genital edema in patients undergoing continuous ambulatory peritoneal dialysis. *Journal of Urology* **134**, 880–884.

Kortekangas-Savolainen, O. & Kiilholma, P. (2007) Treatment of vulvovaginal erosive and stenosing lichen planus by surgical dilatation and methotrexate. *Acta Obstetrica et Gynecologica Scandinavica* **86**, 339–343.

Kranl, C., Zelger, B., Kofler, H. *et al.* (1998) Vulvar & vaginal adenosis. *British Journal of Dermatology* **139**, 128–131.

Kruppa, A., Korge, B., Lasch, J. *et al.* (2000) Successful treatment of Hailey-Hailey disease with a scanned carbon dioxide laser. *Acta Dermato-venereologica* **80**, 53–54.

Kübler, H.C., Kühn, W., Rummel, H.H., Kaufmann, I. & Kaufmann, M. (1987) Zur Karzinoentstehung (Vulvakarzinom) beim Netherton-Syndrom (Ichthyosis, Haaranomalien, atopische Diathese). *Geburtshilfe und Frauenheilkunde* **47**, 742–744.

Kuo, J.H., Smith, L.M. & Berkowitz, C.D. (2002) A hair tourniquet resulting in strangulation and amputation of the clitoris. *Obstetrics and Gynecology* **99**, 939–941.

Kuroda, K., Kojima, T., Fujita, M., Iseki, T. & Shinkai, H. (1995) Unusual cutaneous manifestations of the myelodysplastic syndrome. *British Journal of Dermatology* **133**, 483–486.

Lacey, H.B., Ness, A. & Mandal, B.K. (1992) Vulval ulceration associated with foscarnet. *Genitourinary Medicine* **68**, 182.

Lambiris, A. & Greaves, M.W. (1997) Dyspareunia and vulvodynia: unrecognised manifestations of symptomatic dermographism. *Lancet* **349**, 28.

Landthaler, M., Hohenleutner, U. & Braun-Falco, O. (1990) Acquired lymphangioma of the vulva: palliative treatment by means of laser vaporization carbon dioxide. *Archives of Dermatology* **126**, 967–968.

Lapiere, J.C., Hirsch, A., Gordon, K.B. *et al.* (2000) Botulinum toxin Type A for the treatment of Hailey-Hailey disease. *Dermatological Surgery* **26**, 371–374.

Laplanche, C., Grosshans, E. & Heid, G. (1984) Anorectal ulcerations after prolonged use of suppositories containing dextropopoxyphene. *Annales de Dermatologie et de Vénéréologie* **111**, 347–355.

Lavery, H.A. (1984) Vulval dystrophies: new approaches. *Clinics in Obstetrics and Gynaecology* **11**, 155–169.

Lavery, H.A., Pinkerton, J.H.M., Roberts, S.D., Sloan, J. & Walsh, M. (1985) Dermatomyositis of the vulva–first reported case. *British Journal of Dermatology* **113**, 349–352.

Lebbe, C., Moulonguet-Michau, I., Perrin, P. *et al.* (1992) Steroid-responsive pyoderma gangrenosum with vulvar and pulmonary involvement. *Journal of the American Academy of Dermatology* **27**, 623–625.

le Boit, P.E. (1996) Multinucleated atypia. *American Journal of Surgical Pathology* **20**, 507.

Lee, M.S. & Barnetson, R.S. (1996) Sweet's syndrome associated with Behçet's disease. *Australasian Journal of Dermatology* **37**, 99–101.

Lee Wong, M., Collins, J.S., Nozad, C. & Resnick, D.J. (2008) The diagnosis and treatment of human seminal plasma hypersensitivity. *Obstetrics and Gynecology* **111**, 538–539.

Leibowitch, M., Neill, S., Pelisse, M. & Moyal-Barracco, M. (1990) The epithelial changes associated with squamous carcinoma of the vulva: a review of the clinical, histological and virological findings in 78 women. *British Journal of Obstetrics and Gynaecology* **97**, 1135–1139.

Leppard, B. & Sneddon, I.B. (1975) Milia occurring in lichen sclerosus et atrophicus. *British Journal of Dermatology* **92**, 711–714.

Leung, A.K.C., Robson, W.L.M. & Tay-Uyboco, J. (1993) The incidence of labial fusion in children. *Journal of Paediatrics and Child Health* **29**, 235–236.

Levine, V., Sanchez, M. & Nestor, M. (1992) Localized vulvar pemphigoid in a child misdiagnosed as sexual abuse. *Archives of Dermatology* **128**, 804–806.

Lewis, F.M. & Harrington, C.I. (1994) Squamous cell carcinoma arising in vulval lichen planus. *British Journal of Dermatology* **131**, 703–705.

Lewis, F.M., Harrington, C.I. & Gawkrodger, D.J. (1994a) Contact sensitivity in pruritus vulvae: a common and manageable problem. *Contact Dermatitis* **31**, 264–265.

Lewis, F.M., Gawkrodger, D.J. & Harrington, C.I. (1994b) Colophony: an unusual factor in pruritus vulvae. *Contact Dermatitis* **31**, 119.

Lewis, F.M., Shah, M. & Harrington, C.I. (1996) Vulval involvement in lichen planus: a study of 37 women. *British Journal of Dermatology* **135**, 89–91.

Li, Q., Leopold, K. & Carlson, J.A.(2003) Chronic vulvar purpura: persistent pigmented purpuric dermatitis (lichen aureus) of the vulva or plasma cell (Zoon's) vulvitis? *Journal of Cutaneous Pathology* **30**, 572–576.

Lim, J. & Ng, S.K. (1992) Oral tetracycline rinse improves symptoms of white sponge nevus. *Journal of the American Academy of Dermatology* **26**, 1003–1005.

Lindskov, R. (1984) Acute febrile neurophilic dermatosis with genital involvement. *Acta Dermato-venereologica* **64**, 559–561.

Lipschutz, B. (1913) Über eine eigenartige Geschwürsform des Weiblichen Genitales (ulcus vulvae acutum). *Archiv für Dermatologie und Syphilis (Berlin)* **114**, 363–396.

Lonsdale, R.N. & Gibbs, S. (1998) Pemphigus vulgaris with involvement of the cervix. *British Journal of Dermatology* **138**, 363–365.

Lonsdale-Eccles, A.A. & Velangi, S. (2005) Topical pimecrolimus in the treatment of genital lichen planus: a prospective case series. *British Journal of Dermatology* **153**, 390–394.

Lotan, T.L., Tefs, K., Schuster, V. *et al.* (2007) Inherited plasminogen deficiency presenting as ligneous vaginitis: a case report with molecular correlation and review of the literature. *Human Pathology* **38**, 1569–1575.

Lurie, S., Manor, M. & Hagay, Z.J. (1998) The threat of type IV Ehlers–Danlos syndrome on maternal well-being during pregnancies: early delivery may make a difference. *Journal of Obstetrics and Gynaecology* **18**, 245–248.

Lutterloh, C.H. & Shellenberger, P.L. (1946) Unusual pigmentation developing after prolonged suppressive therapy with quinacrine hydrochloride. *Archives of Dermatology* **53**, 349.

Luxman, D., Cohen, J.R., Gordon, D. *et al.* (1996) Unilateral vulvar edema associated with severe ovarian hyperstimulation syndrome. *Journal of Reproductive Medicine* **41**, 771–774.

Lynch, P.J., Moyal-Barracco, M., Bogliatto, F., Micheletti, L. & Scurry, J. (2007) 2006 ISSVD classification of vulvar dermatoses:

pathologic subsets and their clinical correlates. *Journal of Reproductive Medicine* **52**, 3–9.

Maekawa, Y., Sakazaki, Y. & Hayashibara, T. (1978) Diaper area granuloma of the aged. *Archives of Dermatology* **114**, 382–383.

Malik, M. & Ahmed, A.R. (2005) Involvement of the genital tract in pemphigus vulgaris. *Obstetrics and Gynecology* **106**, 1005–1012.

Marchesoni, D., Mozzanega, B., De Sandre, P. *et al.* (1995) Gynaecological aspects of primary Sjögren's syndrome. *European Journal of Obstetrics, Gynaecology and Reproductive Biology* **63**, 49–53.

Marcoux, C., Bourland, A. & Decroix, J. (1991) Hyperplasie angiolymphoïde avec éosinophilie (HALE). *Annales de Dermatologie et de Vénéréologie* **118**, 217–221.

Marren, P., Wojnarowska, F. & Powell, S. (1992) Allergic contact dermatitis and vulvar dermatoses. *British Journal of Dermatology* **126**, 52–56.

Marren, P., Wojnarowska, F., Venning, V., Wilson, C. & Nayar, M. (1993) Vulvar involvement in autoimmune bullous diseases. *Journal of Reproductive Medicine* **38**, 101–107.

Marren, P., Millard, P., Chia, Y. & Wojnarowska, F. (1994) Mucosal lichen sclerosus/lichen planus overlap syndromes. *British Journal of Dermatology* **131**, 118–123.

Marren, P., Yell, J., Charnock, F.M. *et al.* (1995) The association between lichen sclerosus and antigens of the HLA system. *British Journal of Dermatology* **132**, 197–203.

Marren, P.M., Millard, P.R. & Wojnarowska, F. (1997a) Vulval lichen sclerosus: lack of correlation between duration of clinical symptoms and histological appearances. *Journal of the European Academy of Dermatology and Venereology* **8**, 212–216.

Marren, P., Dean, D., Charnock, M. & Wojnarowska, F. (1997b) The basement membrane zone in lichen sclerosus: an immunohistochemical study. *British Journal of Dermatology* **136**, 508–514.

Martin, J. & Holdstock, G. (1997) Isolated vulval oedema as a feature of Crohn's disease. *Journal of Obstetrics and Gynaecology* **17**, 92–93.

McCalmont, C.S., Leshin, B., White, W.L., Greiss, F.C. & Jorizzo, J.L. (1991) Vulvar pyoderma gangrenosum. *International Journal of Gynecology and Obstetrics* **35**, 175–178.

McDonagh, A.J.G., Gawkrodger, D.J. & Walker, A.E. (1990) White sponge naevus successfully treated with topical tetracycline. *Clinical and Experimental Dermatology* **15**, 152–153.

McLachlin, C.M., Mutter, G.L. & Crum, C.P. (1994) Multinucleated atypia of the vulva. Report of a distinct entity not associated with human papillomavirus. *American Journal of Surgical Pathology* **18**, 1233–1239.

McQueen, J. (1974) Self-inflicted vaginal ulceration treated by infibulation. *Proceedings of the Royal Society of Medicine* **67**, 15–16.

Meffert, J.J. & Grimwood, R.E. (1994) Lichen sclerosus appearing in an old burn scar. *Journal of the American Academy of Dermatology* **31**, 671–673.

Mendonça, C.O. & Griffiths, C.E.M. (2006) Clindamycin and rifampicin combination therapy for hidradenitis suppurativa. *British Journal of Dermatology* **154**, 977–978.

Meneux, E., Paniel, B.J., Pouget, F. *et al.* (1997) Vulvovaginal sequelae in toxic epidermal necrolysis. *Journal of Reproductive Medicine* **42**, 153–156.

Meyrick Thomas, R.H., McGibbon, D.H. & Munro, D.D. (1985) Basal cell carcinoma of the vulva in association with vulval lichen sclerosus et atrophicus. *Journal of the Royal Society of Medicine* **78** (Suppl 2), 16–18.

Meyrick Thomas, R.H., Ridley, C.M., McGibbon, D.H. & Black, M.M. (1988) Lichen sclerosus and autoimmunity – a study of 350 women. *British Journal of Dermatology* **118**, 41–46.

Meyrick Thomas, R.H., Ridley, C.M., McGibbon, D.H. & Black, M.M. (1996) Ano-genital lichen sclerosus in women. *Journal of the Royal Society of Medicine* **89**, 694–698.

Michael, A. & Mayer, C. (2000) Fluoxetine-induced anaesthesia of the vagina and nipples. *British Journal of Psychiatry* **176**, 299.

Michael, A. & Andrews, S. (2002) Paroxetine-induced vaginal anaesthesia. *Pharmacopsychiatry* **35**, 150–151.

Micheletti, L., Preti, M., Bogliatto, F. *et al.* (2000) Vulval lichen planus in the practice of a vulval clinic. *British Journal of Dermatology* **143**, 1349–1350.

Milde, P., Goerz, G. & Plewig, G. (1992) Dowling-Degos disease with exclusively genital manifestations. *Hautarzt* **43**, 369–372.

Montegi, S., Tamura, A., Okada, E. *et al.* (2007) Successful treatment with lymphaticovenular anastomosis for secondary skin lesions of chronic lymphoedema. *Dermatology* **215**, 147–151.

Montes-Romero, J.A., Callejas-Rubio, J.L., Sánchez-Cano, D. *et al.* (2008) Amyloidosis secondary to hidradenitis suppurativa. Exceptional response to infliximab. *European Journal of Internal Medicine*, in press.

Morgan, E.D., Laszlo, J.D.B. & Stumpf, P.G. (1988) Incomplete Behçet's syndrome in the differential diagnosis of genital ulceration and post-coital bleeding: a case report. *Journal of Reproductive Medicine* **33**, 844–846.

Morioko, S., Nakajima, S., Yaguchi, H. *et al.* (1988) Vulvitis circumscripta plasmacellularis treated successfully with interferon alpha. *Journal of the American Academy of Dermatology* **19**, 947–950.

Mortimer, P.S., Dawber, R.P.R., Gales, M.A. & Moore, R.A. (1986a) Mediation of hidradenitis suppurativa by androgens. *British Medical Journal* **292**, 245–248.

Mortimer, P.S., Dawber, R.P.R., Gales, M.A. & Moore, R.A. (1986b) A double-blind cross-over trial of cyproterone acetate in females with hidradenitis suppurativa. *British Journal of Dermatology* **115**, 263–268.

Moschella, S.L. (2007) Is there a role for infliximab in the current therapy of hidradenitis suppurativa? A report of three treated cases. *International Journal of Dermatology* **46**, 1287–1291.

Mottl, H., Rob, L., Stary, J., Kodet, R. & Drahokoupilova, E. (2007) Langerhans cell histiocytosis of vulva in adolescent. *International Journal of Gynecological Cancer* **17**, 520–524.

Moyal-Barracco, M., Lautier-Frau, M., Bechérel, P.A. *et al.* (1993) Lichen plan conjunctival: une observation. *Annales de Dermatologie et de Vénéréologie* **120**, 857–859.

Mulherin, D.M., Sheeran, T.P., Kumararatne, D.S. *et al.* (1997) Sjögren's syndrome presenting in chronic dyspareunia. *British Journal of Obstetrics and Gynaecology* **104**, 1019–1023.

Muram, D. & Gold, S.S. (1993) Vulvar ulcerations in girls with myelocytic leukemia. *Southern Medical Journal* **86**, 293–294.

Nagano, T., Tani, M., Adachi, A. *et al.* (1994) Childhood bullous pemphigoid: immunohistochemical, immunoelectron microscopic and Western blot analysis. *Journal of the American Academy of Dermatology* **39**, 884–888.

Neill, S.M., Smith, N.P. & Eady, R.A.J. (1984) Ulcerative sarcoidosis: a rare manifestation of a common disease. *Clinical and Experimental Dermatology* **9**, 277–279.

Neill, S.M., Tatnall, F.M. & Cox, N.H. (2002) Guidelines for the management of lichen sclerosus. *British Journal of Dermatology* **147**, 640–649.

Newton, J.A., Camplejohn, R.S. & McGibbon, D.H. (1987) A flow cytometric study of the significance of DNA aneuploidy in cutaneous lesions. *British Journal of Dermatology* **117**, 169–174.

Nichols, G.E., Cooper, P.H., Underwood, P.B. & Greer, K.E. (1990) White sponge nevus. *Obstetrics and Gynecology* 76, 545–548.

Niinimäki, A., Kallioinen, M & Oikarinen, A. (1989) Etretinate reduces connective tissue degeneration in lichen sclerosus et atrophicus. *Acta Dermato-venereologica* 69, 439–442.

Nissi, R., Eriksen, H., Risteli, J. & Niemimaa, M. (2007) Pimecrolimus cream 1% in the treatment of lichen sclerosus. *Gynecologic and Obstetric Investigation* 63, 151–154.

Northcutt, A.D. & Vanover, M.J. (1985) Nodular cutaneous amyloidosis involving the vulva. *Archives of Dermatology* 121, 518–521.

Ochiai, T., Honda, A., Morishima, T. *et al.* (1999) Human papillomavirus types 16 and 39 in a vulval carcinoma occurring in a woman with Hailey-Hailey disease. *British Journal of Dermatology* 140, 509–513.

O'Goshi, K., Terui, T. & Tagami, H. (2001) Dowling-Degos disease affecting the vulva. *Acta Dermato-venereologica* 81, 148.

Oikarinen, A., Sandberg, M., Aurskainen, T., Kinnnunen, T. & Kallioinen, M. (1991) Collagen biosynthesis in lichen sclerosus et atrophicus studied by biochemical *in situ* hybridization techniques. *Acta Dermato-venereologica. Supplementum.* 162, 3–12.

Okur, M., Yildirim, A. & Köse, R. (2005) Severe haematoma of the vulva and defloration caused by goring. *European Journal of Obstetrics and Gynaecology and Reproductive Biology* 119, 250–252.

Oprica, C. & Nord, C.E. (2006) Bacteriology of hidradenitis suppurativa. In: Hidradenitis suppurativa (eds G. Jemec, J. Revuz, J. Leyden), pp. 86–94. Springer Verlag, Berlin.

Ormerod, A.D. (2005) Topical tacrolimus and pimecrolimus and the risk of cancer: how much cause for concern? *British Journal of Dermatology* 153, 701–5.

Ormsby, O. & Mitchell, J.H. (1922) Lichen planus atrophicus et sclerosus and kraurosis vulvae. *Archives of Dermatology and Syphilology* 5, 786.

Ostlere, L.S., Tildsley, G. & Holden, C.A. (1996) Lichen sclerosus over a strawberry naevus: a new example of the Koebner phenomenon? [Letter]. *Clinical and Experimental Dermatology* 21, 394–395.

Ozkaya-Bayazit, E. (2003) Specific site involvement in fixed drug eruption. *Journal of the American Academy of Dermatology* 49, 1003–1007.

Pados, G., Vavilis, D., Pantazis, K. *et al.* (2005) Unilateral vulval edema after operative laparoscopy: a case report and literature review. *Fertility and Sterility* 83, 471–473.

Pandolfini, T.L., Cottell, S. & Katta, R. (2001) Pigmented vulvar macules as a presenting feature of the Carney complex. *International Journal of Dermatology* 40, 728–730.

Park, S.B., Cho, K.H., Youn, J.I. *et al.* (1997) Epidermolysis bullosa acquisita in childhood – a case mimicking chronic bullous disease of childhood. *Clinical and Experimental Dermatology* 22, 220–222.

Pass, C.J. (1984) An unusual variant of lichen sclerosus et atrophicus: delayed appearance in a surgical scar. *Cutis* 33, 405–408.

Patterson, J.A.K. & Ackerman, A.B. (1984) Lichen sclerosus et atrophicus is not related to morphea. A clinical and histological study of 24 patients in whom both conditions were reputed to be present simultaneously. *American Journal of Dermatopathology* 6, 323–335.

Pelisse, M. (1996) Erosive vulvar lichen planus and desquamative vaginitis. *Seminars in Dermatology* 15, 47–50.

Pelisse, M., Leibowitch, M., Sedel, D. & Hewitt, J. (1982) Un nouveau syndrome vulvo-vagino-gingival. Lichen plan érosif plurimuqueux. *Annales de Dermatologie et de Vénéréologie* 110, 797–798.

Perrin, L. (1901) Contribution à l'étude de la leucoplasie vulvo-anale, ses rapports avec le kraurosis vulvae, son traitement. *Annales de Dermatologie et de Syphiligraphie* 2, 21–28.

Pescatori, E.S., Engelman, J.C., Davis, G. & Goldstein, I. (1993) Priapism of the clitoris: a case report following trazodone use. *Journal of Urology* 149, 1557–1559.

Petersen, C.S., Brocks, K., Weisman, K., Kobayasi, T. & Thomsen, H.K. (1996) Pretibial epidermolysis bullosa with vulvar involvement. *Acta Dermato-venereologica* 76, 80–81.

Pock, L., Svrcková, M., Macháčková, R. & Hercogová, J. (2006) Pimecrolimus is effective in Fox-Fordyce disease. *International Journal of Dermatology* 45, 1134–1135.

Pokorny, S.F. (1992) Prepubertal vulvovaginopathies. *Obstetrics and Gynecology Clinics of North America* 19, 39–58.

Ponyai, G., Kárpáti, S., Ablonczy, E. *et al.* (1999) Benign familial chronic pemphigus (Hailey-Hailey) provoked by contact sensitivity in two patients. *Contact Dermatitis* 40, 168–169.

Powell, J. (2006) Paediatric vulval disorders. *Journal of Obstetrics and Gynaecology* 26, 596–602.

Powell, J., Wojnarowska, F., Winsey, S. *et al.* (2000) Lichen sclerosus premenarche: autoimmunity and immunogenetics. *British Journal of Dermatology* 142, 481–484.

Prezyna, A.P. & Kalyanaraman, B. (1977) Bowen's carcinoma in vulvovaginal Crohn's disease (regional enterocolitis): report of first case. *American Journal of Obstetrics and Gynecology* 128, 914–915.

Quinn, T.R. & Young, R.H. (1997) Epidermolytic hyperkeratosis in the lower female genital tract: an uncommon stimulant of mucocutaneous papillomavirus infection – a report of two cases. *International Journal of Gynaecological Pathology* 16, 163–168.

Radman, H.M. & Bhagavan, B.S. (1972) Pilonidal disease of the female genitalia. *American Journal of Obstetrics and Gynecology* 114, 271–272.

Raguin, G., Boisnic, S., Souteyrand, P. *et al.* (1992) No evidence for a spirochaetal origin of localized scleroderma. *British Journal of Dermatology* 127, 218–220.

Rainford, D. (1970) Southey's tubes and vulval oedema. *British Medical Journal* 4, 538.

Ramrakha-Jones, V.S., Paul, M., McHenry, P. & Burden, A.D. (2001) Nail dystrophy due to lichen sclerosus? *Clinical and Experimental Dermatology* 26, 507–509.

Rasmussen, H.B., Hagdrup, H. & Schmidt, H. (1986) Psoriasiform napkin dermatitis. *Acta Dermatology Venereology* 66, 534–536.

Rebora, A., Parodi, A. & Marialdo, G. (2002) Basiliximab is effective for erosive lichen planus. *Archives of Dermatology* 138, 1100–1111.

Reed, O.M., Mellette, J.R. & Fitzpatrick, J.E. (1986) Cutaneous lentiginosis with atrial myxomas. *Journal of the American Academy of Dermatology* 15, 398–402.

Rege, V.L. & Shukla, P. (1993) Osteomyelitis presenting as genital sore: a case report. *Genitourinary Medicine* 69, 460–461.

Reyman, L., Milano, A., Demopoulos, R., Mayron, J. & Schuster, S. (1986) Metastatic vulvar ulceration in Crohn's disease. *American Journal of Gastroenterology* 81, 46–49.

Rhodes, A.R., Silverman, R.A., Harrist, T.J. & Perez-Atayde, A.R. (1986) Mucocutaneous lentigines cardiomuco-cutaneous myxomas and multiple blue nevi: the LAMB syndrome. *Journal of the American Academy of Dermatology* 10, 72–82.

Ricard-Rothiot, L., Ruiz-Hernandez, C.E. & Fernandez-Torres, E. (1979) Acquired vaginal atresia in Sjögren's syndrome. *Ginecologyica y Obstetricia de Mexico* 45, 217–222.

Ridley, C.M., Frankman, O., Jones, I.S.C. *et al.* (1989) New nomenclature for vulvar disease: report of the committee on terminology. *American Journal of Obstetrics and Gynecology* 160, 769.

Roberts, D.C., Whitaker, I.S. & Drew, P. (2007) Perineal scalds from drive through restaurants: a public health hazard. *Burns* 33, 258–260.

Robson, K., Maughan, J., Purcell, S. *et al.* (2006) Erosive papulonodular dermatosis associated with topical benzocaine: a report of 2 cases and evidence that granuloma gluteale, pseudoverrucous papules and Jacquet's erosive dermatitis are a disease spectrum. *Journal of the American Academy of Dermatology* 55, S74–S80.

Rocamora, A., Santonja, C., Vives, R. & Varona, C. (1986) Sebaceous gland hyperplasia of the vulva: a case report. *Obstetrics and Gynecology* 68, S63–S65.

Romaguera, C. & Grimalt, F. (1981) Contact dermatitis from a copper containing IUD. *Contact Dermatitis* 7, 163–164.

Roman, L.D., Mitchell, M.D., Burke, T.W. & Silva, E.G. (1991) Unsuspected invasive squamous carcinoma of the vulva in young women. *Gynecologic Oncology* 41, 182–185.

Rosamilia, L.L., Schwartz, J.L., Lowe, L. *et al.* (2006) Vulvar melanoma in a 10-year-old girl in association with lichen sclerosus. *Journal of the American Academy of Dermatology* 54 (Suppl 1), S52–S53.

Rosenzweig, L.B., Brett, A.S., Lefaivre, J.-F. & Vandersteenhoven, J.J. (2005) Hidradenitis suppurativa complicated by squamous cell carcinoma and paraneoplastic neuropathy. *American Journal of the Medical Sciences* 329, 150–152.

Roul, S., Ducombs, G., Leaute-Labreze, C. & Taieb, A. (1998) 'Lucky Luke' contact dermatitis due to the rubber components of diapers. *Contact Dermatitis* 38, 363–364.

Royal College of Paediatrics and Child Health (2008) The physical signs of child sexual abuse. An evidence based review and guidance for best practice. Lavenham Press, Sudbury.

Rubin, A., Buck, D. & MacDonald, M.R. (1989) Ligneous conjunctivitis involving the cervix. *British Journal of Obstetrics and Gynaecology* 96, 1228–1230.

Rudd, N.L., Nimrod, C., Holbrook, K.A. & Byers, P.H. (1983) Pregnancy complications in Type IV Ehlers–Danlos syndrome. *Lancet* 1, 50–53.

Ruiz-Rodriguez, R., Alvarez, J.G., Jaen, P. *et al.* (2002) Photodynamic therapy with 5-aminolaevulinic acid for recalcitrant familial benign pemphigus (Hailey-Hailey disease). *Journal of the American Academy of Dermatology* 47, 740–742.

Rycroft, R.J.G. & Penney, P.T. (1983) Dermatoses associated with brominated swimming pools. *British Medical Journal* 287, 462.

Salem, O.S. & Steck, W.D. (1983) Cowden's disease (multiple hamartoma and neoplasia syndrome). A case report and review of the English literature. *Journal of the American Academy of Dermatology* 8, 686–696.

Samaratunga, H., Strutton, G., Wright, R.G. & Hill, B. (1991) Squamous cell carcinoma arising in a case of vulvitis granulomatosa or vulval variant of Melkersson–Rosenthal syndrome. *Gynecologic Oncology* 47, 263–269.

Sand, C. & Thomsen, H.K. (2003) Topical tacrolimus ointment is an effective therapy for Hailey-Hailey disease. *Archives of Dermatology* 139, 1401–1402.

Schempp, C., Bocklage, H., Lange, R. *et al.* (1993) Further evidence for *Borrelia burgdorferi* infection in morphea and lichen sclerosus et atrophicus confirmed by DNA amplification. *Journal of Investigative Dermatology* 100, 717–720.

Schott, D., Dempfle, C.E., Beck, P. *et al.* (1998) Therapy with a purified plasminogen concentrate in an infant with ligneous conjunctivitis and homozygous plasminogen deficiency. *New England Journal of Medicine* 339, 1679–1686.

Schuster, V. & Seregard, S. (2003) Ligneous conjunctivitis. *Surveys in Ophthalmology* 48, 369–388.

Schwimmer, E. (1878) Die idiopathischen Schleimhaut der Mundhöle; Leukoplakia buccalis. *Vierteljahresschrift für Dermatologie und Syphilis* 5, 53–114.

Scurry, J., Planner, R., Fortune, D.W., Lee, C.S. & Rode, J. (1993a) Ligneous (pseudomembranous) inflammation of the female genital tract. A report of two cases. *Journal of Reproductive Medicine* 38, 407–412.

Scurry, J., Dennerstein, G., Brenan, J. *et al.* (1993b) Vulvitis circumscripta plasmacellularis. A clinicopathological entity? *Journal of Reproductive Medicine* 38, 14–18.

Scurry, J., Dennerstein, G. & Brennan, J. (1995) Angiolymphoid hyperplasia of the vulva. *Australian and New Zealand Journal of Obstetrics and Gynaecology* 35, 347–348.

Sedlacek, T.V., Riva, J.M., Magen, A.B., Mangan, C. & Cunnane, M.F. (1990) Vaginal and vulvar adenosis. An unsuspected side effect of carbon dioxide laser vaporization. *Journal of Reproductive Medicine* 35, 995–1001.

Sehgal, V.H. & Gangwan, O.P. (1986) Genital fixed drug eruptions. *Genitourinary Medicine* 62, 56–58.

Setterfield, J., Bhogal, B., Shirlaw, P. *et al.* (1996a) A comprehensive study of the clinical immunopathological and immunogenetic findings in cicatricial pemphigoid. *British Journal of Dermatology* 135 (Suppl 47), 13.

Setterfield, J., Neill, S., Ridley, M. *et al.* (1996b) The vulvo-vaginal syndrome is associated with the HLA DQB1*0201 allele. *British Journal of Dermatology* 135 (Suppl 47), 43.

Setterfield, J.F., Neill, S.M., Shirlaw, P. *et al.* (2006) The vulvo-vaginal syndrome: a severe subgroup of lichen planus with characteristic clinical features and a novel association with the class II HLA DQB1*0201 allele. *Journal of the American Academy of Dermatology* 55, 98–113.

Shackleford, G.D., Bauer, E.A., Graviss, E.R. & McAlister, W.H. (1982) Upper airway and external genital involvement in epidermolysis bullosa dystrophica. *Radiology* 143, 429–432.

Shelley, W.B. & Crissey, J.T. (1953) *Classics in Clinical Dermatology*, pp. 194–195. Thomas, Springfield, IL.

Shelley, W.B. & Wood, M.G. (1981) Transformation of the common wart into squamous cell carcinoma in a patient with primary lymphoedema. *Cancer* 48, 820–824.

Shono, S., Imura, M., Ota, M. *et al.* (1991) Lichen sclerosus et atrophicus, morphea, and coexistence of both diseases. Histological studies using lectins. *Archives of Dermatology* 127, 1352–1356.

Short, K.A., Kalu, G., Mortimer, P.S. & Higgins, E.M. (2005) Vulval squamous cell carcinoma arising in chronic hidradenitis suppurativa. *Clinical and Experimental Dermatology* 30, 481–483.

Shuttleworth, D., Graham-Brown, G.A.C., Hutchinson, P.E. & Joliffe, D.S. (1985) Cicatricial pemphigoid in D-penicillamine treated patients with arthritis – a report of three cases. *Clinical and Experimental Dermatology* 10, 392–397.

Sideri, M., Origoni, M., Spinaci, L. & Ferrari, A. (1994) Topical testosterone in the treatment of vulvar lichen sclerosus. *International Journal of Gynecology and Obstetrics* 46, 53–56.

Simpkin, S. & Oakley, A. (2007) Clinical review of 202 patients with vulval lichen sclerosus: a possible association with psoriasis. *Australasian Journal of Dermatology* 48, 28–31.

Singer, A., Mansell, M.E. & Neill, S. (1994) Symptomatic vaginal adenosis. *British Journal of Obstetrics and Gynaecology* 101, 633–635.

Sinha, M.R. (1982) Fixed genital drug eruption due to dapsone. A case report. *Leprosy in India* **54**, 152–154.

Slade, D.E.M., Powell, B.W. & Mortimer, P.S. (2003) Hidradenitis suppurativa: pathogenesis and management. *British Journal of Plastic Surgery* **56**, 451–461.

Soini, Y., Paako, P., Vahakangas, K., Vuopala, S. & Lehto, V.-P. (1994) Expression of p53 and proliferating cell nuclear antigen in lichen sclerosus et atrophicus with different histological features. *International Journal of Gynecological Pathology* **13**, 199–204.

Sorrow, J.M. & Hitch, J.M. (1963) Dyskeratosis congenita. *Archives of Dermatology* **88**, 340–347.

Souteyrand, P., Wong, E. & MacDonald, D.M. (1981) Zoon's balanitis (balanitis circumscripta plasmacellularis). *British Journal of Dermatology* **105**, 195–199.

Soyer, T. (2007) Topical estrogen therapy in children: therapeutic or prophylactic? *Journal of Paediatric and Adolescent Gynaecology* **20**, 241–244.

Spiryda, L.B., Laufer, M.R., Soiffer, R.J. *et al.* (2003) Graft versus host disease of the vulva and/or vagina: diagnosis and treatment. *Biology of Blood and Marrow Transplant* **9**, 760–765.

Srebrnik, A., Bar-Nathan, G.A., Ilie, B., Peyser, R. & Brenner, S. (1991) Vaginal ulceration due to lithium carbonate therapy. *Cutis* **48**, 65–66.

Steinkampf, M.P., Reilly, S.D. & Ackerman, A.B. (1987) Vaginal agglutination and hematometra associated with epidermolysis bullosa. *Obstetrics and Gynecology* **69**, 519–521.

Sterry, W. & Schmoll, M. (1985) Contact urticaria and dermatitis from self-adhesive pads. *Contact Dermatitis* **13**, 284–285.

Stratton, P., Turner, M.L., Childs, R. *et al.* (2007) Vulvovaginal graft versus host disease with allogeneic haemopoietic stem cell transplantation. *Obstetrics and Gynecology* **110**, 1041–1049.

Sturkenboom, M.C., Middelbeek, A., de Jong van den Berg, L.T. *et al.* (1995) Vulvo-vaginal candidiasis associated with acitretin. *Journal of Clinical Epidemiology* **48**, 991–997.

Sutton, R.L. (1935) *Diseases of the Skin*, Vol. 2, 9th edn, p. 1386. Mosby, St Louis.

Swann, M.H., Pujais, J.S., Pillow, J. *et al.* (2003) Localised epidermolytic hyperkeratosis of the female external genitalia. *Journal of Cutaneous Pathology* **30**, 379–381.

Sweet, R.D. (1979) Acute febrile neutrophilic dermatosis. *British Journal of Dermatology* **100**, 93–99.

Szymanski, F.J. & Caro, M.R. (1955) Pseudoxanthoma elasticum. Review of its relationship to internal disease and report of an unusual case. *Archives of Dermatology* **71**, 184–189.

Tai, Y.J. & Kelly, R. (2005) Pyoderma gangrenosum complicated by herpes simplex virus infection. *Australasian Journal of Dermatology* **46**, 161–164.

Tan, S.-H., Derrick, E., McKee, P.H. *et al.* (1994) Altered p53 expression and epidermal cell proliferation is seen in vulval lichen sclerosus. *Journal of Cutaneous Pathology* **21**, 316–323.

Tappeiner, J. & Pfleger, L. (1971) Granuloma gluteale infantum. *Hautarzt* **22**, 383–388.

Tatnall, F.M., Barnes, H.M. & Sarkany, I. (1985) Sarcoidosis of the vulva. *Clinical and Experimental Dermatology* **10**, 384–385.

Taussig, F.J. (1929) Leukoplakic vulvitis and cancer of the vulva (etiology, histopathology, treatment, five-year results). *American Journal of Obstetrics and Gynecology* **18**, 472–503.

Taylor, S.C., Baker, E. & Grossman, M.E. (1991) Nodular vulvar amyloid as a presentation of systemic amyloidosis. *Journal of the American Academy of Dermatology* **24**, 139.

Tebruegge, M., Misra, I. & Nerminathan, V. (2007) Is the topical application of oestrogen cream and effective intervention in girls suffering from labial adhesions? *Archives of Diseases in Childhood* **92**, 268–271.

Teresa Sartori, M., Saggiorato, G., Pellati, D. *et al.* (2003) Contraceptive pills induce an improvement in congenital hypoplasminogenemia in two unrelated patients with ligneous conjunctivitis. *Thrombosis and Haemostasis* **90**, 86–91.

Thomson, J. (1986) Etretinate and vulvitis. *Retinoids Today and Tomorrow* **5**, 49.

Tilsley, D.A. & Wilkinson, D.S. (1965) Necrosis and dequalinium. II. Vulval and extra-genital ulceration. *Transactions of the St John's Hospital Dermatological Society* **51**, 49–54.

Trice, L., Bennert, H. & Stubblefield, P.G. (1996) Massive vulvar edema complicating tocolysis in a patient with twins. *Journal of Reproductive Medicine* **41**, 121–124.

Tromovitch, T.A., Jacobs, P.H. & Kem, S. (1964) Acanthosis nigricans-like lesions from nicotinic acid. *Archives of Dermatology* **89**, 222–223.

Tucker, S.C. & Yell, J.A. (1999) Dramatic postcoital vulval laceration and bruising in Ehlers–Danlos syndrome. *British Journal of Dermatology* **140**, 974.

Václavínková, V. & Neumann, E. (1982) Vaginal involvement in familial benign chronic pemphigus (morbus Hailey–Hailey). *Acta Dermato-venereologica* **62**, 80–81.

Vakilzadeh, F. & Kolde, G. (1985) Relapsing linear acantholytic dermatosis. *British Journal of Dermatology* **112**, 349–355.

Valsecchi, R., Bontempelli, M., Rossi, A. *et al.* (1988) HLA-DR and DQ antigens in lichen planus. *Acta Dermato-venereologica* **68**, 77–80.

van Furth, M., van't Wout, J.W., Wertheimer, P.A. & Zwartendijk, J. (1992) Ciprofloxin for treatment of malakoplakia. *Lancet* **339**, 148–149.

van Joost, T., Faber, W.R. & Manuel, H.R. (1980) Drug induced anogenital cicatricial pemphigoid. *British Journal of Dermatology* **102**, 715–718.

van Voorst Vader, P.C., Kardaun, S.H., Tupker, R.A. *et al.* (1988) Orogenital lichenoid (drug) reaction. *British Journal of Dermatology* **118**, 836–838.

Vega Gutierrez, J., Miranda-Romero, A., Martinex, G. *et al.* (2003) Hyperpigmentation mimicking Laugier syndrome, levodopa therapy and Addison's disease. *Journal of the European Academy of Dermatology and Venereology* **17**, 324–327.

Verbov, J.L. (1973) The skin in patients with Crohn's disease and ulcerative colitis. *Transactions of the St John's Hospital Dermatological Society* **59**, 30–36.

Verburg, D.J., Burd, L.I., Hoxtell, E.O. & Merrill, L.K. (1974) Acrodermatitis enteropathica in pregnancy. *Obstetrics and Gynecology* **44**, 233–237.

Vidal, D., Puig, L., Gilaberte, M. & Alomar, A. (2004) Review of 26 cases of classical pyoderma gangrenosum: clinical and therapeutic features. *Journal of Dermatological Treatment* **15**, 146–152.

Viljoen, D.L., Beatty, S. & Beighton, P. (1987) The obstetric and gynaecological implications of pseudoxanthoma elasticum. *British Journal of Obstetrics and Gynaecology* **94**, 884–888.

Virgili, A., Corazzo, M., Bianchi, A., Mollica, G. & Califano, A. (1995) Open study of topical 0.025% tretinoin in the treatment of vulvar lichen sclerosus. *Journal of Reproductive Medicine* **40**, 614–618.

Virgili, A., Lauriola, M.M., Mantovani, L. & Corazza, M. (2007) Vulvar lichen sclerosus: 11 women treated with tacrolimus 0.1% ointment. *Acta Dermato-venereologica* **87**, 69–72.

Virgili, A., Mantovani, L., Lauriola, M.M, Marzola, A. & Corazza, M. (2008) Tacrolimus 0.1% ointment: is it really effective in plasma cell vulvitis? Report of four cases. *Dermatology* **216**, 243–246.

Wagenberg, H.R. & Downham, T.F. (1981) Chronic edema of the vulva: a condition similar to cheilitis granulomatosa. *Cutis* **27**, 526–527.

Walkden, V., Chia, Y. & Wojnarowska, F. (1997) The association of squamous cell carcinoma of the vulva and lichen sclerosus: implications for management and follow-up. *Journal of Obstetrics and Gynaecology* **17**, 551–553.

Wallace, H.J. (1971) Lichen sclerosus et atrophicus. *Transactions of the St John's Dermatological Society* **57**, 9–30.

Warrington, S.A. & de San Lazaro, C. (1996) Lichen sclerosus et atrophicus and sexual abuse. *Archives of Diseases in Childhood* **75**, 512–516.

Weigand, D.A. (1993) Microscopic features of lichen sclerosus et atrophicus in achrocordons: a clue to the cause of lichen sclerosus et atrophicus? *Journal of the American Academy of Dermatology* **28**, 751–754.

Weiler-Mithoff, E.M., Hassall, M.E. & Burd, D.A. (1996) Burns of the female genitalia and perineum. *Burns* **22**, 390–395.

Weiner, K. (1940) Vaginal melanosis caused by bismuth therapy and carcinoma of the cervix. *Archives of Dermatology* **42**, 23.

West, R., Davies, A. & Fenton, T. (1989) Accidental vulval injuries in childhood. *British Medical Journal* **298**, 1002–1003.

Whimster, I.W. (1973) The natural history of endogenous skin malignancy as a basis for experimental research. *Transactions of the St John's Hospital Dermatological Society* **59**, 195–224.

Williams, J.D., Frowen, K.E. & Nixon, R.L. (2007) A contact dermatitis from methyldibromoglutaronitrile in a sanitary pad and review of Australian clinic data. *Contact Dermatitis* **56**, 164–167.

Wishart, J.M. (1973) Reticulosarcoma of the vulva complicating dermatomyositis treated by immunosuppression. *Proceedings of the Royal Society of Medicine* **66**, 330.

Yaghsezian, H., Palazzo, J.P., Finkel, G.C., Carlson Jr, J.A. & Talerman, A. (1992) Primary vaginal adenocarcinoma of the intestinal type associated with adenosis. *Gynecologic Oncology* **45**, 62–65.

Yates, V.M., King, C.M. & Dave, V.K. (1985) Lichen sclerosus et atrophicus following radiation therapy. *Archives of Dermatology* **121**, 1044–1047.

Yu, C.C.-W. & Cook, M.G. (1990) Hidradenitis suppurativa: a disease of follicular epithelium, rather than apocrine glands. *British Journal of Dermatology* **122**, 763–769.

Zaki, I., Dalziel, K.L., Solomonsz, F.A. & Stevens, A. (1997) The under-reporting of skin disease in association with squamous cell carcinoma of the vulva. *Clinical and Experimental Dermatology* **21**, 334–37.

Zamirska, A., Reich, A., Berny-Moreno, J. *et al.* (2008) Vulvar pruritus and burning sensation in women with psoriasis. *Acta Dermatovenereologica* **88**, 132–135.

Zantomio, D., Grigg, A.P., MacGregor, L. *et al.* (2006) Female genital tract graft versus host disease: incidence, risk factors and recommendations for management. *Bone Marrow Transplant* **38**, 567–572.

Zedek, D.C., Langel, D.J. & White, W.L. (2007) Clear-cell acanthoma versus acanthosis: a psoriasiform reaction pattern lacking trichlemmal differentiation. *American Journal of Dermatopathology* **29**, 378–384.

Zoon, J.J. (1955) Balanitis and vulvitis plasmacellularis. *Dermatologica* **111**, 157.

Chapter 6: Vulvodynia

F.M. Lewis & S.M. Neill

Introduction

Chronic vulval pain, soreness or burning (as opposed to itching) has become a frequently encountered complaint. The patient with a pain problem may present to gynaecologists, urologists, genitourinary physicians, paediatricians, dermatologists and psychiatrists, who may have no special expertise in the diagnosis and management of painful dermatological conditions or chronic pain problems such as vulvodynia. Consequently, these patients are not accurately diagnosed even after many of them have been subjected to extensive and invasive investigations. Now the term *vulvodynia* should be reserved for patients with pain localized to the vulva lasting for more than 3 months in the absence of any visible, neurological or inducible disease, i.e. it is essentially a sensory problem. This is to differentiate from those patients with *vulval pain* due to active dermatological disease, i.e. fissures, ulceration or erosions.

History

Vulvodynia, as it is currently known, is not a new entity as there are early descriptions that would now be readily recognized as this condition. In 1888, Skene writes of 'hyperaesthesia' of the vulva:

> Pruritus is absent, and on examination of the parts affected no redness or other external manifestation of the disease is visible. When, however, the examining finger comes in contact with the hyperaesthetic part, the patient complains of pain, which is sometimes so great as to cause her to cry out. Indeed, the sensitiveness is occasionally so exaggerated as to keep the patient from consulting her physician until it becomes absolutely unbearable. Sexual intercourse is equally painful, and becomes in aggravated cases impossible. This affection must not be confounded with vaginismus, or with other conditions of increased sensitiveness of the vulva due to inflammatory conditions.

Thomas and Mundé (1891) also used the term 'hyperaesthesia', writing:

> The disease . . . constitutes, on account of its excessive obstinacy, and the great influence which it obtains over the mind of the patient, a malady of a great deal of importance. It consists in an excessive sensibility of the nerves supplying the mucous membrane of some portion of the vulva; sometimes the area of tenderness is confined to the vestibule, at other times to one labium minus, at others to the meatus urinarius; and again a number of these parts may be affected . . . So commonly is it met with at least that it becomes a matter of surprise that it has not been more generally and fully described . . . No inflammatory action affects the tender surface, no pruritus attends the condition, and physical examination reveals nothing except occasional spots of erythematous redness scattered here and there . . . The slightest friction excites intolerable pain and nervousness; even a cold and unexpected current of air produces discomfort; and any degree of pressure is absolutely intolerable. For this reason sexual intercourse becomes a source of great discomfort, even when the ostium vaginae is large and free from disease . . . it will be observed that her mind is disproportionately disturbed and depressed by this. In some cases it seems to absorb all the thoughts and to produce a state bordering upon monomania.

Kelly (1928) clearly distinguishes the condition from vaginismus, noting 'Exquisitely sensitive deep-red spots in the mucosa of the hymeneal ring are a fruitful source of dyspareunia – tender enough at times to make a vaginal examination impossible.'

Skene, Thomas and Mundé noticed that surgical intervention was ineffective, with Munde recording, 'My observation of the results of caustics and the knife is not such as to inspire me with confidence in them'.

Forty years later, Kelly returned to the idea of localized surgical excision of the tender spots, as he did also of caruncles, but admitted '. . . the hope is greater when the cause lies more obviously in the caruncles'.

It is curious that reports of the painful problem disappeared from the literature for almost a century, emerging again in the 1970s. Were women during the intervening period really free of the problem, were they less articulate, or were their doctors insufficiently interested and attentive? Another strange fact is that Mundé, in 1891, when enlarging

Ridley's The Vulva, 3rd edition. Edited by Sallie M. Neill and Fiona M. Lewis. © 2009 Blackwell Publishing, ISBN: 978-1-4051-6813-7.

and revising the sixth edition of Thomas's textbook, adds a footnote to the section on 'hyperaesthesia': 'I have never seen an instance of this disease, but Dr Thomas assures me of its undoubted occurrence in his practice. Hence I reproduce this section unchanged.'

Over the last 25 years there has been an evolving classification of vulval pain syndromes. In 1982 the International Society for the Study of Vulvovaginal Disease (ISSVD) set up a committee to study the problem (McKay 1984). The term used for the complaint of chronic pain, soreness or burning, when there was no obvious cause for the symptoms, was at the preliminary stage 'the burning vulva syndrome'. It was proposed to continue with the term 'burning vulva syndrome', but to use the term 'vulvodynia' (Latin *vulva*, Greek *odynia* – pain) to describe chronic symptoms, even including those cases in which the cause for the pain was clear, such as an inflammatory dermatosis. In due course, the name 'burning vulva syndrome' was dropped, with 'vulvodynia' remaining as the overall term. In practice, however, 'vulvodynia' tended to be used to refer to the group without an obvious visible cause.

Between that time and the early 1990s, the focus centred on the human papillomavirus and the finding of vestibular papillomatosis as potential causes for the symptoms. Neither of these proposals is now accepted, and vestibular papillomatosis is considered a variant of normal, unrelated to human papillomavirus (Bergeron *et al.* 1990, Moyal-Barracco *et al.* 1990). A second report (McKay *et al.* 1991) noted this point, and listed what was then felt to represent some valid clinical groupings. The most clearly recognized was *vestibulitis*, as defined by the criteria of Friedrich (1987), i.e. severe pain on vestibular touch or attempted vaginal entry, tenderness to pressure localized within the vestibule and physical findings confined to erythema of varying degrees. *Essential vulvodynia*, later termed *dysaesthetic vulvodynia*, was the term used for patients without abnormal physical signs but who complained of constant burning pain in the vulva. *Cyclic vulvitis* or *vulvovaginitis* was used for those patients in whom symptoms were intermittent and often accompanied by erythema of the labia and sensations of swelling. It was again emphasized that these categories were not applicable to cases in which the symptoms were adequately accounted for by an inflammatory condition such as an infection or dermatosis, but confusion reigned.

During the ensuing years, the two subsets vestibulitis and dysaesthetic vulvodynia emerged as being of the greatest significance, and it has been realized that, while generally distinct, they have much in common. When, in the 1970s, attention began to be paid to patients with such symptoms, they were reported under such titles as 'psychosomatic vulvovaginitis' (Dodson & Friedrich 1978).

The classification is still evolving and the ISSVD working party has proposed a new classification (Moyal-Barracco &

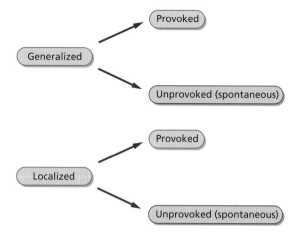

Fig. 6.1 The International Society for the Study of Vulvovaginal Disease 2003 classification of vulvodynia.

Lynch 2004). Vulvodynia is now defined as 'vulval pain in the absence of relevant, visible physical findings, or a specific, clinically identifiable neurologic disorder'. Vulvodynia is further divided into *generalized vulvodynia*, which previously would have been termed dysaesthetic vulvodynia, and *localized vulvodynia*, in which a specific area of the vulva is affected. The most common location for this pain is the vulval vestibule, and so the term *vestibulodynia* has replaced vestibulitis. The removal of the suffix – *itis*, as expressed in vestibulitis, is more logical as there is little evidence of cutaneous inflammation in this entity. The approach of the scientific pain community has been to divide peripheral neuropathic pain into stimulus-evoked pain or stimulus-independent (spontaneous) pain (Woolf & Mannion 1999). Hence, both types of vulvodynia are further subdivided into provoked or unprovoked (spontaneous) pain (Fig. 6.1). In practice, patients will often complain of symptoms which overlap between the two types, and then the diagnosis is not so clear cut.

Complex regional pain syndromes

There have been major advances in our understanding of pain in recent years with the recognition of chronic pain syndromes. Chronic pain is defined as pain lasting more than 3 months. There are now a number of musculoskeletal conditions whose aetiopathology is not understood that have been identified as chronic pain syndromes. These pain syndromes have been further subdivided into two categories causing either diffuse pain, e.g. fibromyalgia, or regional pain, e.g. low back pain and repetitive strain injury. Generalized unprovoked vulvodynia is regarded as a further example of a complex regional pain syndrome.

The physiology of acute and persistent pain

Pain has been defined as 'an unpleasant sensory and emotional experience associated with actual or potential tissue damage, or described in terms of such damage' (International Association for the Study of Pain 1986). Pain has an important role in protecting tissues while they are being repaired after damage. The persistence of pain after such damage despite adequate repair leads to significant physical and mental morbidity. The skin possesses pain receptors – nociceptors – that respond to mechanical, thermal or chemical stimulation. A painful signal is carried to the spinal cord via the dorsal root either by fast, myelinated Aδ fibres transmitting localized, short-lived, sharp pain or by slow, unmyelinated C fibres, which are responsible for the transmission of diffuse, dull, aching pain. The Aδ fibres carry signals predominantly from mechanical nociceptors, whereas the C fibres are sensitive to mechanical, thermal and chemical nociceptors. The cell bodies of the peripheral sensory neurones lie in the dorsal root ganglia and these connect with internuncial neurones in the substantia gelatinosa of the same level. The fibres of the internuncial neurones then cross over the spinal cord to the opposite side and travel up the spinal cord in the lateral spinothalamic columns to the posteroventral nucleus of the thalamus. Signals from the thalamus are then sent to the postcentral gyrus of the parietal lobe where the quality and site of the pain are recognized. Further connections to the frontal, hypothalamic and limbic systems result in a complex mixture of perception, arousal, interpretation, emotion and memory. Transmission is mediated by a large number of neuropeptides including β-endorphin, enkephalin, substance P, calcitonin gene-related peptide, histamine, vasoactive intestinal peptide, somatostatin, serotonin and other catecholamines. The gate theory of pain proposed by Melzack and Wall (1965) explains the processing of pain in the dorsal horn. There are neural mechanisms that control the transmission of pain signals within the dorsal horn by acting like a gate either facilitating or inhibiting the pain impulses that are coming in from the periphery. There is also a descending pathway of neurones to the dorsal horn cells from the brain that can dampen down incoming pain impulses, providing one type of analgesia by 'closing' the gate. Sensations of fine touch and proprioception are carried via Aδ fibres in the afferent nerve, and these fibres synapse with short neurones in the substantia gelatinosa that are inhibitory and can block the transmission of impulses carried by both the Aδ and C fibres, thereby 'closing' the gate. This is the principle behind the use of transcutaneous electric nerve stimulation (TENS). The nervous system is 'plastic' in that it can modulate the type and quantity of neurotransmitters released, the receptor sensitivity can alter and new synapses can be developed. Peripheral and central neurones can become sensitized, leading to an amplification of the signal; this phenomenon is known as 'wind-up'. The affected area may become hyperaesthetic, i.e. hypersensitive to touch, and hyperalgesic, i.e. hypersensitive to painful stimuli. There are two types of mechanical hyperalgesia: stroking hyperalgesia (dynamic hyperalgesia or allodynia) and punctate hyperalgesia. Pain is exceedingly difficult to treat effectively once it has persisted for a year or more (Melzack 1982) and it may become permanent once established.

Persistent pain falls into three groups.

1 *Nociceptive*. This pain is a result of excessive and continuous stimulation of pain receptors due to diseased tissue. The nervous system is intact.

2 *Neuropathic*. Here the pain is a result of damage to the nervous system, e.g. peripheral nerve injury, post-herpetic neuralgia. There is evidence for the influence of many factors on the central and peripheral nervous systems; therefore, making the mediation of neuropathic pain very complex (Holdcroft & Power 2003).

3 *Psychogenic*. No organic basis can be found.

Generalized unprovoked vulvodynia

Generalized vulvodynia describes diffuse vulval pain that occurs without provocation and is usually constant and unremitting, although it may vary in intensity on a day-to-day basis. The pain is usually confined to the vulval area and is usually described as dull and burning with episodes of paroxysmal shooting pain into the pelvis, inner upper thighs or rectal area. There may also be the complaint of even the lightest touch from underwear exacerbating the pain, i.e. allodynia. Generalized vulvodynia tends to occur in the elderly who are not often still sexually active. Those who do have intercourse interestingly deny any dyspareunia.

Patients with generalized vulvodynia seldom give a history of an initiating event, but interestingly it may develop as a sequel in patients with vestibulodynia (provoked localized vulvodynia). These patients frequently have a history of other chronic pain problems, most commonly glossodynia, temporomandibular joint dysfunction, facial or dental neuralgia and chronic low back pain. There are studies to support a reduction in quality of life in patients with vulvodynia (Arnold *et al.* 2006, Tribo *et al.* 2008), many will stop their usual social activities and become housebound and there may be a risk of suicide.

Depression is well recognized in chronic pain and it is difficult to know whether it is a primary cause of the problem or a secondary phenomenon. Its development, after the onset of the pain, is dictated to some extent by the patient's premorbid personality. It is uncertain whether women with generalized vulvodynia have a higher psychiatric morbidity than women with other vulval pathology. One study showed that although there was a higher overall psychiatric prevalence rate in women attending a vulval clinic, similar to that seen in other outpatient clinics, there was not a higher prevalence rate in the vulvodynia group (Jadresic *et al.* 1993). This study did not specify whether the patients had generalized or localized vulvodynia. However, the mean age of the patients was 52.5 years, which is the age most likely to be associated with generalized vulvodynia. Patients with vulvodynia were found to be more anxious and somatizing than women attending a vulval clinic for other vulval pathology (Stewart *et al.* 1994). Although rates of current major depressive disorder symptoms were lower in women with vulvodynia than in other chronic pain patients, comorbidity with these symptoms was related to increased pain severity and reduced general and sexual functioning (Masheb *et al.* 2005).

On examination the vulval skin and architecture are normal and there are no associated abnormal neurological findings. In a study of 17 patients with chronic perineal pain, 13 were found to have sacral meningeal cysts using magnetic resonance imaging (MRI). Ten of these patients went on to surgical treatment of the cysts with resolution of the pain in nine patients (van der Kleft & van Vyve 1991). However, a further study of a group of patients with generalized vulvodynia showed no evidence of sacral cysts on MRI examination of the lumbosacral spine (Lewis & Harrington 1997).

Management

The management is essentially that used in the treatment of other chronic pain syndromes. The topical anaesthetic 5% lidocaine ointment can be used, particularly in those patients whose generalized vulvodynia has followed vulval vestibulodynia or inflammatory dermatosis.

The majority of patients with generalized vulvodynia will need to have treatment directed at the downregulation of either the peripheral or central neuronal wind-up. Medications that block the reuptake of biogenic amines are effective in a significant number of patients. The tricyclic antidepressant amitriptyline is one of the most widely used medications for chronic pain syndromes, exerting an analgesic effect that is believed to be unrelated to its antidepressant action (Davar & Maaciewicz 1989). The exact mechanism of action is unknown. Tricyclic antidepressants are effective in other chronic pain syndromes but there is still limited evidence for the use of the newer serotonin reuptake inhibitors (Saarto & Wiffen 2007). The starting dose of amitriptyline is usually 10 mg each night and the dose is increased by 10 mg increments weekly until there is a response. The dose required may be anywhere between 30 mg and 100 mg a day. The patient should be warned that she will experience a dry mouth and drowsiness. If amitriptyline is too sedating, desipramine or nortriptyline can be used instead.

Anticonvulsants are another group of drugs that have been used to treat neuropathic pain, particularly trigeminal neuralgia and diabetic neuropathic pain; carbamazepine, gabapentin and pregabalin have been used. Again, their mechanism of action is not clear. More recently, gabapentin has been used to treat patients with vulvodynia (Ben-David & Friedman 1999). In a study of 152 patients with generalized vulvodynia, 64% reported a reduction in symptoms of at least 80% during a study period of 30 months (Harris *et al.* 2007). There is one case report of pregabalin, a related drug of gabapentin, being helpful in a patient with long-standing vulvodynia (Jerome 2007).

Unfortunately, a number of patients, particularly those with a long history of well-established pain, remain resistant to all modalities of treatment, and a strategy has to be devised to help them adjust and cope with their chronic pain. Pain clinics in the UK are well established and have management programmes for patients with back pain and pelvic pain syndromes but few as yet have experience with patients with vulvodynia. However, a pain clinic is important for patients with vulvodynia as the anaesthetists who run these clinics are experienced in the use of the medications that are used for other chronic pain syndromes and combinations of various drugs may achieve a positive result. The psychologists who are involved in the pain management programmes of these clinics may be able to offer help to these patients by using cognitive and behavioural techniques, which educate and distract the patient from her pain and help her to achieve the optimal adjustment to coping and living with a chronic pain syndrome. This multidisciplinary approach has been reported to give good results, but these services are scarce. Twenty-seven out of 29 patients reported significant benefit after participation in a programme which included medical evaluation, psychotherapy, physiotherapy and dietary advice (Munday *et al.* 2007). In cases where clinical depression is the primary pathology, referral to a psychiatrist is indicated for a fuller assessment.

There are anecdotal reports of the use of other treatment modalities, including regional nerve blocks, acupuncture (Powell & Wojnarowska 1999), TENS, photodynamic therapy (Zawislak *et al.* 2007) and topical capsaicin, which acts by depleting the C fibres of substance P. The results are inconsistent. Botulinum toxin A blocks the cholinergic innervation of target tissue. In seven women with vulvodynia, the pain score fell from 8.3 to 1.4 after injection (Yoon *et al.* 2007).

With the advent of the worldwide web, there are opportunities for patients to research their problems and patient support groups dedicated to helping these women have been established. The National Vulvodynia Association in the USA and the British Vulval Pain Support Group in the UK are examples of such organizations.

Localized vulvodynia

The commonest area to be affected in localized vulvodynia is the vestibule and is termed vestibulodynia. Much less common is localization of pain to the clitoris – then termed clitorodynia. Vestibulodynia describes pain at the vestibule which is provoked by touch or pressure. If there is no provoking trigger, the patient is usually asymptomatic. A web-based survey of 994 women had a self-reported incidence of vestibular pain in 27.9%, which had lasted longer than 3 months in 1.7% (Reed *et al.* 2004). There was no difference between African American and non-African American women, thereby challenging the perception that vestibulodynia was rare in African and Caribbean women. The incidence of vestibulodynia in an American private gynaecological practice was 15%, but it was also noted in this study that 20% of asymptomatic women had some point tenderness to vestibular touch (Goetsch 1991).

The original triad of symptoms described by Friedrich included entry dyspareunia, vestibular erythema and vestibular tenderness (Friedrich 1987). However, vestibular erythema is a variable entity and is not a reliable diagnostic sign; therefore, it is not necessary to make the diagnosis (Bergeron *et al.* 2001a). The maximal tenderness is usually located at 5 and 7 o'clock in the posterior part of the vestibule close to the hymenal ring, where the major vestibular glands, Bartholin's glands, open on to the surface.

In the majority of patients with vestibulodynia the posterior part of the vestibule mainly is affected, and they therefore complain of discomfort with intercourse or the insertion of tampons. In a small proportion of patients the anterior vestibule is also tender, particularly over the openings of the paraurethral glands. These patients will complain of the additional symptoms of dysuria and strangury and a few are diagnosed as having interstitial cystitis. In fact, there is a definite association of vestibulodynia and interstitial cystitis with a relative risk of 6.9 for vulval pain in patients with interstitial cystitis (Wu *et al.* 2006). This has raised the question as to whether the two conditions could be a disorder of the epithelium derived from the urogenital sinus (McCormack 1990, Fitzpatrick *et al.* 1993).

Unlike those patients with generalized vulvodynia, those with vestibulodynia give a clear history of a precipitating event such as a severe episode of thrush and/or a reaction to an antifungal cream or urinary tract infection. Some patients develop vestibular tenderness after resolution of an inflammatory condition at this site, such as lichen planus. The patients complain of discomfort after using many of the topical medications prescribed for their vulval problem and admit to a history of skin sensitivity at extragenital sites, particularly the face and hands, to highly perfumed soaps and cosmetics. In addition, they describe intolerance to the metal in costume jewellery. However, patch testing rarely reveals relevant positive reactions, which would suggest that the problem may be a low-grade irritant reaction and not an allergic contact problem (Marinoff & Turner 1986). Further studies have shown no role for routine patch testing in these patients (Nunns *et al.* 1997, Petersen 1997). It has also been demonstrated that these women have increased peripheral sensitivity at other sites such as the upper arm or leg (Pukall *et al.* 2002, Giesecke *et al.* 2004). Interestingly, although improvement of superficial dyspareunia was seen with topical lidocaine or electromyographic (EMG) feedback treatment, there was no effect on hypersensitivity elsewhere in 35 women with vestibulodynia (Bohm-Starke *et al.* 2007), thus suggesting that they have an abnormal generalized hypersensitivity.

The human papillomavirus and *Candida* have been suggested as causative agents, as they are frequently associated in the history of the onset of the problem. However, the appropriate treatment for these conditions does not result in the eradication of the symptoms. Furthermore, several sound studies have failed to demonstrate evidence of any of the known human papillomavirus types (Wilkinson *et al.* 1993, Bergeron *et al.* 1994, Prayson *et al.* 1995). Genitourinary screening for other sexually transmitted diseases is invariably negative.

The differential diagnosis of women presenting with vestibular pain includes herpes simplex infection and nymphohymenal tears (Fig. 6.2). There are rare reports of type I allergic reactions to seminal fluid (Halpern *et al.* 1967), or to drugs taken by the male partner that are secreted in

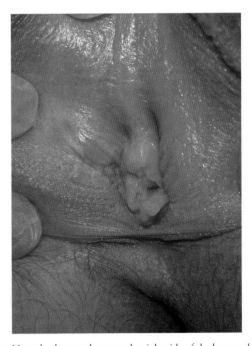

Fig. 6.2 Nympho-hymenal tear on the right side of the hymenal ring.

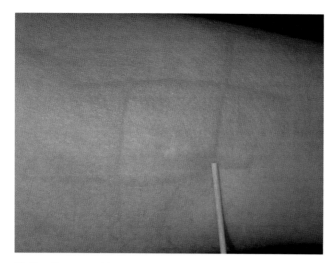

Fig 6.3 Dermographism.

seminal fluid (Schimkat *et al.* 1993), which might mimic the symptoms of vestibulodynia. However, most of these reactions to seminal fluid are urticarial (Poskitt *et al.* 1995) with immediate localized itching, swelling and erythema with associated bronchospasm and angio-oedema and anaphylaxis in rare cases. The history is very important in these cases as usually there is no problem if a condom is used. Dermographism (Fig. 6.3) also has to be excluded, but the history of the sensation of burning and swelling lasts less than an hour.

In early studies, patients with vulvodynia were thought to have psychological issues that may predispose them to pain. Many of the patients are very health-conscious non-smokers who often verge on hypochondriasis as they consult frequently for other problems, the commonest of which include low back pain, migraine, irritable bowel syndrome and lassitude (Lynch 1986). There is initially a strong denial that there could be any underlying stressful problems in their lives either precipitating or exacerbating their vestibulodynia. There are claims that their relationship with their partner is good and the partners are described as supportive and understanding with the additional comment that this state of affairs may not last indefinitely. The majority of patients who are affected with vestibulodynia are probably no more or less abnormal psychologically than any other comparable group but they do have significantly higher anxiety and somatization scores (van Lankveld *et al.* 1996). Another study reported no difference in psychological morbidity between women with vestibulodynia and controls (Reed *et al.* 2000). A study of women with vestibulodynia and their partners showed that they did not differ from controls in global sexual functioning or psychological adjustment (Desrosiers *et al.* 2008). Not surprisingly, partner solicitousness and hostility was associated with higher

levels of pain during intercourse. Although vestibulodynia leads to difficulties with sexual intercourse because of complaints of poor lubrication and dyspareunia, there is no good evidence to date to support that there is marital dissatisfaction in either the patients themselves or their partners (van Lankveld *et al.* 1996). The prevalence of sexual abuse in patients with vestibulodynia is similar to or lower than that of the normal population (Friedrich 1987, Schover *et al.* 1992, Edwards *et al.* 1997). However, the stress, anxiety or depression associated with vestibulodynia can lead to an exacerbation of any underlying psychological or personality disorder, but it also has to be acknowledged that stress and depression arising in the patient's life from other causes may exacerbate and exaggerate pain. It is therefore important to address these problems in case stress is contributing to the perpetuation of their symptoms, as these patients may be offered referral for appropriate professional help if necessary.

The histological changes found include a non-specific mixed inflammatory cell infiltrate without eosinophils, metaplasia of the vestibular glands forming clefts, and no evidence, despite special stains, to demonstrate bacterial or fungal organisms (Pyka *et al.* 1988). Despite the finding of inflammatory cells it is not essentially an inflammatory condition, and a non-specific inflammatory infiltrate has been demonstrated in healthy vestibular tissue (Nylander-Lundqvist *et al.* 1997). Further work has shown a significant increase in the number of intraepithelial nerve endings in women with vestibulodynia as demonstrated by protein gene product (PGP)9.5 immunohistochemistry (Bohm-Starke *et al.* 1998, Tympanidis *et al.* 2003). These free nerve endings were then confirmed to be nociceptors as calcitonin gene-related peptide was the only neuropeptide detected in these superficial nerves (Bohm-Starke *et al.* 1999). The low levels of expression of the inflammatory mediators cyclo-oxygenase 2 and inducible nitric oxide synthase indicate that there is no active inflammation in vestibulodynia (Bohm-Starke *et al.* 2001). Although some changes in cytokine levels have been reported by some authors, no significant increase in expression of the inflammatory markers interleukin 1α, 1β and tumour necrosis factor α was found in vestibular tissue from patients with vestibulodynia (Eva *et al.* 2007). It is difficult to know whether this is cause or effect.

Vestibulodynia remains a syndrome of unexplained aetiology but in the light of what is currently known it is best categorized as a chronic pain syndrome (Bergeron *et al.* 1997). It may occur as a result of peripheral or central sensitization of nociceptors following some painful initiating event, which then leaves the patient with a frictional allodynia. There is now good evidence for the lack of an inflammatory basis for the condition. The anxiety engendered by these symptoms combined with the inevitable strain and stress of the inability to function sexually tends to intensify and reinforce the abnormal sensation of burning.

Management

Spontaneous resolution may occur but is unusual, although one report has cited a remission rate as high as 50% (Peckham et al. 1986). There is no one effective treatment and often the consultation alone may prove to be therapeutic in those with minor symptoms. A careful consultation with an interested physician who clearly recognizes the problem will reassure the anxious patient that she has not been imagining her symptoms and that her condition has at long last been given a name. Further medical measures include the use of a soap substitute in case of a low-grade irritancy problem and the topical local anaesthetic 5% lidocaine ointment. Lidocaine is to be preferred to other local anaesthetics because of the low risk of sensitization. This can be used as required, such as before intercourse, but application of the 5% lidocaine ointment on a cotton wool ball placed in the fourchette overnight on a regular basis can minimize feedback amplification of pain. After a mean of 7 weeks' treatment, 76% were able to have intercourse compared with 36% at baseline (Zolnoun et al. 2003). Topical steroids are unhelpful.

If topical agents have not helped then a trial of a tricyclic antidepressant may be added. As for generalized vulvodynia, the most frequently used is amitriptyline. Once an effective dose is reached the patient remains on the medication for at least 2 months and then the dose is gradually tapered down. The reason for the small doses initially is that many of these patients are very sensitive to the side-effects, which may well be a reflection of their heightened awareness state. Oral steroids have no effect and have no role to play in the treatment of this condition. Calcium citrate tablets and a low oxalate diet proved effective for one woman with vestibulitis (Solomons et al. 1991). However, further studies have failed to show any significant relationship (Baggish et al. 1997, Greenstein et al. 2006, Harlow et al. 2008).

Biofeedback training has been used for vulvodynia, both localized and generalized. A small proportion of women have pelvic floor muscle hypertonia, which results in vaginismus, and successful biofeedback techniques studying pelvic floor muscle function have resulted in improvement in women who have evidence of such muscle dysfunction (Glazer et al. 1995). In a trial of EMG feedback versus topical lidocaine in 46 women, both treatments were found to result in statistically significant improvements in vestibular pain measurements and sexual functioning, but there was no difference between the treatments. Compliance with biofeedback was lower (Danielsson et al. 2006).

Of those women treated by an expert physiotherapist, 71% reported over a 50% reduction in their overall symptoms (Hartmann & Nelson 2001) but the techniques used are wide ranging and not widely accessible.

Behavioural therapy has proved beneficial in one group of patients (Weijmar Schultz et al. 1996), and showed a 30% response in a randomized trial (Bergeron et al. 2001b). However, psychiatric intervention with psychologically normal patients is ineffective and not indicated.

Surgical treatment is reportedly successful in the management of some patients with vestibulodynia, although there is no clear rationale why this should be a therapeutic option in a chronic pain syndrome. In the past, surgical management has included excision of the posterior vestibule with advancement of the vaginal mucosa (Woodruff et al. 1981), perineoplasty (Friedrich 1983, 1987) and vestibuloplasty, which entails incising the distal perimeter of the vestibule, undermining the vestibule and then securing it back into position without any tissue advancement or excision. Perineoplasty has proved to be the more effective of the two procedures (Bornstein et al. 1995). These authors emphasize that surgical success depends on the selection of those patients who fulfil the strict criteria laid down for the definition of vestibulodynia. More recently a simple skinning dissection of the affected tissue in those patients who lose their tenderness to touch after the application of topical lidocaine has been described (Goetsch 1996). This procedure is not mutilating and can be performed under local anaesthetic with a successful outcome that is equal to that reported from the more extensive surgical procedures. However, it should be stressed that any surgical management should be reserved solely for those desperate patients who have failed to improve with all other treatments (Weijmar Schultz et al. 1996). It is also particularly important that these patients have a psychological assessment prior to surgery to ascertain their suitability for such a procedure (Schover et al. 1992). One long-term follow-up study showed that over half the women who had undergone a perineoplasty were still symptomatic and had been psychologically traumatized by their experience (de Jong et al. 1995). These authors felt that surgery was not the answer. Some authors report good results with follow-up to 1 year but women with primary vestibulodynia were less likely to benefit (Bohm Starke & Rylander 2008). Carbon dioxide laser has been reported to be successful in the management of anterior vestibulodynia but follow-up was only for 1 year (Friedrich 1983). Successful treatment with the KTP/Nd:YAG laser has also been claimed to reduce pain but 29% of patients reported no change in their symptoms and 35% went on to vestibulectomy (Leclair et al. 2007).

Reported but as yet unproven treatments for vestibulodynia include intralesional interferons (Kent & Wisniewski 1990, Marinoff & Turner 1992, Bornstein et al. 1993), cromoglycate cream (Nyirjesy et al. 2001), acupuncture (Danielsson et al. 2001), montelukast (Kamdar et al. 2007) and hypnosis (Pukall et al. 2007).

References

Arnold, L.D., Bachmann, G.A., Rosen, R. *et al.* (2006) Vulvodynia: characteristics and associations with co-morbidities and quality of life. *Obstetrics and Gynaecology* 107, 617–624.

Baggish, M.S., Sze, E.H.M. & Johnson, R. (1997) Urinary oxalate excretion and its role in vulvar pain. *American Journal of Obstetrics and Gynecology* 177, 507–511.

Ben-David, B. & Friedman, M. (1999) Gabapentin therapy for vulvodynia. *Anaesthetic Annals* 89, 1459–1462.

Bergeron, C., Ferenczy, A., Richart, R.M. & Guralnick, M. (1990) Micropapillomatosis labialis appears unrelated to human papillomavirus. *Obstetrics and Gynecology* 76, 281–286.

Bergeron, C., Moyal-Barracco, M., Pelisse, M. & Lewin, P. (1994) Vulvar vestibulitis. Lack of evidence for a human papillomavirus etiology. *Journal of Reproductive Medicine* 39, 936–938.

Bergeron, S., Binik, Y.M., Khalifé, S. & Pagidas, K. (1997) Vulvar vestibulitis syndrome: a critical review. *The Clinical Journal of Pain* 13, 27–42.

Bergeron, S., Binik, Y., Khalife, S. *et al.* (2001a) Vulvar vestibulitis syndrome: reliability of diagnosis and evaluation of current diagnostic criteria. *Obstetrics and Gynaecology* 98, 45–51.

Bergeron, S., Binik, Y.M., Khalife, S. *et al.* (2001b) A randomized comparison of group cognitive–behavioural therapy, surface electromyographic biofeedback and vestibulectomy in the treatment of dyspareunia resulting from vulvar vestibulitis. *Pain* 91, 297–306.

Bohm-Starke, N. & Rylander, E. (2008) Surgery for localised, provoked vestibulodynia: a long-term follow-up study. *Journal of Reproductive Medicine* 53, 83–9.

Bohm-Starke, N., Hilliges, M., Falconer, C. & Rylander, E. (1998) Increased intra-epithelial innervation in women with vulvar vestibulitis syndrome. *Gynaecological and Obstetric Investigation* 46, 256–260.

Bohm-Starke, N., Hilliges, M., Falconer, C. & Rylander, E. (1999) Neurochemical characterization of the vestibular nerves in women with vulvar vestibulitis syndrome. *Gynaecological and Obstetric Investigation* 48, 270–275.

Bohm-Starke, N., Falconer, C., Rylander, E. & Hilliges, M. (2001) The expression of cyclooxygenase 2 and inducible nitric oxide synthase indicates no active inflammation in vulvar vestibulitis. *Acta Obstetrica et Gynaecologica Scandinavica* 80, 638–644.

Bohm-Starke, N., Brodda-Jansen, G., Linder, J. & Danielsson, I. (2007) The result of treatment on vestibular and general pain thresholds in women with provoked vestibulodynia. *Clinical Journal of Pain* 23, 598–604.

Bornstein, J., Pascal, B. & Abramovich, H. (1993) Intramuscular B interferon treatment for severe vulvar vestibulitis. *Journal of Reproductive Medicine* 38, 117–120.

Bornstein, J., Zarfati, D., Goldik, Z. & Abramovici, H. (1995) Perineoplasty compared with vestibuloplasty for severe vulvar vestibulitis. *British Journal of Obstetrics and Gynaecology* 102, 652–655.

Danielsson, I., Sjoberg, I. & Ostman, C. (2001) Acupuncture for the treatment of vulvar vestibulitis: a pilot study. *Acta Obstetrica et Gynaecologica Scandinavica* 80, 437–441.

Danielsson, I., Torstensson, T., Brodda-Jansen, G. & Bohm-Starke, N. (2006) EMG biofeedback versus topical lidocaine gel: a randomized study for the treatment of women with vulval vestibulitis. *Acta Obstetrica et Gynaecologica Scandinavica* 85, 1360–1367.

Davar, G. & Maaciewicz, R.J. (1989) Deafferentation pain syndromes. *Neurological Clinics* 7, 289–304.

de Jong, J.M.J., van Lunsen, R.H.W., Robertson, E.A., Stam, L.N.E. & Lammes, F.B. (1995) Focal vulvitis: a psychosexual problem for which surgery is not the answer. *Journal of Psychosomatic Obstetrics and Gynecology* 16, 85–91.

Desrosiers, M., Bergeron, S., Meana, M. *et al.* (2008) Psychosexual characteristics of vestibulodynia couples: partner solicitousness and hostility are associated with pain. *Journal of Sexual Medicine* 5, 418–427.

Dodson, M.G. & Friedrich, E.G. (1978) Psychosomatic vulvovaginitis. *Obstetrics and Gynecology* 51 (Suppl), 23s–25s.

Edwards, L., Mason, M., Phillips, M., Norton, J. & Boyle, M. (1997) Childhood sexual and physical abuse. Incidence in patients with vulvodynia. *Journal of Reproductive Medicine* 42, 135–139.

Eva, L.J., Rolfe, K.J., MacLean, A.B. *et al.* (2007) Is localised, provoked vulvodynia an inflammatory condition? *Journal of Reproductive Medicine* 52, 379–384.

Fitzpatrick, C.C., DeLancey, J.O.L., Elkins, T.E. & McGuire, E.J. (1993) Vulvar vestibulitis and interstitial cystitis: a disorder of urogenital sinus derived epithelium? *Obstetrics and Gynecology* 81, 860–861.

Friedrich, E.G. (1983) The vulvar vestibule. *Journal of Reproductive Medicine* 28, 773–777.

Friedrich, E.G. (1987) Vulvar vestibulitis syndrome. *Journal of Reproductive Medicine* 32, 110–114.

Giesecke, J., Reed, B., Haefner, H.K. *et al.* (2004) Quantitative sensory testing in vulvodynia patients and increased peripheral pain sensitivity. *Obstetrics and Gynaecology* 104, 126–133.

Glazer, H.I., Rodke, G., Swencionis, C., Hertz, R. & Young, A.W. (1995) Treatment of the vulvar vestibulitis syndrome with electromyographic biofeedback of pelvic floor musculature. *Journal of Reproductive Medicine* 40, 283–290.

Goetsch, M.F. (1991) Vulvar vestibulitis: prevalence and historic features in a general gynecologic practice population. *American Journal of Obstetrics and Gynecology* 164, 1609–1616.

Goetsch, M.F. (1996) Simplified surgical revision of the vulvar vestibule for vulvar vestibulitis. *American Journal of Obstetrics and Gynecology* 174, 1701–1707.

Greenstein, A., Militscher, I., Chen, J. *et al.* (2006) Hyperoxaluria in women with vulvar vestibulitis syndrome. *Journal of Reproductive Medicine* 51, 500–502.

Halpern, B.N., Ky, T. & Robert, B. (1967) Clinical and immunological study of an exceptional case of reagenic type sensitisation to human seminal fluid. *Immunology* 12, 2457–2458.

Harlow, B.L., Abenhaim, H.A., Vitonis, A.F. & Harnack, L. (2008) Influence of dietary oxalates on the risk of adult-onset vulvodynia. *Journal of Reproductive Medicine* 53, 171–178.

Harris, G., Horowitz, B. & Borqida, A. (2007) Evaluation of gabapentin in the treatment of generalised vulvodynia, unprovoked. *Journal of Reproductive Medicine* 52, 103–106.

Hartmann, E.H. & Nelson, C. (2001) The perceived effectiveness of physical therapy treatment on women complaining of chronic vulvar pain and diagnosed with either vulvar vestibulitis syndrome or dysaesthetic vulvodynia. *Journal Section of Women's Health* 25, 13–18.

Holdcroft, A. & Power, I. (2003) Management of pain. *British Medical Journal* 326, 635–639.

International Association for the Study of Pain; Subcommittee on Taxonomy (1986) Classification of chronic pain: descriptions of chronic pain syndromes and definitions of pain terms. *Pain* 3 (Suppl), S1–S226.

Jadresic, D., Barton, S., Neill, S., Staughton, R. & Marwood, R. (1993) Psychiatric morbidity in women attending a clinic for vulval problems: is there a higher rate in vulvodynia? *International Journal of STD and AIDS* **4**, 237–239.

Jerome, L. (2007) Pregabalin-induced remission in a 62 year old woman with a 20 year history of vulvodynia. *Pain Research Management* **12**, 212–214.

Kamdar, N., Fisher, L. & MacNeill, C. (2007) Improvement in vulvar vestibulitis with montelukast. *Journal of Reproductive Medicine* **52**, 912–916.

Kelly, H.A. (1928) Dyspareunia. In: *Gynecology* (ed. H.A. Kelly), p. 23. Appleton, New York.

Kent, H.L. & Wisniewski, P.M. (1990) Interferon for vulvar vestibulitis. *Journal of Reproductive Medicine* **12**, 1138–1140.

Leclair, C.M., Goetsch, M.F., Lee, K.K. & Jensen, J.T. (2007) KTP-nd:YAG laser therapy for the treatment of vestibulodynia: a follow-up study. *Journal of Reproductive Medicine* **52**, 53–58.

Lewis, F.M. & Harrington, C.I. (1997) Use of magnetic resonance imaging in vulvodynia. *Journal of Reproductive Medicine* **42**, 169.

Lynch, P. (1986) Vulvodynia: a syndrome of unexplained vulvar pain, psychologic disability and sexual dysfunction. *Journal of Reproductive Medicine* **31**, 773–780.

Marinoff, S.C. & Turner, M.L.C. (1986) Hypersensitivity to vaginal candidiasis or treatment vehicles in the pathogenesis of minor vestibular gland syndrome. *Journal of Reproductive Medicine* **31**, 796–799.

Marinoff, S.C. & Turner, M.L.C. (1992) Vulvar vestibulitis syndrome. *Dermatologic Clinics* **10**, 435–444.

Masheb, R.M., Wang, E., Lozano, C. & Kerns, R.D. (2005) Prevalence and correlates of depression in treatment-seeking women with vulvodynia. *Journal of Obstetrics and Gynaecology* **25**, 786–791.

McCormack, W.M. (1990) Two urogenital sinus syndromes. *Journal of Reproductive Medicine* **35**, 873–876.

McKay, M. (1984) Burning vulva syndrome. Report of the ISSVD task force. *Journal of Reproductive Medicine* **29**, 457.

McKay, M., Frankman, O., Horowitz, B.J. *et al.* (1991) Vulvar vestibulitis and vulvar papillomatosis. Report of the ISSVD Committee on vulvodynia. *Journal of Reproductive Medicine* **36**, 413–415.

Melzack R. (1982) *The Challenge of Pain.* Basic Books, New York.

Melzack, R. & Wall, P.D. (1965) Pain mechanisms: a new theory. *Science* **150**, 971–979.

Moyal-Barracco, M. & Lynch, P.J. (2004) 2003 ISSVD terminology and classification of vulvodynia: a historical perspective. *Journal of Reproductive Medicine* **49**, 772–777.

Moyal-Barracco, M., Leibowitch, M. & Orth, G. (1990) Vestibular papillae of the vulva. Lack of evidence for human papillomavirus etiology. *Archives of Dermatology* **126**, 1594–1598.

Munday, P., Buchan, A., Ravenhill, G. *et al.* (2007) A qualitative study of women with vulvodynia. II. Response to a multidisciplinary approach to management. *Journal of Reproductive Medicine* **52**, 19–22.

Nunns, D., Ferguson, J., Beck, M. & Mandal, D. (1997) Is patch testing necessary in vulval vestibulitis. *Contact Dermatitis* **37**, 87–89.

Nyirjesy, P., Sobel, J.D., Weitz, M.V. *et al.* (2001) Cromolyn cream for recalcitrant idiopathic vulvar vestibulitis: results of a placebo controlled study. *Sexually Transmitted Infections* **77**, 53–57.

Nylander-Lundqvist, E., Hofer, P.-A., Olofsson, J.I. & Sjoberg, I. (1997) Is vulvar vestibulitis an inflammatory condition? A comparison of histological findings in affected and healthy women. *Acta Dermato-venereologica (Stockholm)* **77**, 319–322.

Peckham, B.M., Maki, D.G., Patterson, J.J. & Hafez, G.-R. (1986) Focal vulvitis: a characteristic syndrome and cause of dyspareunia. *American Journal of Obstetrics and Gynecology* **154**, 855–864.

Petersen, C.S. (1997) Lack of contact allergy in consecutive women with vulvodynia. *Contact Dermatitis* **37**, 46–47.

Poskitt, B.L., Wojnarowska, F.T. & Shaw, S. (1995) Semen contact urticaria. *Journal of the Royal Society of Medicine* **88**, 108–109.

Powell, J. & Wojnarowska, F. (1999) Acupuncture for vulvodynia. *Journal of the Royal Society of Medicine* **92**, 579–581.

Prayson, R.A., Stoler, M.H. & Hart, W.R. (1995) Vulvar vestibulitis. A histopathologic study of 36 cases including human papillomavirus in situ hybridization analysis. *American Journal of Surgical Pathology* **19**, 157–160.

Pukall, C.F., Binik, Y.M., Khalife, S. *et al.* (2002) Vestibular tactile and pain thresholds in women with vulvar vestibulitis syndrome. *Pain* **96**, 163–175.

Pukall, C.F., Kandyba, K., Amsel, R. *et al.* (2007) Effectiveness of hypnosis for the treatment of vulvar vestibulitis syndrome: a preliminary investigation. *Journal of Sexual Medicine* **4**, 417–425.

Pyka, R.E., Wilkinson, E.J., Friedrich, E.G. & Croker, B.P. (1988) The histopathology of vulvar vestibulitis syndrome. *International Journal of Gynecological Pathology* **7**, 249–257.

Reed, B.D., Haefner, H.K., Punch, M.R. *et al.*(2000) Psychosocial and sexual functioning in women with vulvodynia and chronic pelvic pain. A comparative evaluation. *Journal of Reproductive Medicine* **45**, 624–632.

Reed, B., Crawford, S., Couper, M. *et al.* (2004) Pain at the vulvar vestibule; a web based survey. *Journal of Lower Genital Tract Disease* **8**, 48–57.

Saarto, T. & Wiffen, P.J. (2007) Antidepressants for neuropathic pain. *Cochrane Database Systematic Review* **4**, CD005454.

Schimkat, H.G., Meynadier, J.M. & Meynadier, J. (1993) Contact urticaria. In: *Vulvovaginitis* (eds P. Elsner & J. Martius), pp. 83–110. Marcel Dekker, New York.

Schover, L.R., Youngs, D.D. & Cannata, R. (1992) Psychosexual aspects of the evaluation and management of vulvar vestibulitis. *American Journal of Obstetrics and Gynecology* **167**, 630–636.

Skene, A.J.C. (1888) Diseases of the external organs of generation. In: *Treatise on Diseases of Women* (ed. A.J.C. Skene), pp. 76–98. Appleton, New York. (1890, H.K. Lewis, London.)

Solomons, C., Melmed, M.H. & Heitler, S.M. (1991) Calcium citrate for vulval vestibulitis. A case report. *Journal of Reproductive Medicine* **36**, 879–882.

Stewart, D.E., Reicher, A.E., Gerulath, A.H. & Boydell, K.M. (1994) Vulvodynia and psychological distress. *Obstetrics and Gynecology* **84**, 587–590.

Thomas, T.G. & Mundé, P.F. (1891) *A Practical Treatise on the Diseases of Women*, p. 143. Lea Brothers, Philadelphia.

Tribo, M.J., Audion, O., Ros, S. *et al.* (2008) Clinical characteristics and psychopathological profile of patients with vulvodynia; an observational and descriptive study. *Dermatology* **216**, 24–30.

Tympanidis, P., Terenghi, G. & Dowd, P. (2003) Increased innervations of the vulval vestibule in patients with vulvodynia. *British Journal of Dermatology* **148**, 1021–1027.

van der Kleft, E. & van Vyve, M. (1991) Chronic perineal pain related to sacral meningeal cysts. *Neurosurgery* **29**, 223–226.

van Lankveld, J.J.D.M., Weijenborg, P.T.M. & Ter Kuile, M.M. (1996) Psychologic profiles of and sexual function in women with vulvar vestibulitis and their partners. *Obstetrics and Gynecology* **88**, 65–70.

Weijmar Schultz, W.C.M., Gianotten, W.L., van der Meijden, W.I. *et al.* (1996) Behavioural approach with or without surgical intervention to the vulvar vestibulitis syndrome: a prospective randomized and non-randomized study. *Journal of Psychosomatic Obstetrics and Gynecology* **17**, 143–148.

Wilkinson, E.J., Guerrero, E., Daniel, R. *et al.* (1993) Vulvar vestibulitis is rarely associated with human papillomavirus infection types 6, 11, 16, or 18. *International Journal of Gynecological Pathology* **28**, 134–141.

Woodruff, J.D., Geandry, R. & Poliakoff, S. (1981) Treatment of dyspareunia and vaginal outlet distortions by perineoplasty. *Obstetrics and Gynecology* **57**, 750–754.

Woolf, C.J. & Mannion, R.J. (1999) Pain: neuropathic pain: aetiology, symptoms, mechanisms and management. *Lancet* **353**, 1959–1964.

Wu, E.Q., Birnbaum, H., Mareva, M. *et al.* (2006) Interstitial cystitis: cost, treatment and co-morbidities in an employed population. *Pharmacoeconomics* **24**, 55–65.

Yoon, H., Chung, W.S. & Shim, B.S. (2007) Botulinum toxin A for the management of vulvodynia. *International Journal of Impotence Research* **19**, 84–87.

Zawislak, A.A., McCarron, P.A., McCluggage, W.G. *et al.* (2007) Novel bioadhesive patch-type system for photodynamic vulvodynia therapy after delivery of 5-aminolaevulinic acid: preliminary evaluation. *Journal of Reproductive Medicine* **52**, 645–653.

Zolnoun, D.A., Hartmann, K.E. & Steege, F. (2003) Overnight 5% lidocaine ointment for treatment of vulvar vestibulitis. *Obstetrics and Gynaecology* **102**, 84–87.

Chapter 7: Psychological and psychiatric aspects of vulval disorders

E.R.L. Williams & J. Catalán

Introduction

Some degree of psychiatric morbidity is common in both men and women seeking help for many physical disorders and in many different medical and surgical settings (see report of the Royal College of Physicians and the Royal College of Psychiatrists 2003), and, thus, the presence of psychological symptoms is not exclusive to vulval complaints. Women are particularly vulnerable to psychiatric disorders. There is significant maternal mortality and morbidity associated with puerperal psychosis, postpartum depression, drug and alcohol misuse (Confidential Enquiry into Maternal and Child Health 2007, NICE 2007).

There is a close association between having physical disorders and the development of psychological symptoms or frank psychiatric disorder (Wells *et al.* 1988). The presence of psychological symptoms does not preclude the existence of a medical condition and vice versa; in practice, they often coexist. The body–mind split is not a helpful model when trying to tease out and understand the aetiological factors, and may get in the way of providing effective help in an integrated, holistic manner. As with all psychological reactions to physical illness there are several factors that contribute to the nature of the psychological response. It is important to consider the reaction to the condition of the patient and the patient's immediate family, friends and healthcare professionals.

The nature of the association between physical and psychological symptoms is a complex one: causality and association are usually unclear. A physical disorder can cause a psychiatric one, as when a diagnosis of cancer leads to severe depression, or a primarily psychiatric condition may present with medical symptoms, as when panic attacks present as chest pain. Even in these instances causality is not always as clear or straightforward as it appears. In other cases, both medical and psychiatric disorders present together. This occurs in functional somatic complaints or medically unexplained symptoms, such as muscle and joint pain (fibromyalgia), tension headache and irritable bowel syndrome. These conditions often lead to multiple and expensive investigations, treatments with a poor evidence base, and sometimes referral to psychiatry (Mayou & Farmer 2002, Fischhoff & Wessely 2003). Throughout the history of medicine there are many examples of conditions which initially lacked a clear physical aetiology and which were labelled psychosomatic, e.g. asthma, peptic ulcer, ulcerative colitis and rheumatoid arthritis. The term psychosomatic was applied when psychological conflict, stress or complex personality traits were thought to be implicated in the aetiology of the disease.

Recognition of the association of physical and psychiatric disorders is now fully accepted in clinical practice, as is the development of specialties such as general hospital psychiatry and health psychology. Consideration of the psychological aspects of any clinical presentation can have many advantages and, we would argue, are integral to all aspects of care. People with psychiatric conditions are more likely to seek help in medical settings. They are frequent attenders at general practice, outpatient clinics and emergency departments, and have a higher rate of hospital admission (Kroenke & Spitzer 1998, Williams *et al.* 2001, Hansen *et al.* 2002). Acknowledging psychological symptoms and factors, and helping to resolve them, is important. Owing to medical advances, conditions that were previously fatal, for example cancer and HIV, can now be managed with long-term treatment. Consequently, there is now evidence that there is a high prevalence of depression and anxiety in people with such disorders. Treatment of the depression and anxiety leads to a better quality of life (Sheard & Maguire 1999, Citron *et al.* 2005, Cohen & Gorman 2008).

This chapter outlines the range of psychological symptoms and psychiatric disorders that women with vulval conditions may develop. Psychological interventions for assessment and management of such psychiatric disorders are discussed below.

Ridley's The Vulva, 3rd edition. Edited by Sallie M. Neill and Fiona M. Lewis. © 2009 Blackwell Publishing, ISBN: 978-1-4051-6813-7.

Women seeking help for vulval complaints, regardless of the aetiology, may also present with symptoms of anxiety, depression and sexual dysfunction. The severity of the psychological symptoms does not necessarily correlate with the severity of the clinical problem (Andersen & Hacker 1983, Jadresic *et al.* 1993, Jensen *et al.* 2003, Fischer 1996, Wojnarowska *et al.* 1997).

A woman's past experience of a disease affecting her or her family will influence her expectations of the current episode. Personality is also important, and those prone to anxiety, depression and obsessional tendencies may react more to their illness, particularly as there may be concerns about loss of control or independence. Clearly, any pre-existing or past psychiatric disorder is also important. The severity of the illness together with the physical symptoms of pain and discomfort and the treatment required will all play a part in the patient's response. Support, or lack of it, from her partner or other relatives and friends will influence the woman's ability to adjust to her illness. The way that healthcare professionals handle the patient is very important in alleviating her concerns. Sympathetic physical examination and discussion of diagnosis and treatment is essential to minimize concerns. Full explanation for the reasons of referral to other departments or agencies should be given. In some areas of medical practice such as oncology and infectious diseases, psychological distress is acknowledged and its detection and treatment is integral to the care of patients.

Psychiatric presentations

Depression and anxiety

Depression is ranked as the fourth global burden of disease by the World Health Organization (Timonen & Liukkonen 2008). Depression and anxiety, which may coexist, are the commonest psychiatric conditions seen in any medical setting. Minor degrees of depression and anxiety may be a normal reaction to illness or other life event. However, if severe, they may be part of a depressive illness, anxiety disorder, posttraumatic stress disorder or obsessive–compulsive disorder.

A common assumption held by healthcare professionals and patients alike is that it is understandable for a person to develop depression in such circumstances as profound illness, and rationalize it by thinking 'I would be depressed in those circumstances'. Regardless of the understandable nature of the reaction, the severity and persistence of the depressive symptoms may warrant treatment. The report of the Royal College of Physicians and Royal College of Psychiatrists (2003) suggests the following questions that may help to elicit the diagnosis of depression:
- Does the person's distress appear to be very severe?
- Is the mood change persistent (i.e. lasting more than 2 weeks)?
- Is there evidence of a failure to adjust to the illness?
- Is the person expressing suicidal ideas?
- Is the person's physical function poorer than expected?
- Is the person's recovery from illness slower than expected, or is rehabilitation difficult?
- Is there poor social interaction (e.g. the patient does not respond to relatives visiting, staff or other patients on the ward)?

Clinical depression has features in several domains: affective (sadness, loss of hope, loss of enjoyment), cognitive (thoughts of worthlessness and death, suicidal ideas, inappropriate guilt, impaired concentration) and somatic (pain, fatigue, insomnia, weight changes). It may be mild, moderate or severe. Infrequently there are psychotic features (delusions, hallucinations). Perhaps the most important feature, which distinguishes the mood disorder from being upset, is the lack of adaptation to the situation and the persistence of symptoms: symptoms must be persistent and last for several weeks, showing little response to happy experiences or good news.

It is not always clear whether anxiety and depression are consequent or coexistent to a physical diagnosis. Profound mood disorders may also be further complicated by other physical problems as lifestyle changes that compromise health, such as smoking and drinking, are used as coping mechanisms. Depression and anxiety may be associated with poor communication skills and dissatisfaction with information and treatment received (Royal College of Physicians and Royal College of Psychiatrists 2003).

The association between pain and depression and anxiety is particularly important, although the direction of causality is not always clear: pain may cause depression and anxiety, and depression and anxiety may, in turn, cause pain to worsen or the report of it to be more pressing.

Very often, depression occurs after a diagnosis of cancer. Those of younger age are more likely to develop problems. This does not preclude older people or those who are pain free of developing such problems but highlights groups in which it is particularly likely. Finally, illnesses that affect the brain, such as multiple sclerosis, Parkinson's disease and stroke, are particularly associated with depression.

Effective interventions are available for depression and anxiety in those with physical illness and so they should not be left untreated (Sheard & Maguire 1999, Citron *et al.* 2005, Cohen & Gorman 2008). Treatment leads to an enhanced quality of life, improving emotional and social function together with physical symptoms such as pain.

Severe depression can lead to ideas of deliberate self-harm and consequent attempted or completed suicide. Suicidal thoughts or intentions are associated with many other psychiatric or psychological problems and are not normally a reaction to physical illness. It is important to ask about these thoughts or intentions and there is no evidence that this questioning is more likely to lead the patient to act upon them. However, identifying these thoughts allows active intervention and treatment. In terminal illness such thoughts may be an expression of desperation and fear about the loss of control or extreme pain. Discussion about how symptoms might be controlled can alleviate this fear and assuage suicidal ideation. If the person has a depressive illness, effective treatment will lead to improved mood and fading out of suicidal thoughts. Suicide may also be committed in the absence of depression, but this is usually carefully planned and thought through over a long period of time. Questions that may help the physician to approach the subject in these situations are as follows (Royal College of Physicians and Royal College of Psychiatrists 2003):

- Thoughts of dying. Step 1: *Are there ever times when you feel you just want to go to sleep and never wake up?*
- Suicidal ideation. If yes to Step 1, Step 2: *Have you thought of harming yourself or taking your own life?*

It is also important to explore the person's consumption of alcohol, as it may be used to modulate feelings of anxiety or depression, and, in turn, contribute to make such feelings worse. Simple questions to elicit alcohol use in the context of depression are:

- *Do you ever have a drink to relieve stress or cheer yourself up?*
- *Have you been drinking more than usual?*
- *Roughly how much have you been drinking?*

Recreational drugs and prescribed medicines, such as analgesics and hypnotics, can also be misused as a way of dealing with uncomfortable or distressing feelings.

Anxiety, like depression, can be a normal human experience, as well as a symptom of underlying mental disorders. Anxiety describes feelings of unease or worry. These feelings may be entirely appropriate, and are adaptive reactions that assist problem-solving. It is only when they become excessive or inappropriate and difficult to control that they are counterproductive and disabling. These persistent worries do not respond to reassurance or may do so for only a limited period.

Anxiety is the principal feature of generalized anxiety disorder (persistent and generalized but not restricted to a particular environment, with motor tension, apprehension and autonomic overactivity). Anxiety symptoms may also be prominent in panic disorder, agoraphobia, social phobia, obsessive–compulsive disorders and post-traumatic stress disorders. Post-traumatic stress disorder is associated with recurrent intrusive thoughts or images of a traumatic experience and may be a feature of the presentation of women who have been sexually abused or raped. As with depression, a past psychiatric history increases the chance of an anxiety disorder developing. Women with obsessive–compulsive disorders may report unwanted thoughts or images that are difficult to resist but have enough insight to recognize that they are their own.

Psychotic illnesses, delirium and drug-induced states

Psychotic disorders such as schizophrenia and bipolar affective disorder (previously known as manic depression) are relatively rare. Delirium is a non-specific term for a disorder caused by localized or systemic pathology affecting brain function. Psychotic symptoms, such as delusions and hallucinations, may also be associated with delirium. Delirium has organic causes such as infection, inflammation or systemic disease. There are also iatrogenic causes, in particular steroids, as well as self-administered recreational drugs or withdrawal from alcohol. Causes of delirium may be difficult to elucidate and are often multifactorial. Typically, such states will resolve rapidly if the underlying cause or causes are treated.

Women with psychotic problems may have sexual hallucinations, but it would be unlikely that these symptoms would be the sole presentation. They are also likely to find these symptoms perplexing or may account for them by delusional explanations. For example, a young woman with schizophrenia complained of orgasmic sensations, which she believed to be the result of intercourse with the devil. She had these hallucinatory sensations during interview much in the same way that people with psychotic disorders may have auditory hallucinations. Delusions and hallucinations are unresponsive to rational argument, the patient refusing to accept explanations that are offered to account for the problem. Vulval symptoms and sexual concerns may lead women with these disorders to present not to psychiatrists but to other healthcare professionals in primary or secondary care. Complaints may initially appear highly plausible, but on closer questioning it becomes apparent that there is an underlying psychotic disorder.

Women with chronic mental health problems such as schizophrenia may experience a decline in their physical health as a result of their mental illness. This may be a consequence of poverty, chaotic lifestyle (with failure to engage in preventative behaviour such as cervical screening or eating a healthy diet) or concomitant drug abuse. However, these patients should be investigated as fully as possible for their presenting complaints. Perhaps the most difficult decision for the healthcare professional being consulted is not whether to perform an examination or investigations but at which point to stop. This may be a decision that should be taken by the most senior, and hence most experienced, member of a team rather than the most junior, which is where such decisions are sometimes made.

Medically unexplained symptoms

A proportion of patients have symptoms which can be described as medically unexplained. This problem is common, especially in primary care. In hospital outpatient clinics, up to half of the patients may have medically unexplained symptoms where there is no detectable pathology (Escobar *et al.* 1987, Russo *et al.* 1994, Bhui & Hotopf 1996, Wessely *et al.* 1997, Gureje *et al.* 1998, Nimnuan *et al.* 2001), or the symptoms may be disproportionate to clinical findings. In patients with this problem, some may have a well-defined psychiatric disorder, whereas others are healthy but with severe anxiety about their health (the 'worried well'). The psychiatric diagnoses that may apply to these patients include somatoform disorders (hypochondriasis and somatization) and conversion disorders.

Somatoform disorders

Patients with somatoform disorders are preoccupied with physical symptoms which cause significant distress and are disproportionate to the mild underlying pathology. This preoccupation is not intentionally produced, nor accounted for by other psychiatric conditions but is precipitated and maintained by psychological factors. Somatoform disorders include hypochondriasis and somatization disorders. In hypochondriasis, better described as health anxiety, the patient is preoccupied with the belief or fear that she has a serious disease and cannot be reassured that this is not the case. In somatization disorder, the patient has a history of at least eight different kinds of symptoms at different body sites. There is always evidence of a link with psychological or emotional factors. Psychogenic pain, the preoccupation with pain when there is no physical disorder, is also a somatoform disorder.

Some medically unexplained symptoms cluster into well-recognized functional somatic syndromes such as chronic pelvic pain, irritable bladder or irritable bowel syndrome. It is important to remember that organic pathology can occur concurrently with medically unexplained symptoms, e.g. a patient with urethral syndrome may develop a coincidental urinary tract infection.

Body dysmorphic disorder is an excessive concern about a trivial or non-existent imperfection that patients then perceive as a serious deformity.

Conversion disorder

Conversion disorder presents with symptoms or deficits that affect voluntary motor or sensory function and would suggest a neurological condition but no organic cause is found.

Health professionals can contribute to the persistence of some of these unexplained symptoms by inappropriate investigations or treatments, which can lead the patient to become concerned about the seriousness of her symptoms and reinforce her health anxiety and illness beliefs (Mayou & Farmer 2002).

There is good evidence that patients with mild disorders of recent onset respond to simple reassurance and explanation. Those with moderate disorders may need brief psychological interventions or psychotropic treatment and those with more chronic and severe conditions may require intensive psychological management or treatment in a specific rehabilitation setting (Royal College of Physicians and Royal College of Psychiatrists 2003).

Factitious disorders and malingering

Factitious disorders in which physical or psychological symptoms are feigned in order to assume the sick role are unusual if there is no obvious reason for gain (Lubbe *et al.* 2000, Schultz *et al.* 2005). Malingering, on the other hand, describes intentionally feigned symptoms in which there is an obvious underlying motivation, such as the desire for compensation. If there are concerns that either are occurring the situation requires careful assessment and documentation as the problem may become a medicolegal issue.

Factitious disorders

These disorders are often missed by health workers, particularly at initial presentation. In factitious disorders, the person deliberately falsifies and creates the physical or mental symptoms to receive medical attention and assume the sick role. In rare cases of a factitious disorder, the patient consults widely, visiting geographically distant hospitals presenting with dramatic and fantastic stories (Munchausen's syndrome). In other cases, generally female, women present their children with the symptoms and signs of a medical problem (Munchausen's by proxy). Typically, patients with a factitious disorder have a history of childhood emotional neglect or abuse, and they frequently have a nursing or paramedical background. Management requires careful evaluation of the physical symptoms to exclude any possible pathology. This may be followed by direct or indirect challenge, providing some form of face-saving exit, together with efforts to provide alternative ways of dealing with their emotional difficulties (Lubbe *et al.* 2000, Schultz *et al.* 2005, Semple *et al.* 2005).

Malingering

In malingering the symptoms are deliberately feigned with a clear underlying motivation. This may be the desire for compensation, the patient may want hospital admission or to be given opiates. Careful assessment and documentation are important to avoid both iatrogenic problems and the risk of medicolegal action. Psychiatric assessment and advice on management may be helpful in factitious disorders and malingering.

Psychological aspects of specific conditions or events

Chronic vulval pain syndromes

Women seeking help for chronic vulval pain are frequently seen in a variety of healthcare settings from dermatology to psychiatry, and they can present a complex diagnostic and management problem.

A chronic vulval pain syndrome (vulvodynia) is defined as a sensation of burning or soreness in the absence of any visible or inducible cause. Two main types of vulvodynia are described. The first one is vestibulodynia (previously termed vestibulitis), and is characterized by the symptoms of entry dyspareunia and vestibular tenderness. The second is generalized vulvodynia, and describes diffuse vulval pain which may or may not be provoked by touch. It is usually constant but varies in intensity sometimes with episodes of exacerbation and radiation of the pain into the pelvic and thigh areas. There can be overlap and some authors have questioned the existence of two distinct syndromes (Smart & MacLean 2003) (see Chapter 6 for more details). There are many areas of uncertainty and therefore of debate about the prevalence, aetiology, physiopathology, treatment and contribution of psychological factors to vulvodynia.

A survey of over 2000 US households reported an incidence of current chronic vulval pain in almost 4%, with a lifetime prevalence close to 10% (Arnold *et al.* 2007). These are much lower figures than reported elsewhere (Bachmann *et al.* 2006a–c). The presence of chronic vulval pain was associated with depression, chronic fatigue syndrome, fibromyalgia and irritable bowel syndrome, as well as reported repeated urinary tract and yeast infections. Overlap with other pain syndromes has been noted by other authors (Wesselmann & Reich 1996, Baranowski *et al.* 1999, Gordon *et al.* 2003, Smart & MacLean 2003, Ness 2005, Arnold *et al.* 2006). It is unclear whether such an overlap is indicative of vulnerable personality traits, differences in perception of pain (Lotery *et al.* 2004) or other mechanisms.

Symptoms of anxiety and depression are not uncommon in women with chronic vulval pain. The question however, is whether anxiety and depression are more common in patients with chronic pain, or whether the pain is a consequence of anxiety or depression. Green and Hetherton (2005) carried out a systematic review of publications on the psychological aspects of vestibulitis (now vestibulodynia). They concluded that there was marked inconsistency between studies, with those carried out in a specialist setting tending to show greater levels of psychological morbidity (anxiety and depression) than controls (Stewart *et al.* 1994, Masheb *et al.* 2002, Wylie *et al.* 2004, Lundqvist & Bergdahl 2005, Latthe *et al.* 2006), while community surveys tended not to show such differences. The authors suggested that confounding factors involved in the process of referral to specialist services might play a part as there would be selection bias, many of these patients having a worse psychological profile as well as more severe physical symptoms. Some authors have argued against regarding vulvodynia as a psychological condition (Bachmann *et al.* 2006a–c).

So it is not surprising to find that women with vulvodynia experience sexual difficulties, including pain during intercourse or when penetration is attempted, avoidance of sexual intercourse, loss of interest and orgasmic difficulties, although non-penetrative sexual activities may not be affected (Van Lankveld *et al.* 1996, Marin *et al.* 2000, Masheb *et al.* 2002, Gordon *et al.* 2003, Reed *et al.* 2003a–c, Green & Hetherton 2005, Arnold *et al.* 2006, Latthe *et al.* 2006).

The possible contribution of childhood sexual abuse to the development of chronic vulval pain has been the subject of research but the evidence is inconclusive. Although some researchers found an association between vestibulodynia and childhood sexual abuse (Friedrich 1987, Goetsch 1991, Jantos & White 1997, Harlow & Stewart 2005), others failed to do so (Edwards *et al.* 1997, Dalton *et al.* 2002, Gordon *et al.* 2003). Other factors that may contribute to these inconsistencies in the literature include sampling and recall bias, and survey technique (use of telephone and questionnaire techniques against face-to-face assessment). The assumption of a history of abuse in all cases of chronic vulvodynia is incorrect, but, in an individual in whom there has been abuse, the disclosure may be relevant and psychological intervention can be therapeutic.

Childhood sexual abuse

A study in primary care in the UK of childhood abuse (at age less than 16 years) reported that 9% of women had had unwanted sexual intercourse and 11% unwanted sexual activities, but not intercourse, and 5% experienced both unwanted sexual intercourse and other unwanted sexual activities. With regards to physical abuse, 5% were severely beaten by a parent or carer on one occasion and 12% severely beaten more than once. In those women beaten on more than one occasion, 21% reported unwanted sexual intercourse and 27% unwanted sexual activities; 2% reported all three forms of abusive experience (Coid *et al.* 2003).

Adverse early experiences, such as childhood sexual abuse, affect the developing brain and may lead to lifelong psychiatric sequelae. Adolescents experiencing a traumatic event after the age of 13 years are less likely to develop depression but may experience post-traumatic stress disorder, whereas children (up to age 12 years) traumatized by abuse are more likely to develop major depression but not post-traumatic stress disorder (Maercker *et al.* 2004). There is a higher risk of developing depressive and anxiety disorders in children and adults because of neurobiological changes (Heim & Nemeroff 2001, Nemeroff 2004). Children and adolescents who have been physically or sexually abused are more likely to experience suicidal thoughts and behaviours than other adolescents, which may be mediated by low self-esteem (Evans *et al.* 2005). They are also more likely to experience other types of psychiatric illness, to have more physical symptoms (both medically explained and unexplained) and to engage in more health-risk behaviours. The more severe the abuse, the more likely they are to have psychological problems in adulthood. Childhood sexual abuse in particular is more likely to result in physical complaints such as chronic pain associated with depression in adult life. They are more likely to become high users of medical care and emergency services. Men and women who have experienced childhood abuse are seen particularly in specialties such as emergency psychiatric care (Arnow 2004).

Sexual assault and rape

It has been suggested that between 10% and 50% of women have experienced some form of sexual assault (Matsakis 1996), with significant increases in the reported incidence in recent years. Although unwanted sexual assault not including sexual intercourse and rape is relatively common, it is not always reported by victims at the time of the assault, and, thus, their psychological consequences may not become obvious for some time. It is likely that greater recognition of the problem of rape and social changes that have shifted the blame from the victim to the perpetrator have both contributed to an increase in the proportion of women prepared to report the attack. Additionally, it is now recognized that there are specific needs of women who have suffered this form of violence. In the immediate aftermath of the sexual assault, some women may be in shock and seemingly unable to show emotion. Others may be acutely distressed and scared, so that the process of assessing the physical impact of the assault, treating the physical trauma, performing investigations and providing emotional support will need to be carried out sympathetically and sensitively. Symptoms of anxiety and depression, insomnia and feelings of self-blame and guilt may be prominent over the following weeks and months.

A proportion of women who have been the victims of rape or sexual assault will develop post-traumatic stress disorder. The features of post-traumatic stress disorder include re-experiencing the traumatic events (recollections, dreams, feelings), avoidance of related reminders, numbing and detachment, and increased arousal (hypervigilance, insomnia, irritability). If these symptoms last more than 3 months, the syndrome becomes chronic, and delayed reactions sometimes appear within 6 months of the trauma. Studies in primary care have found a strong association between sexual assault in adulthood and substance misuse, and rape is associated with depression, anxiety and post-traumatic stress disorder (Coid et al. 2003). In fact, rape has been reported to lead to post-traumatic stress disorder in more than 50% of cases, the highest reported incidence for any traumatic experience (Bisson 2007). General population studies have reported a greater risk of developing post-traumatic stress

disorder rather than major depression in older adolescents after sexual trauma (Maercker et al. 2004).

The comparatively high prevalence of sexual assault and rape in the general population suggests that a significant proportion of women attending clinics seeking help for genital symptoms will have experienced such traumas. In some cases, the sexual trauma may be the explicit reason for consulting, while, in other cases, the woman may feel too ashamed or embarrassed to volunteer details of her previous trauma. Whether or not the traumatic experience is relevant to the presenting symptoms will require sensitive evaluation. Post-traumatic stress disorder usually presents with other psychiatric syndromes, such as depression, anxiety, sexual dysfunction or unexplained pain. It is important to recognize post-traumatic stress disorder as treatment is often effective (see below).

Surgical procedures

Vulvectomy

The psychological consequences of vulvectomy for genital cancer are predictably related to both the diagnosis of cancer and the disfiguring surgery. They include the possible development of depression and other mood disorders, which may contribute to sexual and relationship difficulties. One study found no difference in levels of depression in women undergoing total or partial vulvectomy compared with women having surgery for other forms of cancer (Andersen & Hacker 1983). However, Stellman et al. (1984) found more severe depression following vulvectomy than following hysterectomy. Interestingly, Andreasson et al. (1986) found mood disorders not only in more than half of the women who had had a vulvectomy but also in a similar proportion of their partners.

Sexual dysfunction problems have been well documented in women after vulvectomy (Andersen & Hacker 1983, Moth et al. 1983, Andreasson et al. 1986). This link with mood disorders was clearly shown in the study by Green et al. (2000) involving 41 women who had undergone vulvectomy. They showed that there was an aversion to sexual contact with a reduction in the frequency of sexual contact and sexual interest after surgery. Furthermore, sexual arousal was poor and there was a worsening of body image. The extent of the surgery or the technique used did not seem to correlate with the degree of sexual problems, but the presence of depression was associated with a higher rate of sexual difficulties. Comprehensive assessment of mood and of the sexual and relationship impact of this form of surgery should be the first step towards supporting the woman and her partner.

Other surgical procedures

The performance of episiotomy is subject to trends in practice, and there are reservations about its widespread use without any evidence base (Thakar & Banta 1983). The complications of this procedure include infection, haemorrhage, scarring with anatomical distortion, chronic pain and dyspareunia. Pain syndromes and sexual dysfunction following episiotomy may be associated with mood disorders and relationship difficulties.

Individuals with gender identity disorder or transsexuality may present before or after undergoing sex reassignment. Transsexuals will typically describe a long-standing conviction that their gender identity (I am a man or I am a woman) is at odds with their anatomical sex and will show persistent distress at their birth sex; they will maintain a desire to live and be treated as a member of the opposite sex. Male-to-female transsexuals are 3–4 times more common than female-to-male ones, with a prevalence of 1 in 30 000 for male-to-female and about 1 in 100 000 for female-to-male reassignments. A significant proportion suffer from comorbid psychological disorders, such as depression and anxiety. Sexual self-mutilation is rare. Psychological interventions aimed at changing the core beliefs are ineffective, and sex-reassignment treatment will include real-life testing of the desired gender role, use of sex hormones and surgery. Male-to-female individuals undergo orchidectomy and penectomy with vaginoplasty. Female-to-male surgery involves mastectomy, hysterectomy and salpingo-oophorectomy, but few undertake phalloplasty, as the results are poor (Wylie 2004, Semple *et al.* 2005).

Cosmetic procedures

Cosmetic procedures such as body piercing are currently popular, and can involve the female genitalia, including the labia majora and minora as well as the clitoral hood. Complications include infection, bleeding and scarring, which can interfere with later childbirth. Urethral rupture has also been reported. The motivation for undergoing these procedures is complex, involving an element of fashion, private need and a public social statement. It is important for the health worker coming into contact with pierced individuals who experience complications to be free from prejudice and respect the person's path to her own identity (Stirn 2003).

Requests for genital cosmetic surgery may be related to obvious disfigurement, e.g. hypertrophy which may be congenital or post-traumatic following childbirth. However, it may be wanted purely for aesthetic reasons in the search for a more youthful genital appearance. In other cases, it may be the result of dysmorphophobia, a belief that a part of the body is abnormal or deformed. In such cases, it is unlikely that surgical correction will reassure the patient, who will continue to consult further unless the underlying psychological disorder is addressed.

Female genital mutilation

Female genital mutilation (FGM) is also known as female circumcision or female genital cutting. It involves removal

Table 7.1 Categories of female genital mutilation

Type I	Removal of all or part of the clitoris and its prepuce
Type II	Excision of clitoris, with partial or total removal of labia minora
Type III	All external genitalia excised, vaginal opening closed except for a matchtip-sized hole to allow urine and blood to escape
Type IV	Unclassified. Pricking, piercing, incision, stretching, scraping or other harming procedures on clitoris and or labia

of part or all the female genitalia for no medical indication. There are four categories (WHO 1996), as shown in Table 7.1.

The true extent of FGM is unreliable as self-reporting is low, and so there is probably considerable underestimation of the practice. Furthermore, the risk of complications and mortality may be inaccurate as studies have relied on self-reporting (Elmusharaf *et al.* 2006).

It is estimated that 130 million women are living with the consequences of FGM (WHO 2008) and is practised most commonly in the western, eastern and north-eastern regions of Africa (WHO 1998) and in the Middle East (parts of Oman, the United Arab Emirates and in Yemen) and in other countries such as Indonesia and Malaysia (Isa *et al.* 1999, Population Council 2003). In the UK, it is estimated that there are 3000–4000 new cases every year as FGM continues after emigration to Europe from countries where it is practised (Bosch 2001). In many cultures, there is a decline in the practice (Msuya *et al.* 2002), but, in others, despite legislation, there is not (Hassanin *et al.* 2008).

The consequences of this practice are revealed in two studies showing that there are more psychosexual problems in women who had undergone FGM than in controls. These included dysmenorrhoea (81%), poor lubrication during intercourse (48.5%), lack of sexual desire (45%), less initiative during sex (11%) and decreased satisfaction (49%). Symptoms of sexual dysfunction in this group included reduced intensity (39%) and frequency of orgasm (25%), with 61% reporting a failure to achieve orgasm (el-Defrawi *et al.* 2001). Women who had undergone FGM had significant mental problems such as somatization, anxiety and phobia. Obstetric trauma including tears, episiotomy and delayed labour with consequent fetal distress were more common among circumcised women, which may add to the psychological distress (Elnashar & Abdelhady 2007). The other studies suggest the ability to achieve orgasm is not impaired by FGM and defibulation may relieve intact clitoral tissue. It is important, as with all clinical interactions, to respect the patient's cultural and religious beliefs. Sexual counselling, psychotherapy and support groups may be offered in addition to any medical or surgical interventions that are required (Catania *et al.* 2007). Physicians need to clarify their own legal and ethical responsibility so that patients understand why their request to be resutured after childbirth may be declined.

Sexual dysfunction

Sexual dysfunction describes the various ways in which individuals are unable to participate in a sexual relationship as they would wish. Sexual response is a psychosomatic process involving emotions and thoughts as well as physical responses, and so it is vulnerable to disorders and difficulties affecting all domains. Sexual dysfunction problems are understandably common in women presenting with vulval disorders. (Andersen & Hacker 1983, Huffman 1983, Marin *et al.* 2000, Hallam-Jones *et al.* 2001, Jensen *et al.* 2003, Morris & Mukhopadhyay 2006, Wylie 2007).

The prevalence of female sexual dysfunction has been estimated to be around 40% in the USA and UK. It is reported that 64% have decreased desire, 35% difficulties with orgasm, 31% poor arousal and 26% sexual pain (Hayes *et al.* 2006). Sexual dysfunction is more common in younger women, and they complain of conflict within relationships, poor knowledge of their body, partner sexual dysfunction, poor partner technique, personal psychopathology and a history of trauma, including genital, obstetric and others (Wylie 2007). The medical and psychological aspects of sexual dysfunction are inextricably linked. Sexual dysfunction may be associated with depression as well as heralding serious underlying disease such as renal failure, hypertension, diabetes and multiple sclerosis. Furthermore, the medical treatment of these conditions can affect sexual function, which may lead to poor patient compliance.

Loss of interest in sex may be a symptom of depression, which should resolve when the depression is treated. It may also be secondary to debilitating physical illness, dermatological condition or dyspareunia (Dalziel 1995). In the absence of psychiatric or physical pathology it may arise as a result of relationship problems. Loss of interest in sex may include sexual aversion and lack of sexual enjoyment, so that sexual activity is avoided. In others, sexual responses occur normally and orgasm is experienced but there is still a lack of appropriate pleasure.

In orgasmic dysfunction, orgasm either does not occur or is markedly delayed. In vaginismus, spasm of the pelvic floor muscles that surround the outer part of the vagina causes occlusion of the vaginal opening. In dyspareunia penile entry is either impossible or painful during sexual intercourse and may be attributable to local pathology and should then properly be categorized under the pathological condition, and not as a psychological problem. Entry dyspareunia that occurs in the absence of any recognized pathology is categorized as a sensory disorder that could

also be associated with a psychological problem, e.g. vestibulodynia. This sensory disorder can be a primary problem, but often it is secondary to failure of arousal that may be due to depression in up to 26% cases (Van Lankveld & Grotjohan 2000).

Hypoactive sexual desires

Hypoactive sexual desires occur with many diseases such as renal failure, diabetes, multiple sclerosis, hyperprolactinaemia, bilateral oophorectomy, adrenal disease, neurological disease, psychiatric problems, cerebrovascular disease, Parkinson's disease and head injuries (Basson & Schultz 2007). Drugs may also reduce sexual desire, including antipsychotics, and in schizophrenia this side-effect occurs in over 50% of patients. Antidepressants, especially serotonin serum reuptake inhibitors (SSRIs), cause low desire in 30–50% of women. Other prescribed drugs such as narcotics, beta-blockers, anti-androgens and antiepileptic drugs also have an effect, as do many recreational drugs (Basson & Schultz 2007, Wylie 2007).

Female genital arousal disorder

Decreased lubrication and vaginal congestion are associated with decrease in sexual arousal and a decrease in orgasm. Reduced lubrication occurs with low oestrogen, diabetes or hypertension and in women with mild atheroma of the hypogastric arteries, pudendal arteries or both (Hultgren *et al.* 1999). Vaginal congestion is reduced in women receiving haemo- or peritoneal dialysis, and it persists even after renal transplantation (Toorians *et al.* 1997).

Priapism is persistent erection of the corpora cavernosa due to excessive congestion. It can occur secondary to drug treatment with antidepressants (see Chapter 5). Persistent genital arousal syndrome, a recently recognized disorder, is unwanted, persistent genital congestion with preorgasmic feelings, which is only slightly relieved by orgasm (Leiblum & Nathan 2001). The aetiology is unknown and there is little effective treatment.

Orgasmic dysfunction

Increase in sexual interest is rarely a reason for consulting a health professional, but, when it is encountered, one possible diagnosis to consider is that of a manic episode in the context of a bipolar affective disorder. It may present with absent or delayed orgasm and can occur with upper motor neurone lesions such as multiple sclerosis and spinal cord injury. Low testosterone and drugs may be causative factors, including SSRIs, antipsychotics and anti-androgens. Painful orgasm may occur after the menopause, or with intrauterine devices, pelvic inflammatory disease, endometriosis and pelvic floor dysfunction. Radical hysterectomy does not preclude orgasm nor does weakening of the pelvic floor from vaginal deliveries (Basson & Schultz 2007).

Psychological assessment

Basic communication and clinical assessment

Patients attending general hospitals are usually concerned about their symptoms, likely diagnosis, treatment and prognosis. Such reactions are understandable, and, in the majority of cases, their severity is reduced by good communication between the patient and the clinician. Essential elements of good communication include:

• introducing oneself and explaining the purpose of the appointment and possible further investigations
• listening to the patient's complaints and symptoms
• recognizing and exploring the patient's concerns and worries
• providing information about the clinician's views about what is wrong and what further investigations and treatment may be required
• involving the patient in decisions about her care.

The patients' perception of the doctor as sympathetic and knowledgeable in vulval disorders has been shown to be associated with patient satisfaction, regardless of the clinical outcome (Wojnarowska *et al.* 1997, Smart & MacLean 2003, Munday 2001). Management of sexual dysfunction consists of treating any underlying organic disorder in conjunction with specific management of any sexual dysfunction. The variety of medical and surgical interventions tried and the lack of evidence for their efficacy favour a more psychological approach (Basson & Schultz 2007).

Brief psychological evaluation

Clinicians treating women with vulval problems will be aware of the issues around using chaperones when performing intimate examinations of women. This is particularly important for women with psychological problems as they may be more prone to misinterpreting situations and may appear to have the competence to give consent when in fact they do not. The presence of a chaperone, who must be introduced to the patient at the outset, should be a reassuring sign to them.

The astute clinician can gather much information by listening and watching the patient. Clues to anxiety, sadness, fears about serious illness and impact on relationships and work can all be picked up. These are then confirmed by direct and focused questioning. It should be possible for the physician without any specialist psychiatric training to recognize symptoms of significant psychological disorder, and to take steps for the patient to receive appropriate help (Report of the Royal College of Physicians and Royal College of Psychiatrists 2003).

The following are some of the main areas for assessment.

The degree of concern

Is this out of proportion to the severity of the problem? A strong response may reflect past personal history or experience of a close friend or relative with a serious problem. It may also suggest the presence of a sensitive and anxious personality, or even be a sign of a depression or anxiety disorder.

Negative feelings and thoughts

Persistent feelings of sadness and worry, tearfulness, lack of hope in the future, suicidal thoughts and plans, and disturbed sleep and appetite would point towards the presence of a significant depressive disorder requiring specific intervention. Active suicidal thoughts and plans should always be taken seriously and a psychiatric opinion should be sought urgently.

Symptoms of anxiety

Symptoms of anxiety with both mental manifestations, such as worry or fears of serious illness, and somatic symptoms, such as palpitations, aches and pains, giddiness or unsteadiness, indicate conditions that should be referred for specialist mental health assessment.

Multiple secondary care consultations

A history of multiple serial somatic complaints leading to referral to secondary specialist services, such as cardiology, gastroenterology, neurology or gynaecology, often in the absence of any clear evidence of disease, would suggest a functional somatic syndrome (Mayou & Farmer 2002).

General health and family history

Questions about current or past stresses, as well as a past history of personal or family difficulties, including psychiatric history, must be asked. In addition, enquiry about alcohol consumption and recreational drug use can be introduced as part of the assessment of the patient's coping mechanisms for her health problems.

Subjective complaints about memory problems and objective evidence of poor concentration, short-term memory and orientation would alert the clinician to the presence of an organic brain syndrome requiring further investigation.

In most instances, women with vulval conditions will attend the clinic on their own, despite being involved in an emotional and physical relationship with a partner. Exploring the impact of the vulval condition on her sexual function is an important part of the assessment. Enquiries should be made about changes in sexual interest, willingness to engage in penetrative sex and difficulties with orgasm. The nature of the relationship between the sexual difficulties and the vulval condition may be complex, and it would be important not to make assumptions about the causal direction of the association without careful assessment. On occasions, it may be important to offer the woman the chance of inviting her partner to attend the clinic with her, partly to explain the nature of the problem to the partner and to involve the partner in any therapeutic intervention. This is also a good opportunity to gain a greater understanding of the partner's possible contribution to the situation. This must be negotiated with the patient as she may not wish her partner to be involved.

Examination and investigation of psychosexual problems is worth outlining. It is important for the clinicians involved in the care of the patient to establish who is primarily responsible for a full examination and investigation. It is easy to overlook these basic principles in shared care and to assume incorrectly that they have been performed by the referring doctor.

The clinical examination may cause concern but it is rarely unnecessary; if is done in a sensitive manner, it should not cause distress to the patients and can be reassuring (see Chapter 2). The genital examination should be done to exclude a local pathology and a general examination should exclude any comorbidity, e.g. diabetes, hypertension. Investigations for patients presenting with sexual dysfunction may be indicated (Wylie 2007). These might include full blood count, urea and electrolytes and glucose. Androgen and oestrogen function and prolactin and thyroid levels should be checked in patients with hypoactive sexual desire disorder. In patients with anorgasmia, a full work-up would include a screen for autonomic neuropathy and serum testosterone.

Psychological and psychiatric interventions

Sexual health concerns were found in 99% of women seeking routine gynaecological care (Nusbaum et al. 2000), but over half of patients with a sexual problem fail to ask their physicians for help, even though they would have liked to (Berman et al. 2003). It is worth remembering that only 15% of women with sexual problems in the postnatal period discuss them with healthcare professionals (Barrett et al. 2006), despite childbirth having a major impact on sexual function (Botros et al. 2006).

Understandably, patients with psychotic disorders or delirium may not disclose the problem because of the lack of insight that accompanies the illness. This may be discovered only by direct questioning. If clear evidence of a significant psychiatric disturbance is identified, the patient should be referred to the mental health services by the clinician dealing with the vulval disorder. This will depend on the local resources and care pathways available.

Severe psychiatric disorders, such as major depression or generalized anxiety disorders, need to involve specialists. Many clinicians from specialties other than psychiatry are in general competent in managing people with functional somatic symptoms using simple reassurance and advice (Mayou & Farmer 2002). Specific measures for insomnia

such as sleep hygiene advice can also be discussed, but more complex disorders and conditions requiring specialist psychological or psychopharmacological intervention are more appropriately managed by the hospital mental health services. Liaison psychiatry and health psychology are now well-established services working alongside their medical colleagues in many general hospitals. This development has led to joint working practices to deal with particular groups of patients likely to present with mental health difficulties. Examples of such services include the pain clinic, gynaecology, perinatal care, emergency department, genitourinary medicine, oncology and HIV/AIDS (Peveler et al. 2000).

Individual psychological interventions

A broad range of interventions are used, ranging from brief counselling aimed at exploring traumatic events and helping to choose a course of action, to more specialized therapies, such as cognitive–behaviour therapy (CBT) or analytical techniques. CBT has been shown to be effective in the treatment of mild to moderately severe depression, anxiety disorders, post-traumatic stress disorders, hypochondriasis and health anxiety disorders. Integrating CBT and other individual therapies with general medical intervention has been advocated in the management of vulvodynia and related disorders (Stewart et al. 1994, Katz 1996, Weijmar Schultz et al. 1996, Munday et al. 2001, Wylie 2007).

A short psychoeducational intervention for women with sexual arousal problems following surgery for gynaecological cancer has been developed. This helps with the sexual difficulties and has the additional benefit of improving mood and overall well-being (Brotto et al. 2008).

The treatment of post-traumatic stress disorder includes psychological and psychopharmacological interventions, although there is less well-documented evidence for the latter. However, there is some evidence for the value of SSRI antidepressants, sometimes in combination with olanzapine (Bisson 2007). Trauma-focused CBT and eye movement desensitization and reprocessing (EMDR) have been shown to be effective therapies (Bisson et al. 2007) and self-help books can be of assistance (Matsakis 1996).

Couple therapy

If sexual and emotional difficulties are an important part of the presentation, it is important to include the partner in therapy. In particular, this type of therapy is indicated in cases where there is vaginismus, dyspareunia, loss of interest in sex or phobic avoidance of intimacy and sexual contact (Abramov et al. 1994, Schultz et al. 2005).

Psychopharmacological treatments

The use of antidepressants is indicated for the treatment of severe depression, and for some anxiety disorders (Timonen & Liukkonen 2008). There are several classes of antidepressants in current use, the most popular being the SSRIs, such as citalopram and fluoxetine, and these in general are safe and effective. Tricyclic antidepressants are also used for chronic pain and there is some evidence for their value in vulvodynia (Reed *et al.* 2003a,b). The newer agents such as venlafaxine (serotonin and noradrenaline reuptake inhibitor) have also been used in vulvodynia (Eisen 1995). Anxiolytic medications, such as benzodiazepines, are indicated only for short-term use; for a chronic problem, psychological interventions such as anxiety management or relaxation therapy are more appropriate. Similarly, hypnotics should be used for only brief periods in acute conditions. Unfortunately, psychotropic medication can lead to psychosexual side-effects and this has to be taken into account when prescribing them.

References

Abramov, L., Wolman, I. & David, M.P. (1994) Vaginismus: an important factor in the evaluation and management of vulvar vestibulitis syndrome. *Gynecologic and Obstetric Investigation* 38, 194–197.

Andersen, B.L. & Hacker, N.F. (1983) Psychosexual adjustment after vulvar surgery. *Obstetrics and Gynecology* 62, 457–462.

Andreasson, B., Moth, I., Jensen, S.B. & Bock, J.E. (1986) Sexual function and somatopsychic reactions in vulvectomy operated women and their partners. *Acta Obstetrica et Gynaecologica Scandinavica*, 65, 7–10.

Arnold, L.D., Bachmann, G.A., Rosen, R. *et al.* (2006) Vulvodynia: characteristics and associations with comorbidities and quality of life. *Obstetrics and Gynecology* 107, 617–624.

Arnold, L.D., Bachmann, G.A., Rosen, R. & Rhoads, G.G. (2007) Assessment of vulvodynia symptoms in a sample of US women: a prevalence survey with a nested case control study. *American Journal of Obstetrics and Gynecology* 196, e1–e6.

Arnow, B.A. (2004) Relationships between childhood maltreatment, adult health and psychiatric outcomes, and medical utilization. *Journal of Clinical Psychiatry* 65 (Suppl 12), 10–15.

Bachmann, G., McElhiney, J., Peters, S. & Rosen, R. (2006a) Vulvodynia: real condition, real pain. *Sexuality, Reproduction and Menopause* 4, 71–73.

Bachmann, G.A., Rosen, R., Arnold, L.D. *et al.* (2006b) Chronic vulvar and other gynecologic pain: prevalence and characteristics in a self-reported survey. *Journal of Reproductive Medicine* 51, 3–9.

Bachmann, G.A., Rosen, R., Finn, V.W. *et al.* (2006c) Vulvodynia: a state-of-the-art consensus on definitions, diagnosis and management. *Journal of Reproductive Medicine* 51, 447–456.

Baranowski, A.P., Mallinson, C. & Johnson, N.S. (1999) A review of urogenital pain. *Pain Reviews* 6, 53–84.

Barrett, G., Pendry, E., Peacock, J. *et al.* (2006) Women's sexual health after birth. *British Journal of Obstetrics and Gynaecology* 107, 186–195.

Basson, R. & Schultz, W.W. (2007) Sexual dysfunction. 1. Sexual sequelae of general medical disorders. *Lancet* 369, 409–424.

Berman, L., Berman, J., Felder, S. *et al.* (2003) Seeking help for sexual function complaints: what gynaecologists need to know about the female patient's experience. *Fertility and Sterilisation* 79, 572–576.

Bhui, K.H. & Hotopf, M. (1996) Somatization disorder. *British Journal of Hospital Medicine* 171, 364–370.

Bisson, J. (2007) Post-traumatic stress disorder. *British Medical Journal* 334, 789–793.

Bisson, J., Ehlers, A., Matthews, R., *et al.* (2007) Psychological treatments for chronic treatments for chronic post-traumatic stress disorder. Systematic review and meta-analysis. *British Journal of Psychiatry* 190, 97–104.

Bosch, X. (2001) Female genital mutilation in developed countries. *Lancet* 358.1177–1179.

Botros, S.M., Abramov, Y., Miller, J.J. *et al.* (2006) Effect of parity on sexual function: an identical twin study. *Obstetrics and Gynecology* 107, 765–770.

Brotto, L., Heiman, J., Goff, B. *et al.* (2008) A psychoeducational intervention for sexual dysfunction in women with gynaecological cancer. *Archives of Sexual Behavior* 37, 317–329.

Catania, L., Abdulcadir, O., Puppo, V. *et al.* (2007) Pleasure and orgasm in women with female genital mutilation/cutting. *Journal of Sexual Medicine* 4, 1666–1678.

Citron, K., Brouillette, M.-J. & Beckett, A. (eds) (2005) *HIV and Psychiatry*, 2nd edn. Cambridge University Press, Cambridge.

Cohen, M.G. & Gorman, J.M. (eds) (2008) *Comprehensive Textbook of AIDS Psychiatry*. Oxford University Press, Oxford.

Coid, J., Petruckevitch, A., Chung, W. *et al.* (2003) Abusive experiences and psychiatric morbidity in women primary care attenders. *British Journal of Psychiatry* 183, 332–339.

Confidential Enquiry into Maternal and Child Health. (2007) *Saving Mothers' Lives 2003–2005* (full report). Available from: http://www.cemach.org.uk.

Dalton, V.K., Haefner, H.K., Reed, B.D. *et al.* (2002) Victimization in patients with vulvar dysesthesia/vestibulodynia. Is there an increased prevalence? *Journal of Reproductive Medicine* 47, 829–834.

Dalziel, K.L. (1995) Effect of lichen sclerosus on sexual function and parturition. *Journal of Reproductive Medicine* 40, 351–354.

Edwards, L., Mason, M., Phillips, M. *et al.* (1997) Childhood sexual and physical abuse: incidence in patients with vulvodynia. *Journal of Reproductive Medicine* 42, 135–139.

Eisen, A. (1995) Venlafaxine therapy for vulvodynia. *The Pain Clinic* 8, 365–367.

el-Defrawi, M.H., Lotfy, G., Dandash, K.F. *et al.* (2001) Female genital mutilation and its psychosexual impact. *Journal of Sex and Marital Therapy* 27, 465–473.

Elmusharaf, S., Elhadi, N. & Almroth, L. (2006) Reliability of self reported form of female genital mutilation and WHO classification: cross sectional study. *British Medical Journal* 333, 124–129.

Elnashar, A. & Abdelhady, R. (2007) The impact of female genital cutting on health of newly married women. *International Journal of Gynaecology and Obstetrics* 97, 238–244.

Escobar, J.I., Burnam, M.A., Karno, M. *et al.* (1987) Somatization in the community. *Archives of General Psychiatry* 44, 713–718.

Evans, E., Hawton, K. & Rodham, K. (2005) Suicidal phenomena and abuse in adolescents: a review of epidemiological studies. *Child Abuse and Neglect* 29, 45–58.

Fischer, G.O. (1996) The commonest causes of symptomatic vulvar disease: a dermatologist's perspective. *Australasian Journal of Dermatology* 37, 12–18.

Fischhoff, B. & Wessely, S. (2003) Managing patients with inexplicable health problems. *British Medical Journal* 26, 595–597.

Friedrich, E.G. (1987) Vulvar vestibulitis syndrome. *Journal of Reproductive Medicine* 32, 110–114.

Goetsch, M.F. (1991) Vulvar vestibulitis: prevalence and historic features in a general gynecologic practice population. *American Journal of Obstetrics and Gynecology* 164, 1609–1616.

Gordon, A.S., Panahian-Jand, M., McComb, F. *et al.* (2003) Characteristics of women with vulvar pain disorders: responses to a web-based survey. *Journal of Sex and Marital Therapy* 29, 45–58.

Green, J. & Hetherton, J. (2005) Psychological aspects of vulvar vestibulitis syndrome. *Journal of Psychosomatic Obstetrics and Gynecology* 26, 101–106.

Green, M.S., Naumann, R.W., Elliott, M. *et al.* (2000) Sexual dysfunction following vulvectomy *Gynaecological Oncology* 77, 73–77.

Gureje, O., Von Korff, M., Simon, G.E. & Gater, R. (1998) Persistent pain and well-being: a World Health Organization study in primary care. *Journal of the American Medical Association* 280, 147–151.

Hallam-Jones, R., Wylie, K.R., Osborne-Cribb, J. *et al.* (2001) Sexual difficulties within a group of patients with vulvodynia. *Sexual and Relationship Therapy* 16, 113–126.

Hansen, A., Carr, K. & Jensen, J.T. (2002) Characteristics and initial diagnoses in women presenting to a referral center for vulvovaginal disorders in 1996–2000. *Journal of Reproductive Medicine* 47, 854–860.

Harlow, B.L. & Stewart, E.G. (2005) Adult-onset vulvodynia in relation to childhood violence victimization. *American Journal of Epidemiology* 161, 871–880.

Hassanin, I.M., Saleh, R., Bedaiwy, A.A. *et al.* (2008) Prevalence of female genital cutting in Upper Egypt: 6 years after enforcement of prohibition law. *Reproductive Biomedicine Online* 16 Suppl 1, 27–31.

Hayes, R.D., Bennett, C.M., Fairley, C.K. & Dennerstien, L. (2006) What can prevalence studies tell us about female sexual difficulty and dysfunction? *Journal of Sexual Medicine* 3, 589–595.

Heim, C. & Nemeroff, C.B. (2001) The role of childhood trauma in the neurobiology of mood and anxiety disorders: preclinical and clinical studies. *Biological Psychiatry* 49, 1023–1039.

Huffman, J.W. (1983) Dyspareunia of vulvo-vaginal origin. Causes and management. *Postgraduate Medicine* 73, 287–296.

Hultgren, R., Sjogren, B., Soderberg, M. *et al.* (1999) Sexual function in women suffering from aortoiliac occlusive disease. *European Journal of Vascular and Endovascular Surgery* 17, 306–312.

Isa, A.R., Shuib, R. & Othman, M.S. (1999) The practice of female circumcision among Muslims in Kelantan, Malaysia. *Reproductive Health Matters* 7, 137–144.

Jadresic, D., Barton, S., Neill, S. *et al.* (1993) Psychiatric morbidity in women attending a clinic for vulval problems: is there a higher rate in vulvodynia? *International Journal of STD & AIDS* 4, 237–239.

Jantos, M. & White, G. (1997) The vestibulitis syndrome: medical and psychosexual assessment of a cohort of patients. *Journal of Reproductive Medicine* 42, 145–152.

Jensen, J.T., Wilder, K., Carr, K. *et al.* (2003) Quality of life and sexual function after evaluation and treatment at a referral center for vulvovaginal disorders. *American Journal of Obstetrics and Gynecology* 188, 1629–1637.

Katz, S.R. (1996) The experience of chronic vulvar pain: psychosocial dimensions and the sense of self. *Dissertation Abstracts International: Section B: The Sciences and Engineering* 56, 7048.

Kroenke, K. & Spitzer, R.L. (1998) Gender differences in the reporting of physical and somatoform symptoms. *Psychosomatic Medicine* 60, 150–155.

Latthe, P., Mignini, L., Gray, R. *et al.* (2006) Factors predisposing women to chronic pelvic pain: systematic review. *British Medical Journal* 332, 49–51.

Leiblum, S. & Nathan, S. (2001). Persistent sexual arousal syndrome: a newly discovered pattern of female sexuality. *Journal of Sex and Marital Therapy* 27, 365–380.

Lotery, H.E., McClure, N. & Galask, R.P. (2004) Vulvodynia. *Lancet* 363, 1058–1060.

Lubbe, J., Valiton, A., Pedrazetti, P. *et al.* (2000) Vulvodynia and factitious urticaria. *Annales de Dermatologie et de Venereologie* 127, 377–379.

Lundqvist, E.N. & Bergdahl, J. (2005) Vestibulodynia (former vulvar vestibulitis): personality in affected women. *Journal of Psychosomatic Obstetrics and Gynecology* 26, 251–256.

Maercker, A., Michael, T., Fehm, L. *et al.* (2004) Age of traumatisation as a predictor of post-traumatic stress disorder or major depression in young women. *British Journal of Psychiatry* 184, 482–487.

Marin, M.G., King, R., Sfameni, S. & Dennerstein, G.J. (2000) Adverse behavioral and sexual factors in chronic vulvar disease. *American Journal of Obstetrics and Gynecology* 183, 34–38.

Masheb, R.M., Brondolo, E. & Kems, R.D. (2002) A multidimensional, case-control study of women with self-identified chronic vulvar pain. *Pain Medicine* 3, 253–259.

Matsakis, A. (1996) *I Can't Get Over It: a Handbook for Trauma Survivors*, 2nd edn. New Harbinger Publications, Oakland, CA.

Mayou, R. & Farmer, A. (2002) Functional somatic symptoms and syndromes. *British Medical Journal* 325, 265–268.

Morris, E. & Mukhopadhyay, S. (2006) Dyspareunia in gynaecological practise. *Current Obstetrics and Gynaecology* 16, 226–233.

Moth, I., Andreasson, B., Jensen, S.B. & Bock, J.E. (1983) Sexual dysfunction and somatopsychic reactions after vulvectomy: a preliminary report. *Danish Medical Bulletin* 30, 27–30.

Msuya, S.E., Mbizvo, E., Hussain, A. *et al.* (2002) Female genital cutting in Kilimanjaro, Tanzania: changing attitudes? *Tropical Medicine International Health* 7, 159–165.

Munday, P.E. (2001) Response to treatment in dysaesthetic vulvodynia. *Journal of Obstetrics and Gynaecology* 21, 610–613.

Nemeroff, C.B. (2004) Neurobiological consequences of childhood trauma. *Journal of Clinical Psychiatry* 65 Suppl 1, 18–28.

Ness, T.J. (2005) Pelvic pain in women and men: recent findings. *Current Opinion in Anaesthesiology* 18, 555–562.

NICE. (2007) *Antenatal and Postnatal Mental Health*. National Institute for Health and Clinical Excellence, Clinical Guideline 45.

Nimnuan, C.H., Hotopf, M. & Wessely, S. (2001) Medically unexplained symptoms: an epidemiological study in seven specialities. *Journal Psychosomatic Research* 51, 361–367.

Nusbaum, M.R., Gamble, G., Skinner, B. & Heiman, J. (2000) The high prevalence of sexual concerns among women seeking routine gynaecological care. *Journal of Family Practice* 49, 229–232.

Peveler, R., Feldman, E. & Friedman, T. (eds) (2000) *Liaison Psychiatry: Planning Services for Specialist Settings*. Gaskell, London.

Population Council (2003) Female circumcision in Indonesia: extent, implications and possible interventions to uphold women's health rights. Available from: http://www.popcouncil.org/pdfs/frontiers/reports/Indonesia_FGM.pdf

Reed, B.D., Advincula, A.P., Fonde, K.R. *et al.* (2003a) Sexual activities and attitudes of women with vulvar dysesthesia. *Obstetrics and Gynecology* 102, 325–331.

Reed, B.D., Gorenflo, D.W. & Haefner, H.K. (2003b) Generalized vulvar dysesthesia vs. vestibulodynia: are they distinct diagnoses? *Journal of Reproductive Medicine* 48, 858–864.

Reed, B.D., Haefner, H.K. & Cantor, L. (2003c) Vulvar dysesthesia (vulvodynia): a follow-up study. *Journal of Reproductive Medicine* 48, 409–416.

Royal College of Physicians and Royal College of Psychiatrists (2003) *The Psychological Care of Medical Patients: a Practical Guide*, 2nd edn. CR 108. London, Gaskell.

Russo, J., Katon, W. Sullivan, M. *et al.* (1994) Severity of somatization and its relationship to psychiatric disorders and personality. *Psychosomatics* **35**, 546–556.

Schultz, W.W., Basson, R., Binik, Y. *et al.* (2005) Women's sexual pain and its management. *Journal of Sexual Medicine* **2**, 301–316.

Semple, D., Smyth, R., Burns, J. *et al.* (2005) *Oxford Handbook of Psychiatry*. Oxford, Oxford University Press.

Sheard, T. & Maguire, P. (1999) The effect of psychological interventions on anxiety and depression in cancer patients: results of two meta-analyses. *British Journal of Cancer* **80**, 1770–1780.

Smart, O.C. & MacLean, A.B. (2003) Vulvodynia. *Current Opinion in Obstetrics and Gynecology* **15**, 497–500.

Stellman, R., Goodwin, J., Robinson, J. *et al.* (1984) Psychological effects of vulvectomy. *Psychosomatics* **25**, 779–783.

Stewart, D.E., Reicher, A.E., Gerulath, A.H. & Boydell, K.M. (1994) Vulvodynia and psychological distress. *Obstetrics and Gynecology* **84**, 587–590.

Stirn, A. (2003) Body piercing: medical consequences and psychological motivations. *Lancet* **361**, 1205–1215.

Thakar, S.B. & Banta, H.D. (1983) Benefits and risks of episiotomy: an interpretative review of the English language literature 1860–1980. *Obstetrical and Gynaecological Survey* **38**, 322–338.

Timonen, M. & Liukkonen, T. (2008) Management of depression in adults. *British Medical Journal* **336**, 435–439.

Toorians, A.W., Jansen, F.T., Laan, E. *et al.* (1997) Chronic renal failure in sexually functioning: clinical status versus objectively assessed clinical response. *Nephrology Dialysis Transplantation* **12**, 2654–2663.

Van Lankveld, J.J.D.M. & Grotjohann, Y. (2000) Psychiatric comorbidity in heterosexual couples with sexual dysfunction assessed with the composite international diagnostic interview. *Archives of Sexual Behaviour* **29**, 479–498.

Van Lankveld, J., Weijenborg, P.T.M. & Ter Kuile, M.M. (1996) Psychologic profiles of and sexual function in women with vulvar vestibulitis and their partners. *Obstetrics and Gynecology* **88**, 65–70.

Weijmar Schultz, W.C., Gianotten, W.L., Van der Meijden, W.I. *et al.* (1996) Behavioral approach with or without surgical intervention to the vulvar vestibulitis syndrome: a prospective randomized and non-randomized study. *Journal of Psychosomatic Obstetrics and Gynecology* **17**, 143–148.

Wells, K.B., Golding, J.M. & Burnam, M.A. (1998) Psychiatric disorder in a sample of the general population with and without chronic medical conditions. *American Journal of Psychiatry* **145**, 976–981.

Wesselmann, U. & Reich, S.G. (1996) The dynias. *Seminars in Neurology* **16**, 63–74.

Wessely, S., Chalder, T. Hirsch, S. *et al.* (1997) The prevalence and morbidity of chronic fatigue syndrome: a prospective care study. *American Journal of Public Health* **87**, 1449–1455.

WHO. (1996) *Technical Working Group. Female Genital Mutilation*. World Health Organization, Geneva.

WHO. (1998) *Female Genital Mutilation: an Overview*. World Health Organization, Geneva.

WHO. (2008) *Female Genital Mutilation*. Fact Sheet 241. World Health Organization, Geneva.

Williams, E.R., Guthrie, E., Mackway-Jones, K. *et al.* (2001) Psychiatric status, somatisation, and health care utilization of frequent attenders at the emergency department: a comparison with routine attenders. *Journal of Psychosomatic Research* **50**, 161–167.

Wojnarowska, F., Mayou, R., Simkin, S. & Day, A. (1997) Psychological characteristics and outcome of patients attending a clinic for vulval disease. *Journal of the European Academy of Dermatology and Venereology* **8**, 121–129.

Wylie, K. (2004) Gender related disorders. *British Medical Journal* **329**, 615–617.

Wylie, K. (2007) Assessment and management of sexual problems in women. *Journal of the Royal Society of Medicine* **100**, 547–550.

Chapter 8: Cysts and epithelial neoplasms of the vulva

G.W. Spiegel & E. Calonje

Benign cysts

Epidermoid (tricholemmal, sebaceous, keratinous, epidermal inclusion) cysts

These are the most common cysts in the vulva, as they are elsewhere in the skin. They usually occur in the hair-bearing regions, and may be single or multiple. They present as painless nodular swellings up to 1 cm in diameter. They are frequently tethered to the overlying epidermis, which may have a depression or central pore connecting with the lumen. They are lined by bland orthokeratotic squamous epithelium and filled with laminated keratin. Sebaceous differentiation may be present. Rupture of a cyst may lead to inflammation with a foreign body giant cell response.

Mucinous cysts

Mucinous cysts usually occur in adults, but have been described in adolescents (Junaid & Thomas 1981). They are usually single, but may be multiple, and range from a few millimetres to 3 cm in size (Junaid & Thomas 1981, Oi & Munn 1982). They are most common in the vestibule, where they have been postulated to arise from the obstruction of the minor vestibular ducts (Robboy *et al.* 1978) or the embryological remnants of the urogenital sinus (Oi & Munn 1982). They usually form a subepithelial mass, but may be pedunculated (Hart 1970). The cysts are lined by a single cell layer of bland columnar (endocervical) type mucinous epithelium (Fig. 8.1). Focal squamous metaplasia, reserve cell hyperplasia and ciliated cells may be present, but there is no myoepithelial cell layer or associated rim of smooth muscle (Fu 2002).

Bartholin's cysts

Bartholin's gland cysts are not uncommon and are attributed to a blockage of the transitional cell epithelium-lined duct. They typically occur during the reproductive years and present as 1–10 cm fluctuant cystic swellings that may be

Ridley's The Vulva, 3rd edition. Edited by Sallie M. Neill and Fiona M. Lewis. © 2009 Blackwell Publishing, ISBN: 978-1-4051-6813-7.

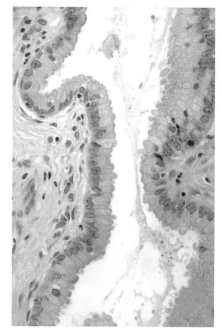

Fig. 8.1 Mucinous cyst lined by a single layer of columnar endocervical-type epithelium.

painful as they are prone to infection and secondary abscess formation (Azzaz 1978). Histologically, the cysts are lined by transitional cell epithelium that frequently has areas of squamous metaplasia that may be extensive. Bartholin's gland acini are present in the wall (Fig. 8.2). In the event of infection or abscess formation, the lining epithelium may be replaced by granulation tissue, but the Bartholin's gland acini should still be present in the wall. The usual treatment is enucleation of the cyst, but incompletely excised cysts may recur. Rarely, a carcinoma of Bartholin's gland may present as a cyst, and repeated recurrences should be completely excised to exclude an occult malignancy.

Anogenital gland cysts

Anogenital glands may undergo cystic dilatation that may be accompanied by apocrine metaplasia. In the absence of apocrine metaplasia, the cysts are lined by an outer myoepithelial cell layer and an inner layer of secretory cells

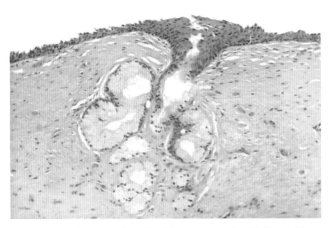

Fig. 8.2 Bartholin's gland cyst lined by transitional epithelium with contiguous mucinous acini.

that have luminal snouts. The secretory cells are positive for oestrogen and androgen receptors, and are often positive for progesterone receptor. However, metaplastic apocrine epithelium in these cysts is negative for oestrogen and progesterone receptors, and the anogenital gland origin of the cyst may be recognized only by a transition from native to metaplastic epithelium or the presence of typical anogenital glands and absence of apocrine glands in the region of the cyst (van der Putte & van Gorp 1995).

Mesonephric-like (Gartner's duct) cysts

Traditionally, these cysts were considered to arise from embryonic remnants of the mesonephric duct, but, since the mesonephric ducts do not extend to the rudimentary vulva during embryogenesis, they are of unknown histogenesis and designated as 'mesonephric-like' cysts. They typically occur on the lateral aspects of the vulva as a blue to red domed cyst and are filled with clear colourless fluid. The cysts are lined by a single cell layer of bland cuboidal epithelium, which may be flattened by the pressure of the cyst contents, overlying a thin layer of smooth muscle.

Mesothelial cyst (cyst of canal of Nuck)

The cysts occur in the upper labia majora in the region of the insertion of the round ligament. They are lined by bland mesothelial cells, and are frequently associated with an inguinal hernia.

Miscellaneous cysts of probable adnexal origin

There are cysts that fail to fit into any of the well-described types. These tend to be less than 1 cm in diameter and have no connection with the overlying epidermis or adnexal structures. The cysts may be lined by bland ciliated, sebaceous-like or apocrine-like cells (Fig. 8.3). Squamous metaplasia may be present. These benign cysts should be reported as a 'benign cyst of probable adnexal origin'.

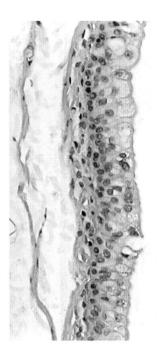

Fig. 8.3 Benign cyst of probable adnexal origin lined by a double cell layer bland epithelium with the inner layer having a vacuolated cytoplasm suggestive of sebaceous differentiation.

Benign squamous non-neoplastic proliferations and neoplastic tumours

Fibroepithelial polyps

Ordinary skin tags are common on the vulva, but characteristic fibroepithelial polyps are relatively rare. They may be associated with pregnancy. The aetiology is not known, but they are probably non-neoplastic. Grossly, they present as either sessile or pedunculated polyps. They have a vascular connective tissue stroma composed of cells derived from the subepithelial stromal cells that line the lower female genital tract from the cervix to the labia minora. The stroma is usually hypocellular and composed of mononucleated stellate cells and multinucleated cells with long tapering cytoplasmic processes and merges with the adjacent non-polypoid stroma. However, occasional tumours are cellular, with the cellularity being greatest at the centre of the polyp (Nucci et al. 2000). Atypical cells may be present, particularly among the multinucleated cells, and there may be occasional mitoses (Fig. 8.4). The overlying squamous epithelium is usually acanthotic (Fig. 8.5) and may be hyperkeratotic or parakeratotic.

Vestibular micropapillomatosis

These are 1–5 mm slender filiform papillae that occur in the region of the introitus. They are usually asymptomatic, although they are occasionally pruritic. They are considered to be a normal variant of the vestibular mucosa (Foster

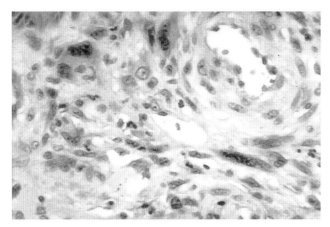

Fig. 8.4 High magnification of atypical stromal cells in fibroepithelial polyp.

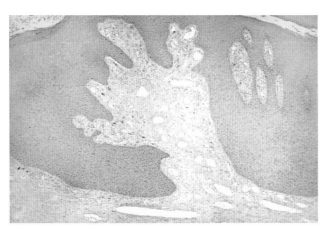

Fig. 8.5 Low magnification of fibroepithelial polyp with mildly cellular stroma and overlying bland acanthotic epithelium.

2002). They are composed of delicate fibrovascular cores lined by bland squamous epithelium that may have a thin layer of keratin. There is an absence of koilocytosis and association with human papillomavirus (Wilkinson *et al.* 1993) (see Chapter 2).

Squamous papillomas

Squamous papillomas are small warty proliferations that appear 'pasted' onto the surface, and usually occur during the late reproductive years to the postmenopausal period in the hair-bearing parts of the vulva. They are rarely greater than 1 cm in greatest dimension. They are composed of papillary acanthotic and hyperkeratotic or parakeratotic proliferations of bland squamous epithelium with normal maturation. They may be variants of warts or seborrhoeic keratoses (see below).

Seborrhoeic keratoses

Like squamous papillomas, these usually form warty proliferations that appear pasted onto the surface, are usually

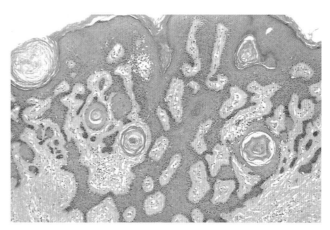

Fig. 8.6 Seborrhoeic keratosis composed of bland basaloid cells with keratin tunnels and pigmented lentiginous pigmented cords.

pigmented and may have a waxy appearance owing to extruded keratin. They are composed of papillary proliferations of small bland basaloid cells that resemble those of normal squamous epithelium and have delicate fibrovascular cores. Melanin pigment is frequently present throughout the proliferation, and the surface is usually hyperkeratotic. Mitoses are absent or rare. Commonly, laminated keratin in apparent cystic spaces, 'keratin tunnels', are present (Fig. 8.6). When irritated, there may be prominent inflammation and atypia that is characterized by mild nuclear atypia and a more squamoid appearance. But unlike squamous carcinoma and vulval intraepithelial neoplasia (VIN), mitotic figures remain confined to the basal layers and atypical mitoses are absent. The proliferation retains its 'pasted' on appearance, there is an absence of atypical parakeratosis and residual keratin tunnels may be present. Occasionally, the proliferation may be 'inverted' with pushing rounded nests of bland basaloid cells with keratin tunnels that may resemble a basal cell carcinoma. However, unlike basal cell carcinomas, the surface epithelium from which the nests originate is a full thickness of bland basaloid cells rather than atypical basaloid cells limited to the basal layer, and mitotic figures are rare or absent.

Verruciform xanthoma

Verruciform xanthoma of the vulva is a rare benign lesion that typically occurs in women of reproductive age. It presents as one or more papillary or cauliflower-like lesions that may be clinically suspected of being a condyloma or VIN (Santa Cruz & Martin 1979). However there is an absence of warty koilocytosis and there is no atypia or abnormal mitotic activity. Histologically, there is acanthosis and focal papillomatosis of bland hyperkeratotic and/or parakeratotic squamous epithelium. The papillary dermis contains characteristic collections of foamy histiocytes that may be cuffed by a pseudoepitheliomatous hyperplastic

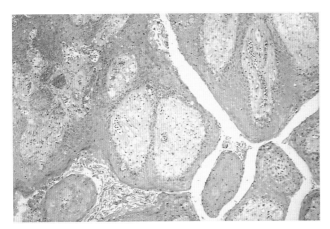

Fig. 8.7 Low magnification of verruciform xanthoma composed of papillary proliferations with foamy histiocytes in cores and lined by bland squamous epithelium.

elongation of the rete pegs (Fig. 8.7). Treatment is by local excision.

Epidermolytic acanthoma (epidermolytic hyperkeratosis)

Two cases of vulval epidermolytic acanthoma have been described in the literature (DeConinck *et al.* 1986, Quinn & Young 1997). However, owing to the possibility that other cases may have been misdiagnosed as warts or un-differentiated VIN, the true frequency is not known. The condition may occur sporadically or be genetically inherited and associated with oral lesions. The lesions form white hyperkeratotic plaques. Histologically, there is a cup-shaped invagination of broad rete pegs of hyperkeratotic epithelium with well-circumscribed borders. Surface papillae are present, but they lack the typical parakeratosis of warts. The basal epithelium lacks atypia, but may have increased mitotic activity relative to the adjacent non-involved epithelium. Abnormal mitoses are absent. Dyskeratotic cells are present in the overlying maturing epithelium and the surface granular cell layer contains coarse keratohyaline granules and corp ronds, dense eosinophilic globoid bodies that are the remnants of the dyskeratotic cells. Although binucleated cells may be present, well-developed warty koilocytes are absent.

Keratoacanthoma

These have classically been considered benign neoplasms, but recently have been classified as indolent low-grade squamous carcinomas that fail to metastasize. They are rare in the vulva, and occur in the hair-bearing portions (Rhatigan & Nuss 1985). Clinically, there is a rapidly growing nodule that usually has a central crater, but may be overlain by intact squamous epithelium. Generally, it is reported that the lesions will enlarge for about 6 weeks and

then regress. However, these lesions are usually excised for histological assessment. A superficial biopsy specimen is inadequate in differentiating the proliferation from a non-neoplastic squamous proliferation or a typical squamous or verrucous carcinoma.

Histologically, there is an exophytic proliferation of squamous epithelium that burgeons into the underlying dermis. A central keratin-filled crater is present that extends from the surface to the central portion of the invading tumour that is composed of nests of mildly atypical squamous cells with a peripheral layer of bland basaloid cells. Mitotic figures may be numerous, but they are limited to the periphery of the nests, and abnormal forms are not present. Unlike squamous carcinomas with a more clinically aggressive course, the invasive margin is smooth and there is often a collarette at the periphery that appears to confine the proliferation, and, unlike verrucous carcinoma, there is an absence of papillomatosis. There is no VIN in the adjacent epithelium. A proliferation with features of a keratoacanthoma should be reported as a low-grade squamous carcinoma with a marginal capacity for lymph node metastases, and should be completely excised.

Condyloma acuminata

Condylomata acuminata are benign neoplasms secondary to infection by human papillomaviruses (HPVs) 6 and 11 (McLachlin *et al.* 1994) that are usually transmitted by sexual contact. They may apparently be transmitted by non-sexual contact in young children (Hammerschlag 1998), and are not always evidence of sexual abuse. Clinically, condylomata acuminata form exophytic cauliflower-like growths on the any area of the vulva and perineum. They may be solitary, multiple or form confluent growths.

Histologically, there are delicate fibrovascular cores lined by acanthotic hyperkeratotic and/or parakeratotic squamous epithelium. There is minimal, if any, atypia. Mitotic figures may be present, but they are limited to basal areas and, by definition, none are atypical, as the latter are indicative of undifferentiated VIN. The acanthotic epithelium may expand the basal rete pegs, but there is no invasion. Warty koilocytes are invariably present in condyloma acuminata, but they may be few (Fig. 8.8). They are composed of cells with large, irregular but otherwise relatively bland nuclei with perinuclear cytoplasmic clearing. Towards the surface the nuclei may be spindled and wavy. Generally, this change is apparent at low magnification. The nuclei appear irregularly arranged, as opposed to the normal basketweave pattern of glycogenated epithelium. In addition, the condensation of the cytoplasm to the periphery of the cells usually creates the appearance of cell walls. However, the warty koilocytes should be bland and have a relatively uniform dark chromatin and similar size. The presence of smudged chromatin, prominent nucleoli and pleomorphism should prompt a

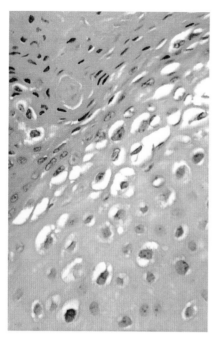

Fig. 8.8 High magnification of superficial bland warty koilocytes in condyloma acuminatum.

search for atypical and superficial mitoses, the hallmarks of undifferentiated VIN. A chronic inflammatory infiltrate may be present, but eosinophils are virtually absent.

If left untreated, most condylomata acuminata regress over months to years, but may persist or increase in size. Spontaneous regression can occur following delivery. Treatment is discussed in Chapter 3. The application of podophyllin may lead to atypia characterized by ballooning of the cells, nuclear enlargement and abnormal appearing mitoses owing to metaphase maturation arrest (Pope *et al.* 1973), but, unlike VIN, there is an absence of significant pleomorphism, abnormal chromatin pattern and atypical mitoses (Wade & Ackerman 1984). Any warty appearing lesions, particularly if they are large, should be biopsied prior to treatment. The presence of vulval condylomata acuminata should also prompt screening of the vagina and cervix since approximately 30–40% of patients will also have lesions at these sites.

Flat condylomata also occur on the vulva, and are misinterpreted by some pathologists as VIN1. Both flat and exophytic condylomata are associated with HPV-6 and -11 (Logani *et al.* 2003). However, they may be difficult to recognize, as well-developed warty koilocytosis is often absent, the proliferations being characterized by mild acanthosis, mild nuclear atypia and parakeratosis and may resemble a seborrhoeic keratosis. By the same token, these features may be present in non-neoplastic inflammation, candidiasis and psoriasis and lead to overdiagnosis of flat condyloma or VIN1 (Micheletti *et al.* 1994, van Beurden

et al. 1999, Logani *et al.* 2003). Immunohistochemical staining by MIB-1 above the parabasal layer has been proposed for distinguishing flat condylomas from non-neoplastic conditions, but in one study only a minority of HPV-positive proliferations had an abnormal MIB-1 staining pattern (Bai *et al.* 2003).

Squamous carcinoma and its precursors

Vulval intraepithelial neoplasia

The precursor of vulval squamous cell carcinoma is VIN, a non-invasive neoplastic replacement of the squamous epithelium. Basically, this presents in two forms:

1 *undifferentiated*, which is described as the usual type and is associated with HPV

2 *differentiated* VIN (or carcinoma *in situ*, simplex type), which is not associated with HPV, occurs in older women and is nearly always associated with lichen sclerosus or epithelial hyperplasia.

These two types have strikingly different histological appearances and follow different clinical courses and will be discussed separately.

Undifferentiated VIN

Traditionally, undifferentiated VIN has been graded as VIN1, VIN2 and VIN3, using the same criteria as for grading cervical intraepithelial neoplasia, but this has now been abandoned (Sideri *et al.* 2005).

Undifferentiated VIN is considered to be a precancerous condition that is composed of a proliferation of markedly atypical cells which occupy greater than one-third of the epithelium and encompasses those types of VIN that have been associated with HPV. While the histological appearance may vary from 'typical Bowenoid', to 'basaloid' or 'warty', evidence points to them all having a similar clinical behaviour. It typically occurs in sexually active women during the reproductive years anywhere on the vulva or perineal region and is usually associated with HPV-16, but occasionally with other high-risk types (van Beurden *et al.* 1995). It is frequently multifocal, and up to two-thirds are associated with cervical intraepithelial neoplasia either concurrently or in the past. Other sites of involvement include the vagina, perianal regions and perineum. There is an increased risk in immunocompromised patients (Sillman *et al.* 1997), and a strong association with smoking.

The clinical presentation is variable. The most common symptom is pruritus, but up to 46% of patients may be asymptomatic with the lesion being discovered during routine cervical screening. The clinical appearance of the lesions can range from hypopigmented to pigmented black, brown, grey or red lesions, which may have a warty, granular or plaque-like appearance (Fig. 8.9a,b). In the mucosal parts

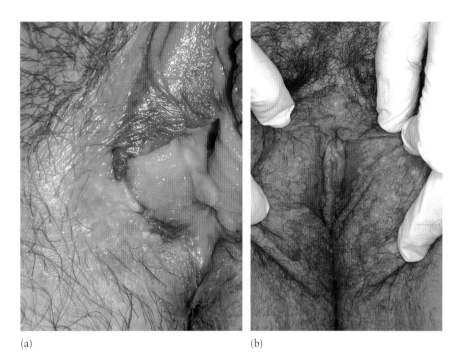

Fig. 8.9 (a) Unifocal warty plaque with surface erosion. (b) Multifocal confluent warty and pigmented lesions.

(a)   (b)

of the vulva, the lesions may be more obvious after the application of acetic acid. They may be unifocal or multi-focal covering much of the vulva. Frequently, there is extension beyond the grossly visible margin that is identified only in the excision specimen.

Histologically, undifferentiated VIN is characterized by a proliferation of atypical squamous cells that is often best appreciated in the basal and parabasal regions where they are markedly atypical, but extends beyond this region with varying degrees of atypia. Generally, the epithelium is acan-thotic with elongation and broadening of the rete pegs. The superficial epithelium frequently contains atypical warty koilocytes. The surface is usually parakeratotic, but may be hyperkeratotic or both, with atypical hyperchromatic enlarged nuclei in the parakeratotic cells or granular cell layer. While there may be glycogenization and decreased atypia in the superficial portions, there is a full-thickness proliferation of abnormal cells. The cells may vary from basaloid to large keratinocytes. The basaloid cells have scant cytoplasm, mildly to moderately enlarged nuclei with hyperchromatic smudged chromatin and fail to undergo maturation beyond the normal parabasal area. Atypical keratinocytes have a variable amount of eosinophilic cyto-plasm and large nuclei with coarse dense and/or vesiculated chromatin with prominent nucleoli, and, regardless of the amount of cytoplasm, there is an increased nuclear–cytoplasmic ratio compared with normal keratinocytes. Frequently, there is a mixture of abnormal basaloid cells and atypical keratinocytes, with the former being present in the lower layers and atypical keratinocytes in the upper

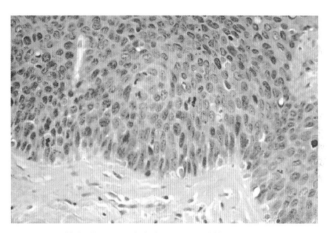

Fig. 8.10 Full-thickness epithelial atypia (undifferentiated VIN, classical type).

layers. Dyskeratotic cells are a common finding among the atypical keratinocytes, and may be present among the basa-loid cells. When composed of predominantly basaloid cells there may be marked melanin pigmentation that frequently spills over into the adjacent non-neoplastic stroma. Mitotic figures are present above the parabasal layer, and may extend throughout the full thickness of the epithelium. Atypical mitoses are usually identified, and their presence alone dis-tinguishes undifferentiated VIN from lesions that may have a condylomatous appearance (Figs 8.10 and 8.11). Not uncommonly, undifferentiated VIN extends into pilose-baceous units, and occasionally into sweat gland ducts. Extension into adnexal structures and tangential sectioning

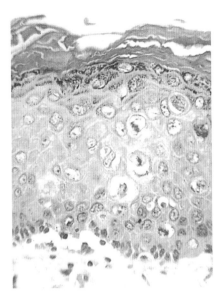

Fig. 8.11 Undifferentiated VIN composed of a full-thickness proliferation of mitotically active atypical large cells, some of which have koilocyte-like clear cytoplasm and overlying hyperkeratosis.

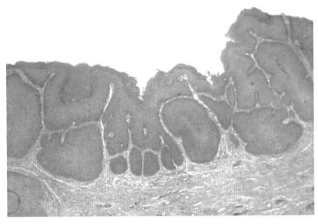

Fig. 8.12 Tangentially sectioned rete pegs of undifferentiated VIN.

of acanthotic epithelium may mimic invasion, but, unlike invasive tumour, the nests retain a lobular configuration and lack the streaming pattern of invasion (Fig. 8.12). Paradoxical maturation to large atypical keratinocytes among the basaloid cells is a 'preinvasive' change that warrants a more careful search for early invasion when not present in the initial planes of completely sectioned specimens or by submitting additional sections in incompletely sectioned large specimens. The adjacent stroma usually has a chronic inflammatory cell infiltrate, but, in the absence of ulceration, eosinophils are usually absent. The presence of more

than three eosinophils per high power field (hpf) or five or more per 10 hpfs in an incisional biopsy specimen and ≥ 20 per hpf or > 50 per 10 hpfs in an excisional specimen should raise the possibility of invasive disease. The presence of intraepithelial eosinophils in incisional and excisional specimens is again indicative of some degree of invasion (Spiegel 2002).

The natural history of undifferentiated VIN is still unknown, and most of the relationship between undifferentiated VIN and the development of invasive squamous carcinoma is based of the frequency of VIN in specimens resected for invasive carcinoma. In studies, full-thickness atypia was present in the epithelium adjacent to the carcinoma in 20–30% of cases (Leibowitch *et al.* 1990). In other studies, approximately 20% of women undergoing total excision of full-thickness atypia and in which the specimens were blocked *in toto* had foci of invasion (Chafe *et al.* 1988, Husseinzadeh & Recinto 1990). It is known that some cases of undifferentiated VIN undergo spontaneous regression, usually multifocal pigmented basaloid VIN in young women, and particularly if associated with pregnancy (Jones & Rowan 2000). Consequently, one is left only with the knowledge that undifferentiated VIN may regress or progress to invasion. One cannot predict those that will regress and those that will progress to invasion if left untreated, nor the duration of the undifferentiated VIN prior to invasion when it eventually occurs (van Seters *et al.* 2005).

The treatment for unifocal undifferentiated VIN is surgical excision. Multifocal disease may be treated by carbon dioxide laser ablation, surgical excision or photodynamic therapy (Hillemans *et al.* 2006). The immune response modifier imiquimod has been reported to achieve complete regression in 26–100% of patients treated (Lavazzo *et al.* 2008, van Seters *et al.* 2008). The recently introduced vaccines against HPV should also be helpful in preventing HPV-associated VIN (Joura *et al.* 2007).

All patients with undifferentiated VIN require long-term follow-up, particularly in women who fail to stop smoking or who are immunocompromised. In pregnant women, if the lesions are multifocal and develop after the onset of pregnancy, it may be possible to simply observe and determine whether there is regression following delivery; however, the patients require careful observation since there is a theoretical possibility that the decreased immune status associated with pregnancy may predispose to progression.

Differentiated VIN (carcinoma *in situ*, simplex type)

Differentiated VIN is a form of carcinoma *in situ* in which significant atypia is confined to the basal layers of the epithelium and studies have reported its presence adjacent to invasive carcinomas in a substantial number of cases, particularly in elderly women. The histological changes can be subtle and are often overlooked. It is found most frequently on a background of a lichen sclerosus or epithelial hyperplasia. To date, there has been no association with HPV infection (Yang & Hart 2000).

The clinical presentation is usually on a background of lichen sclerosus, with development of a small ulcer, hyperkeratotic papule or plaque. Multiple biopsy specimens may be required before the diagnosis is made, and the presence of atypia within a biopsy specimen with lichen sclerosus in an elderly patient is an indication for additional biopsies and frequent follow-up.

Unlike the undifferentiated form of VIN, differentiated VIN is composed of well-differentiated squamous cells with only mild atypia confined to the basal layers and a slight disturbance of maturation. On the surface there is usually hyperkeratosis, and occasionally parakeratosis, but there are mildly atypical nuclei in the granular cell layer or parakeratotic cells. Those in the basal layer have enlarged hyperchromatic nuclei with an increased nuclear–cytoplasmic ratio and the parabasal cells usually have prominent nucleoli. Mitotic figures are present, but are usually confined to the basal layer or adjacent abnormal keratinocytes, and they may be atypical. The immunohistochemical proliferative index marker MIB-1 (Ki-67) is elevated relative to non-neoplastic epithelium with nuclear staining extending beyond the basal epithelium, and the cells may have overexpression of p53 (Yang & Hart 2000). There are usually prominent slender elongations of the rete pegs resembling pseudo-epitheliomatous hyperplasia, but the elongations may be bulbous or absent with minimal simple acanthosis. Early differentiated VIN arising in lichen sclerosus is often thin, but the characteristic abnormal mitotically active basal and parabasal cells are present (Fig. 8.13), and immunohistochemical staining for p53 or MIB-1 may aid diagnosis. Paradoxical maturation with the formation of squamous pearls or pearl-like formations is a hallmark of the disease,

particularly when there is pseudoepitheliomatous hyperplasia-like elongation of the rete pegs (Figs 8.14 and 8.15). Warty koilocytes and a proliferation of abnormal basaloid cells beyond the parabasal area are absent. There is usually a dense chronic inflammatory cell infiltrate in the adjacent

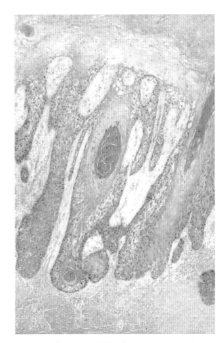

Fig. 8.14 Low magnification of slender elongation of rete pegs with central keratinization in differentiated VIN.

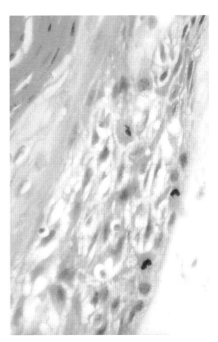

Fig. 8.15 High magnification of mitotically active atypical basal cells adjacent to central keratinization in differentiated VIN.

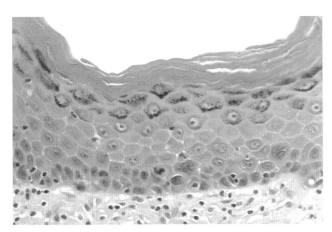

Fig. 8.13 Differentiated VIN showing atypia in the basal and parabasal cell layers in lichen sclerosus.

dermis or stroma. Eosinophils have been reported in the inflammatory infiltrate (Yang & Hart 2000). However, they are virtually absent except in cases associated with ulceration or an adjacent invasive carcinoma, and their presence in a small biopsy specimen should raise the suspicions of an invasive tumour (Spiegel 2002). Squamous carcinomas associated with differentiated VIN are thought to have a higher recurrence rate than those associated with undifferentiated VIN (Hart 2001).

Differentiated VIN is carcinoma *in situ*, simplex type, and is more likely to progress to invasive carcinoma than undifferentiated VIN (Yang & Hart 2000). In one study differentiated VIN was more commonly present in the epithelium adjacent to invasive carcinomas than undifferentiated VIN (Spiegel 2002). The invasive carcinomas associated with differentiated VIN are almost always well to moderately differentiated large-cell keratinizing carcinomas (Kurman *et al.* 1993). Early invasive tumours are usually well differentiated with large bulbous invasive nests that may be difficult to distinguish from tangentially cut differentiated VIN. Features that may be helpful in distinguishing early invasive tumour from differentiated VIN are the presence of small more diffusely invasive nests at the deep periphery, tumour deeper than the adjacent differentiated VIN, and the presence of eosinophils in the adjacent dermis (Spiegel 2002).

Treatment is surgical excision and careful follow-up.

Invasive squamous carcinoma

Vulval squamous carcinoma accounts for 80–95% of vulval malignancies, and approximately 3–8% of gynaecological cancers. Once invasive carcinoma has developed, the outcome is determined by stage rather than histological features of the tumour or antecedent VIN (see Chapter 11).

The overall mean age of women with vulval squamous carcinoma is 66–74 years. There appears to be two backgrounds to the development of vulval squamous cell carcinoma. The more common arises in elderly postmenopausal women, with a background of lichen sclerosus and no known association with HPV. The tumours are usually well to moderately differentiated large-cell keratinizing type. The other background is usually associated with undifferentiated VIN, HPV-16 or -18 related, occurring in younger women with a mean age of 50 years. The tumours in this group are usually moderately to poorly differentiated and non- or poorly keratinizing tumours (Pilotti *et al.* 1996). However, there is overlap; squamous carcinoma arising on a background of lichen sclerosus may be HPV positive, and those arising in younger women in the absence of lichen sclerosus may be HPV negative (Crum *et al.* 1997, van Seters *et al.* 2007). However, the vast majority of patients with lichen sclerosus are unlikely to develop differentiated VIN or invasive carcinoma.

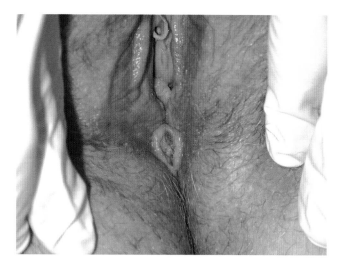

Fig. 8.16 Invasive squamous cell carcinoma arising from a plaque of undifferentiated VIN at the fourchette.

Squamous carcinoma may occur anywhere in the vulva and perineum, but the labia (70%) and clitoris (5–24%) are the most common sites. Approximately 15% of cases occur in the perineal body or posterior fourchette. The most common presentation is a vulval mass, with symptoms of pruritus, bleeding or pain. The tumours may be either exophytic or plaque-like and are frequently ulcerated (Fig. 8.16).

The histology of vulval squamous carcinomas is the same as that of squamous carcinomas elsewhere. They have been classified into various subtypes: large-cell (typical) keratinizing (approximately 65%), basaloid (approximately 30%) and warty (5–10%) (Kurman *et al.* 1993). There are also less common types with tumour giant cells, spindle cells, pseudoglandular, adenoid or acantholytic, and lymphoepitheliomatous features. The tumours have also been traditionally classified into three grades, but grading systems differ. The Gynecologic Oncology Group (GOG) base the grade on the percentage of 'undifferentiated' cells, defined as small cells with scant cytoplasm that form diffusely infiltrative narrow cords and small nests ('spray pattern'). Using this definition, tumours that lack undifferentiated cells are grade 1, those with less than 50% undifferentiated cells are grade 2, and tumours with greater than 50% undifferentiated cells are grade 3 (Sedlis *et al.* 1987). Other grading systems are based on the degree of pleomorphism, nuclear atypia and degree of mitotic activity. However, regardless of the grading system, except for the best and most poorly differentiated tumours, the grading is highly subjective.

Typical large-cell keratinizing carcinomas are characterized by the formation of squamous pearls in the invasive nests and cords. However, the definition of a 'squamous pearl' is not rigorous; some pathologists require only the

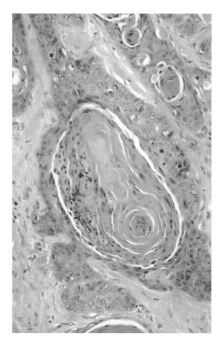

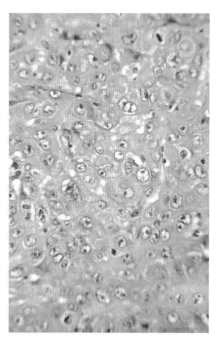

Fig. 8.17 Moderately differentiated large-cell keratinizing carcinoma with keratin pearl rimmed by cells with hyperchromatic nuclei increased nuclear–cytoplasmic ratio unlike well-differentiated carcinoma.

Fig. 8.18 Poorly differentiated large-cell non-keratinizing squamous carcinoma composed of sheets of pleomorphic cells with prominent nucleoli.

presence of central maturation with glycogenated cells, whereas others require the presence of central amorphous keratin or parakeratotic cells. These distinctions are probably of no significance, for most squamous carcinomas with either of these features have a significant portion of malignant cells of easily recognized squamous differentiation. Well-differentiated tumours are composed predominantly of nests of relatively bland squamous cells with central maturation. Amorphous keratin may be conspicuous, constituting most of the tumour. Mitotic figures are infrequent and may be atypical and are usually limited to the periphery of the nests. Most of the tumour appears to have a pushing invasive pattern, but focal areas of diffusely invasive small nests and cords may be present, particularly at the periphery. Moderately differentiated tumours have a greater degree of pleomorphism and nuclear atypia with prominent nucleoli, and a brisk mitotic index. Squamous differentiation in the form of amorphous keratin or central maturation in the invasive nests is less conspicuous than in well-differentiated tumours (Fig. 8.17). Frequently, particularly at the invasive edge, there is a component of diffusely invasive cords and nests composed of small undifferentiated cells. Poorly differentiated carcinomas are composed predominantly of sheets or confluent and anastomosing nests of large cells with marked pleomorphism with prominent nucleoli or diffusely infiltrative cords of small to moderately sized cells with pleomorphic nuclei with dense chromatin

and scant cytoplasm, similar to those at the edge of some moderately differentiated carcinomas (Fig. 8.18). Mitotic figures, often atypical, are usually easily identified, and there is usually an absence of keratinization. The well- and moderately differentiated keratinizing tumours are generally associated with differentiated VIN in the adjacent epithelium, whereas the moderately differentiated non-keratinizing and poorly differentiated carcinomas are usually associated with undifferentiated VIN.

Unlike the more common large-cell squamous carcinomas, basaloid carcinomas usually have scant or no mature appearing squamous elements, and squamous pearls are rare or non-existent. The tumours are composed of infiltrating anastomosing broad islands and cords and/or narrow cords and nests of small atypical basaloid cells with scant cytoplasm, moderately hyperchromatic nuclei with dense chromatin, and a high nuclear–cytoplasmic ratio (Fig. 8.19). Mitotic figures are easily identified, and are often atypical. Maturation of the neoplastic cells, when it is present, is towards the centre of the larger nests or at the surface. The tumours tend to be HPV positive, occur in younger women and are associated with undifferentiated VIN in the adjacent epithelium. Using the GOG grading criteria, these tumours are either grade 2 or 3. The tumours may be misdiagnosed as basal cell carcinomas in small biopsy specimens. However, unlike basal cell carcinomas, the intact surface epithelium has a full thickness of neoplastic cells, there is an absence of peripheral palisading in the invasive element

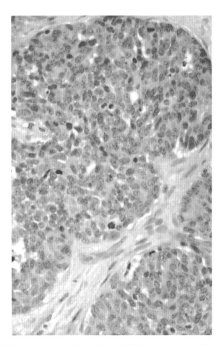

Fig. 8.19 High magnification of basaloid squamous carcinoma composed of cells with hyperchromatic nuclei and increased nuclear–cytoplasmic ratio.

and there is usually a greater degree of atypia and mitotic activity. Specific staining with Ber EP4 (positive in basal cell carcinomas) may be helpful in differentiating the two (Tellechea *et al.* 1993).

Like basaloid carcinomas, so called 'warty' carcinomas are usually HPV positive and occur on a background of undifferentiated VIN that is characterized by large atypical keratinocytes with superficial warty koilocytes (Kurman *et al.* 1993). The tumours have an exophytic surface with condylomatous features, i.e. fibrovascular cores lined by large atypical keratinocytes with superficial warty koilocytosis and prominent parakeratosis, hyperkeratosis or both. The underlying invasive tumour is composed of infiltrating, irregularly shaped nests of large atypical cells which frequently have central maturation. Mitotic figures are easily identified, and are often atypical. Unlike condylomatous carcinomas, the exophytic portion, while having a condylomatous architecture, has a significantly greater degree of atypia and mitotic activity than a typical condyloma acuminatum.

Other variants of squamous carcinoma are uncommon. Adenoid or acantholytic and pseudoglandular variants are composed of nests or cords of variably differentiated squamous cells with central acantholysis to produce mucin-negative gland-like spaces. Unlike rare adenosquamous carcinomas, there is no organization of cells about these spaces to form true glands. The giant cell variant of squamous carcinoma is a poorly differentiated large cell, often keratinizing carcinoma, with scattered multinucleated bizarre neoplastic giant cells. The spindle cell variant is composed of spindle cells that may be mistaken for a sarcoma and may be arranged in interlacing fascicles or in a diffuse sarcomatoid pattern (Fig. 8.20). However, in well-sampled tumours, there are almost always areas of more conventional squamous carcinoma. When absent, particularly in small biopsy specimens, positive staining for cytoplasmic cytokeratin usually leads to the correct diagnosis. Rarely, a squamous carcinoma may have a dense chronic infiltrate that obscures the neoplastic squamous cells. Again, positive staining for cytoplasmic keratin will highlight the neoplastic large squamous cells.

In 1994, the International Society for the Study of Vulvovaginal Disease (ISSVD) adopted the recommendation proposed by Wilkinson *et al.* (1982) that the depth of invasion be from the deepest invasive tumour to the tip of the nearest dermal papilla. An alternative proposal is that the depth of invasion be measured from the deepest tumour to its site of origin from the non-invasive epithelium, which may be a rete peg, and as such would be less than that measured from the nearest dermal papillae (Wells & Jenkins 1994); however, most current studies employ the ISSVD recommendation. In cases where the tumour is ulcerated, the depth of invasion cannot be measured, and only a tumour thickness can be estimated. In this case, one measures the depth of the tumour from the base of the ulcer and adds the estimated depth of the ulcer to arrive at a thickness. For all intents and purposes, ulcerated tumours are assumed to have a depth of invasion greater than 1 mm.

Many histological features in the past have been reported to be prognostic factors. These include the presence or absence of lymphatic/vascular space invasion, the degree of differentiation of the tumour, tumour surface diameter and thickness, the pattern of invasion, the presence of p53, HPV status, and degree of proliferative activity as determined by immunohistochemical staining for MIB-1 (Ki-67). However, to date, in multivariate analyses, only the surgical stage using the Federation Internationale de Gynecologie et d'Obstetrique (FIGO) criteria (Beller *et al.* 2006) has proved to be of prognostic significance and, within stage II, tumours ≤ 5 mm were associated with an increased survival relative to larger tumours (Bryson *et al.* 1991) (see Chapter 11).

Surgery is the standard therapy for vulval squamous carcinoma. The extent of surgery to remove the primary tumour is dependent on its size and depth of invasion and varies from wide local excision for tumours < 2 cm to radical vulvectomy for larger tumours. The extent of lymphadenectomy is dependent on the size of the tumour and its depth of invasion, its location and presence or absence of enlarged lymph nodes by either palpation or imaging (see Chapter 11).

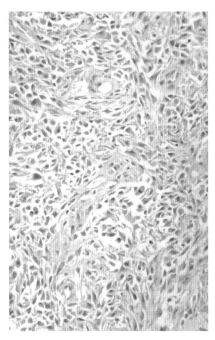

Fig. 8.20 Spindle cell squamous carcinoma composed of interlacing fascicles of atypical spindle cells.

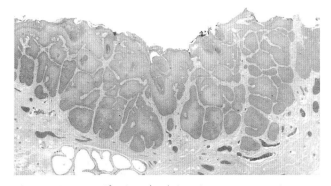

Fig. 8.21 Low magnification of early invasive squamous carcinoma with pushing invasion of variably sized islands of basaloid cells that connect to the surface and have central maturation.

Distinguishing between tangentially cut full-thickness VIN and stage Ia tumours can be difficult and is still the subject of considerable debate. The presence of invasion is usually characterized by small irregular nests of cells that lack the peripheral palisading that is present in the accompanying undifferentiated VIN or streaming large cords and nests that connect with the surface and lack the well-circumscribed insular pattern of tangentially cut elongated rete pegs with undifferentiated VIN (Fig. 8.21). When associated with undifferentiated VIN, the cells have a paradoxically more mature appearance with abundant eosinophilic

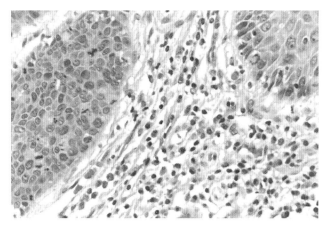

Fig. 8.22 High magnification of inflammatory response with eosinophils to invasive islands of invasive basaloid cells.

cytoplasm, better developed intercellular bridges, and may be associated with the production of keratin. A desmoplastic stromal response may be present. The distinction is more difficult and may be impossible in cases associated with differentiated VIN, since both the invasive and *in situ* elements are composed of mature appearing cells. In these cases, the presence of closely spaced bulbous islands or small nests, rather than solely pseudoepitheliomatous elongated rete pegs, are the clue to invasion. In early invasion associated with both types of VIN, there is often the appearance of, or an increase in, a chronic inflammatory response, and, in one study, an increased number of eosinophils was present (Spiegel 2002) (Fig. 8.22).

Verrucous carcinoma

Verrucous carcinoma is an uncommon indolent form of squamous carcinoma that was first reported in the vulva by Kraus and Perez-Mesa (1966). It tends to occur in post-menopausal women and, in the older literature, was often designated as 'giant condyloma of Buschke–Löwenstein' (Gallousis 1972). Verrucous carcinomas form condylomatous appearing growths that may reach up to 10 cm in greatest dimension and cover most of the vulva (Fig. 8.23). The tumours are typically slow growing. In one series, half of patients gave a history of warts 3–10 years prior to the diagnosis of the carcinoma (Japaze *et al.* 1982).

Histologically, the tumours are composed of an exophytic papillary component with underlying invasive broad bulbous nests. The exophytic portion of the tumour is composed of broad papillations that lack the delicate fibrovascular cores of condylomata acuminata. The surface is usually markedly parakeratotic without atypical nuclei, although areas of bland marked hyperkeratosis may be present (Fig. 8.24). The invasive nests are well rounded and frequently have central keratin or bland parakeratotic cells with a pushing, rather than diffusely infiltrative, margin

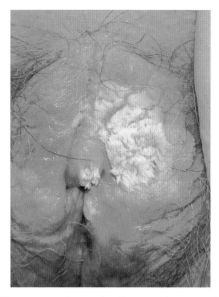

Fig. 8.23 Verrucous carcinoma showing extensive warty plaques on the vulva.

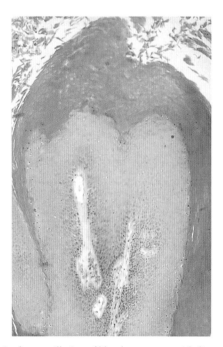

Fig. 8.24 Surface papillation of bland squamous epithelium with overlying hyperkeratosis in verrucous carcinoma.

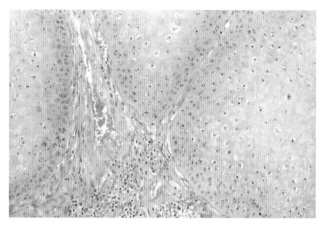

Fig. 8.25 High magnification of pushing broad invasive nests that have minimal atypia in verrucous carcinoma.

and parabasal layers, and atypical forms are absent. Unlike condylomata acuminata and condylomatous carcinomas, well-developed koilocytes are absent. Although warty koilocytes are absent, the tumour has been reported to be associated with HPV-6 or its variants (Ratskar *et al.* 1982, Okagaki *et al.* 1984). There is no evidence of VIN in the adjacent epithelium, although there may be condyloma-like papillations with hyperkeratosis and/or parakeratosis without warty koilocytosis at the periphery of the tumour.

Treatment is by wide local excision without inguinal lymphadenectomy. When inadequately excised, the tumours recur, and, although they rarely, if ever, metastasize, repeated recurrences or delayed primary excision can lead to extensive local destruction that may lead to the death of the patient (Andersen & Sorensen 1988, Gadducci *et al.* 1989). The 5 year survival rate is about 80%. Radiation therapy has been discouraged, since it has been claimed that it may lead to transformation to a more aggressive squamous carcinoma (Lucas *et al.* 1974), but this has not been subsequently confirmed in the vulva in the more recent literature.

The greatest difficulty in diagnosis is that frequently the tumour may be misdiagnosed as a benign condition in a series of superficial small biopsy specimens, as only papillations lined by hyper- or parakeratotic bland epithelium may be present and the true nature of the lesion is not recognized until complete excision is undertaken. Even in these specimens there may be difficulty is distinguishing the tumour from a condyloma acuminatum or a condylomatous carcinoma (see below). The distinction from the former may not be recognized until the tumour recurs, often several times, after incomplete resections. The distinction from the latter is also important, as condylomatous tumours may metastasize to regional lymph nodes. Cases of verrucous carcinoma that have been reported to have metastasized to lymph

that is usually associated with an inflammatory infiltrate (Fig. 8.25). The cells in both components are bland to minimally atypical with a mild degree of nuclear and nucleolar enlargement, the greatest atypia being present in the deeper invasive nests, and undergo a minimally altered maturation sequence. Mitotic figures are rare and limited to the basal

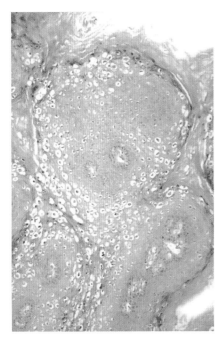

Fig. 8.26 Surface papillations with warty koilocytosis in condylomatous carcinoma.

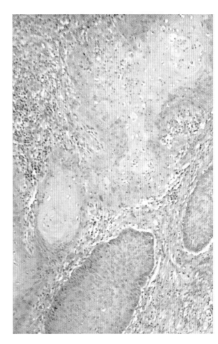

Fig. 8.27 Superficially invasive irregular nests of eosinophilic atypical epithelium in condylomatous carcinoma.

nodes (Vayrynen *et al.* 1981) or distant sites (Stehman *et al.* 1980) may have been misdiagnosed and were truly cases of condylomatous carcinoma.

Condylomatous (warty, verruciform) carcinoma

Condylomatous carcinoma is a low-grade squamous carcinoma that was first described by Ratskar *et al.* (1982). The tumour tends to occur during the late reproductive and early postmenopausal years and is associated with HPV-16 and -18 (Toki *et al.* 1991, Kurman *et al.* 1993). Like condylomata acuminata and verrucous carcinomas, they form exophytic warty growths that can reach a large size.

Histologically, condylomatous carcinomas have an exophytic papillary component and underlying infiltrative nests. The former has fibrovascular cores similar to those of condylomata acuminatum and are usually markedly hyperkeratotic and/or parakeratotic. There is usually mild nuclear enlargement and prominence of the nucleoli, and the granular cell layer or parakeratotic cells may contain enlarged hyperchromatic nuclei. Unlike verrucous carcinomas, well-developed, mildly to moderately atypical warty koilocytes are present in the exophytic papillations (Fig. 8.26). Invasion is usually only a few millimetres and composed of invasive nests that have an appearance of a more conventional well- to moderately differentiated large-cell carcinoma with a diffusely or irregular invasive margin rather than the pushing margin of verrucous carcinoma (Ratskar *et al.* 1982) (Fig. 8.27). Keratinization may be

present in the invasive nests, but it is not cuffed by well-glycogenated bland cells as in verrucous carcinoma. Mitotic figures are more numerous than in verrucous carcinomas, and they are frequently atypical. Unlike verrucous carcinomas, undifferentiated VIN with warty and/or basaloid features is present in the adjacent epithelium (Toki *et al.* 1991, Kurman *et al.* 1993).

The clinical behaviour of condylomatous carcinomas is thought to be intermediate between verrucous carcinomas and well-differentiated large-cell carcinomas. Since lymph node metastases have been reported (Kurman *et al.* 1993), the treatment is the same as for more conventional squamous carcinomas with ipsilateral or bilateral inguinal lymphadenectomy. Presumably, sentinel lymph node dissection may be used in the future.

A major difficulty exists in distinguishing a condylomatous carcinoma from a condyloma acuminatum in a small superficial biopsy specimen. Even in an excisional biopsy specimen of an early carcinoma the distinction may be difficult if the invasive nests are not well developed, and the true nature of the lesion may not be recognized until they recur. Consequently, the presence of significant atypia and the presence of atypical mitoses in any otherwise architecturally typical condylomatous growth should raise the possibility of condylomatous carcinoma.

Basal cell carcinoma

Basal cell carcinomas constitute 2–5% of vulval malignancies, and usually occur in elderly white women (Gibson &

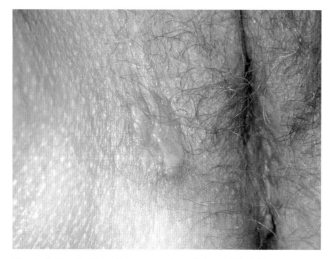

Fig. 8.28 Basal cell carcinoma: pearly nodule on right labium majus.

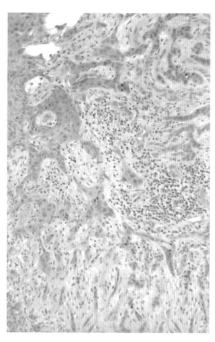

Fig. 8.30 Morphoeic pattern of basal carcinoma of slender infiltrating cords in dense fibrotic stroma.

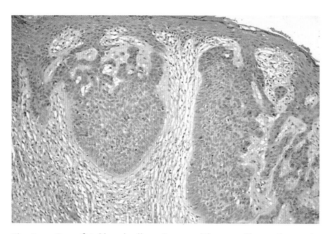

Fig. 8.29 Superficial basal cell carcinoma with nests of hyperchromatic basal cells with peripheral palisading arising from base of epithelium with suprabasal normal maturation.

Ahmed 2001). The labia majora are the most common site (Fig. 8.28), but they may also occur in the fourchette, mons pubis, periurethral region or clitoris. There is wide variation in presentation. They may be nodular or flat, shiny plaques which may be ulcerated. Some are pigmented. Some have been reported in association with lichen sclerosus (see Chapter 5). Grossly, the tumours are usually ≤ 2 cm (Benedet *et al.* 1997), but tumours as large as 10 cm have been reported (Dudzinksi *et al.* 1984).

Histologically, their appearance is identical to those seen elsewhere. The commonest patterns are superficial micronodular and nodular in which multiple invasive nests of variable size appear to bud off or extend from the basal portion of the epithelium (Fig. 8.29), and the morphoea-like pattern in which basaloid cells form cords that elicit a dense fibrotic desmoplastic stroma that may be hyalinized (Fig. 8.30). Gland-like spaces are not uncommon, but tumours with

a predominance of these spaces, the adenomatoid pattern, are uncommon (Feakins & Lowe 1997). The tumour cells closely resemble those of the overlying basal epithelium or periphery of the outer root sheath of hair follicles from which they arise. The cells have scant cytoplasm and small hyperchromatic elongated nuclei. Unlike basaloid squamous carcinomas, there is usually little pleomorphism; while mitotic figures are present, they are usually inconspicuous, and there is characteristic palisading of the nuclei at the periphery of the nests, and an absence of overlying VIN, the intraepithelial neoplastic cells being confined to the basal and parabasal cell layers of the surface epithelium. The stroma frequently has a basophilic myxoid appearance, and there is a variable degree of chronic inflammation. There may be foci of more mature squamous differentiation towards the centres of the nests, but the squamous differentiation is usually either bland or minimally atypical (Fig. 8.31). Occasionally, the squamous element may be prominent with significant pleomorphism or there are invasive nests of the pure squamous element that are identical to pure squamous carcinomas (Breen *et al.* 1975). These tumours are sometimes designated basi-squamous or metatypical basal cell carcinoma, but, as long as they arise from the basal epithelium, they behave as more conventional basal cell carcinomas. The stain Ber EP4 may be helpful in distinguishing between the two (Tellechea *et al.* 1993).

Basal cell carcinomas of the vulva rarely metastasize, but they can cause extensive local destruction. It has been suggested that a tumour thickness > 1 cm, invasion of the

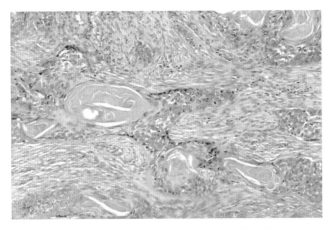

Fig. 8.31 Focal squamous differentiation in basal cell carcinoma.

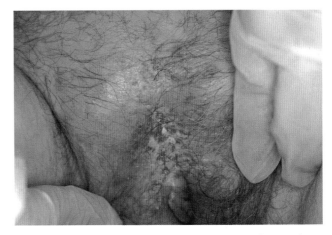

Fig. 8.32 Extramammary Paget's disease: extensive erythema with erosions and areas of hyperkeratosis on the mons pubis and labia.

subcutaneous fat, bleeding or a morphoea-like pattern may increase the likelihood of metastases (Perrone *et al.* 1987). However, as these tumours are uncommon these criteria are of little value in predicting an aggressive behaviour for an individual case. The treatment is local excision with adequate margins (Mulayim *et al.* 2002). Approximately 10–20% will recur when tumour is present at the margins. Either re-excision or careful follow-up with subsequent excision if there is a recurrence is adequate for involved margins.

Extramammary Paget's disease

Paget's disease of the vulva and perineum is defined by the presence of adenocarcinomatous-appearing cells in the epithelium. Paget's disease can be divided into two distinct entities: first, an intraepithelial adenocarcinoma that arises in the vulva and perineum; and second, a pagetoid intra-epithelial spread of a primary carcinoma from an adjacent or contiguous area, most commonly the anorectal region, urethra, uterine cervix, Bartholin's gland or urinary bladder (Lundquist *et al.* 1999).

Primary Paget's disease

Primary Paget's disease is almost exclusively a disease of postmenopausal women, usually older than 60 years. The patients usually present with a history of pruritus that ranges from a few months to up to 30 years, the average being approximately 2 years, but some patients may claim to be asymptomatic. On gross examination, there are multiple, erythematous, eczematoid moderately well-demarcated scaly patches or plaques that are often extensive (Fig. 8.32). Not uncommonly, the patients are treated topically for a non-neoplastic condition, which may provide some temporary relief, and the diagnosis is not established until the patient ultimately fails to respond to therapy and a biopsy is performed.

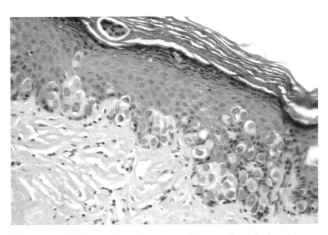

Fig. 8.33 Individual and small clusters of Paget cells with abundant clear cytoplasm and round nuclei in basal epithelium with areas of upward migration.

Histologically, Paget cells have abundant usually clear mucin-positive cytoplasm, and a central large nucleus that often has a prominent nucleolus. Signet ring cells may be present, but usually comprise a minority of neoplastic cells (Gu *et al.* 2005). The cells may occur singly, in small clusters or large nests, the last most commonly being present in the basal portions of the squamous epithelium (Fig. 8.33). The squamous epithelium is often hyperplastic with hyper- or parakeratosis, and, when the Paget cells become confluent, the proliferation may be misinterpreted as undifferentiated VIN in a small biopsy specimen (Fardal *et al.* 1967, Creasman *et al.* 1975). The cells may also be mistaken for melanoma *in situ* or superficial spreading melanoma, but the absence of melanocytic immunohisto-chemical markers and the presence of mucin excludes the diagnosis. While acantholysis in clusters of Paget cells may form gland-like spaces, true gland formation is uncommon

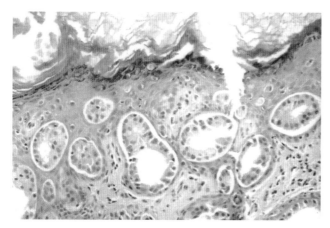

Fig. 8.34 Intraepithelial gland formation by Paget cells.

(Fig. 8.34). The Paget cells often extend individually beyond the margin of the grossly visible lesion, and may extend into the adnexal ducts and pilosebaceous units, but their presence in adnexal glands is uncommon. In approximately 20% of extensively sampled cases, there are foci of invasion. The depth of invasion is usually less than 1 mm and may be multifocal, but deeper invasive carcinomas may occur (Goldblum & Hart 1997, Fanning *et al.* 1999, Ohnishi & Watanabe 2000, Parker *et al.* 2000, Zollo & Zeitouni 2000, Tebes *et al.* 2002). The invasive tumours have a histological appearance identical to invasive mammary duct carcinoma. The extension into adnexal ducts and glands and invasion from the intraepithelial component has often been misdiagnosed as underlying sweat gland carcinoma, particularly in the older literature, and account for most, if not virtually all, cases that were reported to have an underlying sweat gland carcinoma (Helwig & Graham 1963, Koss *et al.* 1968, Creasman *et al.* 1975, Nadji *et al.* 1982, Guldhammer & Nørgaard 1986, Kodama *et al.* 1995, Fanning *et al.* 1999, Parker *et al.* 2000, Zollo & Zeitouni 2000).

The histogenesis of primary Paget's disease is uncertain. Historically, a histogenesis has been ascribed to eccrine and/or apocrine glands and a pluripotent germinative cell in the surface basal epithelium. Neither of these theories accounts for the vast majority of primary Paget's disease in men and women occurring in the genital region, despite the widespread distribution of eccrine glands and a high concentration of apocrine glands in the axilla. Pluripotent germinative cells have never been described or characterized, but presumably they would also have a widespread distribution. On the other hand, evidence is accumulating that the malignant cells arise in the anogenital glands and subsequently spread to the overlying epithelium (van der Putte 1994, van der Putte & van Gorp 1994, Regauer 2006). Anogenital glands are limited to the genital region, and

Paget's disease in the genital regions is histologically identical to that of the breast, like other lesions in the vulva that arise from the anogenital glands. Immunohistochemistry also supports a histogenesis from anogenital glands (see Anogenital gland neoplasms). The tumour cells are diffusely positive for cytokeratin 7 (Onishi & Watanabe 2000), and occasionally have cells positive for oestrogen receptor protein (de Leon *et al.* 2000). While eccrine and apocrine glands and their malignant counterparts may also be positive for these immunohistochemical markers, unlike eccrine and apocrine carcinomas, intraepithelial and invasive Paget cells are negative for epidermal growth factor (EGF) receptor protein (Kikuchi *et al.* 1990), which is present in most eccrine and apocrine carcinomas (Busam *et al.* 1999).

Immunohistochemistry may also play a role in distinguishing primary Paget's disease from pagetoid spread from an adjacent carcinoma. Primary Paget's disease is diffusely positive for cytokeratin 7, but may be focally positive for cytokeratin 20 (Battles *et al.* 1997, Goldblum & Hart 1997, 1998, Smith *et al.* 1997, Crawford *et al.* 1999, Lundquist *et al.* 1999). It is diffusely positive for mucin (MUC)1 and MUC5AC, the former usually greater than the latter (Kuan *et al.* 2001), but may be focally positive for MUC2, and it is usually positive for gross cystic disease fluid protein-15 (GCDFP) (Ordónèz *et al.* 1987, Nakamura *et al.* 1995, Kohler & Smoller 1996, Battles *et al.* 1997, Goldblum & Hart 1997, 1998, Nowak *et al.* 1998, Lundquist *et al.* 1999) and androgen receptor (de Leon *et al.* 2000, Fujimoto *et al.* 2000). Pagetoid spread of anorectal carcinomas is usually diffusely positive for cytokeratin 20, but may also be positive for cytokeratin 7 (Battles *et al.* 1997, Goldblum & Hart 1998, Nowak *et al.* 1998, Lundquist *et al.* 1999, Ohnishi & Watanabe 2000, Kuan *et al.* 2001). It is usually diffusely positive for MUC2 and negative for MUC1 and MUC5AC (Kuan *et al.* 2001) and negative for GCDFP (Battles *et al.* 1997, Goldblum & Hart 1998, Nowak *et al.* 1998, Lundquist *et al.* 1999). Pagetoid spread of urinary system transitional cell carcinoma may be diffusely positive for both cytokeratin 7 and cytokeratin 20 (Goldblum & Hart 1997), is usually positive for cytokeratin 20 (Lundquist *et al.* 1999, Ohnishi & Watanabe 2000) and may be positive for cytokeratin 7 and negative for cytokeratin 20 (Battles *et al.* 1997), but is negative for GCDFP (Battles *et al.* 1997, Goldblum & Hart 1997, Lundquist *et al.* 1999). Immunohistochemistry can also evaluate the extent of disease. Cytokeratin 7 can identify single Paget cells at the periphery, but cannot identify them in adnexal ducts, as they are also positive for cytokeratin 7. Paget cells at the periphery of lesions lack positive staining for EGFP, and this highlights their presence there and in adnexal ducts and glands which stain positively. The stain is also useful in evaluating early invasion, as intraepithelial Paget cells will have an attenuated rim of EGF-positive native squamous basal cells separating them from the underlying stroma (G.W. Spiegel, personal observation).

In the absence of clinically suspicious lymph nodes or documented invasive tumour, the usual treatment of Paget's disease is surgical excision to a depth of 4–6 mm to include the pilosebaceous units and skin adnexal structures. However, approximately 20–40% of cases recur regardless of the histological status of the margins in the plane of section, and cases have been reported to recur in skin flaps that are used to cover the wound (Beecham 1976, de Jonge & Knobel 1988, Misas *et al.* 1990, DiSaia *et al.* 1995). Recurrence in cases with negative margins has been reported to be secondary to multifocal disease; however, there have been no well-documented cases of multifocality, and some ascribe recurrences to serpentiginous spread of disease that is not seen in the plane of section in cases with 'negative margins'. Cases with an invasive element can metastasize to regional lymph nodes; usually the invasion is > 1 mm and the risk of metastases increases with the depth of invasion as with squamous carcinoma, but rare patients with < 1 mm invasion have been reported to develop lymph node metastases (Fine *et al.* 1995, Ewing *et al.* 2004), and in one reported case lymph node and bone metastases occurred in the absence of detected invasion after a vulval recurrence (Cappuccini *et al.* 1997).

In cases where there is invasion, wide local excision, vulvectomy and inguinal lymphadenectomy should be considered, but the treatment needs to be tailored according to the depth of invasion and to the patient's general condition.

The immune modulating cream imiquimod has now been successfully used for non-invasive disease and for recurrences after surgery (Wang *et al.* 2003).

Paget's disease secondary to underlying adjacent carcinoma

The clinical appearance of pagetoid spread of an adjacent carcinoma is almost identical to that of primary Paget's disease, but the distribution is based to a large extent on the site of the primary carcinoma. Pagetoid spread of anorectal carcinoma accounts for 20–50% of cases with Paget's disease in the perianal region and perineum. Spread of urinary tract transitional cell carcinoma tends to be centred on the periurethral region. Rare cases of pagetoid spread from adenocarcinoma of Bartholin's gland (Chamlian & Taylor 1972) and cervix (McKee & Hertogs 1980) have also been reported. In most cases, the primary carcinoma has been diagnosed prior to or synchronously with the development of the pagetoid spread. In occasional cases the spread may be the presenting symptom of the underlying carcinoma and all patients should be thoroughly screened.

Pagetoid spread of anorectal carcinoma to the perianal region has an appearance that can usually be histologically distinguished from primary Paget's disease. Signet ring cells

Table 8.1 Comparison of features of primary Paget's disease and pagetoid spread of anorectal adenocarcinoma

Feature	Primary Paget's	Pagetoid anorectal carcinoma
Signet ring cells	+/–	+++ to +
Extracellular mucin	–	+++ to –
GCDFP	+++ to –	–
Cytokeratin 7	+++	++/–
Cytokeratin 20	+/–	+++ to +
MUC1	+++	+/–
MUC2	+/–	+++
MUC5AC	+++ to +	+/–

are common, and true intraepithelial gland formation that may have central comedo necrosis may be seen (Goldblum & Hart 1998). When invasive tumour is present below the epithelium, gastrointestinal-type malignant glands are present. Extracellular mucin may be present in both the intraepithelial and invasive elements (Williams *et al.* 1976, Wolber *et al.* 1991). The immunohistochemical profile of primary Paget's disease and pagetoid spread of anorectal carcinoma is strikingly different (Table 8.1).

Pagetoid spread of transitional cell carcinoma from the urinary system may be difficult in a small biopsy specimen. Like primary Paget's cells, intraepithelial Paget's cells are round with a central nucleus and have abundant clear cytoplasm. However, the cells are mucin negative (Battles *et al.* 1997) and form clusters that may have central necrosis (Goldblum & Hart 1997). A tumour that is diffusely positive for both cytokeratins 7 and 20 and negative for GCDFP, particularly if it is clinically centred on the periurethral area, should point to a primary in the urinary tract.

The treatment and prognosis of pagetoid spread of a contiguous carcinoma is dependent on the primary tumour. Nevertheless, an attempt should be made to excise the pagetoid spread since it may progress to invasive tumour.

Anogenital glands and neoplasms of anogenital gland origin

Anogenital glands

The presence of ectopic breast tissue in the vulva is well embedded in many textbooks and is based on the assumption that the embryonic milk line extends to the vulva as it does in some mammals. Mammary duct-like structures in the vulva and perineum are often present adjacent to neoplasms that are histologically indistinguishable from mammary benign neoplasms and ductal carcinoma. However, no cases of a rudimentary nipple have been described in the vulva, although it has been described on the inner thigh

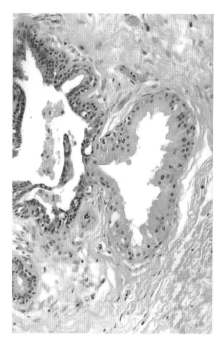

Fig. 8.35 Apocrine metaplasia.

where the embryonic milk line extends after it skirts the vulva (de Cholnoky 1939). van der Putte (1994) terms the presence of vulval ectopic breast tissue a 'phylogenetic and ontogenetic myth'. The tissue that has been described as ectopic breast tissue are the anogenital glands of the vulva, perineum and scrotum and were first described in detail by van der Putte (1994), although their existence had been proposed earlier (Woodruff *et al.* 1971). In the vulva, they are concentrated in the interlabial sulcus and extend to the perineum. By light and electron microscopic criteria they are virtually identical to mammary ducts and are lined by an outer layer of myoepithelial cells and an inner layer of secretory cells and are connected to the surface by a squamous lined duct (see Fig. 1.23). They may undergo apocrine metaplasia (Fig. 8.35), often with cystic dilatation (van der Putte & van Gorp 1995, Offidani & Campanati 1999). They are positive for oestrogen receptors, progesterone receptors and cytokeratin 7, and variably positive for gross cystic disease fluid protein (van der Putte 1994, van der Putte & van Gorp 1994, Offidani & Campanati 1999). It has been reported that the native epithelium is negative for androgen receptors, but that metaplastic apocrine epithelium in the gland is positive (Offidani & Campanati 1999). Consequently, it is to be expected that they can give rise to neoplasms that have an identical counterpart in the breast.

Benign neoplasms of the anogenital glands
Fibroadenomas arising from the anogenital glands of the vulva have the same appearance as those in the breast and have been erroneously reported as arising in vulval ectopic breast tissue (Foushee & Pruitt 1967, Hassim 1969,

Tressara *et al.* 1998). Like their mammary counterpart they are positive for oestrogen and progesterone receptors, and may undergo apocrine metaplasia. A proliferation of anogenital glands may lead to a fibroadenoma that has a histological appearance identical to that of its counterpart in the breast and may undergo lactational change. There may be a prominence of fibrous stroma so that the histology resembles a mammary phyllodes tumour. However, no clinically malignant phyllodes-like tumours have been described in the vulva.

Hidradenoma papilliferum is the vulval counterpart of the mammary intraductal papilloma. An origin from anogenital glands was first proposed by Woodruff *et al.* (1971), who postulated that they arose from a sweat gland with features intermediate between those of eccrine and apocrine glands that was peculiar to the vulva, and dismissed an origin from apocrine glands on the basis of their absence in the axilla, which is a site of numerous apocrine glands.

Hidradenomas usually arise in the interlabial sulcus or in the labium minus or majus adjacent to the sulcus or in the perineum. The tumours tend to occur during the mid-reproductive years and menopause (Offidani & Campanati 1999), and have been usually been described in white women, but this may simply be a reflection of the populations under study. The tumours generally form subepithelial freely mobile and non-tender soft to firm nodules that are usually less than 2 cm in diameter and asymptomatic; however, they may reach a larger size and may be ulcerated with protrusion of red fleshy tissue that may bleed on contact. Often they are long standing with little or no growth, but rapid growth has been reported (Meeker *et al.* 1962), as well as a cyclical change in size (Woodruff *et al.* 1971, Offidani & Campanati 1999). They are usually solitary, but cases of metachronous and synchronous tumours have been described (Woodruff *et al.* 1971). The hidradenomas clinically often appear cystic. Histologically, there are well-formed non-encapsulated subepithelial nodules of acinar–papillary proliferations lined by an outer layer of myoepithelial cells (Konishi *et al.* 1985, Offidani & Campanati 1999), and an inner layer of bland to mildly atypical amphophilic to eosinophilic cuboidal to columnar cells with secretory snouts (Figs 8.36 and 8.37). Rarely, an opening onto the surface may be present. The fibrous stroma is usually scant, but may be prominent. Mitotic figures may be present, but they are usually rare, and atypical mitotic figures are absent. Apocrine metaplasia is frequent (Woodruff *et al.* 1971) (Fig. 8.38). The tumours are positive for cytokeratin 7 and androgen receptor (Offidani & Campanati 1999), and, unlike most tumours of sweat gland origin, are negative for EGF receptor protein. The areas lined by cuboidal to columnar cells are positive for oestrogen and progesterone receptors (Offidani & Campanati 1999) and are usually negative for GCDFP, whereas areas of apocrine metaplasia are negative for oestrogen and progesterone receptors

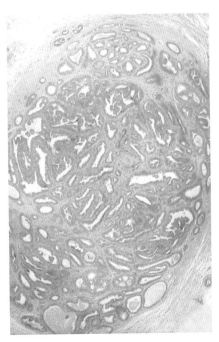

Fig. 8.36 Papillary hidradenoma papilliferum composed predominantly of variably sized tubular glands.

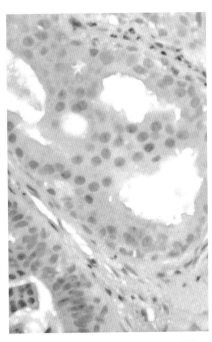

Fig. 8.38 Apocrine metaplasia in hidradenoma papilliferum.

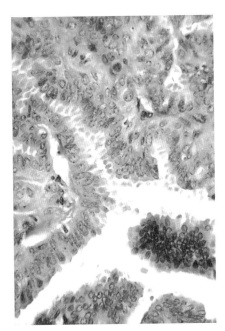

Fig. 8.37 Double cell layer of outer myoepithelial cells and inner secretory cells with secretory snouts in papillary hidradenoma papilliferum.

(Offidani & Campanati 1999) and positive for GCDFP (Mazoujian & Margolis 1988). This profile closely resembles that of the non-neoplastic anogenital glands. Treatment is by local excision.

Anogenital gland carcinoma

Only a few cases of adenocarcinoma attributed to a histogenesis from the anogenital glands appear in the literature (Abbott & Ahmed 2006), although a few others consider the possibility rather than an origin from 'ectopic breast tissue' (Kennedy *et al.* 1997, Ohira *et al.* 2004, Karakov *et al.* 2005).

The tumours form a subepithelial mass in the interlabial sulcus or adjacent labium minus and majus, and occur during the reproductive to postmenopausal years. The tumours have a microscopic appearance identical to that of mammary duct carcinomas and are composed of infiltrating cords, nests and/or tubules of cuboidal cells to rounded malignant cells with a moderate amount of amphophilic to eosinophilic cytoplasm and a central nucleus that often has a prominent nucleolus. Anogenital glands may be present at the periphery, and, in the older literature, these were mistaken for ectopic breast tissue. Like mammary ductal carcinomas, they are usually positive for oestrogen receptor protein, and frequently positive for progesterone receptor protein and GCDFP. However, unlike apocrine gland carcinomas, they are negative for EGF receptor protein (G.W. Spiegel, personal observation). The tumours initially metastasize to the ipsilateral groin lymph nodes. It has not been established whether some eccrine mucinous carcinomas that resemble colloid carcinoma of the breast may also arise from the anogenital glands.

Treatment of adenocarcinomas of anogenital glands is surgical excision and groin lymph node dissection on the ipsilateral side. The resemblance to mammary ductal carcinoma may be so great that a presumptive diagnosis of metastatic mammary carcinoma is made when there is an absence of adjacent anogenital glands. Although the vulva may be a site for metastatic disease, it is rarely a site for the initial presentation of the primary disease. Consequently, when encountering an isolated vulval carcinoma with a histological appearance and immunohistochemical profile identical to that of breast ductal carcinoma, and if metastatic disease is clinically confined to the ipsilateral lymph nodes, a diagnosis of primary anogenital carcinoma is warranted, and subsequent investigations should be limited to staging the patient.

Benign skin adnexal tumours

Syringoma

Syringomas are eccrine sweat gland duct adenomas. They tend to occur in young women, and are rare past the menopause. The patients may present with pruritus, but are more commonly asymptomatic. They may be an incidental finding in specimens resected for other conditions. The tumours form 1–4 mm firm flesh-coloured papules. While they may be solitary, in the vulva they are usually multiple and occur most commonly on the labia majora, but may involve the labia minora (Bal *et al.* 2003, Huang *et al.* 2003).

Histologically, the tumours are composed of small ducts with comma-like tails and may be variably cystically dilated. They are lined by a double layer of bland cells that often appear flattened, and contain periodic acid–Schiff (PAS)-positive diastase-resistant luminal secretions. The stroma is fibrous and may be hyalinized. The proliferating ducts have a random scattered ('shotgun') distribution, and lack the streaming present in adenocarcinomas (Figs 8.39 and 8.40). Rupture of the ducts may elicit a foreign body-type giant cell reaction (Thomas *et al.* 1979). Treatment is ablation and is usually reserved for only severely symptomatic women (Young *et al.* 1980).

Clear cell hidradenoma

These are rare vulval tumours, which like syringomas are believed to arise from eccrine sweat gland ducts. They form solitary 0.5–2 cm subepithelial solid nodules that are usually asymptomatic, but may be tender or pruritic. They are composed of a well-circumscribed collection of closely packed lobules of uniform polygonal cells with small round nuclei and variably clear cytoplasm. Small cysts and tubules may be present within the lobules. There is no connection with the overlying epidermis, although the tumour may extend to the surface and rupture. Mitotic figures are rare. Treatment, if symptomatic, is by local excision.

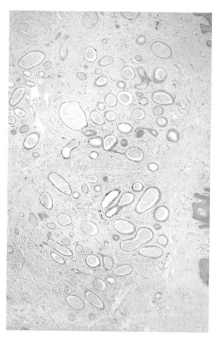

Fig. 8.39 Syringoma composed of randomly placed variably cystic glands in dermis.

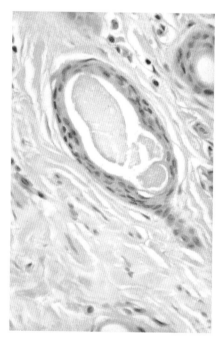

Fig. 8.40 Gland lined by a double cell layer of flattened bland cells, inspissated secretions and comma-like tails.

Trichoepithelioma

These benign tumours of hair follicle origin are located in the dermis and are composed of proliferating nests of bland basaloid cells that surround keratin-filled cystic spaces. They rarely occur in the vulva (Cho & Woodruff 1988).

Hairs are not present, but sebaceous gland differentiation may be seen at the periphery of the nests. Unlike a basal cell carcinoma, the cells are bland, mitotic figures are rare or absent, and there is an absence of an infiltrative border and connection to the basal layer of the overlying epidermis or adjacent hair root sheath.

Trichilemmoma (proliferating trichilemmal tumour, pilar tumour)

These tumours arise from the outer hair root sheath and rarely occur in the vulva (Avinoach *et al.* 1989), but, when they do, they may be confused with squamous carcinoma. The tumours form a spherical mass of lobules of bland squamous epithelium that have an outer rim of bland basaloid cells and a central cystic space filled with amorphous keratin that may undergo calcification. Neither a granular cell layer nor connection with overlying epidermis is present, although the tumour may rupture onto the surface. Unlike squamous carcinoma, the tumours have a non-invasive border, are composed of bland cells, lack associated VIN and the keratin formation is not associated with a granular cell layer.

Sweat gland carcinomas

Apocrine carcinomas

Virtually all cases of apocrine carcinoma of the vulva have been reported in case reports or series of Paget's disease, and most of these are in the older literature. In some of these cases, the reported carcinoma is extension of Paget cells into sweat gland ducts, and, in almost all the others, they are invasive Paget cells. If one accepts the more recently proposed pathogenesis of Paget's disease from anogenital glands, there are rare well-documented cases of vulval apocrine carcinomas, unless those that have a mucinous histology are of apocrine origin (see Eccrine mucinous carcinoma).

Eccrine mucinous carcinoma

Few cases of this distinctive tumour have been reported in the vulva and may be confused with other neoplasms (Karakov *et al.* 2005). Two have had associated neuroendocrine differentiation (Rahilly *et al.* 1995, Grin *et al.* 2008). They have occurred in women from the late reproductive to postmenopausal years. The tumours have an appearance that is virtually identical to that of colloid carcinoma of the breast and are composed of pools of mucin in which there are relatively bland mucin-secreting cells that appear to float in and/or line collections of extracellular mucin. The tumours invade the subepithelial stroma or dermis in a burgeoning fashion (Figs 8.41 and 8.42). Mitotic figures are rare. Based on their clinical behaviour at other sites, they are rarely associated with metastases at presentation, but, when incompletely excised, they tend to recur,

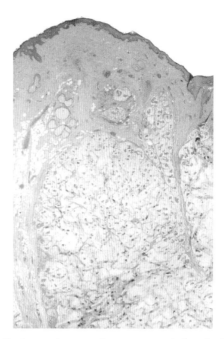

Fig. 8.41 Eccrine mucinous carcinoma composed of pools of mucin with 'floating' epithelium invading dermis and subcutaneous tissue.

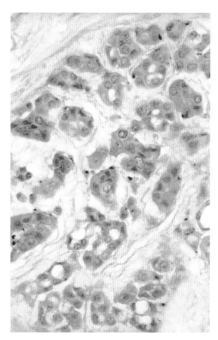

Fig. 8.42 Clusters of mildly atypical cells with focal gland formation 'floating' in mucin in eccrine mucinous carcinoma.

and following several recurrences may metastasize. While these tumours have traditionally been thought to be of eccrine gland origin, their usual occurrence at sites that harbour apocrine glands leads many dermatopathologists to believe that their pathogenesis is probably from these glands (Karakov *et al.* 2005). Owing to their resemblance to mammary colloid carcinoma, they may be mistaken for metastatic tumour from a mammary primary; however, this diagnosis is usually excluded by the absence of metastatic disease elsewhere (see Metastatic carcinoma). On the other hand, the possibility that some vulval eccrine mucinous carcinomas arise from the anogenital glands cannot be excluded (Karakov *et al.* 2005).

Miscellaneous sweat gland carcinomas

Isolated cases of ductal eccrine carcinoma, eccrine porocarcinoma and clear cell hidradenocarcinomas have been reported (Wick *et al.* 1985, Fukuma *et al.* 1986, Messing *et al.* 1993, Massad *et al.* 1996). Microcystic adnexal carcinoma, which is a subset of sebaceous gland carcinomas, has also been described in the vulva (Chiller *et al.* 2000, Buhl *et al.* 2001). These have many of the features of a benign tumour, but behave in an aggressive fashion. Characteristically, collections of small cuboidal and basaloid cells within the dermis form islands, strands, cords and ductal structures. When sought, perineural invasion is often present. Horn cyst formation surrounded by keratinocytes with slight cytological atypia may be present, and the nuclei of peripheral cells surrounding these collections may exhibit pallisading. A small incisional biopsy specimen of these tumours may be misinterpreted as a syringoma; however, unlike syringomas, the tumour forms a mass. Reports of 'mammary lobular carcinoma' arising in 'ectopic breast tissue' have also been reported, but, as this heterotopia does not exist in the vulva, these tumours may also be of sweat gland origin. The general arguments for these tumours being of 'ectopic breast' histogenesis is based on histology and the presence of positive oestrogen or progesterone receptors, but sweat gland tumours are notorious for resembling mammary carcinoma and are frequently positive for oestrogen and progesterone receptors (Busam *et al.* 1999). Consequently, these features and the rarity of vulval sweat gland carcinomas mandate that, when an adenocarcinoma has an unusual appearance or an appearance suggestive of sweat gland origin, a consultation should be sought from an experienced dermatopathologist. Like eccrine mucinous carcinomas, the treatment of these tumours should be based on their behaviour at more common sites.

Bartholin's gland hyperplasia and neoplasms

Bartholin's gland hyperplasia

Hyperplasia of Bartholin's gland was first described in detail by Koenig and Tavassoli (1998) (17 cases), and subsequently 10 cases were reported by Santos *et al.* (2006). In the latter series the patients ranged from 23 to 45 years and the proliferations formed 1.3–4.5 solid, tan, unencapsulated solid masses that were often clinically interpreted as a

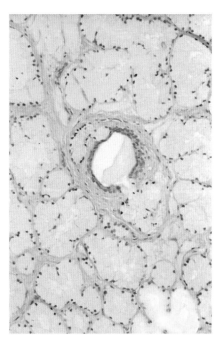

Fig. 8.43 Lobule of closely spaced mucinous acini with central collecting duct.

Bartholin's gland cyst or abscess. Histologically, hyperplasia is characterized by lobular proliferation of densely packed mucinous acini that retains the normal architecture with a central terminal duct among the hyperplastic acini (Fig. 8.43).

Bartholin's gland benign neoplasms

Only rare proliferations have been accepted as benign neoplasms of Bartholin's gland. Koenig and Tavassoli (1998) reported a case of an adenoma and an adenomyoma. In each of these tumours there was a haphazard proliferation of bland acini and terminal ducts, and in the latter there was a fibromuscular stroma. A case of a papilloma has also been reported (Enghardt *et al.* 1993). It was an intracystic focal proliferation of fibrovascular cores lined by columnar to stratified polygonal bland cells with squamous and transitional features.

Carcinoma

Bartholin's gland carcinomas have been reported to constitute 2–7% of vulval malignant tumours. The age at presentation can range from 14 to 91 years with a mean age of 50 years (Leuchter *et al.* 1982). Patients typically present with a 1–6 cm mass (Purola & Widholm 1966). The tumour may be long standing, and, frequently, the mass is clinically interpreted as a Bartholin's gland cyst, and the malignant nature is not recognized until the lesion fails to respond to conservative therapy and recurs. The tumours are solid,

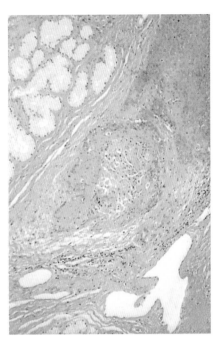

Fig. 8.44 Invasive squamous carcinoma of Bartholin's gland with adjacent mucinous acini.

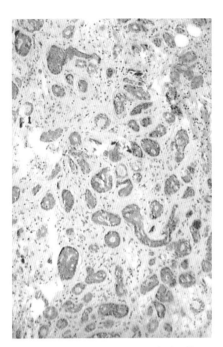

Fig. 8.45 Adenoid cystic carcinoma composed of infiltrating nests punctuated with gland-like spaces containing amorphous eosinophilic material.

grey–white, often have foci of necrosis and haemorrhage, and frequently deeply infiltrate the soft tissue in the region of Bartholin's gland. The tumours are rarely bilateral.

The criteria for a diagnosis of a carcinoma of the Bartholin's gland are lesions arising in the posterior labium majus, histology consistent with that of a Bartholin's gland carcinoma and exclusion of a metastatic tumour (Chamlian & Taylor 1972). Confusingly, there is a wide range of histological features as the tumours may arise from either the mucinous acini or ductal transitional cell epithelium. The presence of residual benign Bartholin's gland adjacent to the tumour, particularly if there is a transition from benign to malignant, is supporting evidence for a histogenesis from Bartholin's gland, but this is rarely the case.

Approximately 40–45% are each adenocarcinomas and squamous carcinomas (Leuchter *et al.* 1982) (Figs 8.44 and 8.45). The remaining tumours are transitional cell carcinomas, anaplastic carcinomas, adenosquamous carcinomas and adenoid cystic carcinomas, the last having a reported frequency of 6–25% of Bartholin gland carcinomas (Copeland *et al.* 1986a,b) and a probable overall frequency of 10–15%. The squamous carcinomas have a histological appearance identical to squamous carcinomas arising elsewhere in the vulva and range from well to poorly differentiated. However, if the tumour is ulcerated and there is no overlying epithelium to assess for the presence or absence of VIN, it may be impossible to establish whether the origin of the tumour is from the Bartholin's gland. The adenocarcinomas may range from well-differentiated with

well-defined acinar-type or tubular glands or papillations to poorly differentiated solid neoplasms (Wahlstrom *et al.* 1978). There can be variable amounts of intracytoplasmic mucin. Rarely, there is pagetoid spread in the adjacent epithelium. Adenosquamous carcinomas contain malignant squamous epithelium and malignant glands or solid areas of mucinous epithelium (Van Nagell *et al.* 1969, Dennefors & Bergman 1980, Wheelock *et al.* 1984). Rare transitional cell carcinomas are composed of proliferations of uniform polygonal cells that frequently line papillary broad fibrovascular cores and resemble those of the urinary tract. Foci of glandular or squamous differentiation may be present, as in the urinary tract (Dodson *et al.* 1970, Wahlstrom *et al.* 1978, Wheelock *et al.* 1984).

With the exception of adenoid cystic carcinoma (see below), the usual treatment of Bartholin's gland carcinoma is vulvectomy and ipsilateral groin lymphadenectomy, with or without adjuvant radiation therapy depending on the extent of spread and adequacy of margins. The overall 5 year survival for these women is 60–80% (Copeland *et al.* 1986a). However, 37–55% of patients with Bartholin's gland carcinoma present with inguinofemoral lymph node metastases, of which 18% will also have pelvic lymph node metastases. For patients with lymph node metastases, the overall survival is approximately 40–50%, and only 18% if more than two nodes are involved (Leuchter *et al.* 1982, Wheelock *et al.* 1984).

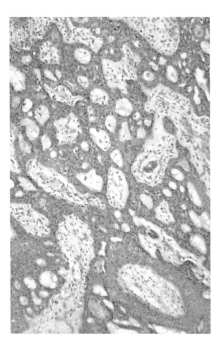

Fig. 8.46 Adenoid cystic carcinoma composed of anastomosing trabeculae with gland-like spaces containing amorphous eosinophilic material.

Adenoid cystic carcinomas involving the posterior labia majora are virtually assumed to be of Bartholin's gland origin. The tumours are composed of uniform small cells with scant cytoplasm and hyperchromatic oval to angulated nuclei that grow in cords, anastomosing trabeculae and nests with sieve-like well-defined rounded spaces. The spaces contain diastase-resistant PAS amorphous basement membrane-like material. The tumours are positive for cytokeratin and S-100 protein (Nadji & Ganjei 1987), the latter being interpreted as myoepithelial cell differentiation. The stroma is fibrous, and there is often a prominent retraction artefact surrounding the nests and cords. The tumours tend to extend along perineural spaces, but lymphatic/vascular space invasion is rarely identified (Fig. 8.46).

Unlike the other histological types of Bartholin's gland carcinoma, adenoid cystic carcinoma uncommonly presents with regional lymph node metastases, and the tumours have a relatively indolent course. They are usually treated with a wide local excision to the deep fascia and ipsilateral groin lymphadenectomy. The local recurrence rate is approximately 25% (Abrao *et al.* 1985), but local and distant recurrences are often late with a mean interval of 8 years (Copeland *et al.* 1986b, Lelle *et al.* 1994). The reported 5 and 10 year survival rates are 71% and 59%, respectively (Copeland *et al.* 1986b); however in one small series, three out of 11 patients died of disease more than 10 years after initial therapy (Lelle *et al.* 1994). Metastases are usually to lung, bone and liver.

Miscellaneous proliferations and neoplasms

Endometriosis

Endometriosis of the vulva is rare. It may occur in scars (Buda *et al.* 2008) and has been postulated to occur secondary to a uterine curettage or implantation of menstrual endometrium into a vulval wound (Duson & Zelenik 1954, Dutta 1987). It typically forms an ill-defined and often painful subepithelial mass, particularly during menses. Histologically, it is composed of characteristic endometrial glands cuffed by endometrial stroma.

Adenocarcinoma

Adenocarcinomas of the vulva arising from the epidermis and not associated with underlying adnexal structures, endometriosis, Paget's disease, anogenital glands, minor vestibular glands or Bartholin's gland are extremely rare. Four cases with a gastrointestinal histology that appear to arise from heterotopic intestinal tissue have been reported (Tiltman & Knutzen 1978, Kennedy & Majmudar 1993, Ghamande *et al.* 1995). The presence of a gastrointestinal-type carcinoma in the vulva should also prompt a search for a primary in the sigmoid colon or rectum and an investigation for metastatic tumour at other sites.

Adenosquamous carcinoma

The criteria for adenosquamous carcinoma are not well established; while the squamous element is usually easily identified, the elements required for adenomatous differentiation are not well defined. The presence of tubuloglandular spaces, particularly if the lumen and lining cells contain mucin, certainly qualifies for adenomatous differentiation (Fig. 8.47), whereas mucin alone is insufficient evidence. In the authors' opinion, in the absence of tubuloglandular spaces, carcinomas with an otherwise squamous appearance that contain intra- and/or extracellular mucin should

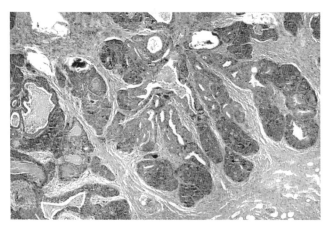

Fig. 8.47 Adenosquamous carcinoma composed of infiltrating islands of squamous epithelium with glandular spaces.

be designated as 'squamous carcinomas with mucin production' and treated as squamous carcinoma. The histogenesis of the latter is not known, but conceivably they may arise from sweat glands, anogenital mammary-like glands, Bartholin's gland and in the perineum from the anal duct glands. While it has been reported that adenosquamous carcinomas are more aggressive than squamous carcinoma, this has not been established owing to the varying criteria for the diagnosis of the entity and the few cases reported (Underwood *et al.* 1978, Bannatyne *et al.* 1989).

Merkel cell carcinoma

Merkel cell carcinomas are highly aggressive neuroendocrine carcinomas which are rare on the vulva (Hierro *et al.* 2000). The American Cancer Society estimates that 3% of Merkel cell carcinomas occur in the vulva with an estimated frequency of approximately 12 cases per year in the USA (Crum 2006). Most of the patients are over 60 years. The tumour usually forms a raised, nodular red to pink mass and is frequently ulcerated or haemorrhagic. The size of the tumour is time dependent, and the lesions may have been present for a few months to up to 2 years, but are usually rapidly growing. The clinical features may mimic a basal cell carcinoma, lymphangioma or haemangioma.

The tumours are located below the surface and infiltrate as sheets and trabeculae of small round to ovoid cells with large nuclei, finely stippled chromatin and inconspicuous nucleoli and scant cytoplasm. Focal squamous and/or glandular differentiation may be present. Superficially, they may resemble a basal cell carcinoma. Unlike basal cell carcinomas they have a high mitotic index, lack peripheral palisading, may have areas of zonal necrosis or form pseudorosettes or Homer-Wright rosettes. They also fail to have continuity with the basal layer of the epithelium or hair follicles, although there may be pagetoid spread. The tumours have a perinuclear dot or crescent pattern of low-molecular-weight cytokeratin immunohistochemical staining, and are frequently positive for the chromogranin and neurone-specific enolase, and less often for synaptophysin, but S-100 protein is absent (Figs 8.48 and 8.49).

Treatment is excision of the primary tumour and ipsilateral lymphadenectomy, often followed by radiation therapy, but the lymphadenectomy probably only offers prognostic information as with vulval melanoma. The tumours tend to recur both locally and distally and have a poor prognosis, even for early stage disease; however, no large-scale studies have been undertaken.

Metastatic carcinoma

It has been reported that 11% of vulval malignancies are either metastatic or direct extension from a non-vulval primary (Dehner 1973). However, vulval metastatic carcinoma is rarely the initial presentation of an occult primary

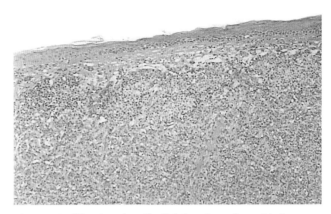

Fig. 8.48 Proliferation of small cells below the surface epithelium.

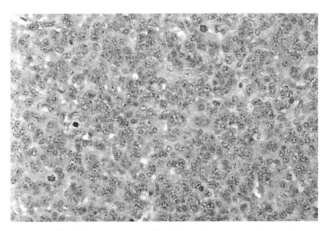

Fig. 8.49 Ill-defined cords of small cells with scant cytoplasm and round vesicular nuclei with inconspicuous nucleoli.

at another site (Mazur *et al.* 1984, Neto *et al.* 2003). The most common primary site is the uterine cervix, followed by the endometrium, ovary and rectum (Dehner 1973, Mazur *et al.* 1984, Neto *et al.* 2003). Overall, the majority of patients have a known primary at the time of presentation and only a very small number have a primary discovered synchronously with the vulval metastasis or afterwards. In those patients with vulval metastases, widespread carcinomatosis is likely. Vulval metastases carry a very poor prognosis and are usually a terminal event.

Vulval metastatic carcinomas involve the dermis alone or the dermis and epidermis, but rarely, if ever, the epidermis alone (Dehner 1973, Neto *et al.* 2003). Lymphatic or vascular space invasion is frequently present, and is usually more prominent below the tumour than between the tumour and epidermis (Dehner 1973). A known history of a primary at another site along with the histology and/or the presence of other metastatic tumour outside the normal lymphatic drainage of the vulva points to the metastatic nature of the lesion. On the other hand, a primary carcinoma may resemble a tumour that is more common at another site, and lead to an erroneous diagnosis of metastatic tumour initiating a time-consuming and expensive search for a non-existent primary. This is particularly the case with anogenital gland carcinomas of the vulva, since, histologically and immuno-histochemically, these tumours are identical to mammary duct carcinomas (see Anogenital gland carcinoma). In cases of a carcinoma with mammary ductal features, and no evidence of metastatic disease at other sites or metastatic disease limited to the inguinal and pelvic lymph nodes, the tumour should be treated as a primary neoplasm, even if there is a past history of breast carcinoma. If the tumour is a mammary metastasis it is almost certainly associated with metastases at other sites and is a terminal event, whereas if the tumour is primary there is a chance for cure.

References

Abbott, J.J. & Ahmed, I. (2006) Adenocarcinoma of mammary-like glands of the vulva: report of a case and review of the literature. *American Journal of Dermatopathology* 28, 127–133.

Abrao, F.S., Marques, A.F., Marziona, F. *et al.* (1985) Adenoid cystic carcinoma of Bartholin's gland: review of the literature and report of two cases. *Journal of Surgical Oncology* 30, 132–137.

Andersen, E.S. & Sorensen, I.M. (1988) Verrucous carcinoma of the female genital tract: report of case and review of the literature. *Gynecologic Oncology* 30, 427–434.

Avinoach, H., Zirkin, H.J. & Glezerman, M. (1989) Proliferating trichilemmal tumor of the vulva: case report and review of the literature. *International Journal of Gynecological Pathology* 8, 163–168.

Azzaz, B.B. (1978) Bartholin's cyst and abscess: a review of treatment of 53 cases. *British Journal of Clinical Practice* 32, 101–105.

Bai, H., Cviko, A., Granter, S. *et al.* (2003) Immunophenotypic and viral (human papillomavirus) correlates of vulvar seborrheic keratosis. *Human Pathology* 34, 559–564.

Bal, N., Aslan, E., Kayaselcuk, F. *et al.* (2003) Vulvar syringoma aggravated by pregnancy. *Pathology and Oncology Research* 9, 196–197.

Bannatyne, P., Elliott, P. & Russell, P. (1989) Vulvar adenosquamous carcinoma arising in a hidradenoma papilliferum, with rapidly fatal outcome: case report. *Gynecologic Oncology* 35, 395–398.

Battles, O.E., Page, D.L. & Johnson, J.E. (1997) Cytokeratins, CEA, and mucin histochemistry in the diagnosis and characterization of extramammary Paget's disease. *American Journal of Clinical Pathology* 108, 6–12.

Beecham, C.T. (1976) Paget's disease of the vulva: recurrence in skin grafts. *Obstetrics and Gynecology* 47, 55s–58s.

Beller, U., Quinn, M.A., Benedet, J.L. *et al.* (2006) Carcinoma of the vulva. *International Journal of Gynecological Obstetrics* 95 (Suppl 1), S7.

Benedet, J.L., Miller, D.M., Ehlen, T.G. & Bertrand, M.A. (1997) Basal cell carcinoma of the vulva: clinical features and treatment results in 28 patients. *Obstetrics and Gynecology* 90, 765–768.

Breen, J.L., Neubecker, R.D., Greenwald, E. & Gregori, C.A. (1975) Basal cell carcinoma of the vulva. *Obstetrics and Gynecology* 46, 122–129.

Bryson, S.C.P., Dembo, A.J., Colgan, T.J. *et al.* (1991) Invasive squamous cell carcinoma of the vulva: defining low and high risk groups

for recurrence. *International Journal of Gynaecological Cancer* 1, 25–31.

Buda, A., Ferrari, L., Marra, C. *et al.* (2008) Vulvar endometriosis in a surgical scar after excision of the Bartholin gland: report of a case. *Archives of Gynecology and Obstetrics* 277, 255–256.

Buhl, A., Landow, S., Lee, Y.C. *et al.* (2001) Microcystic adnexal carcinoma of the vulva. *Gynecologic Oncology* 82, 571–574.

Busam, K.L., Tan, L.K., Granter, S.R. *et al.* (1999) Epidermal growth factor, estrogen, and progesterone receptor expression in primary sweat gland carcinomas and primary and metastatic mammary carcinomas. *Modern Pathology* 12, 786–793.

Cappuccini, F., Tewari Lowell, K.M., Rogers, W. & Disaia, P.J. (1997) Extramammary Paget's disease of the vulva: metastases to the bone marrow in the absence of an underlying adenocarcinoma – case report and literature review. *Gynecologic Oncology* 66, 146–150.

Chafe, W., Richards, A., Morgan, L. & Wilkinson, E.J. (1988) Unrecognized invasive squamous carcinoma in vulvar intraepithelial neoplasia (VIN). *Gynecologic Oncology* 31, 154–165.

Chamlian, D.L. & Taylor, H.B. (1972) Primary carcinoma of Bartholin's gland: a report of 24 patients. *Obstetrics and Gynecology* 39, 489–494.

Chiller, K., Passaro, D., Scheuller, M. *et al.* (2000) Microcystic adnexal carcinoma. Forty eight cases, their treatment, and their outcome. *Archives of Dermatology* 136, 1355–1359.

Cho, D. & Woodruff, J.D. (1988) Trichoepithelioma of the vulva: a report of two cases. *Journal of Reproductive Medicine* 33, 317–319.

Copeland, I.J., Sneige, N., Gershenson, D.M. *et al.* (1986a) Bartholin gland carcinoma. *Obstetrics and Gynecology* 67, 794–802.

Copeland, I.J., Sneige, N., Gershenson, D.M. *et al.* (1986b) Adenoid cystic carcinoma of the Bartholin gland. *Obstetrics and Gynecology* 67, 115–120.

Crawford, D., Nimmo, M., Clement, P.B. *et al.* (1999) Prognostic factors in Paget's disease of the vulva: a study of 21 cases. *International Journal of Gynecological Pathology* 18, 351–359.

Creasman, W.T., Gallager, H.S. & Rutledge, F. (1975) Paget's disease of the vulva. *Gynecologic Oncology* 3, 133–148.

Crum, C.P. (2006) Glandular and other malignancies of the vulva. In: *Diagnostic Gynecologic and Obstetric Pathology* (eds C.P. Crum & K.R. Lee), pp. 149–62. Elsevier, Philadelphia.

Crum, C.P., McLachlin, C.M., Tate, J.E. & Mutter, G. (1997) Pathobiology of vulvar squamous neoplasia. *Current Opinion in Obstetrics and Gynecology* 9, 63–69.

de Cholnoky, T. (1939) Supernumerary breast. *Archives of Surgery* 39, 926–941.

DeConinck, A., Willemsen, M., DeDobbeleer, G. & Roseeuw, D. (1986) Vulvar localization of epidermolytic acanthoma. A light- and electron-microscopic study. *Dermatologica* 172, 276–278.

Dehner, L.P. (1973) Metastatic and secondary tumors of the vulva. *Obstetrics and Gynecology* 42, 47–57.

de Jonge, E.T.M. & Knobel, J. (1988) Recurrent Paget's disease of the vulva after simple vulvectomy and skin grafting: a case report. *South African Medical Journal* 73, 46–47.

de Leon, E.D., Carcangiu, M.L., Prieto, V.G. *et al.* (2000) Extramammary Paget's disease is characterized by the consistent lack of estrogen and progesterone receptors but frequently expresses androgen receptor. *American Journal of Clinical Pathology* 113, 572–575.

Dennefors, B. & Bergman, B. (1980) Primary carcinoma of the Bartholin gland. *Acta Obstetrica et Gynecologica Scandinavica* 59, 95–96.

DiSaia, P.J., Dorion, G.E., Cappuccini, F. & Carpenter, P.M. (1995) A report of two cases of recurrent Paget's disease of the vulva in a split-thickness graft and its possible pathogenesis: labeled 'retrodissemination'. *Gynecologic Oncology* 57, 109–112.

Dodson, M.G., O'Leary, J.A. & Averette, H.E. (1970) Primary carcinoma of Bartholin's gland. *Obstetrics and Gynecology* 35, 578–584.

Dudzinski, M.R., Askin, F.B. & Fowler, W.C. (1984) Giant basal cell carcinoma of the vulva. *Obstetrics and Gynecology* 63, 57s–60s.

Duson, C.K. & Zelenik, J.S. (1954) Vulvar endometriosis apparently produced by menstrual blood. *Obstetrics and Gynecology* 3, 76–79.

Dutta, P. (1987) Vulval endometriosis. *Journal of the Indian Medical Association* 85, 237–238.

Enghardt, M.H., Valente, P.T. & Day, D.H. (1993) Papilloma of Bartholin's gland duct cyst: first report of a case. *International Journal of Gynecological Pathology* 12, 86–92.

Ewing, T., Sawicki, J., Ciaravino, G. & Rumore, G.J. (2004) Microinvasive Paget's disease. *Gynecologic Oncology* 95, 755–758.

Fanning, J., Lambert, H.C.L., Hale, T.M. *et al.* (1999) Paget's disease of the vulva: prevalence of associated vulvar adenocarcinoma, invasive Paget's disease, and recurrence after surgical excision. *American Journal of Obstetrics and Gynecology* 180, 24–27.

Fardal, R.W., Kierland, R.R., Clagett, O.T. *et al.* (1967) Prognosis in cutaneous Paget's disease. *Postgraduate Medicine* 36, 584–593.

Feakins, R.M. & Lowe, D.G. (1997) Basal cell carcinoma of the vulva: a clinicopathologic study of 45 cases. *International Journal of Gynecological Pathology* 16, 319–324.

Fine, B.A., Fowler, L.J., Valente, P.T. & Gaudet, T. (1995) Minimally invasive Paget's disease of the vulva with extensive lymph node metastases. *Gynecologic Oncology* 57, 262–265.

Foster, D.C. (2002) Vulvar disease. *Obstetrics and Gynecology* 100, 145–163.

Foushee, J.H.S. & Pruitt, A.B. Jr. (1967) Vulvar fibroadenoma of supernumerary mammary gland tissue in vulva. *Obstetrics and Gynecology* 29, 819–823.

Fu, S.F. (2002) *Pathology of the Uterine Cervix, Vagina, and Vulva*, 2nd edn. Philadelphia, WB Saunders.

Fujimoto, A., Takata, M., Hatta, N. *et al.* (2000) Expression of structurally unaltered androgen receptor in extramammary Paget's disease. *Laboratory Investigation* 80, 1465–1471.

Fukuma, K., Inoue, S., Tanaka, N. *et al.* (1986) Eccrine adenocarcinoma of the vulva producing isolated α-subunit of glycoprotein hormones. *Obstetrics and Gynecology* 67, 293–296.

Gadducci, A., De Punzio, C., Facchini, V. *et al.* (1989) The therapy of verrucous carcinoma of the vulva. *European Journal of Gynaecological Oncology* 10, 284–287.

Gallousis, S. (1972) Verrucous carcinoma: report of three vulvar cases and review of the literature. *Obstetrics and Gynecology* 40, 502–507.

Ghamande, S.A., Kasznica, J., Griffiths, C.T. *et al.* (1995) Mucinous adenocarcinoma of the vulva. *Gynecologic Oncology* 57, 117–120.

Gibson, G.E. & Ahmed, I. (2001) Perianal and genital basal cell carcinoma, a clinicopathologic review of 51 cases. *Journal of the American Academy of Dermatology* 45, 68–71.

Goldblum, J.R. & Hart, W.R. (1997) Vulvar Paget's disease: a clinicopathologic and Immunohistochemical study of 19 cases. *American Journal of Surgical Pathology* 21, 1178–1187.

Goldblum, J.R. & Hart, W.R. (1998) Perianal Paget's disease: a histologic and immunohistochemical study of 11 cases with and without associated rectal carcinoma. *American Journal of Surgical Pathology* 22, 170–179.

Grin, A., Colgan, T., Laframboise, S. *et al.* (2008) 'Pagetoid' eccrine carcinoma of the vulva: report of an unusual case with review of the literature. *Journal of Lower Female Tract Disease* 12, 134–139.

Gu, M., Ghafari, S. & Lin, F. (2005) Pap smears of patients with extramammary Paget's disease of the vulva. *Diagnostic Cytopathology* 32, 353–357.

Guldhammer, B. & Nørgaard, T. (1986) The differential diagnosis of intraepidermal malignant lesions using immunohistochemistry. *American Journal of Dermatopathology* 8, 295–301.

Hammerschlag, M.R. (1998) Sexually transmitted diseases in sexually abused children: medical and legal implications. *Sexually Transmitted Infections* 74, 167–174.

Hart, W.R. (1970) Paramesonephric mucinous cysts of the vulva. *American Journal of Obstetrics and Gynecology* 107, 1079–1084.

Hart, W.R. (2001) Vulvar intraepithelial neoplasia: historical aspects and current status. *International Journal of Gynecological Pathology* 20, 16–30.

Hassim, A.M. (1969) Bilateral fibroadenoma in supernumerary breasts of the vulva. *Journal of Obstetrics and Gynaecology of the British Commonwealth* 76, 275–277.

Helwig, E.B. & Graham, J.H. (1963) Anogenital (extramammary) Paget's disease: a clinicopathologic study. *Cancer* 16, 387–403.

Hierro, I., Blanes, A., Matilla, A. *et al.* (2000) Merkel cell (neuroendocrine) carcinoma of the vulva. A case report with immunohistochemical and ultrastructural findings and review of the literature. *Pathology Research and Practice* 196, 503–509.

Hillemans, P., Wang, X., Staehle, S. *et al.* (2006) Evaluation of different treatment modalities for vulva intraepithelial neoplasia (VIN): CO_2 laser vaporization, photodynamic therapy, excision and vulvectomy. *Gynecologic Oncology* 100, 271–275.

Huang, Y.H., Chuand, Y.H., Kuo, T.T., *et al.* (2003) Vulvar syringoma: a clinicopathologic study and immunohistologic study of 18 patients and results of treatment. *Journal of the American Academy of Dermatology* 48, 735–739.

Husseinzadeh, N. & Recinto, C. (1999) Frequency of invasive carcinoma in surgically vulvar lesions with intraepithelial neoplasia (VIN 3). *Gynecologic Oncology* 73, 119–120.

Japaze, H., Dinh, T.V. & Woodruff, J.D. (1982) Verrucous carcinoma of the vulva: a study of 24 cases. *Obstetrics and Gynecology* 60, 462–466.

Jones, R.W. & Rowan, D.M. (2000) Spontaneous regression of vulvar intraepithelial neoplasia 2–3. *Obstetrics and Gynecology* 96, 470–472.

Joura, E.A., Leodolter, S., Hernandez-Avila, M. *et al.* (2007) Efficacy of a quadrivalent prophylactic human papillomavirus (types 6,11,16 and 18) L1 virus-like-particle vaccine against high-grade vulva and vaginal lesions: a combined analysis of three randomized clinical trials. *Lancet* 369, 1693–1702.

Junaid, T.A. & Thomas, S.M. (1981) Cysts of the vulva and vagina: a comparative study. *International Journal of Obstetrics and Gynaecology* 19, 239–243.

Karakov, D.V., Suster, S., LeBoit, P.E. *et al.* (2005) Mucinous carcinoma of the skin, primary, and secondary. A clinicopathologic study of 63 cases with emphasis on the morphologic spectrum of primary cutaneous forms: homologies with mucinous carcinomas of the breast. *American Journal of Surgical Pathology* 29, 764–782.

Kennedy, J.C. & Majmudar, B. (1993) Primary adenocarcinoma of the vulva, possibly cloacogenic: a report of two cases. *Journal of Reproductive Medicine* 38, 113–116.

Kennedy, D.A., Hermina, M.S., Xanos, E.T. *et al.* (1997) Infiltrating ductal carcinoma of the vulva. *Pathology Research Practice* **193**, 723–726.

Kikuchi, A., Amagai, M., Hayakawa, K. *et al.* (1990) Association of EGF receptor expression with proliferating cells and of ras p21 expression with differentiating cells in various skin tumors. *British Journal of Dermatology* **123**, 49–58.

Kodama, S., Kaneko, T., Saito, M. *et al.* (1995) A clinicopathologic study of 30 patients with Paget's disease of the vulva. *Gynecologic Oncology* **56**, 63–70.

Koenig, C. & Tavassoli, F.A. (1998) Nodular hyperplasia, adenoma, and adenomyoma of Bartholin's gland. *International Journal of Gynecological Pathology* **17**, 289–294.

Kohler, S. & Smoller, B.R. (1996) Gross cystic disease fluid protein-15 reactivity in extramammary Paget's disease with and without associated internal malignancy. *American Journal of Dermatopathology* **18**, 118–123.

Konishi, I., Fujii, S., Kariya, M. & Mori, T. (1985) Papillary hidradenoma: a light and electron microscopic study of papillary hidradenoma of the vulva. *Acta Obstetrics and Gynecology Japan* **37**, 187–192.

Koss, L.G., Ladinsky, S. & Brockunier, A. Jr. (1968) Paget's disease of the vulva: report of 10 cases. *Obstetrics and Gynecology* **31**, 513–525.

Kraus, F.T. & Perez-Mesa, C. (1966) Verrucous carcinoma: a clinical pathologic study of 105 cases involving oral cavity, larynx and genitalia. *Cancer* **19**, 26–38.

Kuan, S.-F., Montag, A.G., Hart, J. *et al.* (2001) Differential expression of mucin genes in mammary and extramammary Paget's disease. *American Journal of Surgical Pathology* **25**, 1469–1477.

Kurman, R.J., Toki, T. & Schiffman, M.H. (1993) Basaloid and warty carcinomas of the vulva: distinctive types squamous cell carcinoma frequently associated with human papillomavirus. *American Journal of Surgical Pathology* **17**, 133–145.

Lavazzo, C., Pitsouni, E., Athanasiou, S. & Falagas, M.E. (2008). Imiquimod for treatment of vulvar and vaginal intraepithelial neoplasia. *International Journal of Gynecology and Obstetrics* **101**, 3–10.

Leibowitch, M., Neill, S., Pelisse, M. & Moyal-Barracco, M. (1990) The epithelial changes associated with squamous cell carcinoma of the vulva: a review of the clinical, histological, and viral findings in 78 women. *British Journal of Obstetrics and Gynaecology* **97**, 1135–1139.

Lelle, R.J., Davis, K.P. & Roberts, J.A. (1994) Adenoid cystic carcinoma of Bartholin's gland: the University of Michigan experience. *International Journal of Gynecological Cancer* **4**, 145–149.

Leuchter, R.S., Hacker, N.F., Voet, R.I. *et al.* (1982) Primary carcinoma of Bartholin's: a report of 14 cases and a review of the literature. *Obstetrics and Gynecology* **60**, 361–367.

Logani, S., Lu, D., Quint, W.G.V. *et al.* (2003) Low grade vulvar and vaginal intraepithelial neoplasia: correlation of histologic features with human papillomavirus detection and MIB-1 immunostaining. *Modern Pathology* **16**, 735–741.

Lucas, W.E., Benirschke, K. & Lebhertz, T.B. (1974) Verrucous carcinoma of the female genital tract. *American Journal of Obstetrics and Gynecology* **119**, 435–440.

Lundquist, K., Kohler, S. & Touse, R.V. (1999) Intraepidermal cytokeratin 7 expression is not restricted to Paget cells but is also seen in Toker cells and Merkel cells. *American Journal of Surgical Pathology* **23**, 212–219.

Massad, L.S., Bitterman, P. & Clarke-Pearson, D.L. (1996) Metastatic clear cell eccrine hidradenocarcinoma of the vulva: survival after primary excision. *Gynecologic Oncology* **61**, 287–290.

Mazoujian, G. & Margolis, R. (1988) Immunohistochemistry of gross cystic disease fluid protein (GCDFP-15) in 65 benign sweat gland tumors of the skin. *American Journal of Dermatopathology* **10**, 28–35.

Mazur, M.T., Hsueh, S. & Gersell, D.J. (1984) Metastases to the female genital tract: analysis of 325 cases. *Cancer* **53**, 1978–1984.

McKee, P.H. & Hertogs, K.T. (1980) Endocervical adenocarcinoma and vulval Paget's disease: a significant association. *British Journal of Dermatology* **103**, 443–448.

McLachlin, C.M., Kozakewich, H., Craighill, M. *et al.* (1994) Histologic correlates of vulvar human papillomavirus infection in children and young adults. *American Journal of Surgical Pathology* **18**, 728–735.

Meeker, J.H., Neubecker, R.D. & Helwig, E.B. (1962) Hidradenoma papilliferum. *American Journal of Clinical Pathology* **37**, 182–195.

Messing, M.J., Richardson, M.S., Smith, M.T. *et al.* (1993) Metastatic clear-cell hidradenocarcinoma of the vulva. *Gynecologic Oncology* **48**, 264–268.

Micheletti, L., Barbero, M., Preti, M. *et al.* (1994) Vulvar intraepithelial neoplasia of low grade: a challenging diagnosis. *European Journal of Gynecologic Oncology* **15**, 70–74.

Misas, J.E., Larson, J.E., Podczaski, E. *et al.* (1990) Recurrent Paget's disease of the vulva in a split-thickness graft. *Obstetrics and Gynecology* **76**, 543–544.

Mulayim, N., Foster, S.D., Tolgay, O.I. & Babalola, E. (2002) Vulvar basal carcinoma: two unusual presentations and review of the literature. *Gynecologic Oncology* **85**, 532–537.

Nadji, M. & Ganjei, P. (1987) The application of immunoperoxidase techniques in the evaluation of vulvar and vaginal disease. In: *Pathology of the Vulva and Vagina* (ed. E.J. Wilkinson), pp. 239–248. Churchill Livingstone, New York.

Nadji, M., Azorides, M.R., Girtanner, R.E. *et al.* (1982) Paget's disease of the skin: a unifying concept of histogenesis. *Cancer* **50**, 2203–2206.

Nakamura, G., Shikata, N., Shoji, T. *et al.* (1995) Immunohistochemical study of mammary and extramammary Paget's disease. *Anticancer Research* **15**, 467–470.

Neto, A.G., Deavers, M.T., Silva, E.G. & Malpica, A. (2003) Metastatic tumors of the vulva: a clinicopathologic study of 66 cases. *American Journal of Surgical Pathology* **27**, 799–804.

Nowak, M.A., Guerriere-Kovach, P., Pathan, A. *et al.* (1998) Perianal Paget's disease: distinguishing primary and secondary lesions using immunohistochemical studies including gross cystic disease fluid protein-15 and cytokeratin 20 expression. *Archives of Pathology and Laboratory Medicine* **122**, 1077–1081.

Nucci, M.R., Young, R.H. & Fletcher, C.D.M. (2000) Cellular pseudosarcomatous fibroepithelial stromal polyps of the lower female genital tract: an under recognized lesion often misdiagnosed as sarcoma. *American Journal of Surgical Pathology* **24**, 231–240.

Offidani, A. & Campanati, A. (1999) Papillary hidradenoma: immunohistochemical analysis of steroid receptor profile with a focus on apocrine differentiation. *Journal of Clinical Pathology* **52**, 829–832.

Ohira, K., Itoh, K., Osada, K. *et al.* (2004) Vulvar Paget's disease with underlying adenocarcinoma simulating breast carcinoma: case report and review of the literature. *International Journal of Gynecological Cancer* **14**, 1012–1017.

Ohnishi, T. & Watanabe, S. (2000) The use of cytokeratins 7 and 20 in the diagnosis of primary and secondary extramammary Paget's disease. *British Journal of Dermatology* **142**, 243–247.

Oi, R.H. & Munn, R. (1982) Mucous cysts of the vulvar vestibule. *Human Pathology* **13**, 584–586.

Okagaki, T., Clark, B.A., Sachow, K.R. *et al.* (1984) Presence of human papillomavirus in verrucous carcinoma (Ackerman) of the vagina. Immunocytochemical, ultrastructural and DNA hybridization studies. *Archives of Pathology and Laboratory Medicine* **108**, 567–570.

Ordónèz, N.G., Awalt, H. & Mackay, B. (1987) Mammary and extramammary Paget's disease: an immunocytochemical and ultrastructural Study. *Cancer* **59**, 1173–1183.

Parker, L.P., Parker, J.R., Bodurka-Bevers, D. *et al.* (2000) Paget's disease of the vulva: pathology, pattern of involvement, and prognosis. *Gynecologic Oncology* **77**, 183–189.

Perrone, T., Twiggs, L.B., Adcock, L.I. & Dehner, L.P. (1987) Vulvar basal cell carcinoma: an infrequently metastasizing neoplasm. *International Journal of Gynecological Pathology* **6**, 152–165.

Pilotti, S., Dhongi, R., D'Amato, I. *et al.* (1996) Papillomavirus, p53 alteration and primary carcinoma of the vulva. *European Journal of Cancer* **29**, 924–925.

Pope, C., Ingella, H.P. & Strecker, H. (1973) Light and electron microscopic observations following repeated podophyllin benzoin therapy of condyloma acuminata. *Archives of Gynecology* **215**, 417–425.

Purola, E. & Widholm, O. (1966) Primary carcinoma of Bartholin's gland. *Acta Obstetrica et Gynecologica Scandinavica* **45**, 205–210.

Quinn, T.R. & Young, R.H. (1997) Epidermolytic hyperkeratosis in the lower female genital tract: an uncommon stimulant of mucocutaneous papillomavirus infection – a report of two cases. *International Journal of Gynaecology Pathology* **16**, 163–168.

Rahilly, M.A., Beattie, G.J. & Lessells, A.M. (1995) Mucinous eccrine carcinoma of the vulva with neuroendocrine differentiation. *Histopathology* **27**, 82–86.

Ratskar, G., Okagaki, T., Twiggs, L.B. & Clark, B.A. (1982) Early invasive and in situ warty carcinoma of the vulva: clinical, histologic and electron microscopic study with particular reference to viral association. *American Journal of Obstetrics and Gynecology* **143**, 814–820.

Regauer, S. (2006) Extramammary Paget's disease: a proliferation of adnexal origin? *Histopathology* **48**, 341–346.

Rhatigan, R.M. & Nuss, C.R. (1985) Keratoacanthoma of the vulva. *Gynecology Oncology* **21**, 118–123.

Robboy, S.J., Ross, J.S., Prat, J. *et al.* (1978) Urogenital origin of mucinous and ciliated cysts of the vulva. *Obstetrics and Gynecology* **51**, 347–351.

Santa Cruz, D.J. & Martin, S.A. (1979) Verruciform xanthoma of the vulva. *American Journal of Clinical Pathology* **71**, 224–228.

Santos, L.D., Kennerson, A.R. & Killingsworth, M.C. (2006) Nodular hyperplasia of Bartholin's gland. *Pathology* **38**, 223–228.

Sedlis, A., Homesley, H., Bundy, B.N. *et al.* (1987) Positive groin lymph nodes in superficial squamous cell vulvar carcinoma: a Gynecologic Oncology Group study. *American Journal of Gynecology and Obstetrics* **156**, 1159–1164.

Sideri, M., Jones, R.W., Wilkinson, E.J. *et al.* (2005) Squamous vulvar intra-epithelial neoplasia: 2004 modified terminology, ISSVD Vulvar Oncology Sub-committee. *Journal of Reproductive Medicine* **50**; 807–810.

Sillman, F.H., Sentowich, S. & Shaffer, D. (1997) Ano-genital neoplasia in renal transplant patients. *Annals of Transplantation* **2**, 59–66.

Smith, K.J., Tuur, S., Corvette, D. *et al.* (1997) Cytokeratin 7 staining in mammary and extramammary Paget's disease. *Modern Pathology* **10**, 1069–1074.

Spiegel, G.W.(2002) Eosinophils as a marker for invasion in vulvar squamous neoplastic lesions. *International Journal of Gynecological Pathology* **21**, 108–116.

Stehman, F.B., Castaloo, T.W., Charles, E.H. & Lagasse, L. (1980) Verrucous carcinoma of the vulva. *International Journal of Obstetrics and Gynecology* **17**, 523–525.

Tebes, S., Cardosi, R. & Hoffman, M. (2002) Paget's disease of the vulva. *American Journal of Obstetrics and Gynecology* **187**, 281–284.

Tellechea, O., Reis, J.P., Domingues, J.C. & Baptista, A.P. (1993) Monoclonal antibody Ber EP4 distinguished basal-cell carcinoma from squamous cell carcinoma of the skin. *American Journal of Dermatopathology* **15**, 452–455.

Thomas, J., Majmudar, B. & Gorelkin, I. (1979) Syringoma localized to the vulva. *Archives of Dermatology* **115**, 95–96.

Tiltman, A.J. & Knutzen, V.K. (1978) Primary carcinoma of the vulva originating in misplaced cloacal tissue. *Obstetrics and Gynecology* **51**, 30s–33s.

Toki, T., Kurman, R.J., Park, J.S. *et al.* (1991) Probable nonpapillomavirus etiology of squamous carcinoma of the vulva in older women: a clinicopathologic study using in situ hybridization and polymerase chain reaction. *International Journal of Gynecological Pathology* **10**, 107–125.

Tresserra, F., Grases, P.J., Izquierdo, M. & Caranach, M. (1998) Fibroadenoma phyllodes arising in vulvar supernumerary breast tissue: report of two cases. *International Journal of Gynecological Pathology* **17**, 171–173.

Underwood, J.W., Adcock, L.L. & Okagaki, T. (1978) Adenosquamous carcinoma of the skin appendages (adenoid squamous cell carcinoma, pseudoglandular squamous carcinoma, acanthoma of sweat gland of Lever) of the vulva: a clinicopathologic and ultrastructural study. *Cancer* **42**, 1851–1858.

van Beurden, M., ten Kate, F.J., Smits, H.J. *et al.* (1995) Multifocal VIN 111 and multicentric lower genital tract neoplasia is associated with transcriptionally active HPV. *Cancer* **75**, 2879–2884.

van Beurden, M., de Craen, A.J., de Vet, H.C. *et al.* (1999) The contribution of MIB 1 in the accurate grading of vulvar intraepithelial neoplasia. *Journal of Clinical Pathology* **52**, 820–824.

van der Putte, S.C.J. (1994) Mammary-like glands of the vulva and their disorders. *International Journal of Gynecological Pathology* **13**, 150–160.

van der Putte, S.C.J. & van Gorp, L.H.M. (1994) Adenocarcinoma of the mammary-like glands of the vulva: a concept unifying sweat gland carcinoma of the vulva, carcinoma of supernumerary mammary glands and extramammary Paget's disease. *Journal of Cutaneous Pathology* **21**, 157–163.

van der Putte, S.C.J. & van Gorp, L.H.M. (1995) Cysts of mammary-like glands in the vulva. *International Journal of Gynaecological Pathology* **14**, 184–188.

Van Nagell, J.R. Jr, Tweeddale, D.W. & Roddick, J.W. Jr. (1969) Primary acanthoma of Bartholin's gland: report of a case. *Obstetrics and Gynecology* **34**, 87–90.

van Seters, M., van Beurden, M. & de Craen, A.J.M. (2005). Is the assumed natural history of vulvar intraepithelial neoplasia III based on enough evidence? A systematic review of 3322 published patients. *Gynecologic Oncology* **97**, 545–551.

van Seters, M., ten Kate, F.J., van Beurden, M. *et al.* (2007) In the absence of (early) invasive carcinoma, vulvar intraepithelial neoplasia associated with lichen sclerosus is mainly of undifferentiated type: new insights in histology and aetiology. *Journal of Clinical Pathology* **60**, 504–509.

van Seters, M., van Beurden, M., ten Kate, F.J.W. *et al.* (2008) Treatment of vulvar intraepithelial neoplasia with topical imiquimod. *New England Journal of Medicine* **358**, 1465–1473.

Vayrynen, M., Romppanen, T., Koskela, E. *et al.* (1981) Verrucous squamous cell carcinoma of the female genital tract: report of three cases and survey of the literature. *International Journal of Obstetrics and Gynecology* **19**, 351–356.

Wade, T.R. & Ackerman, A.B. (1984) The effects of resin of podophyllin on condyloma acuminatum. *American Journal of Dermatopathology* **6**, 109–122.

Wahlstrom, T., Vesterinen, E. & Saksela, E. (1978) Primary carcinoma of Bartholin's glands: a morphological and clinical study of six cases including a transitional cell carcinoma. *Gynecologic Oncology* **6**, 354–362.

Wang, L.C., Blanchard, A., Judge, D.E. *et al.* (2003) Successful treatment of recurrent extramammary Paget's disease of the vulva with topical imiquimod 5% cream. *Journal of the American Academy of Dermatology* **49**, 769–771.

Wells, M. & Jenkins, M. (1994) Selected topics in the histopathology of the vulva. *Current Diagnostic Pathology* **1**, 41–47.

Wheelock, J.B., Gopelrud, D.R., Dunn, I.T. & Oates, J.F. (1984) Primary carcinoma of the Bartholin gland: a report of two cases. *Obstetrics and Gynecology* **63**, 820–824.

Wick, M.R., Goellner, J.R., Wolfe, J.T. III & Su, W.P.D. (1985) Adnexal carcinomas of the skin. I. Eccrine carcinomas. *Cancer* **56**, 1147–1162.

Wilkinson, E.J., Rico, M.J. & Pierson, K.K.(1982) Microinvasive carcinoma of the vulva. *International Journal of Gynecological Pathology* **1**, 29–39.

Wilkinson, E.J., Guerrero, E., Daniel, R. *et al.* (1993) Vulvar vestibulitis is rarely associated with human papilloma virus infection types 6, 11, 16, or 18. *International Journal of Gynecological Pathology* **12**, 344–349.

Williams, S.L., Rogers, L.W. & Quan, S.H.Q. (1976) Perianal Paget's disease: report of seven cases. *Diseases of the Colon and Rectum* **19**, 30–40.

Wolber, R.A., Dupuis, B.A. & Wick, M.R. (1991) Expression of C-erb-2 oncoprotein in mammary & extramammary Paget's disease. *American Journal of Clinical Pathology* **96**, 243–247.

Woodruff, H. Jr, Dockerty, M.B., Wilson, R.B. & Pratt, J.H. (1971) Papillary hidradenoma of the vulva: a clinicopathologic study of 69 cases. *American Journal of Obstetrics and Gynecology* **110**, 501–508.

Yang, B. & Hart, W.R. (2000) Vulvar intraepithelial neoplasia of the simplex (differentiated) type: a clinicopathological study including analysis of HPV and p53 expression. *American Journal of Surgical Pathology* **24**, 429–441.

Young, A.W. Jr, Herman, E.W. & Torelli, H.M.M.(1980) Syringoma of the vulva; incidence, diagnosis and a cause of pruritus. *Obstetrics and Gynecology* **55**, 515–518.

Zollo, J.D. & Zeitouni, N.C. (2000) The Roswell Park Cancer Institute experience with extramammary Paget's disease. *British Journal of Dermatology* **142**, 59–65.

Chapter 9: Non-epithelial tumours of the vulva

E. Calonje & G.W. Spiegel

Mesenchymal neoplasms

Mesenchymal neoplasms of the vulva are extremely uncommon. They present as enlarging, asymptomatic vulval masses, whose clinical appearance can be very misleading. Benign neoplasms, which are often pedunculated, may become ulcerated and secondarily infected, owing to the effects of local moisture and warmth together with friction from tight underclothing. A benign tumour with an ulcerated surface and secondary infection may produce a reactive enlargement of regional lymph nodes and give the false impression of malignancy.

Accurate identification of most benign neoplasms is not difficult on purely histological grounds, but immunohistochemistry is often used to confirm a diagnosis, particularly when dealing with groups of tumours that have overlapping histological features (i.e. cellular angiofibroma and angiomyofibroblastoma). Malignant mesenchymal neoplasms are often difficult to classify accurately on histological grounds alone and, like malignant soft-tissue tumours presenting elsewhere, require not only an immunohistochemical panel but also more sophisticated techniques such as cytogenetic studies. Specific cytogenetic abnormalities have now been identified in a wide variety of soft-tissue tumours and these studies can be performed in paraffin-embedded material.

Tumours of smooth muscle

Leiomyoma

Vulval leiomyomas are relatively uncommon, and fewer than 120 examples have been documented (Lovelady *et al.* 1941, Palermino 1964, Tavassoli & Norris 1979, Newman & Fletcher 1991, Neri *et al.* 1993, Nielsen *et al.* 1996a), although the majority of such neoplasms now pass unre-

corded. There is no known association with uterine leiomyomas and it is far from clear whether these tumours originate from the smooth muscle of the vulval erectile tissue or from the muscular elements of the round ligament; most arise, however, in the labia majora and leiomyomas limited to the clitoris (Stenchever *et al.* 1973) or Bartholin's gland (Tavassoli & Norris 1979, Katenkamp & Stiller 1980) are distinctly rare.

Vulval leiomyomas occur during the reproductive years and have a tendency to enlarge during pregnancy; their size may also increase in women receiving hormonal treatment and these features, together with their content of progesterone and oestrogen receptors, suggest that they are, to some extent at least, hormone dependent (Siegle & Cartmell 1995). Leiomyomas usually present as well-circumscribed, painless, non-tender nodules or swellings in the labia: they are formed of firm, white, whorled tissue. Local recurrence is exceptional (Guven *et al.* 2005).

Histologically, leiomyomas of the vulva are generally similar to their more commonly occurring counterparts in the uterine body. They have, by definition, well-circumscribed, non-infiltrating margins, show little or no pleomorphism or atypia, and contain fewer than two mitotic figures per 10 high-power fields (Fig. 9.1a,b) (Tavassoli & Norris 1979). Cellular (Kaufman & Gardner 1965), epithelioid (Tavassoli & Norris 1979, Aneiros *et al.* 1982, Newman & Fletcher 1991), symplastic, myxoid (Zhou *et al.* 2006) and neurolemmoma-like variants can all occur at the vulva. It has been suggested that myxoid change is more common in younger women and during pregnancy (Kajiwara *et al.* 2002). The histological criteria, discussed below, for recognizing those vulval smooth-muscle neoplasms that are likely to behave as low-grade leiomyosarcomas are far from absolute (Williams *et al.* 2002). Hence, all tumours require complete local excision and those clearly malignant should be treated with wide local excision (see below).

Leiomyosarcoma

Malignant smooth-muscle neoplasms of the vulva take two forms. One is that of a clearly sarcomatous tumour with

Ridley's The Vulva, 3rd edition. Edited by Sallie M. Neill and Fiona M. Lewis. © 2009 Blackwell Publishing, ISBN: 978-1-4051-6813-7.

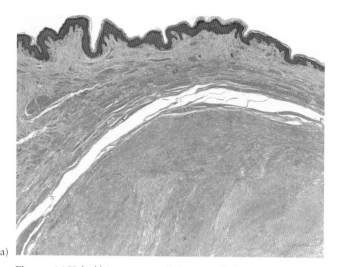

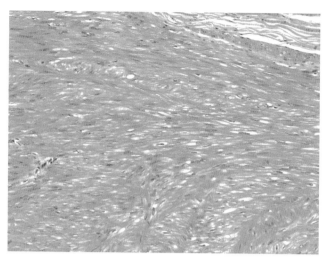

Fig. 9.1 (a) Vulval leiomyoma: well-circumscribed tumour. (b) Vulval leiomyoma: notice bundles of mature smooth muscle.

considerable pleomorphism and mitotic activity while the other closely resembles a leiomyoma but nevertheless behaves in a malignant fashion. The clearly malignant neoplasms may or may not be easily recognizable as being of smooth-muscle origin and in doubtful cases a positive staining reaction for smooth-muscle actin, desmin and H-caldesmon is of considerable diagnostic value.

Leiomyosarcomas of the vulva, showing unmistakable histological evidence of malignancy, are rare (DiSaia *et al.* 1971, Pandhi *et al.* 1975, Audet-Lapointe *et al.* 1980, Guidozzi *et al.* 1987, Lenaz *et al.* 1987, Krag-Moller *et al.* 1990, Kuller *et al.* 1990, Patel *et al.* 1993, Nirenberg *et al.* 1995). These tumours have occurred in women aged from 35 to 84 years, although the mean age at initial presentation was just over 50 years. The history of an enlarging mass is usually less than 12 months and most leiomyosarcomas arise in the labia. Lesions may grow rapidly during pregnancy (Di Gilio *et al.* 2004). In most reported cases initial treatment was by local excision and the true diagnosis was recognized only on histological examination; nearly all patients treated solely by local excision alone have tumour recurrence. Other patients have been treated by radical surgery, often supplemented by radiotherapy or chemotherapy, and about 50% of such patients have died, the length of survival ranging from 6 months to 16 years and death being usually due to pulmonary, hepatic or skeletal metastases.

All the tumours discussed so far are clearly malignant and can be regarded as leiomyosarcomas of high-grade malignancy. Tavassoli and Norris (1979) looked at the question of malignancy in vulval smooth-muscle neoplasms from a quite different viewpoint. They studied 32 vulval neoplasms that were quite clearly of smooth-muscle nature,

and attempted to define criteria for the recognition of those neoplasms which, although not having any obvious potential for metastasis, would tend nevertheless to behave as low-grade leiomyosarcomas and recur locally after initial resection. They concluded that those neoplasms measuring more than 5 cm in diameter, having infiltrating margins and containing more than five mitotic figures per 10 high-power fields are very likely to recur. Furthermore, tumours showing all these three features should be regarded as leiomyosarcomas, irrespective of the degree of cellular atypia. They considered that neoplasms showing any two of these features should be regarded as low-grade leiomyosarcomas.

Nielsen *et al.* (1996a) generally agreed with these criteria but considered the rate of mitotic activity as equal to or more than five per 10 high power fields and added a fourth criterion, namely moderate to severe cytological atypia. They considered that if a tumour had three of the four criteria it should be regarded as a leiomyosarcoma. If only one of these criteria was present the neoplasm should be regarded as a leiomyoma whereas if two were noted the tumour should be classed as an atypical leiomyoma. They considered that both leiomyomas and atypical leiomyomas should be excised conservatively while neoplasms classed by their criteria as leiomyosarcomas should be excised with wide negative margins. Smooth-muscle tumours of the vulva can, however, recur in the absence of all the morphological features suggestive of aggressive behaviour and all leiomyomatous neoplasms should therefore be treated by complete local excision.

A few myxoid leiomyosarcomas of the vulva have been recorded (Salm & Evans 1985, Tjalma & Colpaert 2005), although this is not a particular site of predilection for such neoplasms.

Tumours of striated muscle

Rhabdomyoma

Vulvovaginal rhabdomyomas are well recognized, although there is some dispute as to whether these are a form of fetal rhabdomyoma or represent a specific and discrete entity of genital rhabdomyoma. Most occur in the vagina and only two have arisen at the vulva (Di Sant Agnese & Knowles 1980); one was an incidentally discovered nodule in a 24 year old woman and the other patient presented with a nodule of 3 years' duration in an episiotomy scar. These benign neoplasms, if indeed they are neoplasms rather than hamartomas or examples of reactive hyperplasia, are formed of relatively mature elongated spindle-shaped or strap-like rhabdomyoblasts with distinct cross-striations; these cells are separated from each other by varying amounts of myxoid stroma and collagen and stain positively for desmin, myogenin and MyoD1.

Rhabdomyosarcoma

Three forms of rhabdomyosarcoma are recognized: embryonic, alveolar and pleomorphic. The first two occur principally in children and young adults and the last mainly in adults. Desmin and muscle actin expression serve as markers for rhabdomyosarcomas whereas immunocytochemical demonstration of the *MyoD1* gene product and myogenin are highly specific for striated muscle differentiation (Wesche *et al.* 1995).

Embryonic rhabdomyosarcomas tend to form oedematous polypoidal masses and usually have a myxoid stroma in which pleomorphic spindle-shaped or rounded cells are characteristically widely scattered. Two such neoplasms of the vulva in young children have been reported (James *et al.* 1969, Talerman 1973), although the diagnosis in both cases was not proven. A case of the spindle cell variant of embryonic rhabdomyosarcoma has been reported in an adult woman in a series of cases occurring in adults (Nascimento & Fletcher 2005). In this series, it was suggested that this variant of rhabdomyosarcoma has a more aggressive behaviour than the infantile counterpart.

Alveolar rhabdomyosarcomas are formed principally of rounded cells that are separated into nodules by fibrous septa; central necrosis within these lobules imparts an alveolar pattern to the tumour. Few cases of alveolar rhabdomyosarcoma of the vulva have been reported (Copeland *et al.* 1985, Imachi *et al.* 1991, Bond *et al.* 1994, Ferguson *et al.* 2007), one being confined to the clitoris. Most cases presented in patients aged between 4 and 17 years and rare cases have been diagnosed in adult women. The prognosis is similar to that of alveolar rhabdomyosarcoma presenting elsewhere. It seems that tumours in adults are more aggressive.

Pleomorphic rhabdomyosarcoma is exceptional in the vulva and only one case has been reported (Haroun *et al.* 2007).

Fibroblastic tumours

Prepubertal vulval fibroma

This is a distinctive, rare, recently described lesion that presents as an asymptomatic, slowly growing lesion on the vulva, particularly on the labia majora of prepubertal girls between the ages of 4 and 12 (Iwata & Fletcher 2004). Tumours are submucosal or subcutaneous, infiltrate the subcutaneous tissue and are characterized histologically by a poorly circumscribed, hypocellular mass characterized by myxoid, oedematous or, more frequently, collagenous stroma. Tumour cells are bland and spindle shaped and may stain for CD34. Local recurrence is occasionally seen.

Desmoid tumour

Desmoid tumours are forms of local fibromatosis and, although histologically bland, they can attain a large size, infiltrate neighbouring tissues and recur. They are formed of elongated, slender, spindle-shaped cells, which are separated from each other by abundant collagen. Three cases of desmoid tumour of the vulva have been recorded (Kfuri *et al.* 1981, Allen & Novotny 1997, Ergeneli *et al.* 1999), one of which occurred during pregnancy.

Dermatofibrosarcoma protuberans

Doubt has existed as to the histogenesis and nature of this tumour and it has been classified under the rubric of fibrohistiocytic tumours. It is, however, best considered as a fibroblastic neoplasm of intermediate (low grade) malignancy (Brooks 1994). Only a few cases have been recorded affecting the vulva (Davos & Abell 1976, Soltan 1981, Bock *et al.* 1985, Ghorbani *et al.* 1999, Gökden *et al.* 2003). These tumours have occurred in both pre- and postmenopausal women and usually present as slow-growing, painless, non-tender, mobile lumps, most commonly in the labia majora. They may measure anything up to 8 cm in diameter. The overlying skin may be ulcerated. Histologically (Fig. 9.2a,b), the tumour is infiltrative and formed of plump fibroblastic cells arranged in a distinctly storiform pattern; there is little pleomorphism and mitotic figures are sparse. All patients with vulval dermatofibrosarcoma protuberans have been treated initially by wide local excision, but recurrence occurred, often after a prolonged time interval, in nearly 50% of cases; this sometimes necessitated more radical surgery. There has been one reported instance of metastasis (Soergel *et al.* 1998) but no tumour-related deaths have been recorded. Fibrosarcomatous change was noted in two neoplasms (Leake *et al.* 1991, Ghorbani *et al.* 1999). Cytogenetic studies of dermatofibrosarcoma protuberans typically show a ring chromosome indicative of a 17;22 translocation, an abnormality also found in giant cell fibroblastoma demonstrating that both tumours are part of the same spectrum (Vanni *et al.* 2000, Gökden *et al.* 2003).

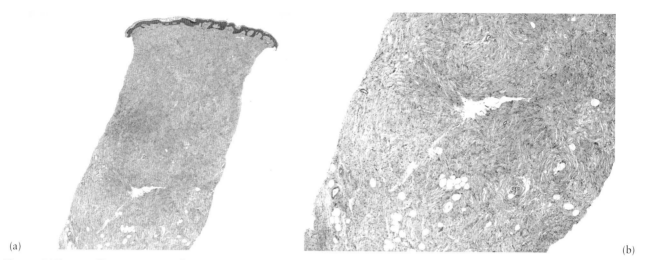

(a)

(b)

Fig. 9.2 (a) Dermatofibrosarcoma protuberans with extensive replacement of the dermis and subcutis. (b) The tumour has infiltrated the subcutaneous tissue in a lace-like pattern.

Only one case of dermatofibrosarcoma protuberans with a giant cell fibroblastoma has been reported in the vulva (Kholová *et al.* 2001). Rare cases demonstrate a variant ring chromosome with cryptic rearrangements of chromosomes 17 and 22. This chromosomal translocation results in an abnormal fusion transcript and involves the collagen type I alpha 1 (*COL1A1*) gene on chromosome 17 and the platelet-derived growth factor B (PDGFB) gene on chromosome 22. This results in autocrine stimulation of PDGFB and platelet-derived growth factor receptor beta (PDGFRB) leading proliferation. Based on this finding imatinib mesylate, a potent inhibitor of a number of protein kinases including the platelet-derived growth factor receptor, has been used with variable success in large unresectable tumours or in those that metastasize.

Fibrosarcoma

The diagnosis of a fibrosarcoma is essentially one of exclusion and it is likely that most, if not all, cases diagnosed as pure fibrosarcomas are examples of other tumours that often have a fibrosarcoma-like growth pattern including synovial sarcoma and malignant peripheral nerve sheath tumour. This has become apparent not only with the use of wide immunohistochemical panels but also with additional techniques such as cytogenetics. Only a few vulval fibrosarcomas have been described (Keller 1951, Woodruff & Brack 1958, DiSaia *et al.* 1971, Davos & Abell 1976, Hall & Amin 1981, Nirenberg *et al.* 1995) and it is far from certain that all these would currently be acceptable as true fibrosarcomas.

Fibrohistiocytic tumours

The concept of fibrohistiocytic tumours has recently undergone considerable criticism and it is widely conceded that none of the neoplasms in this category show true histiocytic differentiation, the term 'fibrohistiocytic' being a misnomer and bringing together a group of heterogeneous lesions, many of which are probably unrelated (Fletcher 1995). Nevertheless, 'fibrohistiocytic' neoplasms will probably continue to be described as such until their true nature is determined.

Dermatofibroma

Vulval dermatofibromas are very rare and similar to lesions occurring elsewhere in the body. They usually occur on the labia majora, are often pedunculated or pendulous, may be superficially ulcerated and can attain a very large size.

Malignant fibrous histiocytoma

Malignant fibrous histiocytoma is a controversial entity which is more likely to represent a 'wastepaper basket' diagnosis, neoplasms classed as such being, in reality, either pleomorphic variants of liposarcoma, leiomyosarcoma or rhabdomyosarcoma, or, in some cases, pleomorphic spindle-cell carcinomas or melanomas (Fletcher 1995). Some authors, while maintaining that malignant fibrous histiocytoma is a distinct entity, albeit of unknown origin, consider the tumour to be greatly overdiagnosed (Brooks 1994). We believe that the group of pleomorphic sarcomas that cannot be classified more accurately should be regarded as high-grade pleomorphic sarcomas rather than as malignant fibrous histiocytomas.

It is not possible to accurately categorize and classify the few examples of vulval malignant fibrous histiocytoma recorded so far in the literature (Davos & Abell 1976, Taylor *et al.* 1985, Santala *et al.* 1987, Elchalal *et al.* 1991, Nirenberg *et al.* 1995). Therefore, they will not be discussed further in this chapter.

Myofibroblastic tumours

Postoperative spindle cell nodule

These, as their name implies, develop within weeks or months of an operative procedure on the vulva and present as a rapidly growing mass (Proppe *et al.* 1984, Manson *et al.* 1995, Micci *et al.* 2007). Histologically, they resemble a fibrosarcoma with sheets of spindle-shaped cells growing in a fascicular pattern and containing many mitotic figures. Despite their alarming appearances these nodules are a form of reactive response to tissue injury and will eventually resolve.

Nodular fasciitis

Only 10 cases of nodular fasciitis of the vulva have been fully documented (Roberts & Daly 1981, Gaffney *et al.* 1982, LiVolsi & Brooks 1987a, O'Connell *et al.* 1997), whereas one case has been briefly alluded to in a review of this lesion (Allen 1972).

The patients with vulval nodular fasciitis have ranged in age from 7 to 51 years, have presented with a short history of a vulval mass and have had mobile subcutaneous nodules that measured 1.5–3.5 cm in diameter. The lesions had the typical histological features of plump fibroblasts arranged in bundles and fascicles set in a myxoid stroma with a mild or moderate lymphocytic infiltrate, intercellular clefts, numerous small blood vessels and a generous sprinkling of mitotic figures; multinucleated osteoclast-like cells may be present. Wide local excision was curative in all cases but there was a local recurrence in one patient in whom excision had been incomplete.

Angiomyofibroblastoma

These neoplasms have a marked predilection for the vulval soft tissues (Fletcher *et al.* 1992, Katenkamp *et al.* 1993, Hisaoka *et al.* 1995, Toti *et al.* 1995, Nielsen *et al.* 1996b). There is some degree of overlap with another recently described entity, cellular angiofibroma, and with aggressive angiomyxoma (see below) (Granter *et al.* 1997, Alameda *et al.* 2006). The patients' ages ranged from 25 to 54 years and they presented with an otherwise asymptomatic vulval mass, nearly always in the labium majus, which had been present for periods ranging from 10 weeks to 8 years. These tumours are well circumscribed, range from 0.5 to 12 cm in diameter and have a partially myxoid appearance on section. Histologically, they are characterized by alternating hypercellular and hypocellular oedematous zones in which abundant blood vessels, predominantly of capillary type, are irregularly distributed (Fig. 9.3). Spindled, plump spindled and oval stromal cells are aggregated around the blood vessels, sometimes forming solid compact foci, or are loosely dispersed in the hypocellular areas: binucleate or multinucleate cells may be present. There is an admixture of

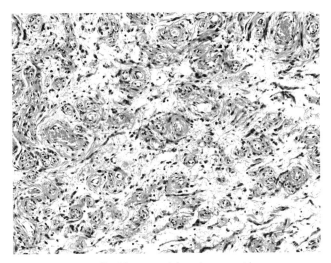

Fig. 9.3 Angiomyofibroblastoma of the vulva: myxoid stroma, numerous small blood vessels and elongated, plump, spindle-shaped cells.

collagen, either as thin wavy strands or as thick bundles. Mitotic figures are exceptional (Takeshima *et al.* 1998) and collections of mature adipocytes may rarely be seen (Laskin *et al.* 1997). The stromal cells stain positively for desmin and oestrogen and progesterone receptors but are negative for cytokeratins and S-100 and are only focally positive or entirely negative for actin and muscle-specific actin. Rare tumours may be positive for CD34.

These tumours are benign but one malignant example has been reported (Nielsen *et al.* 1997). They are cured by local excision. They can, however, be very easily confused with an aggressive angiomyxoma: points of distinction from an aggressive angiomyxoma include the circumscribed borders, greater cellularity, absence of vessels with thick or hyalinized walls, presence of plump stromal cells and the lack of extravasation of erythrocytes. It had previously been thought that positive staining of the stromal cells for desmin was also a distinguishing feature, but it is now recognized that this is not the case (Granter *et al.* 1997).

Cellular angiofibroma

Cellular angiofibroma is a distinctive, relatively rare, benign neoplasm that occurs almost exclusively in the vulva (Nucci *et al.* 1997, Curry *et al.* 2001, Lane *et al.* 2001) and less commonly in the scrotum and inguinal soft tissues of men. In the vulva most cases occur in the labium majus and rarely in the clitoris (Dargent *et al.* 2003). Some cases overlap histologically with angiomyofibroblastoma and a relationship with spindle cell lipoma has been suggested (Laskin *et al.* 1998). Lesions are small, well-circumscribed, subcutaneous and asymptomatic. Histologically, they are characterized by short, bland, spindle-shaped cells with scanty, ill-defined pale pink cytoplasm. Cellularity varies and in the background

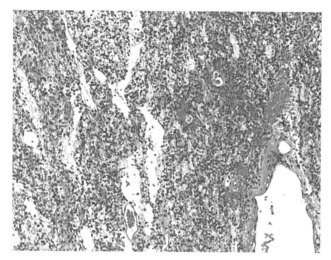

Fig. 9.4 Cellular angiofibroma: rich vascular network and numerous small, bland, somewhat round cells.

there are thin collagen bundles and numerous small- to medium-sized blood vessels (Fig. 9.4). Mitotic figures and cytological atypia are rare. Scattered mononuclear inflammatory cells, mainly lymphocytes, are seen. Degenerative changes are common and consist of haemorrhage, thrombosis, hyalinization and haemosiderin deposition. In myxoid areas, mast cells are present and many tumours contain variable numbers of mature adipocytes. The most consistent immunohistochemical finding is the presence of diffuse positivity for CD34. Muscular markers including actin and desmin tend to be negative but positivity has been reported in male tumours. In a few cases, there is focal positivity for oestrogen and progesterone receptors.

Lesions are benign and local recurrence is exceptional (McCluggage *et al.* 2002). Simple excision is the treatment of choice.

Aggressive angiomyxoma

Although this tumour is not regarded as myofibroblastic but rather as of uncertain histogenesis, it is described here in view of the rare cases that overlap histologically with angiomyofibroblastoma.

These tumours occur in the vulva, perineum and pelvis, most commonly in young patients in their third or fourth decade (Steeper & Rosai 1983, Begin *et al.* 1985, Mandai *et al.* 1990, Elchalal *et al.* 1992, Simo *et al.* 1992, Cheah *et al.* 1993, Skalova *et al.* 1993, Fetsch *et al.* 1996, Granter *et al.* 1997). Occasionally, the tumour may present during pregnancy (Bagga *et al.* 2007). The vulval lesion presents as an enlarging painless mass and the history is usually of only a few months. The neoplasms are nearly always more than 5 cm in diameter, commonly larger than 10 cm and can attain a diameter of 60 cm; they often extend into the pelvis, ischiorectal fossa and retroperitoneum. Some neoplasms are pedunculated. They are smooth, lobulated and, despite their infiltrative nature, may appear deceptively encapsulated; their cut surface has a myxoid appearance. The histological appearance is bland with many blood vessels set in a loose myxoid stroma, which also contains a small population of stellate or thin spindled cells with delicate cytoplasmic processes (Fig. 9.5a,b). The vessels vary in size and frequently some are large with thick muscular or hyalinized walls; others may have an angiomatoid appearance. Extravasation of erythrocytes into the stroma is a frequent finding and there is a variable amount of stromal collagen. Mitotic figures are usually absent. The

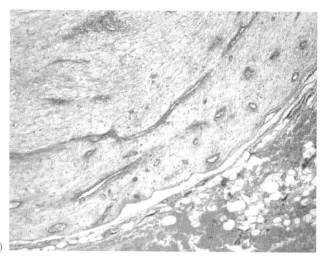

(a)

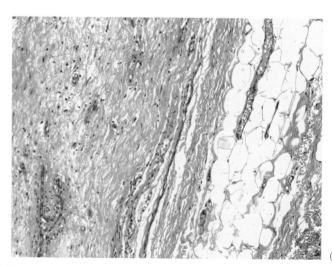

(b)

Fig. 9.5 (a) Aggressive angiomyxoma: hypocellular myxoid lesion in the subcutaneous tissue. (b) Replacement of the fat, and a few bland, spindle-shaped cells in a myxoid stroma.

stromal cells stain positively for vimentin, desmin, smooth-muscle actin and, generally, for oestrogen and progesterone receptors.

The appearances of an aggressive angiomyxoma differ significantly from those of an angiomyofibroblastoma, but Granter et al. (1997) described a few aggressive angiomyxomas that showed a transition, in some areas, to a pattern more characteristic of an angiomyofibroblastoma suggesting a histological spectrum. However, cytogenetic analysis has suggested that, although there is histological overlap in rare cases, both tumours seem to be biologically distinct as in one study about 33% of cases of aggressive angiomyxoma showed rearrangement of the chromatin remodelling gene HMGA2 while no cases of angiomyofibroblastoma or other genital soft-tissue tumours, except for a vaginal leiomyoma, showed rearrangement of this gene (Medeiros et al. 2007). Detection of rearrangement of the HMGA2 gene may be a useful diagnostic test for aggressive angiomyxoma, but this is found in only one-third of cases. The rearrangements of the HMGA2 gene have been described on chromosome 12q15 (Kazmierczak et al. 1995, Nucci et al. 2001). In a single case, a t(5;8)(p15;q22) translocation was described (Tsuji et al. 2007).

Aggressive angiomyxomas infiltrate in such an insidious fashion that complete surgical removal is difficult and recurrences, often repetitive, occur in about 30% of cases, usually within 2 years, although some are delayed for longer periods. Metastases have only rarely been reported (Siassi et al. 1999, Blandamura et al. 2003).

The presence in many of these neoplasms of hormone receptors, and the description of one case in which growth occurred during pregnancy, suggests a possible hormone dependency for at least some aggressive angiomyxomas (Htwe et al. 1995). Some tumours have shown response to gonadotropin-releasing hormone (Fine et al. 2001, McCluggage et al. 2006).

Tumours of fat

Lipoblastoma-like tumour of the vulva

This is a rare, distinctive adipocytic lesion that it is very similar to infantile lipoblastomas occurring elsewhere (Lae et al. 2002, Atallah et al. 2007). Four cases have been reported so far, which occurred in teenagers and young women as well-circumscribed tumours measuring between 3.5 and 10 cm. Lesions are lobulated and consist of slender spindle-shaped cells with eosinophilic cytoplasm and bland nuclei with finely granular chromatin. A prominent myxoid stroma is seen and there is a rich vascular network with a 'chicken wire-like' appearance. Lipoblasts may be seen and tumours mimic a myxoid liposarcoma. All lesions had a benign behaviour.

Spindle cell lipoma

Spindle cell lipoma has only been reported twice in the vulva, and in one case the lesion showed areas of pleomorphic lipoma as seen at other sites (Zahn et al. 2001, Reis-Filho et al. 2002). Both lesions occurred in adult women and had typical histological features with slender spindle-shaped cells with scanty cytoplasm in a myxoid background with wiry collagen, increase in stromal mast cells and variable numbers of mature adipocytes. The spindle-shaped cells are positive for CD34 and the mature adipocytes are positive for S-100.

Lipoma

Benign lipomatous neoplasms of the vulva are relatively common and present either as soft, rounded, lobulated masses or as soft, pedunculated tumours (Kaufman & Gardner 1965, Kehagias et al. 1999). They can, on occasion, be extremely large and attain a diameter of nearly 20 cm. Most vulval lipomas develop from the fatty tissue of the labia majora but examples have been noted of clitoral localization (Haddad & Jones 1960, Van Glabeke et al. 1999). They can occur at any age and one has been described in a neonate (Fukaminzu et al. 1982). Histologically, these neoplasms are formed of mature fat cells, which are often admixed with strands of fibrous tissue.

Liposarcoma

Reports of vulval liposarcoma are extremely rare, with a few reasonably persuasive and fully described accounts of such a neoplasm, most of which represent atypical lipomatous tumours (previously referred to as well-differentiated liposarcoma). One liposarcoma developed in the labium majus of a 29 year old woman (Taussig 1937); despite hemivulvectomy with inguinal and femoral node dissection the patient died 5 months later with pulmonary and skeletal metastases. Brooks and LiVolsi (1987) described a large myxoid liposarcoma in a 15 year old girl that involved the vulva and perineum; following local excision the tumour recurred 20 months later, the patient dying from local disease 31 months after initial presentation. The patient reported by Genton and Maroni (1987) was a 60 year old woman who presented with a slow growing, sharply circumscribed lump in the labium majus; the tumour appeared encapsulated macroscopically and histologically was an atypical lipomatous tumour. The patient was alive and well 10 months later.

Nucci and Fletcher (1998) briefly reported a series of six cases of vulval liposarcomas (atypical lipomatous tumours). The age range of their patients was 28–69 years and the neoplasms, which ranged in size from 0.8 to 8 cm in diameter, presented as slowly enlarging vulval masses, which had been present for between 2 and 5 years. Four of the six tumours had the typical histological appearances of atypical lipomatous tumours (well-differentiated liposarcoma), being distinguished from a lipoma only by some variation in adipocyte cell size, a degree of adipocyte nuclear atypia and the presence of occasional lipoblasts. Two of the neoplasms showed an unusual appearance with an admixture of bland spindle-shaped cells, atypical adipocytes and numerous bivacuolated lipoblasts. All the patients were treated with wide local excision only and follow-up data were available for four cases; three patients were alive and well without recurrence at periods up to 18 months, while one woman, whose tumour was incompletely excised, had recurrence over a 10 year period but was alive and well 31 months after re-excision.

Tumours of vascular tissue

Haemangioma

Haemangiomas of the vulva occur primarily in infancy and childhood. The lesions may be of capillary or cavernous type. Clinically significant haemangiomas of the vulva are uncommon (Lovelady *et al.* 1941, Gerbie *et al.* 1955, Darnalt-Restrepo 1957, Giannone & Avezzi 1959, Gulienetti 1959); such cases are usually reported because the haemangioma is large and unsightly but there can be little doubt that most vulval haemangiomas either pass unrecorded or are insufficiently large for the parents of the child to seek medical aid. Those which have been described have usually been of the cavernous type and have involved the labia, usually unilaterally but sometimes bilaterally. Rare cases present during adult life (Cebesoy *et al.* 2008). Occasionally, the vulva is involved by a large segmental haemangioma (Opie *et al.* 2006). Vascular malformations may also occur rarely in the vulva (Kempinaire *et al.* 1997).

Some cavernous haemangiomas have been localized to the clitoris (Lovelady *et al.* 1941, Haddad & Jones 1960, Kaufmann-Friedman 1978); such lesions produce marked clitoromegaly and may lead to the patient being investigated for an intersex state or for congenital adrenal hyperplasia.

Angiokeratoma

Angiokeratomas are non-neoplastic vascular proliferations that often involve the genitalia. Vulval angiokeratomas are common (Cohen *et al.* 1989) and develop principally in women aged between 20 and 40 years. The majority arise in the labia majora although localization to the clitoris has been described (Yamazaki *et al.* 1992, Yigiter *et al.* 2008). They may be single but are, in 50% of cases, multiple; as many as 24 separate angiokeratomas having been noted in the vulva of one woman (Uhlin 1980). The lesions (Fig. 9.6) usually measure between 2 and 10 mm in diameter and may assume a papular, globular or warty appearance. In the early stages of their development angiokeratomas are commonly cherry red in colour, but as they age their tint darkens to

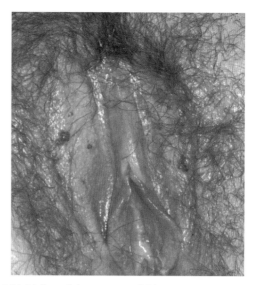

Fig. 9.6 Multiple angiokeratomas on labia majora.

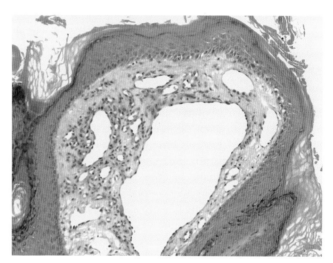

Fig. 9.7 Angiokeratoma of the vulva. Dilated vascular channels in the papillary dermis with mild hyperkeratosis of the overlying epithelium.

brown or black. A possible association with radiotherapy has been suggested (Smith *et al.* 2004). Angiokeratomas may rarely occur on a background of lichen sclerosus (Luzar *et al.* 2009).

Histologically (Fig. 9.7), greatly dilated capillary vessels, often converted into a solitary, sinusoidal vascular channel, are present in the papillary dermis: the overlying epidermis shows a variable degree of hyperkeratosis and acanthosis with elongated rete ridges growing down to surround the dilated vascular channels in the dermis.

Angiokeratomas are usually asymptomatic but may cause pruritus, and bleeding from the lesion is not uncommon; the bleeding is usually of a relatively trivial degree but can occasionally be quite severe. The presence of a black, warty, bleeding lesion can arouse suspicions of a malignant melanoma, which can be rapidly dispelled by histological examination of the locally resected lesion, a procedure that is curative.

Kaposi's sarcoma

The true nature and origin of this tumour is still open to debate, as, although often considered as a vascular neoplasm, it is more probably a multifocal virally induced (human herpesvirus 8) reactive vascular process. Vulval Kaposi's sarcoma appears to have the same gross and histological features as does the lesion elsewhere in the body, although there have been very few reported instances of this tumour involving the vulva. One (Hall *et al.* 1979) arose in a 69 year old woman who had a large, raised, scaling lesion involving the entire right labium majus; satellite nodules were present in the skin of the groin, buttocks and thigh. The patient responded well to chemotherapy but died of renal disease 1 month later; no residual tumour was found at autopsy. LiVolsi and Brooks (1987b) refer briefly to a multifocal Kaposi's sarcoma of the vulva and perineum in an elderly woman; following radiotherapy she was alive 15 years later. A further case of Kaposi's sarcoma involving the vulva mimicking a Bartholin's gland abscess (Laartz *et al.* 2005) and one mimicking a papilloma have been reported (Rajah *et al.* 1990). In a large review of Kaposi's sarcoma occurring in children, 15 cases of anogenital lesions were reported, but it is not stated how many of these, if any, involved the vulva (Ziegler & Katongole-Mbidde 1996).

Epithelioid haemangioendothelioma

This is a malignant vascular tumour that is characterized by cords and nests of large polygonal cells with abundant eosinophilic cytoplasm, some of the cells showing intra-cytoplasmic vacuolation. Tumour cells are surrounded by a myxoid or hyalinized stroma. Immunohistochemically, neoplasms of this type express endothelial markers, particularly CD31 and FLI-1, and many are also positive for cytokeratins; they react negatively for epithelial membrane antigen. Strayer *et al.* (1992) described a neoplasm of this type which presented as a small clitoral nodule, which had been present for a year. After radical vulvectomy and inguinal node dissection the patient was alive and well 27 months later. A further case arising in the labium majus of a young patient was reported by Da Silva *et al.* (2007). Long-term follow-up revealed no evidence of recurrence.

Angiosarcoma

Reports of vulval angiosarcomas have been sparse and rather unsatisfactory. Davos and Abell (1976) described one case in an 83 year old woman; the tumour was treated by local excision and no follow-up information was provided. Bo *et al.* (1976) also reported a vulval angiosarcoma, although this diagnosis was not convincingly supported by the illustrations of the histology. The only fully described

and acceptable case was reported by Nirenberg *et al.* (1995); the tumour arose in an 87 year old woman, formed an ulcerated, poorly circumscribed, bluish mass measuring 8 cm in diameter, and histologically was composed of irregular vascular channels lined by plump to cuboidal endothelial cells that focally formed solid nests. This neoplasm was treated by wide excision and radiotherapy but metastasized to bone and led to the patient's death within 2 years.

Tumours of lymphatic origin

Lymphangiomas

Two types of lymphangioma can occur in the vulva. The more common is the lesion known as lymphangioma simplex or lymphangioma circumscriptum, which may rarely be congenital (Vlastos *et al.* 2003, Roy *et al.* 2006) or more commonly acquired and presents as localized groups of small thin-walled vesicles (Abu-Hamad *et al.* 1989, Akimoto *et al.* 1993, Harwood & Mortimer 1993, Ghaemmaghami *et al.* 2008); microscopically, these consist of irregular dilated lymphatic channels, which may communicate with deeper lymphatic cisterns. Lesions typically develop after surgery or radiotherapy for cervical carcinoma but may arise spontaneously in the absence of predisposing factors. Lesions may also occur in association with tuberculosis of inguinal lymph nodes (Amouri *et al.* 2007). Some assume a warty appearance because of reactive acanthosis of the overlying epithelium and resemble viral warts (Sah *et al.* 2001, Al Aboud *et al.* 2003). Lymphangioma circumscriptum is treated by laser therapy or local excision. Lymphaticovenular anastomosis (Motegi *et al.* 2007), carbon dioxide laser (Smith *et al.* 1999) and sclerotherapy (Ahn *et al.* 2006) have also been reported as alternative therapies. A case not responding to multiple conventional therapies was treated with radiotherapy with good results (Yildiz *et al.* 2008).

The second, less common type is the cavernous lymphangioma. These present as soft, compressible masses, usually in the labia minora but sometimes involving the entire vulva, and can attain a considerable bulk (Lovelady *et al.* 1941, Kaufman & Gardner 1965, Brown & Stenchever 1989, Forsnes 2002). Lymphangiomas of this type usually occur in childhood, and local excision can be curative, but complete removal is not always easy to achieve and recurrence may occur.

Tumours of perivascular cells

Glomus tumour

This benign neoplasm, derived from modified smooth-muscle cells in the walls of arteriovenous anastomoses involved in temperature regulation, presents as a small blue–red, tender nodule and histologically consists of clusters of blood vessels surrounded by cuffs of glomus cells. Vulval glomus tumours are very rare and only a handful of cases have been reported. Kohorn *et al.* (1986) reported a histologically confirmed lesion on the left labium minus causing severe introital dyspareunia and long-standing vulval pain in a woman aged 45 years, and Katz *et al.* (1986) reported a similar lesion at the same site in a woman aged 29 years. Sonobe *et al.* (1994) reported a further two cases, one in the clitoris and the other in the periurethral area. Local excision is curative.

Neural tumours

Neurofibroma

A modest number of vulval neurofibromas have been described; a few of these were solitary lesions in women with no other features of von Recklinghausen's disease (Venter *et al.* 1981), but most have occurred in patients with clear-cut evidence of generalized neurofibromatosis. Vulval neurofibromas have also been described as one component of a localized neurofibromatosis of the female genitourinary tract (Gersell & Fulling 1989).

In some instances the tumours have been confined to the labia (Miller 1979, Friedrich & Wilkinson 1985), but in others the clitoris has been the site of a plexiform neurofibroma, the resulting clitoromegaly in some instances being an isolated phenomenon but in others being associated with labial tumours (Haddad & Jones 1960, Kenny *et al.* 1966, Labardini *et al.* 1968, Messina & Strauss 1976, Greer & Pederson 1981, Schepel & Tolhurst 1981, Ravikumar & Lakshmanan 1983). Not surprisingly, patients, usually children, with clitoral enlargement due to a plexiform neurofibroma tend to be initially diagnosed as cases of intersex, this being particularly the case if accompanying labial tumours are incorrectly taken to be testes. Clitoral neurofibromas in neurofibromatosis type 1 are probably more common than previously reported (Sutphen *et al.* 1995). A case of plexiform neurofibroma in the clitoris has been associated with neurofibromatosis type 2 (Yüksel *et al.* 2003).

A solitary neurofibroma of the vulva is adequately treated by local excision but in many cases of neurofibromatosis the large number of lesions limits surgical treatment to those which are large or painful; unfortunately, the poorly delineated nature of these neoplasms means that surgical removal is often incomplete and that recurrences are common.

Schwannoma

Schwannomas are benign tumours that arise from peripheral nerve sheaths, and a few involving the vulva have been reported. They arise most commonly in the labia (Bryan 1955, Bianco & Samuel 1958, Dini 1959, Yamashita *et al.* 1996), with a few localized to the clitoris (Migliorini & Amato 1978, Llaneza *et al.* 2002). Schwannomas of the vulva show the admixture of Antoni A and B areas characteristic of these neoplasms in other sites. A few plexiform schwannomas arising in the labia (Santos *et al.* 2001, Agaram *et al.* 2005) and in the clitoris (Chuang *et al.* 2007, Yegane *et al.* 2008) have been reported and have not been associated with neurofibromatosis type 2. The case reported by Yegane *et al.* (2008) was congenital.

Malignant peripheral nerve sheath tumour (malignant schwannoma)

These are extremely rare vulval tumours and few reasonably convincing examples have been recorded (Davos & Abell 1976, Terada *et al.* 1988, Lambrou *et al.* 2002, Maglione *et al.* 2002). Two cases appeared to have arisen in a pre-existing solitary neurofibroma and two appeared *de novo*.

Granular cell tumour

This neoplasm is currently thought to show a Schwannian line of differentiation and occurs with modest frequency at the vulva (Altaras *et al.* 1985, Raju & Naraynsingh 1987, Majmudar *et al.* 1990, Wolber *et al.* 1991, Guenther & Shum 1993, Horowitz *et al.* 1995). It represents one of the more common soft-tissue tumours in the vulva. Between 5% and 16% of all granular cell tumours occur in the vulva (Levavi *et al.* 2006). In most instances, the vulval lesion has been an isolated occurrence but, occasionally, it has formed one component of a syndrome in which multiple granular cell tumours arise, either sequentially or synchronously, in various parts of the body (Gifford & Birch 1973, Majmudar *et al.* 1990). The vulval neoplasms can occur at any age but are rare in childhood (Cohen *et al.* 1999). They usually arise in the labia, although some have been confined to the clitoris (Doyle & Hutchinson 1968, Degefu *et al.* 1984, Wolber *et al.* 1991, Laxmisha & Thappa 2007). A case of granular cell tumour presenting in an episiotomy scar has been reported (Murcia *et al.* 1994).

The tumour, which develops in the dermis or immediately subcutaneous tissue, presents as a slow-growing, painless, non-tender lump or nodule; the history usually extends over months or years and the tumour rarely exceeds 4 cm in diameter. The lump is commonly mobile but some tumours situated in the upper dermis show skin tethering. The elevated, overlying skin may be depigmented and occasionally ulcerated. The tumour is poorly circumscribed and yellowish or yellow–grey on section.

Histologically, the neoplasm is formed of rounded or polygonal cells with indistinct margins, central vesicular nuclei and abundant, coarsely granular cytoplasm. There is little pleomorphism and mitotic figures are either absent or extremely sparse. The tumour cells are usually arranged in ribbons or clumps, which are separated from each other. Sometimes, a desmoplastic reaction can largely engulf the tumour cells, which then appear as scattered nests set in a dense fibrous stroma. In the case of those granular cell tumours set in the dermis, the overlying squamous epithelium often shows a pronounced pseudoepitheliomatous hyperplasia, which is not infrequently misdiagnosed as a squamous cell carcinoma. The neoplastic cells stain positively, but weakly, with periodic acid–Schiff stain (PAS) both before and after diastase, and stain strongly for S-100, neurone-specific enolase and NKI-C3.

The majority (98%) of granular cell tumours are benign (the rare exceptions are discussed below) and the patient is cured by local excision, which has to be wide because of the common occurrence of groups of tumour cells beyond the apparent macroscopic limits of growth. Tumours that histologically have an infiltrative rather than a pushing margin are more likely to recur locally (Althausen *et al.* 2000).

Malignant granular cell tumour

Only a handful of malignant granular cell tumours of the vulva have been reported (Robertson *et al.* 1981, Schmidt *et al.* 2003, Ramos *et al.* 2000). In some of these cases, tumours were histologically benign and behaved aggressively. This reflects the difficulty in establishing a histological diagnosis of malignancy in granular cell tumours.

Paraganglioma

Only one paraganglioma of the vulva has been reported (Colgan *et al.* 1991); this presented as a painful, small subepithelial nodule in the labium minus in a 58 year old woman, was cured by local excision and was thought to arise from a peripheral component of the parasympathetic nervous system.

Ewing's sarcoma

Only a handful of genuine cases of peripheral Ewing's sarcoma/neuroectodermal tumour have been described in the vulva (Vang *et al.* 2000a, Takeshima *et al.* 2001, McCluggage *et al.* 2007, Fong *et al.* 2008). The clinical features are non-specific and immunohistological studies demonstrate that tumour cells are usually positive for CD99 and FLI-1.

Mesenchymal tumours of uncertain origin

Epithelioid sarcoma

This is a neoplasm of unknown histogenesis. Tumours classed as epithelioid sarcomas have rarely been reported as occurring in the vulva (Piver *et al.* 1972, Gallup *et al.* 1976, Hall *et al.* 1980, Ulbright *et al.* 1983, Tan *et al.* 1989). Cases of epithelioid sarcoma occurring in proximal sites including the vulva have been described as 'proximal' type variants (Guillou *et al.* 1997, Hasegawa *et al.* 2001) and it is clear that cases of the so-called extrarenal rhabdoid tumour occurring in the vulva represent examples of this variant of epithelioid sarcoma (Argenta *et al.* 2007). This type of epithelioid sarcoma has a more aggressive behaviour with earlier metastasis.

The vulval lesions tend to occur in relatively young women as a slowly enlarging, painless, nodular mass, most commonly in the labium majus; the length of the history varies from 2 to 24 months. Histologically, vulval neoplasms are composed of sheets of plump epithelioid cells with large nuclei and frequent intracytoplasmic rhabdoid inclusions (Fig. 9.8a,b). Areas of necrosis surrounded by tumour cells and simulating granulomas as typically described classic epithelioid sarcoma are not a common feature. The tumours show consistent positivity for cytokeratins

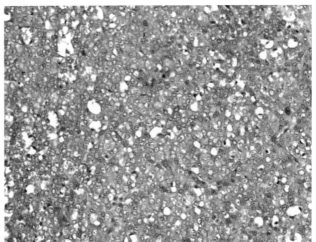

(a)   (b)

Fig. 9.8 (a) Vulval epithelioid sarcoma: sheets of tumour cells often without the central necrosis typically seen in epithelioid sarcoma elsewhere. (b) Large, pleomorphic epithelioid cells which, in some cases, have rhabdoid inclusions.

and epithelial membrane antigen and up to 50% stain for CD34.

Alveolar soft-part sarcoma

The histogenesis of this neoplasm remains obscure despite the presence of positivity for markers of skeletal muscle differentiation. The tumour has a characteristic organoid, pseudoalveolar arrangement of large, rounded or polygonal cells with central nuclei, distinct limiting membranes and abundant granular eosinophilic cytoplasm; it contains PAS-positive, diastase-resistant granules and crystalline rods. Alveolar soft-part sarcoma occurs rarely on the vulva, only two cases having been recorded (Kondratiev & Kurillov 1971, Shen *et al.* 1982); one patient was apparently cured by radical vulvectomy and the other had recurrence after local excision.

Non-mesenchymal, non-epithelial neoplasms

Melanocytic lesions and neoplasms

Lentigo simplex, melanocytic naevi

The term 'melanosis', when applied to the vulva, is often used to describe both patchy or diffuse hyperpigmentation. Idiopathic vulval melanosis is characterized by increased basal layer melanin pigmentation and deposition of melanin in dermal macrophages and is discussed in Chapter 5. Pigmented vulval macules may present in the context of geno-dermatoses, including Carney complex (Pandolfino *et al.* 2001), Laugier–Hunziker syndrome and Dowling–Degos disease (see Fig. 5.7). In the last it may be the only cutaneous manifestation of the disease (O'Goshi *et al.* 2001). When the increase in pigmentation of basal cells is associated with elongation of the rete pegs the lesion is classified as lentigo simplex (Fig. 9.9). Lentigines are the most common pigmented lesions of the vulva and occur as dark-brown macules, measuring 1–5 mm in diameter on the labia minora and around the introitus.

Vulval naevi are relatively uncommon (Fischer & Rogers 2000) and have been found in 2.3% of women (Rock *et al.* 1990) (Fig. 9.10). Intradermal, compound and junctional naevi occur at this site and although it has been claimed that the junctional type predominates this has not always been the case (Christensen *et al.* 1987, Rollason 1992). On occasions, lesions are quite dark and may mimic melanoma (Makino *et al.* 2007). Spitz naevi have also been described (Hulagu & Erez 1973). Naevi can coexist with lichen sclerosus and, both clinically and histologically, these lesions may mimic melanoma (Carlson *et al.* 2002).

A proportion of vulval naevi in women show atypical features (Friedman & Ackerman 1981) and are regarded

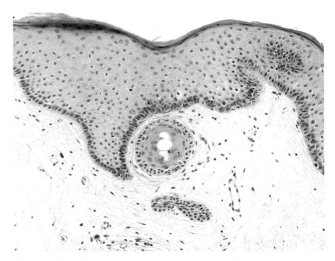

Fig. 9.9 Vulval lentigo: increased pigmentation of basal cells and dendritic processes of melanocytes can be seen.

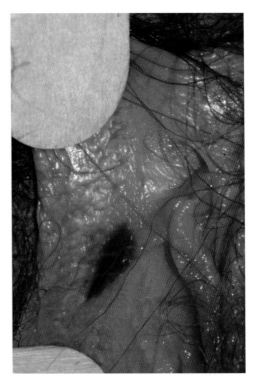

Fig. 9.10 Vulval naevus: well-circumscribed dark-brown macule on right labium minus.

as atypical melanocytic naevi of the genital type or just as atypical genital naevi (Gleason *et al.* 2008). These include the presence of large epithelioid (or sometimes spindled) intraepidermal melanocytes with retraction artefact or cellular discohesion. Cytological atypia may be present and tend to be variable (Fig. 9.11). Nests of tumour cells show

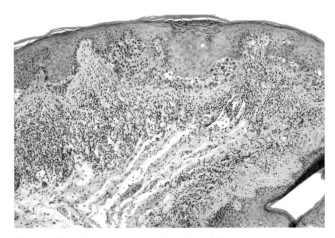

Fig. 9.11 Vulval naevus: atypical histological features may be seen including architectural disorder and some degree of cytological atypia (courtesy of Dr Phillip McKee).

variation in size and shape and focal confluence. Melanocytes in these lesions contain eosinophilic cytoplasm a single nucleolus. A band of dense eosinophilic fibrosis is not uncommonly seen in the superficial dermis. A dermal component is often present and consists of variably sized intradermal melanocytic nests. Mitotic figures are exceptional. Hair shafts and sweat gland ducts are commonly involved. Focal upward migration may be seen. In these lesions there is, however, an overall symmetry with cellular maturation in the deep dermis. Such lesions should not be regarded as variants of the so-called 'dysplastic' naevus as has been suggested in the past (Christensen *et al.* 1987, Pierson 1987, Rollason 1992).

Malignant melanoma

Malignant melanoma of the vulva constitutes between 2% and 4% of all female melanomas. It is the second commonest vulval malignancy (Wechter *et al.* 2004) and has been variously estimated to account for between 3.6% and 10% of malignant vulval neoplasms (Chung *et al.* 1975, Morrow & DiSaia 1976, Silvers & Halperin 1978, Pierson 1987, Bradgate *et al.* 1990, Rollason 1992). It is thought that about 10% arise in pre-existing vulval naevi (Curtin & Morrow 1992). A population-based study estimated that the ratio of vulval to skin melanoma was 1:71 (Stang *et al.* 2005).

Vulval malignant melanoma is exceptional in prepubertal girls (Egan *et al.* 1997) and has been recorded in association with lichen sclerosus (Hassanein *et al.* 2004) (see also Chapter 5). After puberty the incidence of melanoma rises steadily to reach a peak in the sixth and seventh decades. A recent study found a 15% family history of malignant melanoma (Wechter *et al.* 2004). Patients usually present with a relatively short history of, most commonly, a lump,

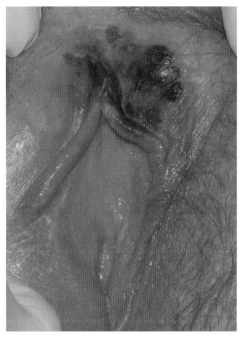

Fig. 9.12 Extensive flat vulval melanoma with elevated areas.

although there may also be complaints of bleeding, pain or itching. In some series the tumours have been predominantly central, i.e. involving the labia minora or the clitoris (Morrow & Rutledge 1972, Podratz *et al.* 1983), but others have found an equal incidence of lateral (i.e. involving labia majora) and central neoplasms (Phillips *et al.* 1982, Jaramillo *et al.* 1985). A large retrospective study in Sweden has shown that the clitoris and labia majora were the most common sites while 46% arose in glabrous skin, 12% developed in hairy skin and 35% involved both areas (Ragnarsson-Olding *et al.* 1999). In this study, melanomas arose in pre-existing naevi only in hairy skin. The melanoma may be flat, elevated, nodular or polypoidal (Fig. 9.12) and is often ulcerated (Fig. 9.13); the colour ranges from brown to bluish-black but some in this site are amelanotic and bear a close macroscopic resemblance to a squamous cell carcinoma. In various series vulval melanomas have been more commonly of the superficial spreading type, but in others the nodular type has predominated (Bouma *et al.* 1982, Landthaler *et al.* 1985, Itala *et al.* 1986, Johnson *et al.* 1986) whereas both the mucosal lentiginous and neurotropic forms have been prominent in yet others (Benda *et al.* 1986, Blessing *et al.* 1991, Ragnarsson-Olding *et al.* 1999). Cytogenetic studies in a handful of vulval melanomas have shown complex karyotypic aberrations involving multiple chromosomes, particularly chromosome 1 (Micci *et al.* 2003).

The 5 year survival rate for patients with a malignant melanoma of the vulva has ranged from 13% to 54% with

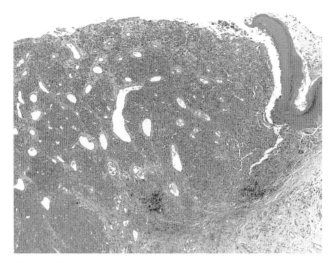

Fig. 9.13 Ulcerated nodular melanoma.

a mean of about 30–35% (Pack & Oropeza 1967, Chung *et al.* 1975, Phillips *et al.* 1982, Podratz *et al.* 1983, Benda *et al.* 1986, Itala *et al.* 1986, Woolcot *et al.* 1988, Blessing *et al.* 1991, Piura *et al.* 1992, Ragnarsson-Olding *et al.* 1993, Scheistroen *et al.* 1995, Raber *et al.* 1996). Five year survival is not synonymous with cure, for recurrences and metastases can occur at any time up to 13 years after primary treatment (Bouma *et al.* 1982, Podratz *et al.* 1983), and the 10 year survival rate is significantly lower than that noted at 5 years (Bradgate *et al.* 1990).

Melanomas of the vulva are staged in the same way as squamous cell carcinomas at this site but the prognostic value of clinical stage in malignant melanoma is still open to debate. There seems little difference in survival rates between stage I and stage II cases (5 year survival 60–70%) and the outlook is agreed to be universally gloomy for patients with stage IV disease; some have also found stage III tumours to be associated with a very poor prognosis (Jaramillo *et al.* 1985, Bradgate *et al.* 1990) while others have been unable to show that the prognosis for such neoplasms is any worse than for tumours in earlier stages (Phillips *et al.* 1982, Podratz *et al.* 1983).

The diameter of a melanoma appears to be of little prognostic importance but it has been maintained that laterally sited tumours have a better prognosis than those which are centrally placed (Podratz *et al.* 1983, Johnson *et al.* 1986), although it has been suggested that this is true only if the central neoplasms involve the urethra or vagina (Morrow 1981). Localization of the tumour to the clitoris has been noted as having a poor prognosis (Scheistroen *et al.* 1995). The traditional belief that superficial spreading melanomas have a better prognosis than their nodular counterparts has been upheld in some series (Podratz *et al.* 1983, Itala *et al.* 1986, Johnson *et al.* 1986) but not in others (Chung *et al.*

1975, Bradgate *et al.* 1990). Other histological features, such as cell type, degree of atypia and number of mitotic figures, are not generally thought to be of prognostic value, although Bradgate *et al.* (1990) found that tumours containing epithelioid-type cells were associated with an unusually poor outlook. DNA non-diploidy emerged as a major prognostic indicator of poor survival in women with vulval melanomas (Scheistroen *et al.* 1995, 1996).

For melanomas confined to the vulva, histological microstaging is thought to be prognostically important (Dunton *et al.* 1995). Some have found Clark's levels (Clark *et al.* 1969), which define depth of tumour invasion in terms of dermal planes, to be of considerable prognostic significance (Phillips *et al.* 1982, Podratz *et al.* 1983), but the value of this technique is limited by the fact that most vulval melanomas are already stage IV, or worse, at presentation (Rollason 1992). Chung's modification of Clark's levels (Chung *et al.* 1975) has the same disadvantage (Blessing *et al.* 1991). The Breslow technique measures tumour thickness and there is widespread agreement that tumour thickness is a dominant prognostic factor, melanomas less than 0.76 mm in thickness having an excellent prognosis and subsequent survival rates beyond this plummeting with increasing thickness (Phillips *et al.* 1982, Podratz *et al.* 1983, Jaramillo *et al.* 1985, Ragnarsson-Olding *et al.* 1999, Verschraegen *et al.* 2001, Wechter *et al.* 2004). The value of Breslow microstaging has, however, not been confirmed in older studies (Piura *et al.* 1992, Scheistroen *et al.* 1996). A further study has suggested that, although tumour thickness is predictive of lymph node involvement, it is not a significant predictor of survival (Raspagliesi *et al.* 2000). In this study, the number of lymph nodes involved was the most powerful predictor of survival.

Malignant melanoma has traditionally been treated by radical vulvectomy and node dissection but it has not been shown that the results following radical surgery are any better than those achieved by wide local excision (Davidson *et al.* 1987, Rose *et al.* 1988, Bradgate *et al.* 1990); there is therefore an increasing move towards purely local surgery, certainly for thin lesions (Tasseron *et al.* 1992, Trimble *et al.* 1992, Look *et al.* 1993, Dunton *et al.* 1995). It has been suggested that a 1 cm margin is adequate for melanomas less than 1 mm and a 2 cm margin for melanomas between 1 and 4 mm (Irvin *et al.* 2001).

There are no large studies evaluating the role of sentinel lymph node biopsy in vulval melanoma (Wechter *et al.* 2004, Avhan *et al.* 2008). It has been suggested that, as with melanomas occurring elsewhere in the skin, the procedure is useful to identify patients with occult metastasis. However, it has also been suggested that the procedure may increase the risk of in-transit metastases in patients with thick melanomas (de Hullu *et al.* 2002). Clearly, larger studies are necessary.

Germ cell neoplasms

Yolk sac tumours

Yolk sac (endodermal sinus) tumours of the vulva are rare and only a handful have been fully documented (Ungerleider *et al.* 1978, Flanagan *et al.* 1997, Traen *et al.* 2004). It is assumed, but certainly not proven, that these neoplasms arise from germ cells which, during embryogenesis, have gone astray during their migration from the yolk sac to the developing gonad.

Yolk sac tumours of the vulva have had exactly the same appearance as their more commonly occurring ovarian counterparts and have arisen in infants, children and young adults. The patients present with a short history, usually of only a few months, of a painless, enlarging vulval mass, usually in the labium majus but in one case confined to the clitoris.

Lymphoma and leukaemia

The vulva can be the site of an apparently primary extranodal lymphoma or may rarely be the site of involvement by a systemic lymphoma (Schiller & Madge 1970, Egwuatu *et al.* 1980, Vang *et al.* 2000b). The vulva seems to be the least common site in the female genital tract to be involved by lymphoma (Kosari *et al.* 2005). Most of the reported cases have been non-Hodgkin's B cell lymphomas (Buckingham & McClure 1955, Iliya *et al.* 1968, Wishart 1973, Bagella *et al.* 1990, Bai & Sun 1995, Lagoo & Robboy 2006, Cheng *et al.* 2007) but there have also been occasional examples of Hodgkin's disease (Hahn 1958) and of post-transplantation T-cell lymphoma (Kaplan *et al.* 1993). There has been one case of an immunoblastic lymphoma of the vulva arising in an HIV-positive woman (Kaplan *et al.* 1996). Of the B cell non-Hodgkin's lymphomas involving the vulva, lymphoplasmacytic lymphoma appears to be somewhat more common (Kosari *et al.* 2005). Cutaneous T cell lymphoma involving the vulva is exceptional particularly as a primary process (Vang *et al.* 2000b). It is worth remembering that, occasionally, some conditions such as lichen sclerosus may histologically mimic a cutaneous T cell lymphoma (Citarella *et al.* 2003).

Presentation of a myeloid leukaemia with vulval ulceration of uncertain nature (Muram & Gold 1993) or as a granulocytic sarcoma of the vulva has also been recorded (Gardaise *et al.* 1974, Joswig & Joswig-Priewe 1974, Laricchia *et al.* 1977).

References

Abu-Hamad, A., Provencher, D., Ganjei, P. & Penalver, M. (1989) Lymphangioma circumscripta of the vulva: case report and review of the literature. *Obstetrics and Gynecology* 73, 496–499.

Agaram, N.P., Praksh, S., & Antonescu, C.R. (2005) Deep-seated plexiform schwannoma: a pathologic study of 16 cases and comparative analysis with the superficial variety. *American Journal of Surgical Pathology* 29, 1042–1048.

Ahn, S.J., Chang, S.E., Choi, J.H. *et al.* (2006) A case of unresectable lymphangioma circumscriptum of the vulva successfully treated with OK-432 in childhood. *Journal of the American Academy of Dermatology* 55, S106–107.

Akimoto, K., Nogita, T. & Kawashima, M. (1993) A case of acquired lymphangioma of the vulva. *Journal of Dermatology* 20, 449–451.

Al Aboud, K., Al Hawsawi, K., Ramesh, V. *et al.* (2003) Vulval lymphangiomata mimicking genital warts. *Journal of the European Academy of Dermatovenereology* 17, 684–685.

Alameda, F., Munné, A., Baró, T. *et al.* (2006) Vulvar angiomyxoma, aggressive angiomyxoma, and angiomyofibroblastoma: an immunohistochemical and ultrastructural study. *Ultrastructural Pathology* 30, 193–195.

Allen, P.W. (1972) Nodular fasciitis. *Pathology* 4, 9–26.

Allen, M.V. & Novotny, D.B. (1997) Desmoid tumor of the vulva associated with pregnancy. *Archives of Pathology and Laboratory Medicine* 121, 512–514.

Altaras, M., Jaffe, R., Bernheim, J. & Ben Aderet, M. (1985) Granular cell myoblastoma of the vulva. *Gynecologic Oncology* 22, 352–355.

Althausen, A.M., Kowaiski, D.P., Ludwig, M.E. *et al.* (2000) Granular cell tumors: a new clinically important histologic finding. *Gynecologic Oncology* 77, 310–313.

Amouri, M., Masmoudi, A., Boudaya, S. *et al.* (2007) Acquired lymphangioma circumscriptum of the vulva. *Dermatology Online Journal* 13, 10.

Aneiros, J., Garcia del Moral, R., Beltran, E. & Nogales, F.F. (1982) Epithelioid leiomyoma of the vulva. *Diagnostic Gynecology and Obstetrics* 4, 351–355.

Argenta, P.A., Thomas, S. & Chura, J.C. (2007) Proximal-type epithelioid sarcoma vs. malignant rhabdoid tumor of the vulva: a case report, review of the literature, and an argument for consolidation. *Gynecologic Oncology* 107, 130–135.

Atallah, D., Rouzier, R., Chamoun, M.L. *et al.* (2007) Benign lipoblastomalike tumor of the vulva: report of a case affecting a young patient. *Journal of Reproductive Medicine* 52, 223–224.

Audet-Lapointe, P., Paquin, F., Guerard, M.J. *et al.* (1980) Leiomyosarcoma of the vulva. *Gynecologic Oncology* 10, 350–355.

Avhan, A., Celik, H. & Dursun, P. (2008) Lymphatic mapping and sentinel lymph node biopsy in gynecological cancers: a critical review of the literature. *The World Journal of Surgical Oncology* 20, 53.

Bagella, M.P., Fadda, G. & Cherchi, P.L. (1990) Non-Hodgkin's lymphoma: a rare primary vulvar localization. *European Journal of Gynaecologic Oncology* 11, 153–156.

Bagga, R., Keepanasserl, A., Suri, V. & Nijhawan, R. (2007) Aggressive angiomyxoma of the vulva in pregnancy: a case report and review of management options. *Medscape General Medicine* 24, 16.

Bai, P. & Sun, J. (1995) Primary malignant lymphoma of the female genital tract: clinical analysis of 15 cases. *Chinese Journal of Obstetrics and Gynecology* 30, 614–617.

Begin, L.R., Clement, P.B., Kirk, M.E. *et al.* (1985) Aggressive angiomyxoma of pelvic soft parts: a clinicopathological study of nine cases. *Human Pathology* 16, 621–628.

Benda, J.A., Platz, C.E. & Anderson, B. (1986) Malignant melanoma of the vulva: a clinical-pathologic review of the 16 cases. *International Journal of Gynecological Pathology* 5, 202–216.

Bianco, R. & Samuel, S. (1958) Neurilemmoma della vulva. *Tumori* 44, 326–336.

Blandamura, S., Cruz, J., Faure Vergara, L. *et al.* (2003) Aggressive angiomyxoma: a second case of metastasis with patient's death. *Human Pathology* **34**, 1072–1074.

Blessing, K., Kernohan, N.M., Miller, I.D. & Al Nafussi, A.L. (1991) Malignant melanoma of the vulva; clinicopathological features. *International Journal of Gynecological Cancer* **1**, 81–87.

Bo, A.V., Bianchi, G., Kron, J.B. & Miglioli, P. (1976) Si un caso ad eccezionale sopravvenza di sarcoma della vulva. *Minerva Ginecologica* **28**, 145–149.

Bock, J.E., Andreasson, B., Thorn, A. & Holck, S. (1985) Dermatofibrosarcoma protuberans of the vulva. *Gynecologic Oncology* **20**, 129–135.

Bond, S.J., Seibel, N. & Kapur, S. (1994) Rhabdomyosarcoma of the clitoris. *Cancer* **73**, 1884–1886.

Bouma, J., Weening, J.J. & Elders, A. (1982) Malignant melanoma of the vulva: report of 18 cases. *European Journal of Obstetrics and Gynecology and Reproductive Biology* **13**, 237–251.

Bradgate, M.G., Rollason, T.P., McConkey, C. & Powell, J. (1990) Malignant melanoma of the vulva: a clinico-pathological study of 30 women. *British Journal of Obstetrics and Gynaecology* **97**, 124–133.

Brooks, J.S.J. (1994) The spectrum of fibrohistiocytic tumours with special emphasis on malignant fibrous histiocytoma. *Current Diagnostic Pathology* **1**, 3–12.

Brooks, J.S.J. & LiVolsi, V.A. (1987) Liposarcoma presenting on the vulva. *American Journal of Obstetrics and Gynecology* **156**, 73–75.

Brown. J.V. & Stenchever, M.A. (1989) Cavernous lymphangioma of the vulva. *Obstetrics and Gynecology* **73**, 877–879.

Bryan, W.E. (1955) Neurilemmoma of the vulva. *Journal of Obstetrics and Gynaecology of the British Empire* **62**, 949–950.

Buckingham, J.C. & McClure, H.J. (1955) Reticulum cell sarcoma of the vulva: report of a case. *Obstetrics and Gynecology* **6**, 138–143.

Carlson, J.A., Mu, X.C., Slominski, A. *et al.* (2002) Melanocytic proliferations associated with lichen sclerosus. *Archives of Dermatology* **138**, 77–87.

Cebesoy, F.B., Kutlar, I. & Aydin, A. (2008) A rare mass formation of the vulva: giant cavernous hemangioma. *Journal of Low Genital Tract Diseases* **12**, 35–37.

Cheah, P.L., Looi, L.M. & Sivanesaratnam, V. (1993) Aggressive angiomyxoma of the vulva with an unusual vascular finding. *Pathology* **25**, 250–252.

Cheng, M.H., Chao, H.T. & Wang, P.H. (2007) Vulvar metastasis as the initial presentation of non-Hodgkin's lymphoma: a case report. *Journal of Reproductive Medicine* **52**, 1065–1066.

Christensen, W.N., Friedman, K.J., Woodruff, J.D. & Hood, A.F. (1987) Histological characteristics of vulvar nevocellular nevi. *Journal of Cutaneous Pathology* **14**, 87–91.

Chuang, W.Y., Yeh, C.J., Jung, S.M. & Hsueh, S. (2007) Plexiform schwannoma of the clitoris. *Acta Pathologica, Mcrobiologica et Immunlogica Scandinavica* **115**, 889–890.

Chung, A.F., Woodruff, J.M. & Lewis, J.L. (1975) Malignant melanoma of the vulva: a report of 44 cases. *Obstetrics and Gynecology* **45**, 638–646.

Citarella, L., Massone, C., Kerl, H. & Cerroni, L. (2003) Lichen sclerosus with histopathologic features simulating early mycosis fungoides. *American Journal of Dermatopathology* **25**, 463–465.

Clark, W.H., Jr, From, L., Bernadino, E.A. & Mihm, M.C. (1969) Histogenesis and biologic behaviour of primary human malignant melanoma of the skin. *Cancer Research* **29**, 705–727.

Cohen, P.R., Young, A.W., Jr, & Tovell, H.M. (1989) Angiokeratoma of the vulva: diagnosis and review of the literature. *Obstetrical and Gynecological Survey* **44**, 339–346.

Cohen, Z., Kapuller, Y., Maor, E. & Mares, A.J. (1999) Granular cell tumor (myoblastoma) of the labia major: a rare benign tumor in childhood. *Journal of Pediatric and Adolescent Gynecology* **12**, 155–156.

Colgan, T.J., Dardick, I. & O'Connell, G. (1991) Paraganglioma of the vulva. *International Journal of Gynecological Pathology* **10**, 203–208.

Copeland, L.J., Sneige, N., Stringer, A. *et al.* (1985) Alveolar rhabdomyosarcoma of the female genitalia. *Cancer* **56**, 849–856.

Curry, J.L., Olejnik, J.L. & Wojcik, E.M. (2001) Cellular angiofibroma of the vulva with DNA ploidy analysis. *International Journal of Gynecological Pathology* **20**, 200–203.

Curtin, J.P. & Morrow, C.P. (1992) Melanoma of lower female genital tract. In: *Gynecologic Oncology*, 2nd edn (ed. M. Coppleson), pp. 1059–1068. Churchill Livingstone, Edinburgh.

Dargent, J.L., de Saint Aubain, N., Galdón, M.G. *et al.* (2003) Cellular angiofibroma of the vulva: a clinicopathological study of two cases with documentation of some unusual features and review of the literature. *Journal of Cutaneous Pathology* **30**, 405–411.

Darnalt-Restrepo, E. (1957) Hemangiomas de la vulva et de la vagina. *Revista Columniana de Obstetricia* **8**, 272–276.

Da Silva, B.B., Lopes-Costa, P.V., Furtado-Veloso, A.M. & Borges, R.S. (2007) Vulval epithelioid hemangioendothelioma. *Gynecologic Oncology* **105**, 539–541.

Davidson, T., Kissin, M. & Westbury, G. (1987) Vulvo-vaginal melanoma: should radical surgery be abandoned? *British Journal of Obstetrics and Gynaecology* **94**, 473–476.

Davos, I. & Abell, M.R. (1976) Soft tissue sarcomas of vulva. *Gynecologic Oncology* **4**, 70–86.

Degefu, S., Dhurandhar, H.N., O'Quinn, A.G. & Fuller, P.N. (1984) Granular cell tumor of the clitoris in pregnancy. *Gynecologic Oncology* **19**, 246–251.

de Hullu, J.A., Hollema, H., Hoekstra, H.J. *et al.* (2002) Vulval melanoma: is there a role for sentinel lymph node biopsy? *Cancer* **94**, 486–491.

Di Gilio A.R., Cormio, G., Resta, L. *et al.* (2004) Rapid growth of myxoid leiomyosarcoma of the vulva during pregnancy: a case report. *International Journal of Gynecological Cancer* **14**, 172–175.

Dini, S. (1959) Rare osservazione di neurinoma del piccolo labbro vulvare. *Archivo de Becchi* **29**, 867–875.

DiSaia, P.J., Rutledge, F. & Smith, J.P. (1971) Sarcomas of the vulva: a report of 12 patients. *Obstetrics and Gynecology* **38**, 180–184.

Di Sant Agnese, P.A. & Knowles, D.M. (1980) Extracardiac rhabdomyoma: a clinicopathological study and review of the literature. *Cancer* **46**, 780–789.

Doyle, W.F. & Hutchinson, J.R. (1968) Granular cell myoblastoma of the clitoris. *American Journal of Obstetrics and Gynecology* **100**, 589–590.

Dunton, C.J., Kautzy, M. & Hanau, C. (1995) Malignant melanoma of the vulva: a review. *Obstetrical and Gynecological Survey* **50**, 739–746.

Egan, C.A., Bradley, R.R., Logsdon, V.K., *et al.* (1997) Vulvar melanoma in childhood. *Archives of Dermatology* **133**, 345–348.

Egwuatu, V.E., Ejeckam, G.C. & Okaro, J.M. (1980) Burkitt's lymphoma of the vulva: a case report. *British Journal of Obstetrics and Gynaecology* **87**, 827–830.

Elchalal, U., Dgani, R., Zosmer, A. *et al.* (1991) Malignant fibrous histiocytoma of the vagina and vulva successfully treated by combined chemotherapy and radiotherapy. *Gynecologic Oncology* 42, 91–93.

Elchalal, U., Lifshitz-Mercer, B., Dgani, R. & Zalel, Y. (1992) Aggressive angiomyxoma of the vulva. *Gynecologic Oncology* 47, 260–262.

Ergeneli, M.H., Demirhan, B. & Duran, E.H. (1999) Desmoid tumor of the vulva: a case report. *Journal of Reproductive Medicine* 44, 748–750.

Ferguson, S.E., Gerald, W., Barakat, R.R. *et al.* (2007) Clinicopathologic features of rhabdomyosarcoma of gynecologic origin in adults. *American Journal of Surgical Pathology* 31, 382–389.

Fetsch, J.F., Laskin, W.B., Lefkowitz, M. *et al.* (1996) Aggressive angiomyxoma: a clinicopathologic study of 29 female patients. *Cancer* 78, 79–90.

Fine, B.A., Munoz, A.K., Litz, C.E. & Gershenson, D.M. (2001) Primary medical management of recurrent aggressive angiomyxoma of the vulva with a gonadotropin-releasing hormone agonist. *Gynecologic Oncology* 81, 120–122.

Fischer, G. & Rogers, M. (2000) Vulval disease in children: a clinical audit of 130 cases. *Pediatric Dermatology* 17, 1–6.

Flanagan, C.W., Parker, J.R., Mannel, R.S. *et al.* (1997) Primary endodermal sinus tumor of the vulva: a case report and review of the literature. *Gynecologic Oncology* 66, 515–518.

Fletcher, C.D.M. (1995) Soft tissue tumors. In: *Diagnostic Histopathology of Tumors* (ed. C.D.M. Fletcher), pp. 1043–1096. Churchill Livingstone, Edinburgh.

Fletcher, C.D.M., Tsang, W.Y.W., Fisher, C. *et al.* (1992) Angiomyofibroblastoma of the vulva: a benign neoplasm distinct from aggressive angiomyxoma. *American Journal of Surgical Pathology* 16, 373–382.

Fong, Y.E., López-Terrada, D. & Zhai, Q.J. (2008) Primary Ewing sarcoma/peripheral primitive neuroectodermal tumor of the vulva. *Human Pathology* 39, 1535–9.

Forsnes, E.V. (2002) Cavernous lymphangioma of the vulva. A case report. *Journal of Reproductive Medicine* 47, 1041–1043.

Friedman, R.J. & Ackerman, A.B. (1981) Difficulties in the histological diagnosis of melanocytic nevi on the vulvae of premenopausal women. In: *Pathology of Malignant Melanoma* (ed. A.B. Ackerman), pp. 119–127. Masson, New York.

Friedrich, E.G. & Wilkinson, E.J. (1985) Vulvar surgery for neurofibromatosis. *Obstetrics and Gynecology* 65, 135–138.

Fukaminzu, H., Matsumoto, K., Inoue, K. & Moriguchi, T. (1982) Large vulvar lipoma. *Archives of Dermatology* 118, 447.

Gaffney, E.F., Majmudar, B. & Bryan, J.A. (1982) Nodular (pseudo-sarcomatous) fasciitis of the vulva. *International Journal of Gynecological Pathology* 1, 307–312.

Gallup, D.G., Abell, M.R. & Morley, G.W. (1976) Epithelioid sarcoma of the vulva. *Obstetrics and Gynecology* 48, 14s–17s.

Gardaise, J., Marie, M. & Bertrand, G. (1974) Chlorome à localizations génitales multiples. *Semaine des Hôpitaux de Paris* 51, 609–616.

Genton, G.Y. & Maroni, E.S. (1987) Vulval liposarcoma. *Archives of Gynaecology* 240, 63–66.

Gerbie, A.B., Hirsch, M.R. & Greene, R.R. (1955) Vascular tumors of the female genital tract. *Obstetrics and Gynecology* 6, 499–507.

Gersell, D.J. & Fulling, K.H. (1989) Localized neurofibromatosis of the female genitourinary tract. *American Journal of Surgical Pathology* 13, 873–878.

Ghaemmaghami, F., Karimi Zarchi, M. & Mousavi, A. (2008) Major labiectomy as surgical management of vulvar lymphangioma circumscriptum: three cases and a review of the literature. *Archives of Gynecology and Obstetrics* 278, 57–60.

Ghorbani, R.P., Malpica, A. & Ayala, A.G. (1999) Dermatofibrosarcoma protuberans of the vulva: clinicopathologic and immunohistochemical analysis of four cases, one with fibrosarcomatous change, and review of the literature. *International Journal of Gynecological Pathology* 18, 366–373.

Giannone, R. & Avezzi, G. (1959) Emangioma cavernose della vulva. *Rivista Italiana de Ginecologia* 53, 471–479.

Gifford, R. & Birch, H.W. (1973) Granular cell myoblastoma of multicentric origin involving the vulva: a case report. *American Journal of Obstetrics and Gynecology* 117, 184–187.

Gleason, B.C., Hirsch, M.S., Nucci, M.R. *et al.* (2008) Atypical genital nevi. A clinicopathologic analysis of 56 cases. *American Journal of Surgical Pathology* 32, 51–57.

Gökden, N., Dehner, L.P., Zhu, X. & Pfeifer, J.D. (2003) Dermatofibrosarcoma protuberans of the vulva and groin: detection of COL1A1-PDGFB fusion transcripts by RT-PCR. *Journal of Cutaneous Pathology* 30, 190–195.

Granter, S.R., Nucci, M.R. & Fletcher, C.D.M. (1997) Aggressive angiomyxoma: reappraisal of its relationship to angiomyofibroblastoma in a series of 16 cases. *Histopathology* 30, 1–10.

Greer, D.M. & Pederson, W.C. (1981) Pseudo-masculinization of the clitoris. *Plastic and Reconstructive Surgery* 68, 787–788.

Guenther, L. & Shum, D. (1993) Granular cell tumor of the vulva. *Pediatric Dermatology* 10, 153–155.

Guidozzi, F., Sadan, U., Koller, A.B. & Marks, S.R. (1987) Combined chemotherapy and irradiation therapy after radical surgery for leiomyosarcoma of the vulva: a case report. *South African Medical Journal* 71, 327–328.

Guillou, L, Wadden, C., Coindre, J.M. *et al.* (1997) 'Proximal-type' epithelioid sarcoma, a distinctive aggressive neoplasm showing rhabdoid features. Clinicopathologic, immunohistochemical, and ultrastructural study of a series. *American Journal of Surgical Pathology* 21, 130–146.

Gulienetti, R. (1959) Haemangiomata of the external genitals. *British Journal of Plastic Surgery* 12, 228–233.

Guven, S., Esinler, D., Salman, M.C. *et al.* (2005) Recurrent vulval leiomyoma in a postmenopausal patient mimicking vulval carcinoma. *Journal of Obstetrics and Gynaecology* 25, 732–733.

Haddad, H.M. & Jones, W.H. (1960) Clitoral enlargement simulating pseudohermaphroditism. *American Journal of Diseases of Children* 99, 282–287.

Hahn, G.A. (1958) Gynecologic considerations in malignant lymphoma. *American Journal of Obstetrics and Gynecology* 75, 673–683.

Hall, J.S.E. & Amin, U.F. (1981) Fibrosarcoma of the vulva: case reports and discussion. *International Surgery* 86, 185–187.

Hall, D.J., Burns, J.C. & Goplerud, D.R. (1979) Kaposi's sarcoma of the vulva: a case report and brief review. *Obstetrics and Gynecology* 54, 478–483.

Hall, D.J., Grimes, M.M. & Goplerud, D.R. (1980) Epithelioid sarcoma of the vulva. *Gynecologic Oncology* 9, 237–246.

Haroun, S.A., Elnaiem, E.A., Zaki, Z.M. & Adam, I. (2007) Aggressive rhabdomyosarcoma of the vulva in a young Sudanese woman. *Saudi Medical Journal* 28, 461–462.

Harwood, C.A. & Mortimer, P.S. (1993) Acquired lymphangiomata mimicking genital warts. *British Journal of Dermatology* 129, 334–336.

Hasegawa, T., Matsuno, Y., Shimoda, T. *et al.* (2001) Proximal-type epithelioid sarcoma: a clinicopathologic study of 20 cases. *Modern Pathology* 14, 655–663.

Hassanein, A.M., Mrstik, M.E., Hardt, N.S. *et al.* (2004) Malignant melanoma associated with lichen sclerosus in the vulva of a 10-year-old. *Pediatric Dermatology* 21, 473–476.

Hisaoka, M., Kouho, H., Aoki, T. *et al.* (1995) Angiomyofibroblastoma of the vulva: a clinicopathologic study of seven cases. *Pathology International* 45, 487–492.

Horowitz, I.R., Copas, P. & Majmudar, B. (1995) Granular cell tumors of the vulva. *American Journal of Obstetrics and Gynecology* 173, 1710–1713.

Htwe, M., Deppisch, L.M. & Saint Julien, J.S. (1995) Hormone-dependent aggressive angiomyxoma of the vulva. *Obstetrics and Gynecology* 86, 697–699.

Hulagu, C. & Erez, S. (1973) Juvenile melanoma of the clitoris. *Journal of Obstetrics and Gynaecology of the British Commonwealth* 80, 89–91.

Iliya, F.A., Muggia, F.M., O'Leary, J.A. & King, T.M. (1968) Gynecologic manifestations of reticulum cell sarcoma. *Obstetrics and Gynecology* 31, 266–269.

Imachi, M., Tsukamoto, N., Kamura, T. *et al.* (1991) Alveolar rhabdomyosarcoma of the vulva: report of two cases. *Acta Cytologica* 35, 345–349.

Irvin, W.P., Jr, Legallo, R.L., Stoler, M.H. *et al.* (2001) Vulvar melanoma: a retrospective analysis and literature review. *Gynecologic Oncology* 83, 457–465.

Itala, J., DiPaola, G.R., Gomez-Rueda, N. *et al.* (1986) Melanoma of the vulva: the experience at Buenos Aires University. *Journal of Reproductive Medicine* 31, 836–838.

Iwata, Y. & Fletcher, C.D.M. (2004) Distinctive prepubertal vulval fibroma. A hitherto unrecognized mesenchymal tumor of prepubertal girls: analysis of 11 cases. *American Journal of Surgery and Pathology* 28, 1601–1605.

James, G.B., Guthrie, W. & Buchan, A. (1969) Embryonic sarcoma of the vulva in an infant. *Journal of Obstetrics and Gynaecology of the British Commonwealth* 76, 458–461.

Jaramillo, B.A., Gansel, P., Averette, H.E. *et al.* (1985) Malignant melanoma of the vulva. *Obstetrics and Gynecology* 66, 398–401.

Johnson, T.L., Kumar, N.B., White, C.D. & Morley, G.W. (1986) Prognostic features of vulvar melanoma: a clinicopathologic analysis. *International Journal of Gynecological Pathology* 5, 110–118.

Joswig, E.H. & Joswig-Priewe, H. (1974) Retikulumzellsarcom im Bereich der Vulva und Vagina. *Zentralblatt für Gynäkologie* 96, 1040–1043.

Kajiwara, H., Yasuda, M., Yahata, G. *et al.* (2002) Myxoid leiomyoma of the vulva: a case report. *Tokai Journal of Experimental and Clinical Medicine* 27, 57–64

Kaplan, M.A., Jacobson, M.O., Ferry, J.A. & Harris, N.L. (1993) T-cell lymphoma of the vulva in a renal allograft recipient with associated hemophagocytosis. *American Journal of Surgical Pathology* 17, 842–849.

Kaplan, E.G., Chadburn, A. & Caputo, T.A. (1996) HIV-related primary non-Hodgkin's lymphoma of the vulva. *Gynecologic Oncology* 61, 131–138.

Katenkamp, D. & Stiller, D. (1980) Unusual leiomyoma of the vulva with fibroma-like pattern and pseudoelastin formation. *Virchows Archives A, Pathological Anatomy and Histopathology (Berlin)* 388, 361–368.

Katenkamp, D., Kosmehl, M., Mentzel, T. & Reinke, J. (1993) Das Angiomyofibroblastom (AMFB) der Vulva und Paravaginalregion: eine neue Entitat. *Pathologie* 14, 131–137.

Katz, V.L., Askin, F.B. & Bosch, B.D. (1986) Glomus tumor of the vulva: a case report. *Obstetrics and Gynecology* 67, 43s–45s.

Kaufmann-Friedman, K. (1978) Hemangioma of clitoris: confused with adreno-genital-syndrome: a case report. *Plastic and Reconstructive Surgery* 62, 452–454.

Kaufman, R.H. & Gardner, H.L. (1965) Benign mesodermal tumors. *Clinical Obstetrics and Gynecology* 8, 953–981.

Kazmierczak, B., Wanschura, S., Meyer-Bolte, K. *et al.* (1995) Cytogenetic and molecular analysis of an aggressive angiomyxoma. *American Journal of Pathology* 147, 580–585.

Kehagias, D.T., Smymiotis, V.E., Karvounis, E.E. *et al.* (1999) Large lipoma of the vulva. *European Journal of Obstetric and Gynecologic Reproductive Biology* 84, 5–6.

Keller, J. (1951) Fibrosarcoma of labium vulvae. *Canadian Medical Association Journal* 64, 574–576.

Kempinaire, A., De Raeve, I., Rosseeuw, D. *et al.* (1997) Capillary-venous malformation in the labia majora in a 12-year-old girl. *Dermatology* 194, 405–407.

Kenny, F.M., Fetterman, G.H. & Preeyasombat, C. (1966) Neurofibromata simulating a penis and labioscrotal gonads in a girl with von Recklinghausen's disease. *Pediatrics* 37, 956–959.

Kfuri, A., Rosenhein, N., Durfman, H. & Goldstein, P. (1981) Desmoid tumor of the vulva. *Journal of Reproductive Medicine* 26, 272–273.

Kholová, L., Ryska, A. & Dedic, K. (2001) Composite tumor consisting of dermatofibrosarcoma protuberans and giant cell fibroblastoma associated with intratumoral endometriosis. Report of a case. *Pathology Research and Practice* 197, 263–267.

Kohorn, E.I., Merino, M.J. & Goldenhersh, M. (1986) Vulvar pain and dyspareunia due to glomus tumor. *Obstetrics and Gynecology* 67, 41s–42s.

Kondratiev, L.N. & Kurillov, A.L. (1971) Soft tissue alveolar sarcoma of the vulva. *Arkhiv Patologii (Moscow)* 33, 80–82.

Kosari, F., Daneshbod, Y., Parwaresch, R. *et al.* (2005) Lymphomas of the female genital tract: a study of 186 cases and review of the literature. *American Journal of Surgical Pathology* 29, 1512–1520.

Krag-Moller, L.B., Nygaard-Nielsen, M. & Trolle, C. (1990) Leiomyosarcoma vulvae. *Acta Obstetrica et Gynecologica Scandinavica* 68, 187–189.

Kuller, J.A., Zucker, P.K. & Peng, T.C. (1990) Vulvar leiomyosarcoma in pregnancy. *American Journal of Obstetrics and Gynecology* 162, 164–166.

Laartz, B.W., Cooper, C., Degryse, A. & Sinnott, J.T. (2005) Wolf in sheep's clothing: advanced Kaposi sarcoma mimicking vulvar abscess. *Southern Medical Journal* 98, 475–477.

Labardini, M.M., Kallet, H.A. & Cerny, J.C. (1968) Urogenital neurofibromatosis simulating an intersex problem. *Journal of Urology* 98, 627–632.

Lae, M.E., Pereira, P.F., Keeney, G.L. & Nascimento A.G. (2002) Lipoblastoma-like tumour of the vulva: report of three cases of a distinctive mesenchymal neoplasm of adipocytic differentiation. *Histopathology* 40, 505–509.

Lagoo, A.S. & Robboy, S.J. (2006) Lymphoma of the female genital tract: current status. *International Journal of Gynecological Pathology* 25, 1–21.

Lambrou, N.C., Mirhashemi, R., Wolfson, A. *et al.* (2002) Malignant peripheral nerve sheath tumor of the vulva: a multimodal treatment approach. *Gynecologic Oncology* 85, 365–371.

Landthaler, M., Braun-Falco, D., Richter, K. *et al.* (1985) Maligne Melanoma der Vulva. *Deutsche Medizinische Wochenschrift* 110, 789–794.

Lane, J.E., Walker, A.N., Mullis, E.N. Jr *et al.* (2001) Cellular angiofibroma of the vulva. *Gynecological Oncology* 81, 326–329.

Laricchia, R., Wierdis, T., Loiudice, L. *et al.* (1977) Neoformazione vulvare (mieloblastoma) come prima manifestazione di una leucemia acuta mieloblastica. *Minerva Ginecologica* 29, 957–961.

Laskin, W.B., Fetsch, J.F. & Tavasoli, F.A. (1997) Angiomyofibroblastoma of the female genital tract analysis of 17 cases including a lipomatous variant. *Human Pathology* 28, 1046–1055.

Laskin, W.B., Fetsch, J.F. & Mostofi, F.K. (1998) Angiomyofibroblastoma-like tumor of the male genital tract: analysis of 11 cases with comparison to female angiomyofibroblastoma and spindle cell lipoma. *American Journal of Surgical Pathology* 22, 6–16.

Laxmisha, C. & Thappa, D.M. (2007) Granular cell tumor of the clitoris. *Journal of the European Academy of Dermatology and Venereology* 21, 392–393.

Leake, J.F., Buscema, J., Cho, K.R. & Currie, J.L. (1991) Dermatofibrosarcoma protuberans of the vulva. *Gynecologic Oncology* 41, 245–249.

Lenaz, M.P., Nguyen, T.C. & Hewett, W.J. (1987) Leiomyosarcoma of the vulva. *Connecticut Medicine* 51, 705–706.

Levavi, H., Sabah, G., Kaplan, B. *et al.* (2006) Granular cell tumor of the vulva: six new cases. *Archives of Gynecology and Obstetrics* 273, 246–249.

LiVolsi, V.A. & Brooks, J.J. (1987a) Nodular fasciitis of the vulva: a report of two cases. *Obstetrics and Gynecology* 69, 513–516.

LiVolsi, V.A. & Brooks, J.J. (1987b) Soft tissue tumors of the vulva. In: *Pathology of the Vulva and Vagina* (ed. E.J. Wilkinson), pp. 209–238. Churchill Livingstone, New York.

Llaneza, P., Fresno, F. & Ferrer, J. (2002) Schwannoma of the clitoris. *Acta Obstetricia et Gynecologica Scandinavica* 81, 471–472.

Look, K.Y., Roth, L.M. & Sutton, G.P. (1993) Vulvar melanoma reconsidered. *Cancer* 72, 143–146.

Lovelady, S.B., McDonald, J.R. & Waugh, J.M. (1941) Benign tumors of vulva. *American Journal of Obstetrics and Gynecology* 42, 309–313.

Luzar, B., Neill, S. & Calonje, E. (2009) Vulvar angiokeratoma in association with lichen sclerosus. *Journal of Cutaneous Pathology*, in press.

Maglione, M.A., Tricarico, O.D. & Calandria, L. (2002) Malignant peripheral nerve sheath tumor of the vulva. A case report. *Journal of Reproductive Medicine* 47, 721–724.

Majmudar, B., Castellano, P.Z., Wilson, R.W. & Siegel, R.J. (1990) Granular cell tumors of the vulva. *Journal of Reproductive Medicine* 35, 1008–1014.

Makino, E., Uchida, T., Matsushita, Y. *et al.* (2007) Melanocytic nevi clinically simulating melanoma. *Journal of Dermatology* 34, 52–55.

Mandai, K., Moriwaki, S. & Motoi, M. (1990) Aggressive angiomyxoma of the vulva: report of a case. *Acta Pathologica Japonica* 40, 927–934.

Manson, C.M., Hirsch, P.J. & Coyne, J.D. (1995) Post-operative spindle cell nodule of the vulva. *Histopathology* 26, 571–574.

McCluggage, W.G., Perenyei, M. & Irwin, S.T. (2002) Recurrent cellular angiofibroma of the vulva. *Journal of Clinical Pathology* 55, 477–479.

McCluggage, W.G., Jamieson, T., Dobbs, S.P. & Grey, A. (2006) Aggressive angiomyxoma of the vulva: dramatic response to gonadotropin-releasing hormone agonist therapy. *Gynecologic Oncology* 100, 623–625.

McCluggage, W.G., Sumathi, V.P., Nucci, M.R. *et al.* (2007) Ewing family of tumours involving the vulva and vagina: report of a series of four cases. *Journal of Clinical Pathology* 60, 674–680.

Medeiros, F., Erickson-Johnson, M.R., Keeney, G.L. *et al.* (2007) Frequency and characterization of HMGA2 and HMGA1 rearrangements in mesenchymal tumours of the lower genital tract. *Genes Chromosomes and Cancer* 46, 981–990.

Messina, A.M. & Strauss, R.G. (1976) Pelvic neurofibromatosis. *Obstetrics and Gynecology* 47, 63s–66s.

Micci, F., Texeira, M.R., Scheistroen, M. *et al.* (2003) Cytogenetic characterization of tumors of the vulva and vagina. *Genes Chromosomes and Cancer* 38, 137–148.

Micci, F., Haugum, L., Abeler, V.M. *et al.* (2007) Trisomy 7 in postoperative spindle cell nodule. *Cancer Genetics and Cytogenetics* 174, 147–150.

Migliorini, A. & Amato, A. (1978) In tema de patologia neoplastica della vulva: rara caso di neurinoma del clitoride. *Minerva Ginecologica* 30, 543–545.

Miller, G.C. (1979) Neurofibromatosis affecting the vulva: case report. *Military Medicine* 144, 542–543.

Morrow, C.P. (1981) Melanoma of the female genital tract. In: *Gynaecologic Oncology* (ed. M. Coppleston), pp. 784–793. Churchill Livingstone, Edinburgh.

Morrow, C.P. & DiSaia, P.J. (1976) Malignant melanoma of the female genitalia: a clinical analysis. *Obstetrical and Gynecological Survey* 31, 233–271.

Morrow, C.P. & Rutledge, F.N. (1972) Melanoma of the vulva. *Obstetrics and Gynecology* 39, 745–752.

Motegi, S., Tamura, A., Okada, E., *et al.* (2007) Successful treatment with lymphaticovenular anastomosis for secondary skin lesions of chronic lymphedema. *Dermatology* 215, 147–151.

Muram, D. & Gold, S.S. (1993) Vulvar ulceration in girls with myelocytic leukemia. *Southern Medical Journal* 86, 293–294.

Murcia, J.M., Idoate, M., Laparte, C. & Baldonado, C. (1994) Granular cell tumor of vulva on episiotomy scar. *Gynecological Oncology* 53, 248–250.

Nascimento, A.F. & Fletcher, C.D. (2005) Spindle cell rhabdomyosarcoma in adults. *American Journal of Surgery and Pathology* 29, 1106–1113.

Neri, A., Peled, Y. & Braslavski, D. (1993) Vulvar leiomyoma. *Acta Obstetricia et Gynecologica Scandinavica* 72, 221–222.

Newman, P.L. & Fletcher, C.D.M. (1991) Smooth muscle tumours of the external genitalia: a clinicopathological analysis of a series. *Histopathology* 18, 523–529.

Nielsen, G.P., Rosenberg, A.E., Koerner, F.C. *et al.* (1996a) Smooth muscle tumors of the vulva: a clinicopathological study of 25 cases and review of the literature. *American Journal of Surgical Pathology* 20, 779–793.

Nielsen, G.P., Rosenberg, A.E., Young, R.H. *et al.* (1996b) Angiomyofibroblastoma of the vulva and vagina. *Modern Pathology* 9, 284–291.

Nielsen, G.P., Young, R.H., Dickersin, G.R. *et al.* (1997) Angiomyofibroblastoma of the vulva with sarcomatous transformation ('angiomyofibrosarcoma'). *American Journal of Surgical Pathology* 21, 1104–1108.

Nirenberg, A., Ostor, A.G., Slavin, J. *et al.* (1995) Primary vulvar sarcomas. *International Journal of Gynecological Pathology* 14, 55–62.

Nucci, M.R. & Fletcher, C.D.M. (1998) Liposarcoma (atypical lipomatous tumors) of the vulva: a clinicopathologic study of six cases. *International Journal of Gynecological Pathology* **17**, 17–23.

Nucci, M.R., Granter, S.R. & Fletcher, C.D. (1997) Cellular angiofibroma: a benign neoplasm distinct from angiomyofibroblastoma and spindle cell lipoma. *American Journal of Surgical Pathology* **21**, 636–644.

Nucci, M.R., Weremowicz, S., Neskey, D.M. *et al.* (2001) Chromosomal translocation t(8;12) induces aberrant HMGIC expression in aggressive angiomyxoma of the vulva. *Genes Chromosomes and Cancer* **32**: 172–176.

O'Connell, J.X., Young, R.H., Nielsen, G.P. *et al.* (1997) Nodular fasciitis of the vulva: a study of six cases and literature review. *International Journal of Gynecological Pathology* **16**, 117–123.

O'Goshi, K., Terui, T. & Tagami, H. (2001) Dowling-Degos disease affecting the vulva. *Acta Dermato-venereologica* **81**, 148.

Opie, J.M., Chow CW., Ditchfield M. & Bekhor, P.S. (2006) Segmental haemangioma of the lower limb with skeletal overgrowth. *Australian Journal of Dermatology* **47**, 198–203.

Pack, G.T. & Oropeza, R.A. (1967) A comparative study of melanoma and epidermoid carcinoma of the vulva: a review of 44 melanomas and 58 epidermoid carcinomas (1930–1965). *Reviews in Surgery* **24**, 305–324.

Palermino, D.A. (1964) Leiomyoma of the vulva: report of a case. *Obstetrics and Gynecology* **24**, 301–302.

Pandhi, R.K., Beci, T.R. & Dhawar, I.K. (1975) Leiomyosarcoma of the labium majus with extensive metastases. *Dermatologica* **150**, 70–74.

Pandolfino, T.L., Cotell, S. & Katta, R. (2001) Pigmented vulval macules as a presenting feature of the Carney complex. *International Journal of Dermatology* **40**, 728–730.

Patel, S., Kapadia, A., Desai, A. & Dave, K.S. (1993) Leiomyosarcoma of the vulva. *European Journal of Gynaecologic Oncology* **14**, 406–407.

Phillips, G.L., Twiggs, L.B. & Okagaki, T. (1982) Vulvar melanoma: a microstaging study. *Gynecological Oncology* **14**, 80–88.

Pierson, K.K. (1987) Malignant melanomas and pigmented lesions of the vulva. In: *Pathology of the Vulva and Vagina* (ed. E.J. Wilkinson), pp. 155–179. Churchill Livingstone, New York.

Piura, B., Egan, M., Lopes, A. & Monaghan, J.M. (1992) Malignant melanoma of the vulva: a clinicopathologic study of 18 cases. *Journal of Surgical Oncology* **50**, 234–240.

Piver, M.S., Tsukada, Y. & Barlow, J. (1972) Epithelioid sarcoma of the vulva. *Obstetrics and Gynecology* **40**, 839–842.

Podratz, K.C., Gaffey, T.A., Symmonds, R.E. *et al.* (1983) Melanoma of the vulva: an update. *Gynecologic Oncology* **16**, 153–168.

Proppe, K.H., Scully, R.E. & Rosai, J. (1984) Postoperative spindle cell nodules of the genitourinary tract resembling sarcomas: a report of eight cases. *American Journal of Surgical Pathology* **8**, 101–108.

Raber, G., Mempel, V., Jackish, C. *et al.* (1996) Malignant melanoma of the vulva. Report of 89 patients. *Cancer* **78**, 2353–2358.

Ragnarsson-Olding, B., Johansson, H., Rutqvist, L.E. & Ringborg, U. (1993) Malignant melanoma of the vulva and vagina: trends in incidence and distribution, and long term survival among 245 consecutive cases in Sweden 1960–1984. *Cancer* **71**, 1893–1897.

Ragnarsson-Olding, B.K., Kanter-Lewensohn, L.R., Lagerlof, B. *et al.* (1999) Malignant melanoma of the vulva in a nation wide, 25-year study of 219 Swedish females: clinical observations and histopathologic features. *Cancer* **86**, 1273–1293.

Rajah, S.B., Moodley, J., Pudifin, D.J. *et al.* (1990) Kaposi's sarcoma associated with acquired immunodeficiency syndrome presenting as a vulval papilloma. *South African Medical Journal* **77**, 585–586.

Raju, G.C. & Naraynsingh, V. (1987) Granular cell tumours of the vulva. *Australian and New Zealand Journal of Obstetrics and Gynaecology* **27**, 349–352.

Ramos, P.C., Kapp, D.S., Longacre, T.A. & Teng, N.N. (2000) Malignant granular cell tumor of vulva in a 17-year-old: case report and literature review. *International Journal of Gynecologic Cancer* **10**, 429–434.

Raspagliesi, F., Ditto, A., Paladini, D. *et al.* (2000) Prognostic indicators in melanoma of the vulva. *Annals of Surgical Oncology* **7**, 738–742.

Ravikumar, V.R. & Lakshmanan, D. (1983) A solitary neurofibroma of the clitoris masquerading as an intersex. *Journal of Pediatric Surgery* **18**, 617.

Reis-Filho, J.S., Milanezi, F., Soares, M.F. *et al.* (2002) Intradermal spindle cell/pleomorphic lipoma of the vulva: case report and review of the literature. *Journal of Cutaneous Pathology* **29**, 59–62.

Roberts, W. & Daly, J.W. (1981) Pseudosarcomatous fasciitis of the vulva. *Gynecologic Oncology* **11**, 383–386.

Robertson, A.J., McIntosh, W., Lamont, P. & Guthrie, W. (1981) Malignant granular cell tumour (myoblastoma) of the vulva: a report of a case and review of the literature. *Histopathology* **5**, 69–79.

Rock, B., Hood, A.F. & Rock, J.A. (1990) Prospective study of vulvar nevi. *Journal of the American Academy of Dermatology* **22**, 104–106.

Rollason, T.P. (1992) Malignant melanoma and related lesions of the lower female genital tract. In: *Advances in Gynaecological Pathology* (eds D. Lowe & H. Fox), pp. 119–143. Churchill Livingstone, Edinburgh.

Rose, P.G., Piver, M.S., Tsukada, Y. & Lau, T. (1988) Conservative therapy for melanoma of the vulva. *American Journal of Obstetrics and Gynecology* **159**, 52–55.

Roy, K.K., Agarwal, R., Agarwal, S. *et al.* (2006) Recurrent vulval congenital lymphangioma circumscriptum: a case report and literature review. *International Journal of Gynecological Cancer* **16**, 930–934.

Sah, S.P., Yadav, R. & Rani, S. (2001) Lymphangioma circumscriptum of the vulva mimicking genital wart: a case report and review of literature. *Journal of Obstetrics and Gynaecology Research* **27**, 293–296.

Salm, R. & Evans, D.J. (1985) Myxoid leiomyosarcoma. *Histopathology* **9**, 159–169.

Santala, M., Suonio, S., Syrjanen, K. *et al.* (1987) Malignant fibrous histiocytoma of the vulva. *Gynecologic Oncology* **27**, 121–126.

Santos, L.D., Currie, B.G. & Killingsworth, M.C. (2001) Case report: plexiform schwannoma of the vulva. *Pathology* **33**, 526–531.

Scheistroen, M., Trope, C., Kaern, J. *et al.* (1995) Malignant melanoma of the vulva: evaluation of prognostic factors with emphasis on DNA plody in 75 patients. *Cancer* **75**, 72–80.

Scheistroen, M., Trope, C., Kaern, J. *et al.* (1996) Malignant melanoma of the vulva FIGO stage I: evaluation of prognostic factors in 43 patients with emphasis on DNA ploidy and surgical treatment. *Gynecologic Oncology* **61**, 253–258.

Schepel, S.J. & Tolhurst, D.E. (1981) Neurofibromata of clitoris and labium majus simulating a penis and testicle. *British Journal of Plastic Surgery* **34**, 221–223.

Schiller, H.M. & Madge, G.E. (1970) Reticulum cell sarcoma presenting as a vulvar lesion. *Southern Medical Journal* **63**, 471–472.

Schmidt, O., Fleckenstein, G.H., Gunawan. B. *et al.* (2003) Recurrence and rapid metastasis formation of a granular cell tumor of the vulva. *European Journal of Obstetrics, Gynecology and Reproductive Biology* 106, 219–221.

Shen, T.-J., D'Ablaing, G. & Morrow, C.P. (1982) Alveolar soft part sarcoma of the vulva: report of first case and review of literature. *Gynecologic Oncology* 13, 120–128.

Siassi, R.M., Papadopoulos, T. & Matzel, K.E. (1999) Metastasizing aggressive angiomyxoma. *New England Journal of Medicine* 341, 1772.

Siegle, J.C. & Cartmell, L. (1995) Vulvar leiomyoma associated with estrogen/progestin therapy: a case report. *Journal of Reproductive Medicine* 40, 58–59.

Silvers, D.H. & Halperin, A.J. (1978) Cutaneous and vulvar melanoma: an update. *Clinical Obstetrics and Gynecology* 21, 1117–1118.

Simo, M., Zapata, C., Esquius, J. & Domingo, J. (1992) Aggressive angiomyxoma of the female pelvis and perineum: report of two cases and review of the literature. *British Journal of Obstetrics and Gynaecology* 99, 925–927.

Skalova, A., Michal, M., Husek, K. *et al.* (1993) Aggressive angiomyxoma of the pelvioperoneal region: immunohistological and ultrastructural study of seven cases. *American Journal of Dermatopathology* 15, 446–451.

Smith, H., Genesen, M.C. & Feddersen, R.M. (1999) Dermal lymphangiomata of the vulva and laser therapy: a case report and literature review. *European Journal of Gynaecological Oncology* 20, 373–378.

Smith, B.L., Chu, P. & Weinberg, J.M. (2004) Angiokeratoma of the vulva: possible association with radiotherapy. *Skinmed* 3, 171–172.

Soergel, T.M., Doering, D.L. & O'Connor, D. (1998) Metastatic dermatofibrosarcoma of the vulva. *Gynecologic Oncology* 71, 320–324.

Soltan, M.H. (1981) Dermatofibrosarcoma protuberans of the vulva. *British Journal of Obstetrics and Gynaecology* 88, 203–205.

Sonobe, H., Ro, J.Y., Ramos, M. *et al.* (1994) Glomus tumor of the female external genitalia: a report of two cases. *International Journal of Gynecological Pathology* 13, 359–364.

Stang, A., Streller, B., Eisinger, B. & Jöckel, K.H. (2005) Population-based incidence rates of malignant melanoma of the vulva in Germany. *Gynecologic Oncology* 96, 216–221.

Steeper, T. & Rosai, J. (1983) Aggressive angiomyxoma of the female pelvis and perineum. *American Journal of Surgical Pathology* 7, 463–476.

Stenchever, M.A., McDivett, R.W. & Fisher, J.A. (1973) Leiomyoma of the clitoris. *Journal of Reproductive Medicine* 2, 75–76.

Strayer, S.A., Yum, M.N. & Sutton, G.P. (1992) Epithelioid hemangioendothelioma of the clitoris: a case report with immunohistochemical and ultrastructural findings. *International Journal of Gynecological Pathology* 11, 234–239.

Sutphen, R., Galan-Gomez, E. & Kousseff, B.G. (1995) Clitoromegaly in neurofibromatosis. *American Journal of Medical Genetics* 55, 325–330.

Takeshima, Y., Shinkoh, Y. & Inai, K. (1998) Angiomyofibroblastoma of the vulva: a mitotically active variant? *Pathology International* 48, 292–296.

Takeshima, N., Tabata, T., Nishida, H. *et al.* (2001) Peripheral primitive neuroectodermal tumor of the vulva: report of a case with imprint cytology. *Acta Cytologica* 45, 1049–1052.

Talerman, A. (1973) Sarcoma botyroides presenting as a polyp on the labium majus. *Cancer* 32, 994–999.

Tan, G.W., Lim-Tan, S.K. & Salmon, Y.M. (1989) Epithelioid sarcoma of the vulva. *Singapore Medical Journal* 30, 308–310.

Tasseron, E.W., van der Esch, E.P., Hart, A.A. *et al.* (1992) A clinicopathological study of 30 melanomas of the vulva. *Gynecologic Oncology* 46, 170–175.

Taussig, F.J. (1937) Sarcoma of the vulva. *American Journal of Obstetrics and Gynecology* 33, 1017–1026.

Tavassoli, F.A. & Norris, H.J. (1979) Smooth muscle tumors of the vulva. *Obstetrics and Gynecology* 53, 213–217.

Taylor, R.N., Bottles, K. & Miler, T.R. (1985) Malignant fibrous histiocytoma of the vulva. *Obstetrics and Gynecology* 66, 145–148.

Terada, K.Y., Schmidt, R.W. & Roberts, J.A. (1988) Malignant Schwannoma of the vulva: a case report. *Journal of Reproductive Medicine* 33, 969–972.

Tjalma, W.A. & Colpaert, C.O. (2005) Myxoid leiomyosarcoma of the vulva. *Gynecologic Oncology* 96, 548–551.

Toti, R., Danti, M. & Fruscella, L. (1995) Angiomiofibroblastoma della vulva: presentazione di un caso clinico. *Minerva Ginecologica* 47, 51–53.

Traen, K., Logghe, H., Maertens, J. *et al.* (2004) Endodermal sinus of the vulva: successfully treated with high-dose chemotherapy. *International Journal of Gynecological Cancer* 14, 998–1003.

Trimble, E.L., Lewis, J.L., Jr, Williams, E.L. *et al.* (1992) Management of vulvar melanomas. *Gynecologic Oncology* 45, 254–258.

Tsuji, T., Yoshinaga, M., Inomoto, Y. *et al.* (2007) Aggressive angiomyxoma of the vulva with a sole t(5;8)(p15;q22) chromosome change. *International Journal of Gynecological Pathology* 26, 494–496.

Uhlin, S.R. (1980) Angiokeratoma of the vulva. *Archives of Dermatology* 116, 112–113.

Ulbright, T.M., Brokaw, S.A., Stehman, F.B. & Roth, L.M. (1983) Epithelioid sarcoma of the vulva: evidence suggesting a more aggressive behaviour than extra-genital epithelioid sarcoma. *Cancer* 52, 1462–1469.

Ungerleider, R.S., Donaldson, S.S., Warnke, R.A. & Wilbur, J.R. (1978) Endodermal sinus tumor: the Stanford experience and the first reported case arising in the vulva. *Cancer* 41, 1627–1634.

Vang, R., Taubenberger, J.K., Mannion, C.M. *et al.* (2000a) Primary vulvar and vaginal extraosseus Ewing's sarcoma/peripheral neuroectodermal tumor: diagnostic confirmation with CD99 immunostaining and reverse transcriptase-polymerase chain reaction. *International Journal of Gynecological Pathology* 19, 103–109.

Vang, R., Medeiros, L.J., Malpica, A. *et al.* (2000b) Non-Hodgkin's lymphoma involving the vulva. *International Journal of Gynecological Pathology* 19, 236–242.

Van Glabeke, E., Audry, G., Hervet, F. *et al.* (1999) Lipoma of the preputium clitoridis in neonate: an exceptional abnormality different from ambiguous genitalia. *Pediatric Surgery International* 15, 147–8.

Vanni, R., Faa, G., Detton, T. *et al.* (2000) A case of dermatofibrosarcoma protuberans of the vulva with a COL1A1/PDGFB fusion identical to a case of giant cell fibroblastoma. *Virchows Archives* 437, 95–100.

Venter, P.F., Rohm, G.F. & Slabber, C.F. (1981) Giant neurofibromas of the labia. *Obstetrics and Gynecology* 57, 128–130.

Verschraegen, C.F., Benjapibal, M., Supakarapongkul, W. *et al.* (2001) Vulvar melanoma at the M.D. Anderson Cancer Center: 25 years later. *International Journal of Gynecological Cancer* 11, 359–364.

Vlastos, A.T., Malpica, A. & Follen, M. C. (2003) Lymphangioma circumscriptum of the vulva: a review of the literature. *Obstetrics and Gynecology* 101, 946–954.

Wechter, M.E., Gruber, S.B., Haefner, H.K. *et al.* (2004) Vulvar melanoma: a report of 20 cases and review of the literature. *Journal of the American Academy of Dermatology* **50**, 554–562.

Wesche, N.A., Fletcher, C.D.M., Dias, P. *et al.* (1995) Immuno-histochemistry of MyoD1 in adult pleomorphic soft tissue sarcomas. *American Journal of Surgical Pathology* **19**, 261–269.

Williams N.P., Williams E. & Fletcher H. (2002) Smooth muscle tumours of the vulva in Jamaica. *West Indian Medical Journal* **51**, 228–231.

Wishart, J. (1973) Reticulosarcoma of the vulva complicating azathio-prine-treated dermatomyositis. *Archives of Dermatology* **108**, 563–564.

Wolber, R.A., Talerman, A., Wilkinson, E.J. & Clement, P.B. (1991) Vulvar granular cell tumors with pseudocarcinomatous hyperplasia: a comparative analysis with well-differentiated squamous carcinoma. *International Journal of Gynecological Pathology* **10**, 59–66.

Woodruff, J.D. & Brack, C.B. (1958) Unusual malignancies of the vulvo-urethral region: a report of twelve cases. *Obstetrics and Gynecology* **12**, 677–686.

Woolcot, R.J., Henry, R.J.W. & Houghton, C.R.S. (1988) Malignant melanoma of the vulva: Australian experience. *Journal of Reproductive Medicine* **33**, 699–702.

Yamashita, Y., Yamada, T., Ueki, K. *et al.* (1996) A case of vulvar schwannoma. *Journal of Obstetrics and Gynaecology* **22**, 31–34.

Yamazaki, M., Hiruma, M., Trie, H. & Ishibashi, A. (1992) Angiokeratoma of the clitoris: a subtype of angiokeratoma vulvae. *Journal of Dermatology* **19**, 553–555.

Yegane, R.A., Alaee, M.S. & Khanicheh E. (2008) Congenital plexi-form schwannoma of the clitoris. *Saudi Medical Journal* **29**, 600–602.

Yigiter, M., Arda, I.S., Tosun, E. *et al.* (2008) Angiokeratoma of the clitoris: a rare lesion in an adolescent girl. *Urology* **71**, 604–606.

Yildiz, F., Atahan, I.L., Ozyar, E. *et al.* (2008) Radiotherapy in congen-ital vulvar lymphangioma circumscriptum. *International Journal of Gynecological Cancer* **18**, 556–559.

Yüksel, H., Odabasi, A.R., Kafkas, S. *et al.* (2003) Clitoromegaly in type 2 neurofibromatosis: a case report and review of the literature. *European Journal of Gynaecological Oncology* **24**, 447–451.

Zahn, C.M., Kendall, B.S. & Liang, C.Y. (2001) Spindle cell lipoma of the female genital tract. A report of two cases. *Journal of Reproductive Medicine* **46**, 769–772.

Zhou J., Ha B.K., Schubeck D. & Chung-Park M. (2006) Myxoid epithelioid leiomyoma of the vulva: a case report. *Gynecological Oncology* **103**, 342–345.

Ziegler, J.L. & Katongole-Mbidde, E. (1996) Kaposi's sarcoma in childhood: an analysis of 100 cases from Uganda and relationship to HIV infection. *International Journal of Cancer* **65**, 200–203.

Chapter 10: Surgical procedures in benign vulval disease

B.J. Paniel & R. Rouzier

Introduction

A wide range of clinical conditions can affect the vulva, including both congenital and acquired abnormalities. Severe congenital abnormalities may be corrected as soon as possible. Variations of the normal vulval anatomy, such as hypertrophy of the labia minora, may require correction to improve self-confidence and quality of life. Acquired abnormalities are the consequence of trauma or scarring dermatoses and require specific management to restore the integrity and function of the vulva.

Female pseudohermaphroditism

The commonest cause of female pseudohermaphroditism is congenital adrenal hyperplasia. Female pseudohermaphroditism is a condition characterized by various degrees of virilization of the external genitalia in a patient with female internal genitalia and karyotype (XX). These children should always be reared as a female because if the uterus, tubes and ovaries are present they can become fertile women and bear children later in life. A five-stage classification by Prader (1954) is used to represent different degrees of virilization, where on a scale of 1 to 5 (I–V) the genitalia can be scored from slightly virilized (e.g. mildly enlarged clitoris) to indistinguishable from a male. Most classical cases of children with 21-hydroxylase deficiency are born with Prader IV genitalia.

The rationale for early reconstruction includes avoiding complications from anatomic anomalies, satisfactory outcomes, minimizing family concern and distress, and decreasing the risks of stigmatization and gender-identity confusion of atypical genital appearance (Houk et al. 2006). Adverse outcomes have led experts to recommend a delay in genital surgery to an age when patients themselves can

Ridley's The Vulva, 3rd edition. Edited by Sallie M. Neill and Fiona M. Lewis. © 2009 Blackwell Publishing, ISBN: 978-1-4051-6813-7.

give consent. Age-specific preparatory procedures, including coping-skill training and behaviour therapy, are psychologically beneficial. The goals of genital surgery are to maximize anatomy to enhance sexual function and partnering.

Feminizing genital surgery involves reconstruction of the external genitalia and exteriorization of the vagina, with early separation of the vagina and urethra. Clitoral reduction may be considered in cases of severe virilization. Vaginal dilatation is not recommended during childhood. Refinement or improvement is generally necessary at puberty. Procedures should emphasize functional cosmetic appearance and be designed to preserve erectile function and innervation. Vaginoplasty should be performed in the teenage years; each of the techniques (self-dilatation, skin or bowel substitution) has specific advantages and disadvantages, and all carry potential for scarring that would require modification before sexual function.

The operation is performed in two stages. The first stage is a perineoplasty, which is done to open up the vulva and vagina. The simplest perineotomy consists of separating the adherent labia majora in the midline. This operation is suitable for Prader stages II and III (Prader 1954) in which the urogenital sinus is close to the perineal skin (Fig. 10.1a–c). Normal childbirth may be possible later. A V–Y plastic operation (Fortunoff et al. 1964) can be used for Prader stages III and IV in which the urogenital sinus is situated deep inside. An inverted U-shaped incision is made as shown in Fig. 10.2a, which is then undermined to free a flap (Fig. 10.2b). A perineotomy is extended as a midline incision to the posterior vaginal wall. The flap that is created is then used to fill the defect (Fig. 10.2c). Normal vaginal delivery in the future may be possible, but a caesarean section is often preferred so that the good cosmetic result of the procedure can be preserved. A transperineal operation has been described by Hendren (1977), which is done to bring the vagina down. It is reserved for those rare patients who are highly masculinized and when the vagina opens into the urethra.

The second stage is the reduction of the clitoral hypertrophy. There are numerous procedures that have been

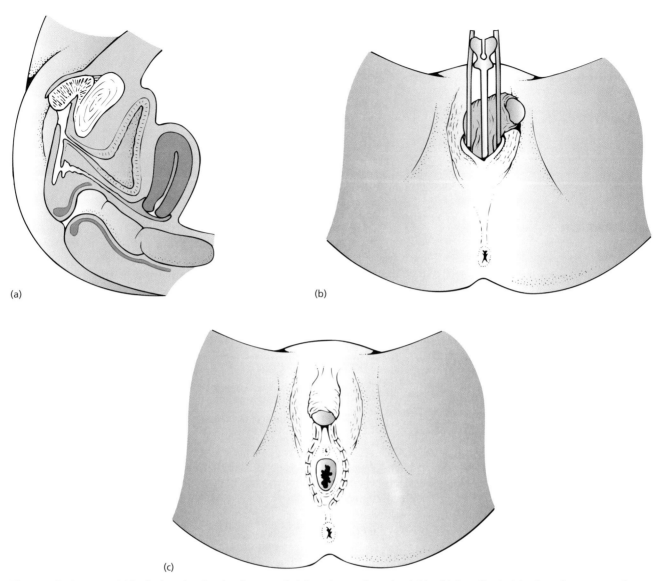

(a)

(b)

(c)

Fig. 10.1 Perineotomy. (a) Sagittal section showing the urogenital sinus close to the perineal skin. (b) A median incision is made to open up the sinus. (c) Mucocutaneous suture after sinus has been opened.

described including excision, embedding or excision with a ventral or a dorsal flap. The most satisfactory procedure (Ferry *et al.* 1977) consists of freeing the clitoris from its dorsal and ventral attachments and then resecting the inferior two-thirds of the corpora cavernosa preserving the dorsal vasculoneural bundle. The preservation of dorsal neurovascular bundles and ventral urogenital cutaneous pedicles is important for an optimal aesthetic and functional result of clitoroplasties (Papageorgiou *et al.* 2000). The cavernosa arteries are clamped and sutured; after a cuneiform resection, the glans clitoris is attached to the symphysis pubis and the preserved clitoral hood is lowered and used to cover the raw surfaces and to refashion the labia minora. A medial incision is made 1 month later to divide the large clitoral hood into two labia minora.

Male pseudohermaphroditism

Male pseudohermaphroditism is defined broadly as incomplete masculinization of the external genitalia in a male (46XY) karyotype. The appearance of the external genitalia in these patients depends on the cause, and ranges from mild hypospadias with some clitoral hypertrophy to a completely female phenotype. Male pseudohermaphroditism can be caused by one of many defects, but mainly by a defect in testosterone synthesis. In the case of male pseudohermaphroditism when the sex assignment is going to be female, the feminizing genitoplasty is similar to that described for female pseudohermaphroditism, but in addition an artificial vagina has to be constructed either by instrumental dilatation of the vaginal dimple according to

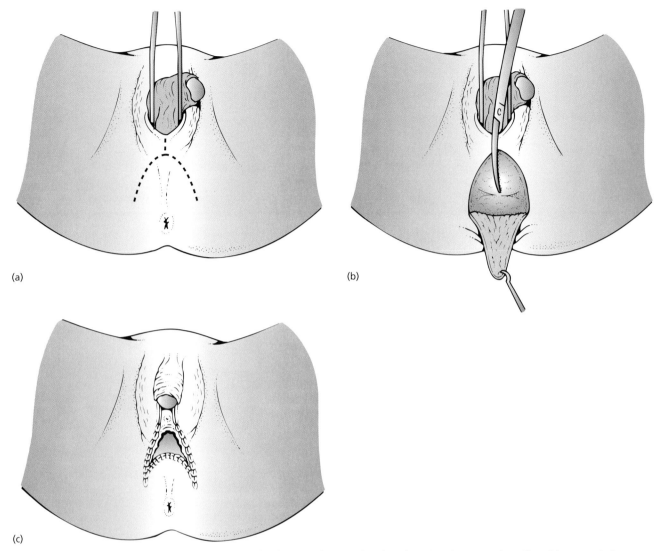

(a)

(b)

(c)

Fig. 10.2 Posterior cutaneous flap. (a) Urogenital sinus deeply situated: inverted U-shaped incision. Apex near the orifice of the urogenital sinus base near the anal margin. (b) Dissection of the perineal cutaneous flap followed by a median perineotomy. (c) The flap is used to fill the triangular defect.

Frank's method (Frank 1938) or by surgical means. The testes need to be removed because of the risk of malignant changes later in life. Nowadays, laparoscopy allows the straightforward identification and removal of gonads. All abnormal ductal structures must be removed as this increases the chance of resecting unidentified gonads. Genitoplasty, according to the social sex, can be performed in the same procedure (Dénes *et al.* 2005).

Bladder exstrophy

Bladder exstrophy is a complex anomaly involving the urinary, genital and intestinal tracts and the musculoskeletal system. Management of bladder exstrophy presents several challenges, beginning with initial repair using the more conventional staged approach or the recently repopularized complete primary repair technique. Major goals in the management of bladder exstrophy are preservation of normal kidney function, close observation for development of adequate bladder function including urinary continence, and provision of acceptable cosmesis and function of the external genitalia. Bladder exstrophy occurs predominantly in females. The vulva has a characteristic appearance where the mons pubis is flattened or depressed, both the labia minora and majora diverge, and the clitoris is bifid. At puberty the growth of pubic hair is split into two halves that extend out towards the inguinal area. A medial perineotomy is done to widen the narrowed introitus. This correction will allow future sexual intercourse. Unfortunately, the

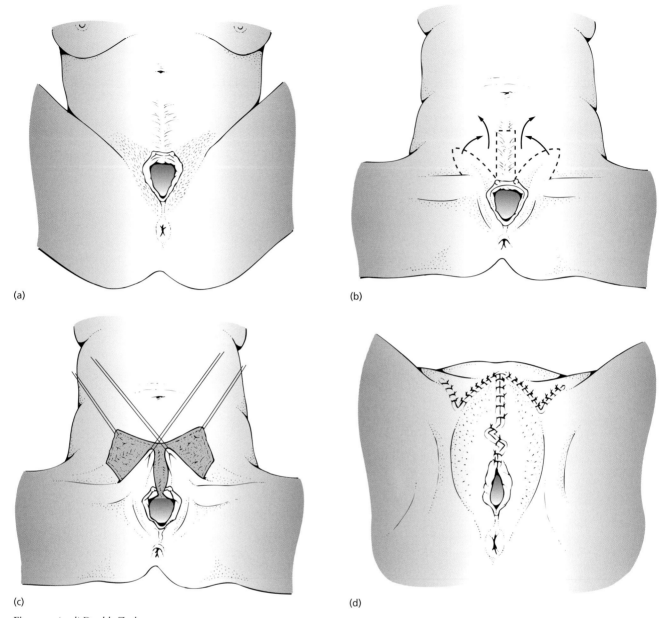

(a)

(b)

(c)

(d)

Fig. 10.3 (a–d) Double Z-plasty.

procedure may be complicated by genital prolapse. A simple clitoridoplasty brings together the divided clitoris. A double Z-plasty (Erich 1959), however, gives a result that looks more like a normal vulva. In this procedure (Fig. 10.3a–d) two inguinal triangular flaps covered with hair are exchanged with two medial hairless triangular flaps; the hair-bearing mons pubis is thus reconstructed and the vulva closed.

Labia minora hypertrophy

Hypertrophy of the labia minora is not a congenital malformation but a developmental anomaly. It is never seen in prepubertal girls, in whom the labia minora are tiny or not developed. The abnormality may be uni- or bilateral, symmetrical or asymmetrical and of varying degrees. It is usually asymptomatic, but sometimes there is a complaint of irritation particularly with exercise and later in life the enlargement may interfere with sexual intercourse. However, the majority of patients complain for cosmetic reasons. In a series of 163 patients requesting reduction of the labia minora, the reasons for requesting surgery were aesthetic concerns (87%), discomfort with clothing (64%), discomfort with exercise (26%) and entry dyspareunia (43%) (Rouzier et al. 2000). Labial reduction can be achieved by one of three procedures as outlined below.

Complete nymphectomy

The labia minora are spread out but not stretched. An incision is made on the outer surface from the point where the labium minus divides to encircle the clitoris. The line of the incision runs along the interlabial sulcus and ends where the labium minus merges into the inner aspect of the labium majus ending before the posterior lateral labial commissure. The incision on the inner aspect of the labium minus matches that already made on the outside border and is down to the level of Hart's line or slightly higher than the level on the opposite edge to enable eversion of the final suture. The labium minus is then amputated by joining the two incisions and cutting across the vascular fibroelastic body of the labium minus (Fig. 10.4a–d). The incision is completed either with a scalpel or scissors. Haemostasis is achieved to avoid a haematoma. The free edges are sutured with 3.0 or 4.0 absorbable suture with interrupted or running stitches. Any remaining stitches are removed 15 days later and the patients are warned that they will initially experience transient sensations produced by the inner surface of the labia majora in apposition.

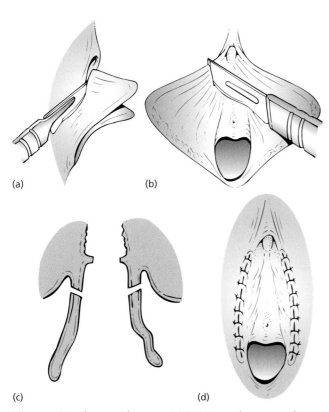

Fig. 10.4 Complete nymphectomy. (a) Incision on the outer surface; (b) incision on the inner aspect; (c) incision is slightly higher than the level on the opposite edge to enable eversion of the primal suture; (d) suturing of edges.

Subtotal nymphectomy

This procedure was first described by Hodgkinson and Hait (1984). The incision starts at the glans clitoris just below where the labia minora divide and finishes where the labia minora merge into the tissue a little way from the fourchette. This curved incision leaves a labium minus that has a maximum breadth of 1 cm, and a free edge that is pink and not pigmented. However, in normal women with small labia minora the free borders of the labia are very often not pigmented. The labia are sutured with interrupted stitches or by oversewing with colourless absorbable thread 4.0. There is no special postoperative care required.

Reduction nymphoplasty

This procedure results in the most natural-looking labia minora in that the resulting free edges of the labia minora are pigmented, which more closely resembles the normal. In addition, there is preservation of the two main functions of the labia minora, i.e. first to provide a lubricated smooth surface to facilitate intercourse and second to protect the inner aspects of the vulva by virtue of their natural apposition (Paniel *et al.* 1985).

Each labium minus is laid out but not stretched and a pair of Kocher forceps is placed along the length and the base of the labium minus near the interlabial sulcus. Another pair is placed at an angle of approximately 90° to the first pair, demarcating two labial segments, which should be of identical dimensions in order to avoid any asymmetry (Fig. 10.5a). Each labial segment may have a base smaller than its length because of its rich blood supply. After incising along the forceps with the scalpel, haemostasis is achieved using coagulating forceps (Fig. 10.5b). The superior labial segment is gently spread out and the edges are joined by one or two stitches at exactly the same levels, without trying to cover the entire raw edge, in order to avoid unwanted tension. The segments are sutured in three planes by fine stitches using 4.0 thread (Fig. 10.5c). A buried running stitch joins the fibroelastic body of the minora. A running suture or separate sutures ensure approximation of the outer and inner edges. Inevitably, there is a formation of dog-ears, which can be resected or may be left to flatten out with time. Postoperative care consists of simple cleansing twice daily. Any residual stitches are removed 3 weeks later, under local anaesthetic if necessary.

Other procedures have been described including wedge nymphectomy with or without a 90° Z-plasty (Alter 1998, Giraldo *et al.* 2004, Munhoz *et al.* 2006), and de-epithelialized reduction of labiaplasty (Choi & Kim 2000).

Vulval trauma

There are various causes of vulval trauma.

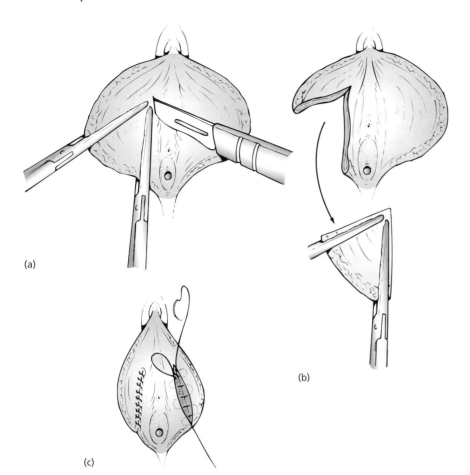

(a)

(b)

(c)

Fig. 10.5 Reduction nymphoplasty. (a) Two pairs of Kocher forceps are placed demarcating the labial segment to be excised. (b) Excision of the large inferior segment. (c) Suture of the smaller anterior segment in three planes.

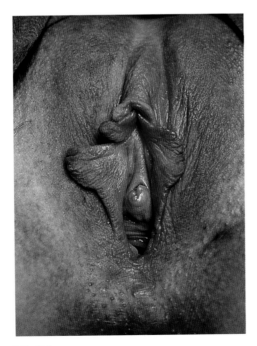

Fig. 10.6 Radial tear.

Obstetric trauma: vulval tears

This is not infrequent and occurs on the vulva or perineum during delivery. These may be anterior around the meatus or clitoris and are usually unilateral. They frequently bleed and may need pressure or suturing to achieve haemostasis. Lateral tears of the labia minora are simple grazes, which cause pain only when urine is passed. Usually they heal spontaneously but sometimes the healing of a torn mucosa may lead to subsequent formation of mucous cysts. Radial tears (Fig. 10.6), labia minora perforations (Fig. 10.7) and labial detachment (Fig. 10.8) are also possible complications and can be easily repaired by excision and suturing in the three planes as described above.

Surgical trauma

Postprolapse repair

Sometimes a surgical procedure undertaken to correct one problem gives rise to another. A good example of this is the vaginal narrowing that can occur after a prolapse repair. This occurs after a posterior colpoperineorrhaphy has been carried out and the vagina is thought to be

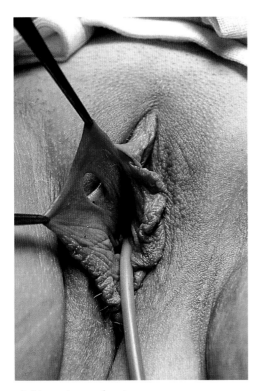

Fig. 10.7 Labium minus perforation.

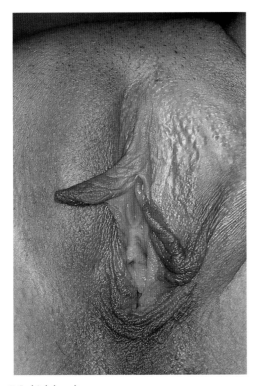

Fig. 10.8 Labial detachment.

sufficiently adequate at the time, as it often is. However, it may become narrow later because of the atresia that develops at the time of the menopause when oestrogen diminishes. There may be eventual stenosis of the vaginal opening that can give rise to dyspareunia or even apareunia.

Treatment is straightforward and involves a median perineotomy, i.e. Fenton's operation, which can be done under local anaesthesia, epidural or general anaesthesia (Fig. 10.9a–d).

A median incision is made using either a scalpel or a pair of scissors running from the hymenal ring to the perineal body, simultaneously cutting through the vestibule. The perineal area is opened up and it is now important to free the vaginal wall and perineal skin by undermining on either side of the incision with a pair of blunt, curved dissecting scissors, particularly at each extremity to enable mobilization of the tissues without tension. If the perineal body has become fibrosed because of previous surgery it is important to free the right and left sides with a cuneiform incision in order to make it more supple and facilitate suturing. Good haemostasis is essential to prevent haematoma formation. The longitudinal incision is then sutured transversely. A tacking stitch is placed centrally. The edges may develop dog-ears, which can be easily resected. Suturing is done with absorbable thread 3.0 and gradually the areas are sewn together, working from the ends towards the centre.

There is very little postoperative discomfort. Sometimes a slight dehiscence occurs; this means longer healing but fortunately does not affect the long-term results. Any residual sutures are removed 3–4 weeks later. Sexual intercourse can then be resumed but postmenopausal women are advised to use oestrogen therapy. The outcome of this operation is usually very satisfactory.

Post vulvectomy

There are several surgical procedures available to correct the introital stenosis that may follow either simple or radical vulvectomy. The Z-plasty is frequently used to correct postoperative scarring and the results are usually good. The annular constriction of the vaginal opening is eliminated and the gusset effect gives it a certain elasticity (Fig. 10.10a–d). In cases of introital stenosis following vulvectomy, a Z-plasty (Scott *et al.* 1963, Wilkinson 1971) is performed on one side. An incision is made into the introital opening measuring approximately 2.5 cm. The other two incisions of identical length form 60° angles, one of the incisions running into the introital opening and the other into the perineal skin. The pieces defined in this way are dissected with skin hooks to prevent crushing. They are then switched and stitched together. A mirror-image Z-plasty is made on the opposite side. An indwelling bladder catheter is inserted and a vaginal tampon is left in place for 24–48 hours.

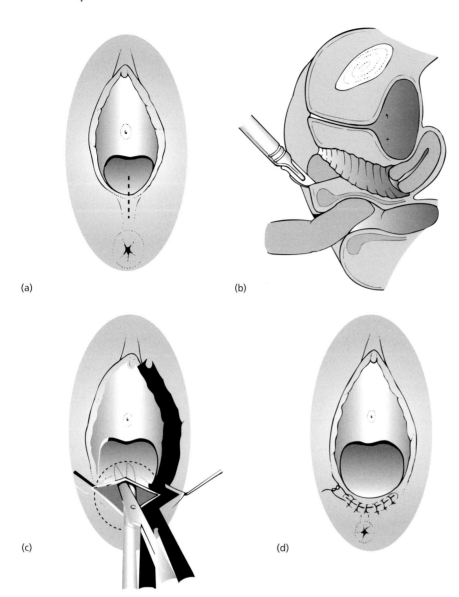

(a)

(b)

(c)

(d)

Fig. 10.9 Median perineotomy (Fenton's operation). (a) and (b) Longitudinal incision running from the hymenal ring to the perineal skin and cutting into the perineal body; (c) undermining the vaginal wall and perineal skin; (d) transverse suturing (Paniel *et al.* 1985).

A unilateral or bilateral transposition flap taken from the labium majus is suitable for stenosis of the vaginal opening and of the lower end of the vagina (Patterson & Rhodes 1958). The operation starts with a lateral or posterolateral incision resembling an extended episiotomy, which creates a triangular defect. A cutaneous full-thickness triangular flap is then drawn out on the labium majus to cover the defect (Fig. 10.11a–c).

The cutaneous and the mucosal edges are then carefully sutured. The non-dissected angle separating the flaps from the raw surfaces stays in place. It inevitably raises itself in a dog-ear, which usually flattens with time because of the elasticity of the surrounding skin. The edges of the donor site are closed by simple approximation after having undermined the edges. If the correction of the stenosis is insufficient the procedure should be repeated on the opposite side at the same time as the operation or it can be done later. Postoperatively a suitable vaginal tampon is left in place for 24–48 hours to apply a light compression on the flap in its new position to avoid the development of a haematoma. The completed skin graft has a very small risk of retraction, but in such a case the aesthetic considerations should yield precedence to the functional result and the patient should be warned about this. The use of Y–V advancement or a 'maple leaf' is also possible for mild and moderate strictures with 98% success rate (Reid 1997).

After incision and drainage of Bartholin's abscess

The incision and drainage of a Bartholin's abscess through the interlabial sulcus can result in either partial detachment

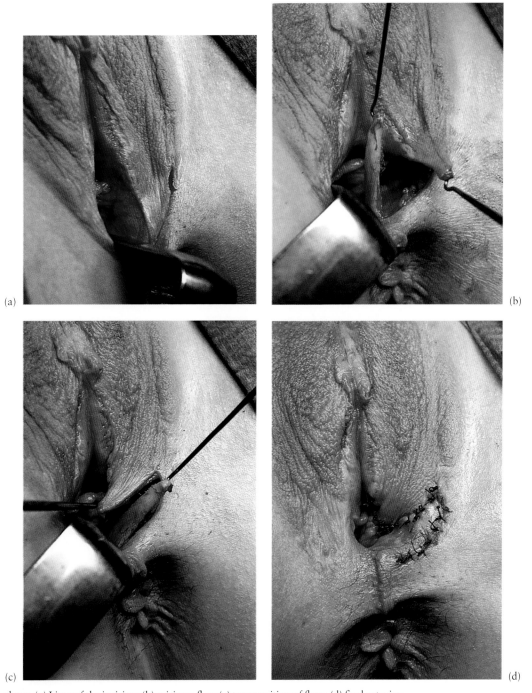

Fig. 10.10 Z-plasty. (a) Lines of the incision; (b) raising a flap; (c) transposition of flaps; (d) final suturing.

of a labium minus or the development of a fistulous track, which oozes mucus. The treatment consists of removal of Bartholin's duct and gland and then resuturing the labium minus. To avoid this complication, it is preferable to make the incision in the nymphohymenal sulcus.

After laser therapy

The complications following carbon dioxide ablation of condyloma acuminata and vulval intraepithelial neoplasia (VIN) include synechiae formation of the labia minora and vestibule. These secondary adhesions are very common

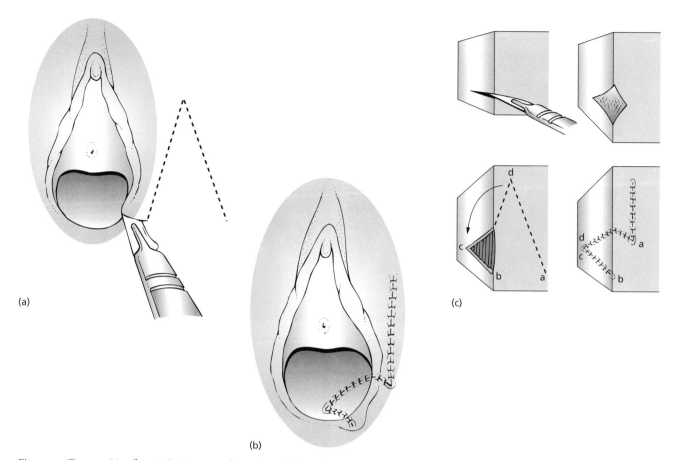

(a)

(b)

(c)

Fig. 10.11 Transposition flap. (a) Incision to make a triangular flap. (b) Positioning and suturing. (c) The procedure in three dimensions.

after lasering of lesions in the fourchette, fossa navicularis and vestibule. The partly fused labia tear apart during sexual intercourse, causing dyspareunia. To avoid this complication, it is recommended that in the case of bilateral lesions only one side is treated at a time. If the fourchette or fossa navicularis are involved with VIN it is preferable to deal with the problem surgically followed by reconstruction using the posterior vaginal wall.

Postcoital fissures

Hymeneal fissures

These occur in young nulliparous women and are one cause of superficial dyspareunia (Michlewitz 1986). Postcoital bleeding and the precise site of pain correspond to the areas of the hymenal tears of first intercourse and serve to make the diagnosis. The areas of scarring can fissure during vaginal examination, particularly if there is any tension on the hymenal ring (i.e. opening a vaginal speculum to take a cervical smear) or during sexual intercourse particularly with a change of partner.

These fissures are arranged in a radial fashion around the

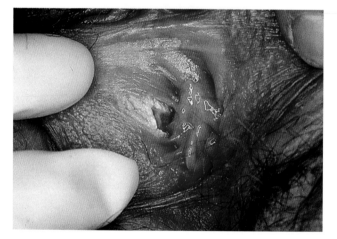

Fig. 10.12 Hymenal fissure (courtesy of M. Moyal-Barracco).

hymenal ring usually between 3 and 4 and 8 and 9 o'clock (Fig. 10.12). They may be uni- or bilateral and look like linear erosions. They can extend from the hymenal ring into the vagina or nymphohymenal sulcus. They may go unnoticed and it is important to try to display the hymen well;

this is done by grasping the labia between the thumb and index finger and stretching them gently out and down.

The fissures heal rapidly in a few days after intercourse, leaving behind a pale scarred site, which refissures at each intercourse. Avoiding intercourse even for long periods does not prevent recurrence. Spontaneous cure does occur but may take a long time.

The treatment entails the excision of the fissures sagittally and resuturing the edges of the vestibular and vaginal mucosa transversely. The procedure is most suitable for removing the scarred area, which is particularly vulnerable to the tension that is exerted at the time of sexual intercourse. The radial incisions are made with a scalpel blade or a pair of scissors, each at 60°, cutting lightly into the mucosa above and below and deeply into the base of the fibrous insertion of the hymen. At 5 and 7 o'clock, care is taken to avoid the excretory ducts of the Bartholin's glands. At 11 and 1 o'clock near the urethral meatus, the incisions are made deeper to ensure dissociation of the meatus from the hymen and to avoid the development of postcoital recurrent cystitis. Interrupted stitches are made using fine absorbable thread, and are placed transversely to achieve haemostasis. Sexual intercourse can be resumed a month postoperatively when healing is complete. It is important to reassure the patient beforehand to lessen her apprehension.

Fossa navicularis fissures

These fissures are a cause of secondary superficial dyspareunia (Michlewitz 1986). Following penetration the patient senses vulval tearing, sometimes accompanied by bleeding, and this may be followed for several days by spontaneous localized burning of the vulva, often triggered by micturition. These symptoms return with each intercourse and understandably lead to difficulties with sexual relations; the patient eventually dreads and avoids intercourse. On gently examining the vulva the fissure can be seen the length of the posterior vestibule in the midline (Fig. 10.13) running from the hymen to the fourchette. Sometimes after intercourse there will be a very fine white scar, which may be only faintly visible but with a more thorough examination it may readily split open. There is no evidence of lichen sclerosus or lichen planus but in some cases the delicate epithelium of the fossa navicularis has been damaged following previous treatment of lesions in this area with carbon dioxide laser, liquid nitrogen or electrocoagulation. Reducing the frequency of sexual intercourse and the use of bland emollients may help, but, if these measures fail, surgical treatment has to be considered. Quadrilateral excision of the vestibular mucosa including the fissure with dissection and cleavage of the posterior vaginal wall for 2–3 cm is required. This provides a flap of vaginal wall that can be used to fill in the defect, and the tissue can be sutured without tension.

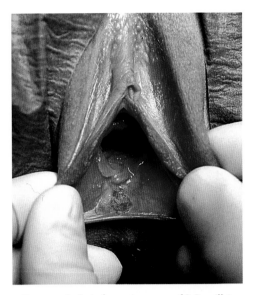

Fig. 10.13 Fossa navicularis fissure (courtesy of S. Berville).

Hymenorrhaphy

It is technically feasible to repair the hymen after forced or consensual sexual activity. This is done using a vaginal flap, or by suture in three planes, after excision of the membrane from 3 o'clock to 9 o'clock.

Female genital mutilation

After clitoridectomy no worthwhile reconstruction is possible. Infibulation or pharaonic circumcision, as practised in Mali, Sudan and the Horn of Africa, consists of removal of the labia minora and suturing with acacia spines after freshening of the edges, with or without a clitoridectomy. A little hole, which is made by leaving a small stick of wood in place while suturing, remains open in front of the posterior commissure to allow urine and menstrual blood to flow out. Surgical correction consists of separating the labia minora along the midline and then suturing their free borders so that a nearly normal appearance can be obtained. This will allow normal sexual function and vaginal delivery later in life.

Reconstruction procedures have been recently reported (Fig. 10.14a–f). The skin covering the stump is resected and the clitoris identified. The suspensory ligament is sectioned in order to mobilize the stump, the scar tissue is removed from the extremity and the clitoral tissue is repositioned at the glans' normal site. Colles fascia is sutured below the new glans and absorbable sutures are used to fix the glans to the skin. In a series of 453 patients, a visible clitoral mass could be restored in 87% of cases and a real improvement in clitoral function was obtained in 75% of the patients 4–6 months postoperatively (Foldes & Louis-Sylvestre 2006).

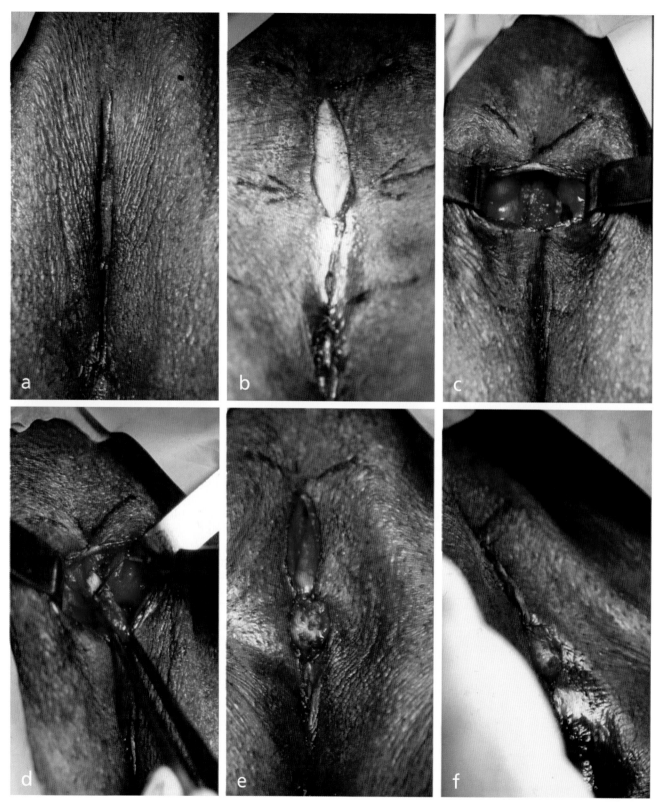

Fig. 10.14 Surgical clitoral repair after ritual excision. (a) Preoperative aspect of female genital mutilation. (b) Median skin incision of the upper half of the clitoral area (also corresponds to the upper half of the pubic symphysis). (c) Dissection of the ascending part of the clitoral body. (d) Section of the suspensory ligament preserving the tunica to spare the dorsal nerve which fans out extensively around the dorsal and lateral parts of the clitoral body. (e) After resection of the fibrous clitoral scar facing the middle of the pubic symphysis, suture of the exteriorized (5 mm) clitoral body. (f) Providing a pseudoclitoral glans.

Labial adhesions

Labial adhesions are relatively common and they are acquired and not congenital (Guillarme *et al.* 1995). The condition is usually asymptomatic but there is often parental concern. If the children are symptomatic they present with dysuria, urinary tract infections and vulval irritation. On inspection and parting of the labia majora, the vulva appears flat as the free edges of the inner aspects of the vulva are adherent one upon the other. This join is seen as a fine line running anteroposteriorly and the adherence may be complete or partial. There is always a small opening at the level of the urethral meatus. Medical management includes the use of bland emollients and topical oestrogen. Success rates range from 50% to 79% but recurrence rates are high (between 41% and 53%) (Muram 1999, Schober *et al.* 2006) (see Chapter 5).

It is particularly important to reassure the parents that labial adhesions are a common and harmless phenomenon that usually resolves spontaneously. This strong reassurance may well diffuse their anxiety and avoid surgical intervention in those asymptomatic children in whom the abnormality has been noted by chance. For a long time it was common practice to separate the adhesions either manually or instrumentally after cleansing the skin. The former technique involved placing a thumb on each labium majus and quickly splitting the adhesion by applying firm but gentle pressure in an outward and downward direction (Fig. 10.15a). The second technique involved passing either a lubricated hollow sound or forceps into the opening of the adhesion (Fig. 10.15b). The adhesion is then broken down. These manoeuvres left torn edges on either side of the vulva with little or no bleeding and frequent applications of an emollient, with or without an antibiotic, were used to help healing and prevent resealing. Although the separation of the labia by these techniques was very effective, further adhesions were common. Despite the use of local anaesthesia this digital and instrumental separation was physically and psychologically traumatic for the child. Furthermore, the child's mother was usually present during the procedure and was distressed herself. For these reasons, the above procedures have now been abandoned.

Nowadays, surgical division of the adhesions is carried out under a general anaesthetic. The two main reasons for intervention are symptomatic children and parental pressure. The pressure usually comes from the mother who is anxious that her daughter may have sexual problems later in life.

Sequelae of lichen sclerosus

Surgical intervention in lichen sclerosus is indicated only for the postinflammatory sequelae of the disease.

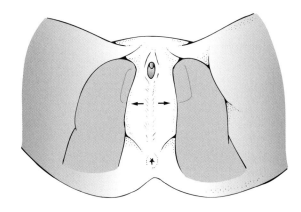

(a)

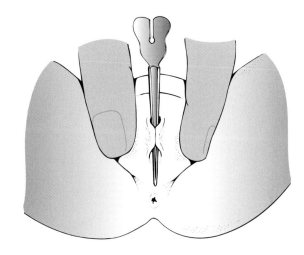

(b)

Fig. 10.15 Labial adhesions. (a) Digital separation; (b) instrumental separation.

Introital stenosis

Vulvoperineoplasty

Vulvoperineoplasty is indicated on the rare occasions when there is introital stenosis following lichen sclerosus (Paniel *et al.* 1984a,b). Patients present with either dyspareunia or apareunia. The procedure involves:

1 wide dissection and mobilization of the posterior wall of the vagina

2 reduction of the height of the perineal body

3 advancement and eversion of the posterior vaginal wall (Fig. 10.16a–g).

The patient is placed in the lithotomy position and, under general anaesthetic or epidural, the procedure begins as for a posterior colpoperineorrhaphy. A marker thread is passed through the posterior extremity of each labium minus. By lifting and stretching out the two threads the mucocutaneous junction can be seen and the initial incision is made along this line. A triangular flap of perineal skin that has

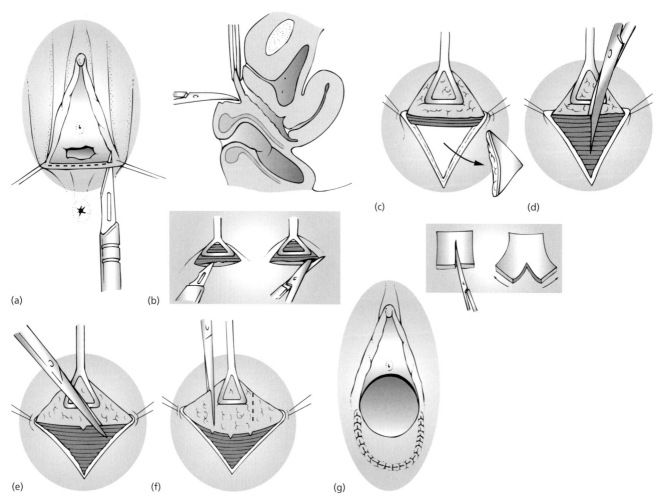

Fig. 10.16 Vulvoperineoplasty. (a) Mucocutaneous incision; (b) dissection of the posterior vaginal wall; (c) excision of a triangular patch of perineal skin; (d and e) radial incision of the fibrous perineal body to reduce its height; (f) individualization of a vaginal flap; (g) the vaginal flap is drawn down, making a cover for the perineal defect, and sutured.

often been involved in the disease process is excised together with the subcutaneous tissue. The base of the triangle is represented by a border of tissue made by the initial vulval incision. The summit of the triangle is always situated close to the anal margin.

The edge of the vestibular mucosa is lifted by a pair of dissecting forceps stretching out the tissue so that the blade can delicately undermine the area. Ring forceps then replace the dissecting forceps and are held in the left hand between the thumb and index finger while the extended third and fourth fingers of this hand are placed under the vaginal wall to facilitate the dissection. The dissection is done freely and widely with the blade or scissors without ever losing contact with the lower vaginal wall. In this way, the rectovaginal plane of cleavage is reached. The division is done digitally for 6–7 cm just to the vicinity of the pouch of Douglas. The fibrous perineal body now exposed is incised medially just near the anal sphincter. If the vaginal opening

is not sufficiently wide, two paramedian incisions are made. The completion of the radial incisions is effected by digital dissection. The height of the fibrous perineal body is thus reduced.

A posterior vaginal flap is then made and brought down. The posterior vaginal wall is incised longitudinally on both sides of the ring forceps at the level of the lateral gutters of the vagina for 3–4 cm, taking care to avoid the ductal openings of the Bartholin's glands. The lower extremity of the vaginal flap, which was grasped and damaged by the pressure of the ring forceps, is then excised. The thin vaginal epithelium, which is supple and well vascularized, is then easily drawn down to the exterior, making a perfect cover for the perineal defect. A small median sagittal incision is made on the inferior edge of the flap to improve the laxity on either side. The suturing must be done without tension and the best way to achieve this is by using interrupted absorbable sutures 3.0. This leaves a widened introitus that will eventually be able to withstand the trauma of coitus. Both sides of the flap as well as the mucocutaneous edges are brought together by interrupted sutures. There are small lateral vestibular defects, which are left to heal spontaneously.

An appropriately sized tampon wrapped in paraffin gauze is left in place for 24 hours together with an indwelling urinary catheter. The pressure exerted by the tampon prevents haematoma formation under the flap.

The procedure takes a trained surgeon 25–45 minutes. Healing is usually straightforward and the patient may be discharged 24–48 hours later once the local discomfort is controlled. Any sutures that have not dissolved spontaneously are removed 2–3 weeks postoperatively. The operation not only successfully restores the introitus to an adequate size but also leaves an area that is not attacked later by lichen sclerosus. The vaginal epithelium that now covers this site seems to remain unaffected, as has been shown by biopsies carried out up to 15 years later. The patient should not discontinue the use of the topical steroids. Success rates of this procedure are high: perineoplasty improved dyspareunia in 45 out of 50 patients (90%) and quality of sexual intercourse in 43 out of 50 patients (86%) in a series reported by Rouzier et al. (2002). None of the risk factors evaluated (duration of lichen sclerosus, age, previous topical steroid therapy, previous perineotomy, time since surgery and histological features) were associated with failure of perineoplasty in this series.

Adhesions

Postinflammatory adhesions due to lichen sclerosus are usually localized to the fourchette, labia minora or clitoral prepuce.

Fourchette adhesions

These usually consist of synechiae, which tear during sexual intercourse or on clinical examination. There may be light bleeding when they are disrupted and patients often complain of dyspareunia. The adhesions reform after healing and tear again with further disturbance. The treatment is simple, consisting of a median perineotomy, i.e. Fenton's operation. This is done under local or general anaesthesia by incising the adhesion, perineal skin, vestibular mucous membrane and the summit of the perineal body. The mucosal edges are undermined and sutured transversely using interrupted stitches of 3.0 Vicryl.

Labia minora adhesions

Extensive labial synechiae or a fused vulva are rare findings, usually occurring in postmenopausal women. The appearance is similar to that seen after ritual infibulation when there is only a small orifice posteriorly. The synechiae are freed and the edges are sutured with fine absorbable thread. It is important to apply a topical steroid postoperatively to prevent refusion.

Clitoral adhesions

The clitoris is frequently buried in lichen sclerosus and, although this is often symptomless, many patients prefer the area to be freed for aesthetic reasons. The adhesions are delicately incised and then, using a probe, the hood is freed from the glans.

Prevention of re-adhesion is achieved either by resection of a fragment of the clitoral hood in the shape of a tricorn hat, which everts the free edge (Fig. 10.17a), or by excision of the clitoral hood, which is the equivalent to a circumcision (Fig. 10.17b).

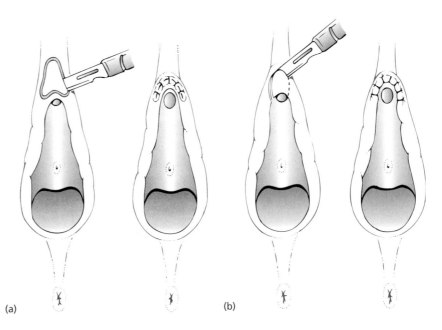

Fig. 10.17 Prevention of re-adhesion. (a) Resection of a segment of the clitoral hood in the shape of a tricorn. (b) Circumcision.   (a)   (b)

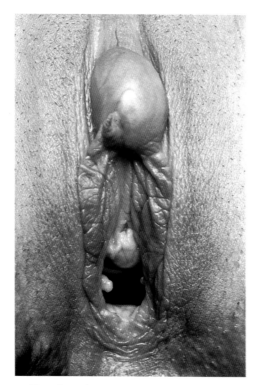

Fig. 10.18 Clitoral pseudocyst.

Sometimes periclitoral adhesion results in a pseudocyst containing smegma, which can lead to a misdiagnosis of a tumour or cyst (Fig. 10.18). It may be complicated by secondary infection with fistula formation. The only treatment that can be offered is subtotal or total circumcision.

Lichen planus and other bullous and erosive diseases

Vulvovaginal adhesions

Vulvovaginal adhesions are associated with several erosive mucosal diseases, which result in scarring and adhesions of the vagina, vestibule or labia minora. These erosive diseases include lichen planus, cicatricial pemphigoid (mucous membrane pemphigoid), toxic epidermal necrolysis, Stevens–Johnson syndrome and graft-versus-host disease.

The active inflammatory dermatosis is treated medically. Surgery is required only for symptomatic postinflammatory adhesions. In the vulva, the localized scarring results in burial of the clitoris, labial adhesions or introital stenosis. The buried glans clitoris is freed surgically and then removal of the clitoral hood can be done to prevent recurrence. Anterior and posterior fusion are divided by sagittal incisions followed by transverse suturing. The adhesions of the fourchette can be corrected by a procedure similar to a median perineotomy.

If there is vestibular stenosis without vaginal wall involvement a perineoplasty may be performed. In those cases with associated vulvovaginal involvement, the healthy surrounding skin of the perineal area is used for reconstruction by carrying out an inverse V–Y plasty. This procedure is identical to that used by Fortunoff to open the urogenital sinus in cases of sexual ambiguity. A V-shaped flap is made on the perineal skin. The apex is at the top of the fourchette and the base lies flush with the anal margin. It is advisable to ensure that the length of the base is equal to the length of the flap so as not to compromise the vascularization. The flap is then dissected from the apex to the base, taking

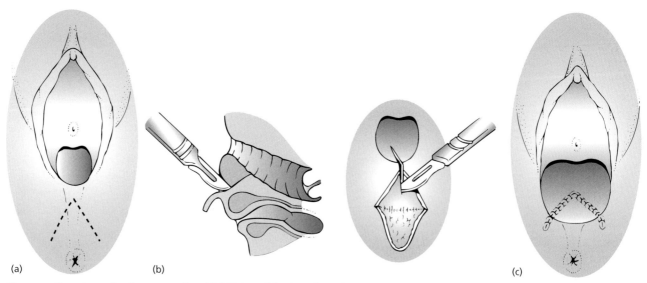

(a)   (b)   (c)

Fig. 10.19 Posterior perineal cutaneous flap. (a) A V-shaped flap is made on the perineal skin. (b) The perineal body is reduced by radial incisions and digital dissection. (c) The perineal flap covers the triangular defect and is sutured with 3.0 or 4.0 Vicryl.

care to preserve a suitable thickness and fatty support. The perineal body is reduced by radial incisions and by digital dissection. The posterior wall of the vagina is then incised along the median line. The gaping sides of the incision allow the recovery of a normal calibre for the introitus and lower vagina. After haemostasis the cutaneous flap is pulled up into the interior of the vaginal conduit to fit into the triangular defect caused by the perineotomy, and the tissue is then sutured with Vicryl 3.0 or 4.0 (Fig. 10.19a–c). A tampon for haemostasis is left in place for 24 hours.

Vaginal adhesions alone have various clinical aspects but the problem most frequently encountered is partial fusion of the anterior and posterior walls of the vagina along the lateral edges. This produces a concentric narrowing of the vagina. Sometimes a small speculum can be passed but otherwise the adhesions may result in the appearance of a funnel-shaped narrowing with a small opening at its apex through which the secretions and menstrual blood can flow out. Rarely a complete adhesion may cause retention of the menstrual flow. The first stage of the procedure is removal of the adhesion with a blade or a blunt instrument, following the line of the fusion, keeping a finger in the rectum and an indwelling catheter in the urethra. The areas underlying the adhesions are haemorrhagic with little or no mucosal covering. The second stage involves the prevention of refusion by placing in the vagina a prosthetic device identical to that used after the surgical treatment of vaginal aplasia. The device is changed every 8–10 days and then daily for 4–8 weeks. As epithelialization is progressing the device is worn only at night and when epithelialization is nearly complete frequent sexual intercourse or the use of a 35 mm vaginal dilator several times daily is encouraged. To prevent further adhesions the device or dilator can be coated in a topical corticosteroid. Other authors use tacrolimus (Kennedy & Galask 2007). The patient should nevertheless be made aware of the risk of recurrence.

References

Alter, G.J. (1998) A new technique for aesthetic labia minora reduction. *Annals of Plastic Surgery* **40**, 287–290.

Choi, H.Y. & Kim, K.T. (2000) A new method for aesthetic reduction of labia minora (the deepithelialized reduction of labioplasty). *Plastic and Reconstructive Surgery* **105**, 419–22.

Dénes, F.T., Cocuzza, M.A., Schneider-Monteiro, E.D. *et al.* (2005) The laparoscopic management of intersex patients: the preferred approach. *BJU International* **95**, 863–867.

Erich, J.B. (1959) Plastic repairs of the female perineum in a case of exstrophy of the bladder. *Mayo Clinic Proceedings* **34**, 235–237.

Ferry, C., Sgro, J.C. & Solente, J.J. (1977) Résection de l'organe péno-clitoridien conservant le gland avec son innervation, chez les interseés à vocation féminine: bases anatomiques et technique opératoire. *Revue Française d'Endocrinologie Clinique, Nutrition et Métabolisme* **18**, 247–254.

Foldes, P. & Louis-Sylvestre, C. (2006) Results of surgical clitoral repair after ritual excision: 453 cases. *Gynecology Obstetrics and Fertility* **34**, 1137–1141.

Fortunoff, S.J., Lattimer, J.K. & Edson, M. (1964) Vaginoplastic technique for female pseudohermaphrodites. *Surgery Gynecology and Obstetrics* **118**, 545–548.

Frank, R.T. (1938) Formation of an artificial vagina without operation. *American Journal of Obstetrics and Gynecology* **35**, 1053–1055.

Giraldo, F., González, C. & de Haro, F. (2004) Central wedge nymphectomy with a 90-degree Z-plasty for aesthetic reduction of the labia minora. *Plastic and Reconstructive Surgery* **113**, 1820–1825.

Guillarme, P., Haddad, B., Touboul, C. & Paniel, B.J. (1995) Coalescence des petites lèvres. *Références en Gynécologie Obstétrique* **3**, 245–250.

Hendren, W.H. (1977) Surgical management of urogenital sinus abnormalities. *Journal of Pediatric Surgery* **12**, 339–357.

Hodgkinson, D.J. & Hait, G. (1984) Aesthetic vaginal labioplasty. *Plastic and Reconstructive Surgery* **74**, 414–416.

Houk, C.P., Hughes, I.A., Ahmed, S.F. & Lee, P.A. Writing Committee for the International Intersex Consensus Conference Participants. (2006) Summary of consensus statement on intersex disorders and their management. *International Intersex Consensus Conference Pediatrics* **118**, 753–757.

Kennedy, C.M. & Galask, R.P. (2007) Erosive vulvar lichen planus: retrospective review of characteristics and outcomes in 113 patients seen in a vulvar specialty clinic. *Journal of Reproductive Medicine* **2**, 43–47.

Michlewitz, H. (1986) Laser ablation of hymeneal fissures. *Journal of Reproductive Medicine* **31**, 63–64.

Munhoz, A.M., Filassi, J.R., Ricci, M.D. *et al.* (2006) Aesthetic labia minora reduction with inferior wedge resection and superior pedicle flap reconstruction. *Plastic and Reconstructive Surgery* **118**, 1237–1247.

Muram, D. (1999) Treatment of prepubertal girls with labial adhesions. *Journal of Pediatric and Adolescent Gynecology* **12**, 67–70.

Paniel, B.J. Truc, J.B., Robichez, B. & Poitout, P. (1984a) Vulvo-perinéoplastie. *Presse Médicale* **13**, 1895–1898.

Paniel, B.J., Berville-Levy, S. & Moyal-Barracco, M. (1984b) La vulvopérinéoplastie. *Journal de Gynécolgie, Obstétrique et Biologie de la Reproduction* **31**, 91–99.

Paniel, B.J., Truc, J.B., Robichez, B. *et al.* (1985) Chirurgie des lésions bénignes de la vulve. *Encyclopédie Medicochirurgicale*. Techniques Chirurgicales Gynocologie. Elsevier, Paris.

Papageorgiou, T., Hearns-Stokes, R., Peppas, D. & Segars, J.H. (2000) Clitoroplasty with preservation of neurovascular pedicles. *Obstetrics and Gynecology* **96**, 821–823.

Patterson, T.J.S. & Rhodes, P. (1958) Treatment of stenosis of the vagina by a thigh flap. *Journal of Obstetrics and Gynaecology of the British Empire* **65**, 481–482.

Prader, A. (1954) Der genitalbefund beim Pseudohermaphroditismus des kongenitalen adrenogenital syndroms. Morphologie, Haüfigkeit, Entwicklung und Vererbung der verschiedenen genital formen. *Helvetica Paediatrica Acta* **9**, 231.

Reid, R. (1997) Local and distant skin flaps in the reconstruction of vulvar deformities. *American Journal of Obstetrics and Gynecology* **177**, 1372–1383.

Rouzier, R., Louis-Sylvestre, C., Paniel, B.J. & Haddad, B. (2000) Hypertrophy of labia minora: experience with 163 reductions. *American Journal of Obstetrics and Gynecology* **182**, 35–40.

Rouzier, R., Haddad, B., Deyrolle, C., *et al.* (2002) Perineoplasty for the treatment of introital stenosis related to vulvar lichen sclerosus. *American Journal of Obstetrics and Gynecology* **186**, 49–52.

Schober, J., Dulabon, L., Martin-Alguacil, N., *et al.* (2006) Significance of topical estrogens to labial fusion and vaginal introital integrity. *Journal of Pediatric and Adolescent Gynecology* **19**, 337–339.

Scott, J.W., Gilpin, C.R. & Vence, C.A. (1963) Vulvectomy, introital stenosis and Z plasty. *American Journal of Obstetrics and Gynecology* **85**, 132–133.

Wilkinson, E.J. (1971) Introital stenosis and Z plasty. *Obstetrics and Gynecology* **38**, 638–640.

Chapter 11: Management of vulval cancers

R. Rouzier & B.J. Paniel

Introduction

Vulval cancer accounts for approximately 4% of all gynae-cological malignancies and 1% of all cancers in women (Ghurani & Penalver 2001). Invasive squamous cell carcinoma (SCC) accounts for 90% of all vulval malignancies. Radical surgery was the cornerstone treatment until the 1990s (Hacker 1999, Marsden & Hacker 2001). It results in 5 year survival rates around 70%, but the morbidity rate is also high. In the last 20 years, surgery has been tailored to the individual patient to reduce complications, particularly in those with limited disease. This has not had an impact on the survival rates, but the morbidity and quality of life have improved (Ghurani & Penalver 2001). This is particularly important in view of the alarming rise in the incidence of human papillomavirus (HPV)-related vulval squamous cell carcinoma in young women (Jones et al. 1997, Joura et al. 2000, Judson et al. 2006).

Vulval cancer is rare, so most studies to assess surgical outcomes are retrospective and there have been no formal prospective, randomized studies (level I, according to the Cochrane Collaboration) to compare radical with modified radical surgery. Existing studies have instead been retrospective, comparing the outcomes between patients who were treated according to a less radical protocol with those treated more radically (level III). This chapter will outline the modifications needed in the surgical management of patients with vulval cancer, according to stage of disease.

Epidemiology and pathogenesis

The incidence of vulval SCC is 1–2/100 000 (Hacker 2005). The median age is 72 years. The number of patients with vulval cancer is expected to increase because of the rise in the ageing population. About 90% of vulval cancers are squamous cell carcinoma, and the remaining 10% include malignant melanoma, basal cell carcinoma, adenocarcinoma of Bartholin's glands and invasive extramammary Paget's disease (Finan & Barre 2003).

There appear to be two distinct aetiologies for vulval SCC (Hording et al. 1993, van Beurden et al. 1998, Sutton et al. 2008). The first of these is a non-HPV-related chronic scarring skin condition such as lichen sclerosus or lichen planus. The second, and less common, is HPV-related vulval intraepithelial neoplasia (VIN; two-thirds to full thickness epithelial atypia) (Sideri et al. 2005). The other term for two-thirds to full thickness VIN is classical VIN. HPV16 has been associated with the majority of cases of classical VIN (van Beurden et al. 1998). Judson et al. (2006) have reported a 411% increase in HPV-related VIN from 1973 to 2000, which corresponds with the 20% rise in invasive SCC seen in the same period. It also correlates with the reported rise in HPV infection observed in a population-based study in Norway (Iversen & Tretli 1998). The increase in VIN has occurred mainly in women under 65 years, with a peak incidence in the 40–49 year old age group with a steady decrease thereafter. The increased incidence of screening, detection and reporting both by the patient and by the physician may also explain the increase of VIN. In 30% of patients with untreated cervical intraepithelial neoplasia, there is a progression to invasive cervical cancer in 5–20 years, with a gradual decline in incidence after that time. On the other hand, HPV-related VIN increases exponentially with age. Other factors must therefore be involved, one explanation being that over half of vulval cancers have been reported in non-HPV-related epithelial disorders such as lichen sclerosus (Borgno et al. 1988, Rouzier et al. 2001). It would appear that progression of multifocal HPV-related VIN has a very small incidence of progression to invasive cancer (van Seters et al. 2005). It has been suggested that treatment of HPV-related VIN reduces the risk of invasion (Jones et al. 2005).

The commonest presenting sign of vulval cancer is a vulval ulcer or mass. Common symptoms include localized pruritus, bleeding, pain, discharge or urinary tract symptoms

Ridley's The Vulva, 3rd edition. Edited by Sallie M. Neill and Fiona M. Lewis. © 2009 Blackwell Publishing, ISBN: 978-1-4051-6813-7.

(Podratz *et al.* 1983, Rosen & Malmstrom 1997, Ghurani & Penalver 2001). The chronic vulval disease often predates malignant change by many years. A delay of up to a year in 50% of patients has been noted (Podratz *et al.* 1983, Ghurani & Penalver 2001). This delay can be due to either late reporting of change by the patient or failure to recognize the problem by the physician.

Anatomy

One of the most challenging aspects in the management of vulval cancer is the lack of uniformity in the terms used in the literature to describe the surgical procedures employed in the management of vulval SCC. This was demonstrated by a survey of gynaecological oncologists to assess the extent of groin dissection used for early vulval cancer (Levenback *et al.* 1996). At least three surgical procedures were commonly performed and, moreover, three different terms were used to describe them. Such inconsistency may lead to confusion and poorer management. Micheletti *et al.* (1998) have proposed a clarification of the terminology in an effort to standardize care.

Anatomy of the vulva
As reported by Micheletti *et al.* (1998), the external borders of the vulva are represented anteriorly by the mons pubis, laterally by the genitocrural folds and posteriorly by the perineum (Fig. 11.1a). The internal borders are represented by the hymenal ring. Between the external and internal borders of the vulva, the clitoral prepuce, the interlabial folds and the fourchette are other important landmarks. The portion of the vulva that begins at the hymenal ring and extends outward to the internal side of the labia minora, upward to the frenulum of the clitoris and downward to include the fourchette is defined as the vestibule. The location of a vulval tumour is important as it will determine whether the lymph nodes have to be removed on one or both sides.

The deeper anatomy is important from a surgical point of view because removal of tissues underlying the vulval skin will make the difference between radical and non-radical surgery. The vulva is superficially covered by the skin where most vulval cancers arise. The majority of the skin is keratinized, stratified, squamous epithelium with the exception of the vestibule, which is mucosa-covered in non-keratinized stratified squamous epithelium (see Chapter 1).

The floor of the vulval region is represented by the inferior fascia of the urogenital diaphragm or perineal membrane, which becomes the femoral fascia in the thigh. Between the skin and the inferior fascia of the urogenital diaphragm is the subcutaneous fat, divided into a superficial portion and a deep portion by the superficial fascia. Several structures lie within the deepest part of the subcutaneous tissue, which include, from the top downward, the body of the clitoris, the membranous urethra, the corpora cavernosa, the ischiocavernosi muscles, the bulbospongiosi muscles, Bartholin's glands, the transversus perinei superficialis muscle and the perineal body (Fig. 11.1b).

Anatomy of the groin
A knowledge of groin anatomy is essential as nodal involvement is an important part of the staging of vulval cancer (Fig. 11.1c). In the late 1980s, groin node dissection was determined by tumour depth. Failure to carry out a lymphadenectomy when indicated worsens the prognosis (van der Velden *et al.* 1996, Rhodes *et al.* 1998, Rouzier *et al.* 2001, 2006). The more detailed anatomy of the groin has been clarified by Borgno *et al.* (1990). They reported the topographic distribution of groin lymph nodes in female cadavers and demonstrated that the femoral nodes were always situated within the openings of the fascia lata, especially at the fossa ovalis. Moreover, they found that there were no lymph nodes distal to the lower margin of the fossa ovalis beneath the fascia lata. Their interpretation of these findings was that a complete femoral lymphadenectomy does not require removal of the fascia lata. It was also shown that the superficial circumflex iliac vessels were easily seen and could act as the lateral surgical landmark, beyond which there should be no inguinal lymph nodes, and that the lymphadenectomy should cease at that point (Micheletti *et al.* 2002). The most lateral superficial inguinal lymph node does not rise above the medial margin of the sartorius muscle, or far lateral to the point where the superficial circumflex iliac vessels cross the inguinal ligament. This modified surgery leaves fatty tissue lateral to these vessels intact, thereby preserving some of the lymphatic channels. This decreases the postoperative incidence of a wound seroma and chronic lymphoedema in the longer term. This important finding has influenced the refinement of the surgical technique used for groin dissection (Micheletti *et al.* 1990). A further study has confirmed that lymphadenectomy with preservation of the fascia lata and saphenous vein has indeed decreased the postoperative morbidity and, moreover, it has been reassuring that the outcome has not been jeopardized (Rouzier *et al.* 2003).

The next step in the management of vulval SCC is the concept of sentinel node biopsy. The proposal is that a tumour metastasis spreads first to one draining lymph node, namely the sentinel node, and therefore the presence of metastases in this node indicates the need for removal of the nodes in the whole nodal basin (Cabanas 1977). Sentinel lymph node biopsy may be currently used as a tool for further staging in melanoma, breast cancer and vulval carcinoma, but further trials are awaited before this will be routine practice.

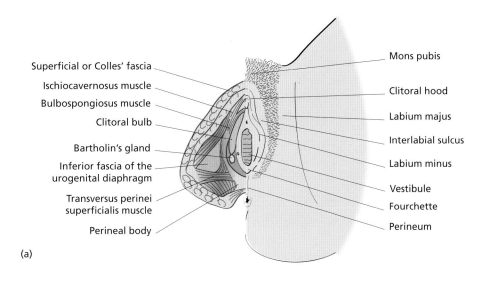

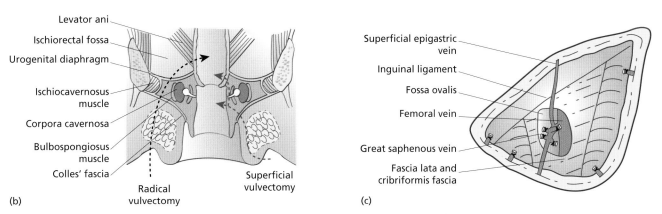

Fig. 11.1 Anatomy of the vulva and groin. (a) External and deep anatomy. (b) Coronal view of the female pelvis: radical (black dashed line) and simple vulvectomy (red dashed line). (c) Groin anatomy.

Staging

The system of classification described by the International Federation of Gynecology and Obstetrics (FIGO) was originally based on anatomical extent of disease, as determined by clinical examination. Over the years, most staging systems for gynaecological cancers have been replaced with a combined clinical and surgical staging system. Vulval cancer has been surgically staged since 1988 (Shepherd 1989), and now the final staging is decided on histopathological evaluation of the vulval tumour together with that of the lymph nodes if excised.

The FIGO and TNM classifications are virtually identical. The TNM Prognostic Factor Project Committee has deferred to the FIGO Committee on Gynecologic Oncology for questions on staging (Shepherd 1995, Benedet *et al.* 2000). The TNM system describes the anatomical extent of disease based on the assessment of three primary components

(Table 11.1), in which **T** refers to the extent of the primary tumour, **N** to the presence or absence and extent of regional lymph node metastases, and **M** to the presence or absence of distant metastases. The combined TNM and FIGO systems are shown in Table 11.2 (Shepherd 1995). If the lesion is 2 cm or less in diameter and depth of stromal invasion is less than 1 mm on wedge biopsy, complete excision of the lesion must be undertaken to allow serial sectioning to assess the depth of invasion accurately. The FIGO Committee on Gynecologic Oncology measures the depth of stromal invasion from the epithelial–stromal junction of the adjacent dermal papilla to the deepest point of invasion by the tumour.

Staging is important. The morbidity associated with groin node dissection is high, and therefore it is tempting to avoid it. However, lack of lymph node resection has been repeatedly shown to worsen survival, and one of the largest series showed that it was an independent predictor of poorer 5 year survival (Rhodes *et al.* 1998, Rouzier *et al.*

Table 11.1 TNM staging system for vulval cancer

Primary tumour (T)	
T1	Lesions 2 cm or less in size confined to the vulva or perineum
1A	Stromal invasion no greater than 1.0 mm[a]
1B	Stromal invasion greater than 1.0 mm[a]
T2	Tumour confined to the vulva and/or perineum or more than 2 cm in the greatest dimension
T3	Tumour of any size with: (i) adjacent spread to the lower urethra and/or the vagina or anus and/or (ii) unilateral regional lymph node metastasis
T4	Tumour invading any of the following: upper urethra, bladder mucosa, rectal mucosa, pelvis
Regional lymph nodes (N)[b]	
NX	Regional lymph nodes cannot be assessed
N0	No regional lymph node metastasis
N1	Unilateral regional lymph node metastasis
N2	Bilateral regional lymph node metastases
Distant metastasis (M)	
MX	Distant metastasis cannot be assessed
M0	No distant metastasis
M1	Distant metastasis

[a] The depth of invasion is defined as the measurement of the tumour from the epithelial–stromal junction of the adjacent most superficial dermal papilla to the deepest point of invasion.
[b] Pathological assessment.

Table 11.2 Staging system for vulval cancer of the International Federation of Gynecology and Obstetrics (FIGO)

Stage I	Lesions 2 cm or less in size confined to the vulva or perineum No nodal metastasis	T1N0M0
Stage IA	Lesions 2 cm or less in size confined to the vulva or perineum and with stromal invasion no greater than 1.0 mm[a] No nodal metastasis	T1AN0M0
Stage IB	Lesions 2 cm or less in size confined to the vulva or perineum and with stromal invasion greater than 1.0 mm[a] No nodal metastasis	T1BN0M0
Stage II	Tumour confined to the vulva and/or perineum or more than 2 cm in the greatest dimension No nodal metastasis	T2N0M0
Stage III	Tumour of any size with: (i) adjacent spread to the lower urethra and/or the vagina or anus and/or (ii) unilateral regional lymph node metastasis	T1–2N1M0 T3N0–1M0
Stage IVA	Tumour invades any of the following: upper urethra, bladder mucosa, rectal mucosa, pelvic bone and/or bilateral regional node metastasis	T1–3N2M0 T4N0–2M0
Stage IVB	Any distant metastasis including pelvic lymph nodes	M1

[a] The depth of invasion is defined as the measurement of the tumour from the epithelial–stromal junction of the adjacent most superficial dermal papilla to the deepest point of invasion.

2001). Studies have shown that between 43% and 80% of women with vulval cancer do not have a lymphadenectomy (van der Velden *et al.* 1996, Rhodes *et al.* 1998, Rouzier *et al.* 2001, van der Velden & Ansink 2001). The failure to perform lymph node resection is inappropriate for a frankly invasive tumour as that tumour cannot be staged accurately. The effect on survival is critical even for women older than 70 (Rouzier *et al.* 2001). Women with vulval cancer should now be managed by trained gynaecological oncologists in a multidisciplinary setting. In the past, women may have had inadequate management in general gynaecology units, owing to the lack of experience when not handling large numbers of cases of vulval malignancy (van der Velden *et al.* 1996).

Diagnosis and investigations

Diagnosis should be confirmed by biopsy prior to definitive treatment: an incisional wedge biopsy under local anaesthesia in the outpatient setting is usually sufficient. Ideally, the biopsy should include some surrounding normal tissue. Multiple biopsies may be indicated if there are many suspicious areas as vulval cancer may be multifocal. In addition, the work-up should include a cervical smear, colposcopy of the cervix and vagina as HPV-related vulval cancer may be associated with multisite intraepithelial neoplasia. For large tumours, preoperative computed tomography (CT) scans of the pelvis and groins may demonstrate enlarged lymph nodes, and routine full blood count, biochemical profile and chest radiograph are important as the results may modify treatment options.

Surgical procedures

Resection of the primary tumour

A more conservative approach has evolved over the last 20 years as radical vulvectomy and bilateral inguinofemoral lymphadenectomy have a high physical and sexual morbidity, despite providing good long-term survival (Hacker 1999). Conservative resections have become the standard treatment for some subsets of patients, without changing outcome (Stehman *et al.* 1992a). Surgery may differ in terms of either extent or depth of skin removal. The terms and definitions of various surgeries and indications are shown in Table 11.3. The amount of skin removed is dependent on the extent of neoplastic and preneoplastic lesions whereas the depth of resection (radicality) depends on the degree of infiltration of the tumour.

Since the beginning of the last century, the standard treatment of patients even with early vulval cancer was radical surgery. Towards the end of the century, it was found that surgery could be limited in early tumours to local excisions with minimal resection margins. This practice was validated by a prospective study conducted by the Gynecological Oncology Group (Stehman *et al.* 1992a), and further retrospective studies, as reported in Table 11.4, have shown the procedure to be appropriate (Burrell *et al.* 1988, Lin *et al.* 1992, Farias-Eisner *et al.* 1994, Burke *et al.* 1995, de Hullu *et al.* 2002). However, the numbers of patients included in these studies were low and the control groups consisted of historical controls in which bias may have been introduced because of different radiation therapy techniques. Studies with contemporary control groups may also be biased in the selection of patients for treatment, i.e. total vulvectomy would have been reserved for larger tumours. A study demonstrated that fatal recurrences occurred at either the resection site or groin more commonly in patients in whom the wide local excision and lymphadenectomy were performed through separate incisions (de Hullu *et al.* 2002). Interestingly, this did not shorten survival, probably owing to a lack of power.

The radical nature of a vulvectomy is defined by both depth of resection and lateral margins. The depth of resection will be superficial if tissues beneath the vulval skin are not removed or radical if they are removed. The levels of resection that are taken to perform either radical or

Table 11.3 Surgery for vulval lesions

Name of surgical procedure	Alternative name	Description of surgical excision	Indication
Extent of skin removal			
Local excision		Removal of the lesion with a lesion-free margin of at least 0.5–1 cm of clinically normal skin	T *in situ*–T1
Partial vulvectomy	Anterior, lateral, posterior vulvectomy (or combination), hemivulvectomy or modified radical vulvectomy	Removal of a portion of the vulva according to the mode of incision, a free margin of 1–2 cm of clinically normal skin is recommended	T1–T2
Total vulvectomy	Radical vulvectomy	Removal of the entire vulva	T2–T4
Depth of surgery			
Superficial vulvectomy	Skinning vulvectomy	Removal of only the skin, leaving *in situ* the underlying fatty tissue and fascial structures	T *in situ*
Simple vulvectomy		Removal of the skin along with the fatty tissue lying on the superficial fascia	T1A
Deep vulvectomy	Radical vulvectomy	Removal of the vulva and fatty tissue from the surface to the urogenital diaphragm	T1B–T4

Table 11.4 Outcome of patients treated with total radical vulvectomy compared with partial radical vulvectomy (modified radical vulvectomy)

Author (year)	Total vulvectomy			Partial vulvectomy		
	n	Recurrence (%)	Death (%)	*n*	Recurrence (%)	Death (%)
Burrell *et al.* (1988)	14	21	7	28	0	0
Stehman *et al.* (1992a)	98	8	17[a]	121	16	12[a]
Hoffman *et al.* (1992)	45	4.4[b]	–	52	2.2[b]	–
Lin *et al.* (1992)	70	9–13[b]	–	12	17[b]	–
Farias-Eisner *et al.* (1994)	18	–	Stage I: 0 Stage II: 25	56	–	Stage I: 0 Stage II: 10
Burke *et al.* (1995)	–	–	–	76	12	5
Magrina *et al.* (1998)	134	15.9	23.8	91	17.9	24
Maggino *et al.* (2000)	403	36.4	–	80	40	–
Rouzier *et al.* (2002)	134	20[b]	34	81	23.5[b]	20
de Hullu *et al.* (2002)	168	19.9	–	85	33.3	–

[a] Death from any cause.
[b] Local recurrence only.
–, not reported.

superficial vulvectomy are shown in Fig. 11.1b. Radical vulvectomies are used for invasive cancer (Fig. 11.2), whereas superficial vulvectomies are used for *in situ* disease (Fig. 11.3).

Initially, the management recommended for an invasive vulval carcinoma included a 1–2 cm margin (Hacker 1999). Heaps *et al.* (1990) reported that local control after radical vulvectomy was achieved in 100% of cases when a 1 cm margin of normal skin was included in the surgical specimen, but if the margin was less than 8 mm there was an associated 50% local recurrence rate. A later study showed the relative risks of local relapse were 3.35 in patients with a normal tissue margin of less than 1 cm and 2.86 in patients with positive margins (Rouzier *et al.* 2002). Partial vulvectomies with specific modified incisions are recommended and may provide the required margins (Micheletti *et al.* 1998). de Hullu *et al.* (2002) showed that surgical margins were inadequate in 50% of the patients treated with partial vulvectomy. Despite the intended surgical margin of 1 cm, on histological examination, only 50% had tumour-free margins measuring ≤ 8 mm. This may be partly due to shrinkage during fixation. Based on this finding, these authors then recommended changing the surgical margins from 1 to 2 cm. In partial radical vulvectomy, modification of the extent of surgical resection applies only to medial and lateral limits. The depth of the dissection must be the same as in total radical vulvectomy, extending from the skin to the level of the urogenital diaphragm. This requires the resection of the bulbocavernosus muscle, which covers the vestibular bulb (clitoral bulb) and the Bartholin's gland.

Vulval carcinoma arises from pre-existing dermatoses in 90% of patients, namely lichen sclerosus or classical HPV-related VIN (Borgno *et al.* 1988, Rouzier *et al.* 2001).

Preserving vulval skin may be controversial in lichen sclerosus as further SCCs may develop as a result of field change. However, with VIN, the common practice is to remove the tumour and surrounding preneoplastic skin with a 5–10 mm margin. If there is residual VIN at a site away from the original tumour, this requires simple excision or skinning vulvectomy if extensive. Close follow-up for life is required in all cases.

Groin procedures

En bloc approach and separate incisions

The standard approach for radical vulvectomy and bilateral groin node dissection was traditionally through a butterfly incision. This was based on the work of Stoekel, Taussig and Way, each of whom reported survival advantage through radical resection (Stoekel 1930, Taussig 1931, 1935, Way 1948). The introduction of inguinofemoral lymphadenectomy via separate incisions was introduced in the 1960s (Byron *et al.* 1962). The rationale was that dissemination to the inguinofemoral lymph nodes does not occur in continuity but by embolization; therefore, the normal intervening skin between the vulvectomy and lymphadenectomy can be left. Preservation of this tissue decreased the postoperative wound breakdown and lymphoedema of the legs (Hacker *et al.* 1981, Helm *et al.* 1992, Lin *et al.* 1992, Hopkins *et al.* 1993, Burke *et al.* 1995). However, tumour recurrences in the skin bridge occasionally have been reported, even in node-negative patients (Christopherson *et al.* 1985, Schulz & Penalver 1989, Rose 1999). The technique and extent of lymphadenectomy have further evolved since the 1980s. Originally, inguinofemoral lymphadenectomy was performed without preservation of the fascia lata, but,

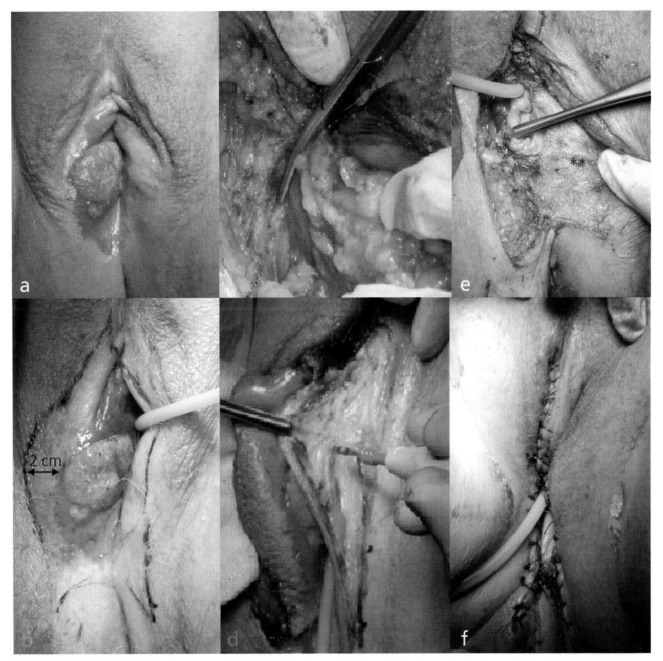

Fig. 11.2 Surgical treatment of an invasive vulval carcinoma arising in a context of lichen sclerosus. (a) A 4 cm exophytic lesion with typical signs of lichen sclerosus. (b) Drawing of the resection limits: a 2 cm margin is considered. (c) Radical left hemivulvectomy: the resection is extended to the level of the urogenital diaphragm – the bulbospongiosus muscle is clamped near the pelvic bone and resected. (d) Superficial right hemivulvectomy: the skin and the superficial layer of fat is resected. (e) Appearance after resection; *vagina, **areolar and fatty tissue of the labia majora. (f) Appearance after suturing.

because of the high morbidity, sartorius transposition was introduced. Unfortunately, this was associated with high rates of postoperative morbidity, such as wound lympho-cyst, dehiscence and infection, and the longer term issue of lymphoedema. To overcome these problems, superficial inguinal lymphadenectomy was performed but no deep femoral nodes were removed (DiSaia *et al.* 1979). Other authors removed preferentially those nodes internal to the superficial epigastric vein, the great saphenous vein and the femoral vein (Rouzier *et al.* 2003). This procedure had been initially used in penile cancer, and was based on reports of the obligatory drainage of lymph and hence metastases to a

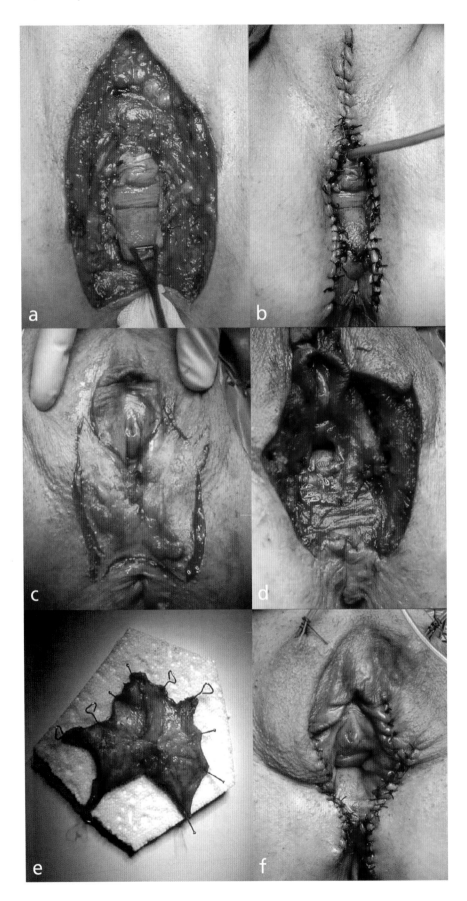

Fig. 11.3 Examples of radical vulvectomy. (a) Total radical vulvectomy. (b) Appearance after suturing. (c) Surgical treatment of an invasive vulval carcinoma located on the fourchette. (d) Appearance following resection. (e) Surgical specimen. (f) Final appearance after suturing.

sentinel inguinofemoral node at the superficial epigastric vein (Cabanas 1977). This technique was abandoned owing to the failure to find positive sentinel nodes in penile cancer and the poor results in vulval cancer. It has been suggested by anatomists that deep femoral lymphadenectomy could be performed without removing the fascia lata, because femoral nodes are always situated medially to the femoral vein (Borgno et al. 1990, Micheletti et al. 1990). This led surgeons to perform inguinal and medial femoral lymphadenectomy (Fig. 11.4). At the same time, it was proposed to spare the great saphenous vein. These latter modifications of lymphadenectomy greatly reduce morbidity while the number of nodes removed is similar to the inguinofemoral lymphadenectomy (Rouzier et al. 2003). This procedure is now considered as the standard groin lymphadenectomy.

Unilateral or bilateral inguinofemoral lymphadenectomy

The lateral vulva and labia drain to the ipsilateral nodes, whereas median structures of the vulva have a bilateral drainage, as demonstrated by Iversen and Aas (1983) and other authors (Burger et al. 1996). Iversen and Aas (1983) injected ^{99m}Tc-labelled colloid into different areas of the vulva in patients with cervical cancer and measured the radioactivity in the groins and pelvis with a scintillation camera. They showed that the clitoris, the anterior part of the vulva and the perineum had a bilateral lymph drainage. In all the other areas, the majority of the radioactivity was found in the ipsilateral lymph nodes. A small amount of radioactivity was recorded in the contralateral nodes in 67% of the patients. The clinical experience in patients with a lateral tumour supports these findings as contralateral lymph node metastases are rare if the ipsilateral nodes are not involved. van der Velden (1996) found that 19 out of 489 patients (3.9%) with a lateral vulval tumour and negative ipsilateral lymph nodes did have positive contralateral lymph nodes. If the tumour was less than 2 cm wide, the incidence of contralateral lymph node metastases was only 0.9% (de Hullu & van der Zee 2006).

In a prospective study conducted by the Gynaecology Oncology Group, contralateral groin node metastases were found in 3 out of 107 patients (2.8%) (Stehman et al. 1992a). Considering the morbidity of an inguinofemoral lymphadenectomy and the low risk of contralateral metastases, it is now generally accepted that it is sufficient to perform an unilateral groin procedure in patients with a T1/T2 laterally placed tumour. The definition of a median tumour is controversial as Iversen and Aas (1983) showed that the medial part of the labia minora has a bilateral drainage, so this area was considered to be the dividing line to define a medial or lateral tumour. However, this margin may be impossible to define in diseases such as lichen sclerosus that have altered vulval anatomy. Most authors would define a

lateral tumour as one which is greater than 1 cm from the midline (Benedet et al. 2000). If there are ipsilateral lymph node metastases the normal lymph flow may be interrupted and alternative channels come into play, and contralateral lymph node metastases may occur as a consequence. If ipsilateral lymph node metastases have been identified, there is an argument as to whether the contralateral groin needs to be treated, either by dissection or by irradiation. The recommendation of FIGO is that patients should receive bilateral pelvic and groin irradiation (Benedet et al. 2000), but the Society of Obstetricians and Gynecologists of Canada recommends a contralateral lymphadenectomy (Faught 2006).

Sentinel node procedure

Recently, sentinel node evaluation and mapping has been developed for the evaluation of the inguinal nodes (Fig. 11.4). This is done by injection of a blue dye and/or a radioactive colloid into the vulval tumour. Subsequently, the 'hot' and/or 'blue' nodes are identified, removed and analysed to determine whether metastases are present. A complete dissection is undertaken only if a sentinel node is positive. If the sentinel node is negative, the remaining lymph nodes are left. The procedure is based on the assumption of an orderly sequential drainage to the nodes, as has been accepted for breast and melanoma. In a series of 21 patients, the sentinel node was detected in 86% by using a blue dye only (Levenback et al. 1994, 2001). Further studies in 59 patients using a combined technique of blue dye and lymphoscintigraphy identified sentinel nodes in 95 groins (de Hullu et al. 2000). Ninety-five groins then underwent complete dissection, with a median yield of 12 nodes per groin. The 95 groins contained 139 sentinel nodes. Twenty-seven groins from 20 patients were node positive, and 68 were node negative. The false negative rate was 0%. In the 102 nodes negative by routine sectioning, four were positive on further sectioning augmented with immunohistochemistry. This combined technique was considered to be superior to the blue dye alone. The value of blue dye in combination with lymphoscintigraphy has been emphasized by other authors and should be recommended as the optimal technique (Stehman & Look 2006, Hauspy et al. 2007, Moore et al. 2008). The complication rate and morbidity of sentinel node mapping technique are low with the exception of a 1–2% risk of anaphylaxis to the dye. A review of the main series published is reported in Table 11.5. The detection rate was 92%, and the positive predictive value was 99%. The technique is limited by the fact that a sentinel node is not always identifiable, especially in midline tumours that may drain bilaterally. In one series, lymphoscintigraphy and intraoperative identification suggested a unilateral drainage of the tumour with sentinel nodes localized in only one groin for 13 out of 17 patients with

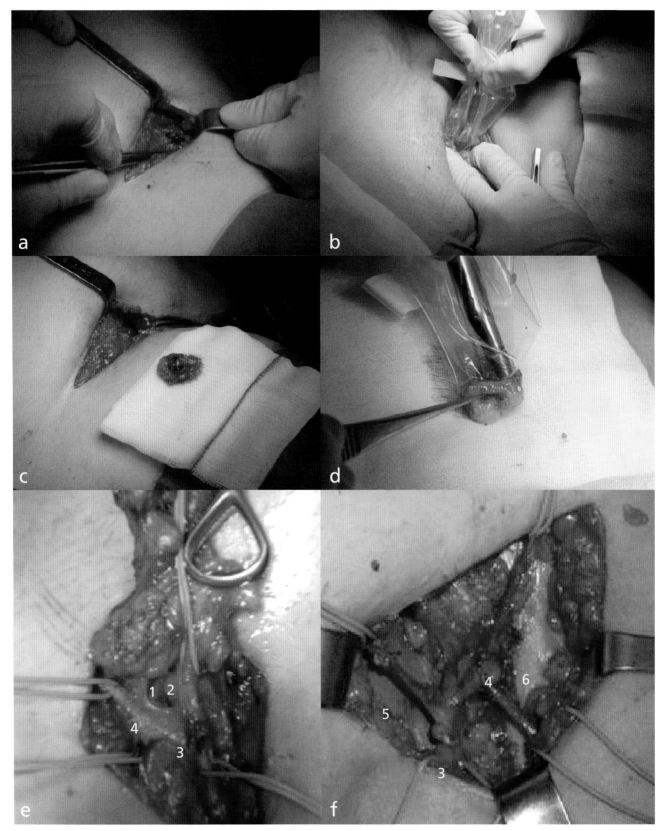

Fig. 11.4 Sentinel lymph node identification and lymphadenectomy. (a and c) Identification of a 'blue' node. (b and d) Identification of a 'hot' node. (e, right side; f, left side) Example of conservative inguinofemoral lymphadenectomies: 1, femoral vein; 2, superficial epigastric vein; 3, saphenous vein; 4, iliac circumflex vein and accessory saphenous vein; 5, long adductor muscle; and 6, sartorius muscle.

Table 11.5 Studies on the accuracy of the sentinel lymph node procedure in vulval cancer

Author (year)	Number of patients	Tracer[a]	Identification rate (%)	False negative cases
Ansink et al. (1999)	51	B	56	2
De Cicco et al. (2000)	37	R	100	0
de Hullu et al. (2000)	59	C	100	0
Levenback et al. (2001)	52	B	88	0
Sliutz et al. (2002)	26	C	100	0
Moore et al. (2003)	21	C	100	0
Puig-Tintoré et al. (2003)	26	C	96	0
Louis-Sylvestre et al. (2006)	17	C	100	0 (+3)
Merisio et al. (2005)	20	C	100	1 (+1)

[a] B, blue dye; R, radioactive; C, combined.

midline tumours (Louis-Sylvestre et al. 2006). Among these 13 patients, three groins with no sentinel node identified in fact contained massively metastatic nodes. They concluded that the unilateral finding of a sentinel node in tumours of the midline does not preclude a metastatic node in the other groin and therefore bilateral lymph node dissection should be the recommended treatment for these patients. Step sectioning may show metastases in nodes considered negative on frozen section, necessitating a second procedure. There are anecdotal reports of false negative sentinel nodes owing to blockage of lymphatic channels by the tumour with a reroute of the drainage to nodes other than the sentinel nodes.

Van der Zee et al. (2008) reported the safety and clinical advantage of the sentinel node procedure in early vulval cancer. In a study of 403 patients with T1/T2 (< 4 cm) tumours, inguinofemoral lymphadenectomy was omitted if the sentinel node was found to be negative. The patients were followed up 2 monthly for at least 2 years and were removed from the trial if there was a groin recurrence. Two hundred and fifty-nine patients had a negative sentinel node (median follow-up time, 35 months), six groin recurrences were diagnosed (2.3%) and the 3 year survival rate was 97%. The short- and long-term morbidity was less after removal of the sentinel node alone then after sentinel node removal and inguinofemoral lymphadenectomy. This large series would suggest that sentinel node removal for histological assessment should become standard treatment in patients with early stage disease. However, the training of the personnel to perform these procedures has yet to be defined and standardized.

Guidelines for management according to staging

Treatment guidelines for vulval cancer according to stage of disease are outlined in Table 11.6. The risk of disease recurrence is low after partial radical vulvectomy in which surgical margins of 1 cm are obtained, providing there is a solitary tumour and no background preneoplastic lesions. En bloc vulvectomies may still be required to treat patients with FIGO stage IV disease. Patients with tumour size less than 4 cm may benefit from sentinel lymph node biopsy. More advanced disease may require the additional approach of chemoradiation as preliminary studies have been encouraging. However, a randomized study still favours surgery as the treatment of choice (Maneo et al. 2003).

Adjuvant treatment

Close surgical margins

Postoperative radiation may be used for close surgical margins (< 5 mm), if further excision is not possible (Faul et al. 1997). However, in one study, it was shown that local control was better in patients with positive margins than in those with narrow margins (Rouzier et al. 2002). This finding may be explained by the additional radiotherapy received by those with positive margins. In some cases, the positive margin may be treated with a radioactive implant (brachytherapy), but this technique requires experience to avoid an excessive risk of necrosis (Blake 2003). Another alternative is electron beam therapy targeted at the operation site after the wound has healed (Blake 2003). Inoperable tumours probably require 60–70 Gy to achieve local control, although a wide variety of chemoradiation schedules are currently under investigation (van Doorn et al. 2006).

Management of pelvic and groin nodes

Pelvic nodes

Systematic pelvic lymphadenectomy was abandoned after the results of a trial of 114 patients randomized to either pelvic radiation or pelvic node resection (Homesley et al.

Table 11.6 Surgical or alternative recommendations for vulval cancer according to FIGO* stage

Stage		Standard treatment	Option
o	Cancer *in situ*	Superficial partial vulvectomy	CO_2 laser or imiquimod
I	Lesions ≤ 2 cm in size, confined to the vulva or perineum, no nodal metastasis		
IA	Stromal invasion ≤ 1.0 mm	Superficial partial vulvectomy	If unfavourable features (neural or vascular invasion), consider more radical excision
IB	Stromal invasion > 1.0 mm	Radical partial vulvectomy + sentinel lymph node procedure or lymphadenectomy	
II	Lesions > 2 cm in size, confined to the vulva or perineum, no nodal metastasis	Radical partial/total vulvectomy + sentinel lymph node procedure (≤ 4 cm) lymphadenectomy	
III	Tumour of any size with adjacent spread to the lower urethra, vagina or anus and/or unilateral regional lymph node metastasis	Radical total vulvectomy + bilateral lymphadenectomy	Preoperative chemoradiation or chemoradiation only
IVA	Tumour invading the upper urethra, bladder mucosa, rectal mucus, or pelvic bone and/or bilateral regional node metastases	Radical or en bloc vulvectomy + lymphadenectomy	Preoperative chemoradiation or chemoradiation only

* International Federation of Gynecology and Obstetrics.

1986) showed that the survival rate was better in the pelvic radiation group ($P = 0.03$). Fixed ulcerated nodes or more than two positive nodes were poor prognostic indicators. The 2 year survival rate was 68% for the radiation treatment arm and 54% for the surgical arm. Pelvic radiation therapy has therefore become the standard treatment for patients with positive groin nodes, especially if the nodes are fixed or multiple. Based on the low incidence of metastatic pelvic lymph nodes in patients with negative inguinofemoral nodes, there is no rationale for routine pelvic lymphadenectomy in these patients. This trial did not assess the results of pelvic irradiation after pelvic lymphadenectomy, especially in patients with metastatic nodes at imaging. Survival might be improved by the removal of enlarged, bulky pelvic nodes (> 2 cm on CT scanning) prior to radiotherapy (Homesley *et al.* 1986, Hacker 2005), as it is theoretically possible that the radiotherapy fails to penetrate these very large nodes. It is unlikely that this combined approach will be beneficial as the prognosis of patients with pelvic nodal involvement is so poor. The new imaging techniques such as positron electron transmission (PET) scanning will improve the detection of pelvic and distant metastatic disease and give more accurate staging.

Groin nodes

The Gynecological Oncology Group started a study in which patients were randomized to either groin lymph node dissection or primary groin radiation (Stehman *et al.* 1992b).

The study was closed prematurely as there was an increased recurrence rate in the radiation group. In a Cochrane review (van der Velden & Ansink 2001), the conclusion was that, independent of the radiation dose, the recurrence rate of tumours was higher in those treated with radiotherapy.

Based on these and other studies, certain recommendations have been established for the management of enlarged lymph nodes in the groin (Benedet *et al.* 2000). Resection of all enlarged groin nodes should be performed, and frozen section histological assessment diagnosis obtained at the time of operation. If nodes are negative, full inguinal–femoral lymphadenectomy should be performed. If nodes are positive, both lymphadenectomy and radiation are required. A complete lymphadenectomy is not necessary in these circumstances because of the chronic lymphoedema associated with extensive surgery and radiation. Other authors recommend complete inguinofemoral lymphadenectomy whatever the status of groin nodes and radiation therapy in the cases in which nodal involvement (macrometastasis > 10 mm, extracapsular spread and two or more micrometastases) is found on histological examination. A further study has shown that adjuvant radiotherapy may improve the disease-specific survival of patients who were single node positive and who underwent a less extensive lymph node resection (≤ 12 nodes removed) (Parthasarathy *et al.* 2006). In a retrospective study (Hyde *et al.* 2007), 40 patients were treated either by a full inguinofemoral lymphadenectomy or debulking of the clinically involved inguinal lymph nodes. All patients received adjuvant radiotherapy to the groins. There was no difference in groin recurrence rate expressed as groin recurrence-free survival. In a univariate analysis, both overall and disease-free survivals were better in the group of patients treated by nodal debulking. However, multivariate analysis showed other variables such as extracapsular growth were independent predictors for survival whereas the method of surgical dissection for the groin had no independent impact on survival.

If, on the full histopathological examination, metastases are found in the sentinel node that was negative on frozen section, further surgery, i.e. full inguinofemoral lymphadenectomy, is required. Trials are awaited comparing adjuvant chemoradiation with complete lymphadenectomy in patients with positive sentinel nodes.

Radiation therapy

Radiation therapy is the first-line adjuvant therapy after surgery in cases of metastatic groin nodes. However, in cases in which there are ulcerated or fixed groin nodes, these should be biopsied first to obtain histological confirmation of metastases. The nodes can then be treated initially with radiation and, when feasible, resected afterwards (Fig. 11.4).

The dose of radiation is determined by the extent of regional disease and any residual tumour (Benedet *et al.* 2000). After a groin dissection with microscopic inguinal metastases, 50 Gy in 1.8–2.0 Gy fractions is usually sufficient. However, if there are multiple positive nodes or if there is evidence of extracapsular extension, higher doses up to 60 Gy may be given. Gross residual disease may require doses of 60–70 Gy. The radiation fields should include the inguinofemoral nodal area and at least the lower pelvic nodes below the sacroiliac joints. Special attention must be paid to adequate coverage of the inguinal nodes and CT-based assessment helps to ensure this.

Combined photon and electron techniques are often used to treat the regional nodes to avoid damaging the femoral heads. Bulky disease can be boosted with appositional electron fields selected to provide an adequate dose both on the surface and to deeper tumour or nodes. The role of concurrent chemotherapy is currently under investigation.

Neoadjuvant or exclusive chemoradiation

Traditionally, the treatment of squamous carcinoma of the anus was abdominoperineal resection of the rectum and permanent colostomy formation. However, surgery for SCC of the anus has been abandoned as primary therapy since the discovery that a combined chemotherapy and radiotherapy regimen could produce equivalent or better results without the necessity to sacrifice the anal sphincter (Flam *et al.* 1996). A similar approach to the treatment of SCC of the uterine cervix has been evolving (Eifel 2000). The superiority of combined radiotherapy and chemotherapy over radiotherapy alone has been demonstrated in randomized controlled trials for anal cancers. Similarities shared by vulval and anal carcinomata in terms of pathogenesis, particularly with regard to the oncogenic HPV, have led investigators to consider the combined radiochemotherapy regimens for the treatment of vulval cancer. Late stage or recurrent vulval cancer has been treated with infusions of 5-fluorouracil and mitomycin C combined with external-beam radiotherapy (Whitaker *et al.* 1990). Unfortunately, the side-effects are a problem as patients develop mucositis, leading to dysuria and generalized pelvic discomfort because there is only a small difference between the therapeutic dose and the toxic dose of radiation in the vulvovaginal area. This may necessitate an indwelling catheter or temporary stoma to ease the discomfort, but occasionally the treatment may have to be intermittent. Results show 31–55% complete response, questioning the need for surgery (Thomas *et al.* 1989, Berek *et al.* 1991, Koh *et al.* 1993, Eifel *et al.* 1995, Wahlen *et al.* 1995, Grigsby *et al.* 1996, Landoni *et al.* 1996, Lupi *et al.* 1996, Moore *et al.* 1998, Montana *et al.* 2000, Gerszten *et al.* 2005). Unfortunately, success rates remain substantially less than those reported with anal tumours. Despite the encouraging preliminary studies of chemoradiation, a randomized study favours primary surgery (Maneo *et al.* 2003).

If it is possible to resect the primary lesion with clear surgical margins and without sphincter damage, primary surgical excision is desirable (Benedet *et al.* 2000). Chemoradiation and limited surgery should be reserved for those tumours in which primary surgery would result in the need for either a bowel or urinary stoma.

Conclusion

Vulval carcinoma is still a rare tumour which can be cured if diagnosed and managed appropriately at an early stage. The last 20 years have seen major changes in the surgical management with individualization of treatment based on the tumour stage. The surgical approach for the primary tumour is now more conservative and there are various options for the management of lymph nodes. If strict criteria are laid down to define the extent of surgery for both the primary lesion and the regional lymph nodes, this will not only offer the optimum treatment but also reduce the physical and psychological morbidity for the patient.

References

Ansink, A.C., Sie-Go, D.M., van der Velden, J. *et al.* (1999) Identification of sentinel lymph nodes in vulvar carcinoma patients with the aid of a patent blue V injection: a multicenter study. *Cancer* **86**, 652–656.

Benedet, J.L., Hacker, N.F., Ngan, H.Y.S. *et al.* (2000) *Staging Classifications and Clinical Practice Guidelines of Gynaecologic Cancers.* Available from: www.figo.org/docs/staging_booklet.pdf.

Berek, J.S., Heaps, J.M., Fu, Y.S., Juillard, G.J. & Hacker, N.F. (1991) Concurrent cisplatin and 5-fluorouracil chemotherapy and radiation therapy for advanced-stage squamous carcinoma of the vulva. *Gynecologic Oncology* **42**, 197–201.

Blake, P. (2003) Radiotherapy and chemoradiotherapy for carcinoma of the vulva. *Clinical Obstetrics and Gynaecology* **17**, 649–661.

Borgno, G., Micheletti, L., Barbero, M. *et al.* (1988) Epithelial alterations adjacent to 111 vulvar carcinomas. *The Journal of Reproductive Medicine* **33**, 500–502.

Borgno, G., Micheletti, L., Barbero, M. *et al.* (1990) Topographic distribution of groin lymph nodes. A study of 50 female cadavers. *The Journal of Reproductive Medicine* **35**, 1127–1129.

Burger, P.M., Hollema, H. & Bouma, J. (1996) The side of groin node metastases in unilateral vulvar carcinoma. *International Journal of Gynecological Cancer* **6**, 318–322.

Burke, T.W., Levenback, C., Coleman, R.L. *et al.* (1995) Surgical therapy of T1 and T2 vulvar carcinoma: further experience with radical wide excision and selective inguinal lymphadenectomy. *Gynecologic Oncology* **57**, 215–220.

Burrell, M.O., Franklin, E.W., 3rd, Campion, M.J. *et al.* (1988) The modified radical vulvectomy with groin dissection: an eight-year experience. *American Journal of Obstetrics and Gynecology* **159**, 715–722.

Byron, S.C., Lamb, E.J., Yonemoto, R.H. & Kase, S. (1962) Radical inguinal node dissection in the treatment of cancer. *Surgery Gynecology Obstetrics* **114**, 401–408.

Cabanas, R.M. (1977) An approach for the treatment of penile carcinoma *Cancer* **39**, 456–466.

Christopherson, W., Buchsbaum, H.J., Voet, R. & Lifschitz, S. (1985) Radical vulvectomy and bilateral groin lymphadenectomy utilizing separate groin incisions: report of a case with recurrence in the intervening skin bridge. *Gynecologic Oncology* **21**, 247–251.

De Cicco, C., Sideri, M., Bartolomei, M. *et al.* (2000) Sentinel node biopsy in early vulvar cancer. *British Journal of Cancer* **82**, 295–299.

de Hullu, J.A. & van der Zee, A.G. (2006) Surgery and radiotherapy in vulvar cancer. *Critical Reviews in Oncology/Hematology* **60**, 38–58.

de Hullu, J.A., Hollema, H., Piers, D.A. *et al.* (2000) Sentinel lymph node procedure is highly accurate in squamous cell carcinoma of the vulva. *Journal of Clinical Oncology* **18**, 2811–2816.

de Hullu, J.A., Hollema, H., Lolkema, S. *et al.* (2002) Vulvar carcinoma. The price of less radical surgery *Cancer* **95**, 2331–2338.

DiSaia, P.J., Creasman, W.T. & Rich, W.M. (1979) An alternate approach to early cancer of the vulva. *American Journal of Obstetrics and Gynecology* **133**, 825–832.

Eifel, P.J. (2000) Chemoradiation for carcinoma of the cervix: advances and opportunities. *Radiation Research* **154**, 229–236.

Eifel, P.J., Morris, M., Burke, T.W. *et al.* (1995) Prolonged continuous infusion cisplatin and 5-fluorouracil with radiation for locally advanced carcinoma of the vulva. *Gynecologic Oncology* **59**, 51–56.

Farias-Eisner, R., Cirisano, F.D., Grouse, D. *et al.* (1994) Conservative and individualized surgery for early squamous carcinoma of the vulva: the treatment of choice for stage I and II (T1-2N0-1M0) disease. *Gynecologic Oncology* **53**, 55–58.

Faught, W. (2006) *Management of Squamous Cell Cancer of the Vulva.* Available from: http://www.sogc.org/guidelines/documents/180E-CPG-July2006.pdf.

Faul, C.M., Mirmow, D., Huang, Q. *et al.* (1997) Adjuvant radiation for vulvar carcinoma: improved local control. *International Journal of Radiation Oncology, Biology, Physics* **38**, 381–389.

Finan, M.A. & Barre, G. (2003) Bartholin's gland carcinoma, malignant melanoma and other rare tumours of the vulva. *Clinical Obstetrics and Gynaecology* **17**, 609–633.

Flam, M., John, M., Pajak, T.F. *et al.* (1996) Role of mitomycin in combination with fluorouracil and radiotherapy, and of salvage chemoradiation in the definitive nonsurgical treatment of epidermoid carcinoma of the anal canal: results of a phase III randomized intergroup study. *Journal of Clinical Oncology* **14**, 2527–2539.

Gerszten, K., Selvaraj, R.N., Kelley, J. & Faul, C. (2005) Preoperative chemoradiation for locally advanced carcinoma of the vulva. *Gynecologic Oncology* **99**, 640–644.

Ghurani, G.B. & Penalver, M.A. (2001) An update on vulvar cancer. *American Journal of Obstetrics and Gynecology* **185**, 294–299.

Grigsby, P.W., Graham, M.V., Perez, C.A. *et al.* (1996) Prospective phase I/II studies of definitive irradiation and chemotherapy for advanced gynecologic malignancies. *American Journal of Clinical Oncology* **19**, 1–6.

Hacker, N.F. (1999) Radical resection of vulvar malignancies: a paradigm shift in surgical approaches. *Current Opinion in Obstetrics and Gynecology* **11**, 61–64.

Hacker, N.F. (2005) Vulvar cancer. In: *Practical Gynecologic Oncology*, 4th edn (eds J.S. Berek and N.F. Hacker), pp. 585–602. Williams & Wilkins, Philadelphia.

Hacker, N.F., Leuchter, R.S., Berek, J.S. *et al.* (1981) Radical vulvectomy and bilateral inguinal lymphadenectomy through separate groin incisions. *Obstetrics and Gynecology* **58**, 574–579.

Hauspy, J., Beiner, M., Harley, I. *et al.* (2007) Sentinel lymph node in vulvar cancer. *Cancer* **110**, 1015–1023.

Heaps, J.M., Fu, Y.S., Montz, F.J. *et al.* (1990) Surgical-pathologic variables predictive of local recurrence in squamous cell carcinoma of the vulva. *Gynecologic Oncology* **38**, 309–314.

Helm, C.W., Hatch, K., Austin, J.M. *et al.* (1992) A matched comparison of single and triple incision techniques for the surgical treatment of carcinoma of the vulva. *Gynecologic Oncology* **46**, 150–156.

Hoffman, M.S., Roberts, W.S., Finan, M.A. *et al.* (1992) A comparative study of radical vulvectomy and modified radical vulvectomy for the treatment of invasive squamous cell carcinoma of the vulva. *Gynecological Oncology* **45**, 192–197.

Homesley, H.D., Bundy, B.N., Sedlis, A. & Adcock, L. (1986) Radiation therapy versus pelvic node resection for carcinoma of the vulva with positive groin nodes. *Obstetrics and Gynecology* **68**, 733–740.

Hopkins, M.P., Reid, G.C. & Morley, G.W. (1993) Radical vulvectomy. The decision for the incision. *Cancer* **72**, 799–803.

Hording, U., Kringsholm, B., Andreasson, B. *et al.* (1993) Human papillomavirus in vulvar squamous-cell carcinoma and in normal vulvar tissues: a search for a possible impact of HPV on vulvar cancer prognosis. *International Journal of Cancer* **55**, 394–396.

Hyde, S.E., Valmadre, S., Hacker, N.F. *et al.* (2007) Squamous cell carcinoma of the vulva with bulky positive groin nodes: nodal debulking versus full groin dissection prior to radiation therapy. *International Journal of Gynecological Cancer* **17**, 154–158.

Iversen, T. & Aas, M. (1983) Lymph drainage from the vulva. *Gynecologic Oncology* **16**, 179–189.

Iversen, T. & Tretli, S. (1998) Intraepithelial and invasive squamous cell neoplasia of the vulva: trends in incidence, recurrence, and survival rate in Norway. *Obstetrics and Gynecology* **91**, 969–972.

Jones, R.W., Baranyai, J. & Stables, S. (1997) Trends in squamous cell carcinoma of the vulva: the influence of vulvar intraepithelial neoplasia. *Obstetrics and Gynecology* **90**, 448–452.

Jones, R.W., Rowan, D.M. & Stewart, A.W. (2005) Vulvar intraepithelial neoplasia: aspects of the natural history and outcome in 405 women. *Obstetrics and Gynecology* **106**, 1319–1326.

Joura, E.A., Losch, A., Haider-Angeler, M.G. *et al.* (2000) Trends in vulvar neoplasia. Increasing incidence of vulvar intraepithelial neoplasia and squamous cell carcinoma of the vulva in young women. *The Journal of Reproductive Medicine* **45**, 613–615.

Judson, P.L., Habermann, E.B., Baxter, N.N. *et al.* (2006) Trends in the incidence of invasive and in situ vulvar carcinoma. *Obstetrics and Gynecology* **107**, 1018–1022.

Koh, W.J., Wallace, H.J., 3rd, Greer, B.E. *et al.* (1993) Combined radiotherapy and chemotherapy in the management of local-regionally advanced vulvar cancer. *International Journal of Radiation Oncology, Biology, Physics* **26**, 809–816.

Landoni, F., Maneo, A., Zanetta, G. *et al.* (1996) Concurrent preoperative chemotherapy with 5-fluorouracil and mitomycin C and radiotherapy (FUMIR) followed by limited surgery in locally advanced and recurrent vulvar carcinoma. *Gynecologic Oncology* **61**, 321–327.

Levenback, C., Burke, T.W., Gershenson, D.M. *et al.* (1994) Intraoperative lymphatic mapping for vulvar cancer. *Obstetrics and Gynecology* **84**, 163–167.

Levenback, C., Morris, M., Burke, T.W. *et al.* (1996) Groin dissection practices among gynecologic oncologists treating early vulvar cancer. *Gynecologic Oncology* **62**, 73–77.

Levenback, C., Coleman, R.L., Burke, T.W. *et al.* (2001) Intraoperative lymphatic mapping and sentinel node identification with blue dye in patients with vulvar cancer. *Gynecologic Oncology* **83**, 276–281.

Lin, J.Y., DuBeshter, B., Angel, C. & Dvoretsky, P.M. (1992) Morbidity and recurrence with modifications of radical vulvectomy and groin dissection. *Gynecologic Oncology* **47**, 80–86.

Louis-Sylvestre, C., Evangelista, E., Leonard, F. *et al.* (2006) Interpretation of sentinel node identification in vulvar cancer. *Gynecologie, Obstetrique et Fertilite* **34**, 706–710.

Lupi, G., Raspagliesi, F., Zucali, R. *et al.* (1996) Combined preoperative chemoradiotherapy followed by radical surgery in locally advanced vulvar carcinoma. A pilot study. *Cancer* **77**, 1472–1478.

Maggino, T., Landoni, F., Sartori, E. *et al.* (2000) Patterns of recurrence in patients with squamous cell carcinoma of the vulva. A multicenter CTF Study. *Cancer* **89**, 116–122.

Magrina, J.F., Gonzalez-Bosquet, J., Weaver, A.L., *et al.* (1998) Primary squamous cell cancer of the vulva: radical versus modified radical vulvar surgery. *Gynecological Oncology* **71**, 116–121.

Maneo, A., Landoni, F., Colombo, A. *et al.* (2003) Randomized study between neoadjuvant chemoradiotherapy and primary surgery for the treatment of advanced vulvar cancer. *International Journal of Gynecological Cancer* **13** (Suppl 1 PL 19), 6.

Marsden, D.E. & Hacker, N.F. (2001) Contemporary management of primary carcinoma of the vulva. *Surgical Clinics of North America* **81**, 799–813.

Merisio, C., Berretta, R., Gualdi, M. *et al.* (2005) Radioguided sentinel lymph node detection in vulvar cancer. *International Journal of Gynaecological Cancer* **15**, 493–497.

Micheletti, L., Borgno, G., Barbero, M. *et al.* (1990) Deep femoral lymphadenectomy with preservation of the fascia lata. Preliminary report on 42 invasive vulvar carcinomas. *The Journal of Reproductive Medicine* **35**, 1130–1133.

Micheletti, L., Preti, M., Zola, P. *et al.* (1998) A proposed glossary of terminology related to the surgical treatment of vulvar carcinoma. *Cancer* **83**, 1369–1375.

Micheletti, L., Levi, A.C., Bogliatto, F. *et al.* (2002) Rationale and definition of the lateral extension of the inguinal lymphadenectomy for vulvar cancer derived from an embryological and anatomical study. *Journal of Surgical Oncology* **81**, 19–24.

Montana, G.S., Thomas, G.M., Moore, D.H. *et al.* (2000) Preoperative chemo-radiation for carcinoma of the vulva with N2/N3 nodes: a gynecologic oncology group study. *International Journal of Radiation Oncology, Biology, Physics* **48**, 1007–1013.

Moore, D.H., Thomas, G.M., Montana, G.S. *et al.* (1998) Preoperative chemoradiation for advanced vulvar cancer: a phase II study of the Gynecologic Oncology Group. *International Journal of Radiation Oncology, Biology, Physics* **42**, 79–85.

Moore, R.G., DePasquale, S.E., Steinhoff, M.M. *et al.* (2003) Sentinel node identification and the ability to detect metastatic tumor to inguinal lymph nodes in squamous cell cancer of the vulva. *Gynecological Oncology* **89**, 475–479.

Moore, R.G., Robison, K., Brown, A.K. *et al.* (2008) Isolated sentinel lymph node dissection with conservative management in patients with squamous cell carcinoma of the vulva: a prospective trial. *Gynecologic Oncology* **109**, 65–70.

Parthasarathy, A., Cheung, M.K., Osann, K. *et al.* (2006) The benefit of adjuvant radiation therapy in single-node-positive squamous cell vulvar carcinoma. *Gynecologic Oncology* **103**, 1095–1099.

Podratz, K.C., Symmonds, R.E., Taylor, W.F. & Williams, T.J. (1983) Carcinoma of the vulva: analysis of treatment and survival. *Obstetrics and Gynecology* **61**, 63–74.

Puig-Tintoré, L.M., Ordi, J., Vidal-Sicart, S. *et al.* (2003) Further data on the usefulness of sentinel lymph node identification and ultrastaging in vulvar squamous cell carcinoma. *Gynecological Oncology* **88**, 29–34.

Rhodes, C.A., Cummins, C. & Shafi, M.I. (1998) The management of squamous cell vulval cancer: a population based retrospective study of 411 cases. *British Journal of Obstetrics and Gynaecology* **105**, 200–205.

Rose, P.G. (1999) Skin bridge recurrences in vulvar cancer: frequency and management. *International Journal of Gynecological Cancer* **9**, 508–511.

Rosen, C. & Malmstrom, H. (1997) Invasive cancer of the vulva. *Gynecologic Oncology* **65**, 213–217.

Rouzier, R., Morice, P., Haie-Meder, C. *et al.* (2001) Prognostic significance of epithelial disorders adjacent to invasive vulvar carcinomas. *Gynecologic Oncology* **81**, 414–419.

Rouzier, R., Haddad, B., Plantier, F. *et al.* (2002) Local relapse in patients treated for squamous cell vulvar carcinoma: incidence and prognostic value. *Obstetrics and Gynecology* **100**, 1159–1167.

Rouzier, R., Haddad, B., Dubernard, G. *et al.* (2003) Inguinofemoral dissection for carcinoma of the vulva: effect of modifications of extent and technique on morbidity and survival. *Journal of the American College of Surgeons* **196**, 442–450.

Rouzier, R., Preti, M., Haddad, B. *et al.* (2006) Development and validation of a nomogram for predicting outcome of patients with vulvar cancer. *Obstetrics and Gynecology* **107**, 672–677.

Schulz, M.J. & Penalver, M. (1989) Recurrent vulvar carcinoma in the intervening tissue bridge in early invasive stage I disease treated by radical vulvectomy and bilateral groin dissection through separate incisions. *Gynecologic Oncology* 35, 383–386.

Shepherd, J.H. (1989) Revised FIGO staging for gynaecological cancer. *British Journal of Obstetrics and Gynaecology* 96, 889–892.

Shepherd, J.H. (1995) Staging announcement, FIGO staging of gynaecologic cancers cervical and vulva. *International Journal of Gynaecological Cancer* 5, 319.

Sideri, M., Jones, R.W., Wilkinson, E.J. *et al.* (2005) Squamous vulvar intraepithelial neoplasia: 2004 modified terminology, ISSVD Vulvar Oncology Subcommittee. *The Journal of Reproductive Medicine* 50, 807–810.

Sliutz, G., Reinthaller, A., Lantzsch, T. *et al.* (2002) Lymphatic mapping of sentinel nodes in early vulvar cancer. *Gynecological Oncology* 84, 449–452.

Stehman, F.B. & Look, K.Y. (2006) Carcinoma of the vulva. *Obstetrics and Gynecology* 107, 719–733.

Stehman, F.B., Bundy, B.N., Dvoretsky, P.M. & Creasman, W.T. (1992a) Early stage I carcinoma of the vulva treated with ipsilateral superficial inguinal lymphadenectomy and modified radical hemivulvectomy: a prospective study of the Gynecologic Oncology Group. *Obstetrics and Gynecology* 79, 490–497.

Stehman, F.B., Bundy, B.N., Thomas, G. *et al.* (1992b) Groin dissection versus groin radiation in carcinoma of the vulva: a Gynecologic Oncology Group study. *International Journal of Radiation Oncology, Biology, Physics* 24, 389–396.

Stoekel, W. (1930) Zur therapie des vulva karzinoms. *Zentralblatt für Gynakologie* 1, 47–71.

Sutton, B.C., Allen, R.A., Moore, W.E. & Dunn, S.T. (2008) Distribution of human papillomavirus genotypes in invasive squamous carcinoma of the vulva. *Modern Pathology* 21, 345–354.

Taussig, F.J. (1931) *Disease of the Vulva*. Appleton-Century-Croft, New York.

Taussig, F.J. (1935) Primary cancer of the vulva, vagina and female urethra: five-year results. *Surgery Gynecology Obstetrics* 60, 477–478.

Thomas, G., Dembo, A., DePetrillo, A. *et al.* (1989) Concurrent radiation and chemotherapy in vulvar carcinoma. *Gynecologic Oncology* 34, 263–267.

van Beurden, M., ten Kate, F.W., Tjong-A-Hung, S.P. *et al.* (1998) Human papillomavirus DNA in multicentric vulvar intraepithelial neoplasia. *International Journal of Gynecological Pathology* 17, 12–16.

van der Velden, J. (1996) Some aspects of the management of squamous cell carcinoma of the vulva. Thesis. Amsterdam, The Netherlands.

van der Velden, J. & Ansink, A. (2001) Primary groin irradiation vs primary groin surgery for early vulvar cancer. *Cochrane Database of Systematic Reviews* 4, CD002224.

van der Velden, J., van Lindert, A.C., Gimbrere, C.H. *et al.* (1996) Epidemiologic data on vulvar cancer: comparison of hospital with population-based data. *Gynecologic Oncology* 62, 379–383.

Van der Zee, A.G., Oonk, M.H., De Hullu, J.A. *et al.* (2008) Sentinel node dissection is safe in the treatment of early-stage vulvar cancer. *Journal of Clinical Oncology* 26, 884–889.

van Doorn, H.C., Ansink, A., Verhaar-Langereis, M. & Stalpers, L. (2006) Neoadjuvant chemoradiation for advanced primary vulvar cancer. *Cochrane Database of Systematic Reviews* 3, CD003752.

van Seters, M., van Beurden, M. & de Craen, A.J. (2005) Is the assumed natural history of vulvar intraepithelial neoplasia III based on enough evidence? A systematic review of 3322 published patients. *Gynecologic Oncology* 97, 645–651.

Wahlen, S.A., Slater, J.D., Wagner, R.J. *et al.* (1995) Concurrent radiation therapy and chemotherapy in the treatment of primary squamous cell carcinoma of the vulva. *Cancer* 75, 2289–2294.

Way, S. (1948) The anatomy of the lymphatic drainage of the vulva, and its influence on the radical operation for carcinoma. *Annals of the Royal College Surgeons of England* 3, 187–209.

Whitaker, S.J., Kirkbride, P., Arnott, S.J. *et al.* (1990) A pilot study of chemo-radiotherapy in advanced carcinoma of the vulva. *British Journal of Obstetrics and Gynaecology* 97, 436–442.

Index

Page numbers in *italics* represent figures, those in **bold** represent tables.

A

abscess, Bartholin's gland, 75
acanthosis nigricans, 99
acetowhite tissue, 37
acquired dyskeratotic leukoplakia, 131
acrodermatitis enteropathica, 91, *91*
Actinomyces
  A. genercseriae, 77
  A. israelii, 77
actinomycosis, 77
acute febrile neutrophilic dermatosis, 93
aciclovir, 57
adenocarcinoma, 192
adenosquamous carcinoma, 192–3, *192*
adhesions, 235–6
  clitoral, 235–6, *235*
  fourchette, 235
  labial, 131–2, *132*, 235
    surgical repair, 233, *233*
  vulvovaginal, 236–7, *236*
aggressive angiomyxoma, 204–5, *204*
allergic contact dermatitis, 113
  children, 132–3
alopecia areata, 104
alveolar soft-part sarcoma, 210
ambiguous external genitalia, 9–11
  female pseudohermaphroditism, 10–11,
    221–2, *222*
  gonadal differentiation disorders, 9–10
  male pseudohermaphroditism, 11, 222–3,
    223
amoebiasis, 72–3, *73*
amyloidosis, 94, *94*
anal stenosis, 13
anal triangle, 18
anatomy, 13–20, 240–1, *241*
  groin, 240
  vulva, 240
  see also individual organs
androgens
  exogenous, 11
  fetal, 11
  maternal, 11
angiokeratoma, 206–7, *206*
angiolymphoid hyperplasia with eosinophilia,
  128
angiomyofibroblastoma, 203, *203*

angiosarcoma, 207
anogenital mammary-like glands, 13, 23,
  185–6, *186*
  benign neoplasms, 186–7
  carcinoma, 187–8
  cysts, 168–9
antidepressants, 164–5
anxiety, 156–7
aphthous ulceration, recurrent, 97, *97*, 98
apocrine carcinoma, 189
apocrine miliaria, 101
apocrine sweat glands, 9
arousal, 27
atopic eczema, 112
azithromycin, 54, 55

B

bacterial infections, 74–7
  corynebacteria, 75–6
  Gram-positive cocci, 74–5
  mycobacteria, 76–7
  sexually transmitted, 48–55
  see also individual conditions
bacterial vaginosis, 48–9, *48*
Bacteroides, 44
Bartholin's abscess, 51, 75, 168, *169*
  post-drainage repair, 228–9
Bartholin's glands, 15, *15*
  benign neoplasms, 190
  carcinoma, 190–2, *191*, *192*
  hyperplasia, 190, *190*
basal cell carcinoma, 181–3, *182*, *183*
Basidiobolas, 74
Behçet's syndrome, 96–7, *97*
benign adnexal skin tumours, 188–9
benign familial chronic pemphigus,
  87–8, *88*
  variants, 88
biopsy, 39–40
Birbeck granules, 24
bladder exstrophy, 12
  reconstruction, 223–4, *224*
blood tests, 40
Borrelia burgdorferi, 79
breast development, 26
Brugia
  B. malayi, 71
  B. timori, 71
bullous (blistering) diseases, 107–10
  in children, 134

bullous congenital ichthyosiform erythroderma,
  88
bullous pemphigoid, 107, *107*, *108*
  in children, 134
Buschke–Lowenstein tumour, 59

C

canal of Nuck, cysts of, 169
Candida, 45
  C. albicans, 46
  C. glabrata, 46
  C. krusei, 46
  C. parapsilosis, 46
  C. tropicalis, 46
carcinoma
  adenosquamous, 192–3, *192*
  anogenital mammary-like glands, 187–8
  apocrine, 189
  Bartholin's glands, 190–2, *191*, *192*
  basal cell, 181–3, *182*, *183*
  condylomatous (warty), 181, *181*
  eccrine mucinous, 189–90, *189*
  Merkel cells, 193, *193*
  metastatic, 193–4
  squamous, 176–9, *176–9*
  sweat glands, 189–90
  verrucous, 179–81, *180*
  see also tumours; vulval cancers
Carnegie stages, 2–7, *2–7*
Carney complex, 210
carunculae myrtiformes, 15
ceftriazone, 55
cellular angiofibroma, 203–4, *204*
cellulitis, 75
  children, 80–1, *81*
cervical intraepithelial neoplasia (CIN), 58,
  59
cervical mucus, 28
cervix, 26
chaperones, 35, 37
chemoradiation, 251
children
  allergic contact dermatitis, 132–3
  bullous (blistering) diseases, 134
  bullous pemphigoid, 134
  cellulitis, 80–1, *81*
  cicatricial pemphigoid, 134
  genital herpes, 80, *80*
  genital warts, 60–1
  infections, 79–81

non-infective, non-neoplastic lesions,
    131–4
    seborrhoeic dermatitis, 133
    sexual abuse, 134, 159–60
    traumatic lesions, 134
    vulva, 37–8
    see also infants
Chlamydia trachomatis, 49–50
chromhidrosis, 101
chromoblastomycosis (chromomycosis), 74
chronic vulval pain syndromes see vulvodynia
cicatricial pemphigoid, 108, 108
    in children, 134
ciprofloxacin, 55
clear cell hidradenoma, 188
clitoral bulbs, 14
clitoris, 8, 13, 14–15
    adhesions, 235–6, 235
    pseudocyst, 236
    structural defects, 12
clitoroplasty, 222, 222
cloacal exstrophy, 12
cloacal membrane, 3, 4
clotrimazole, 47
clue cells, 48
coitus, 27–8
complex regional pain syndromes, 146–7
condyloma acuminata, 59, 60, 171–2, 172
condylomata lata, 53
condylomatous (warty) carcinoma, 181, 181
congenital adrenal hyperplasia, 1
consultation, 35–7
    examination, 35, 37
    history, 35, 36
    investigations, 39–40
    management, 40–1
conversion disorder, 158
corynebacterial infection, 75–6
Corynebacterium
    C. diphtheriae, 76
    C. minutissimum, 75
cosmetic procedures, 161
co-trimoxazole, 55
couple therapy, 164
Cowden's disease, 90
Crohn's disease, 92–3, 92, 93
cryotherapy, 61
cultural sensitivity, 34
cyclic vulvitis, 146
cysts
    anogenital glands, 168–9
    Bartholin's, 51, 168, 169
    benign, 168–9
    of canal of Nuck, 169
    epidermoid, 168
    Gartner's ducts, 169
    mesonephric-like, 169
    mesothelial, 169
    mucinous, 168, 168
    vaginal, 12
    see also individual types
cytology, 40
cytomegalovirus, 79

D
Darier's disease, 86–7, 87
    variants, 88
delirium, 157
depression, 156–7
dermatofibroma, 202
dermatofibrosarcoma protuberans, 201–2, 202
dermatomyositis, 96
dermis, 24–5
    barrier function, 25
    lymphatic system, 24
    nerve supply, 24–5
    vascular system, 24
dermographism, 150
desmoid tumour, 201
diethylcarbamazine, 71
diloxanide furonate, 73
diphtheria, cutaneous, 76
donovanosis, 55
Dowling–Degos syndrome, 90, 90, 210
doxycycline, 54, 55
drug-induced states, 157
drug reactions, 104–7
dyskeratosis congenita, 88

E
eccrine miliaria, 101
eccrine mucinous carcinoma, 189–90, 189
eccrine sweat glands, 9
echinococcosis (hydatid disease), 72
Echinococcus
    E. granularis, 72
    E. multilocularis, 72
econazole, 47
ectoparasite infestation, 62–3, 63
    pubic lice, 63, 63
    scabies, 62–3, 63
ectopic breast tissue, 185–6, 187
eczema, 112–14, 113
    atopic, 112
    irritant/allergic, 112–13
Ehlers–Danlos syndrome, 89
embryology, 1–9
    early female embryogenesis (Carnegie stages),
        2–7, 2–7
    epithelial development, 8–9
    sexual determination and differentiation, 1–2
emollients, 41
endometriosis, 192
Entamoeba histolytica, 72
Enterobius vermicularis, 71, 80
epidermoid cysts, 168
epidermolysis bullosa, 86, 87
epidermolysis bullosa aquisita, 107–8
epidermolytic acanthoma/hyperkeratosis, 88,
    171
Epidermophyton floccosum, 73
epispadias, 12
epithelioid haemangioendothelioma, 207
epithelioid sarcoma, 209–10, 209
epithelium, 22–4, 22, 23
    development, 8–9
Epstein–Barr virus, 78, 78

erythrasma, 75–6, 76
erythromycin, 54, 75
Escherichia coli, 75
Ewing's sarcoma, 209
examination, 35, 37
    cultural sensitivity, 34
    findings, 37–8
    historical aspects, 34
    normal variants, 38–9, 39
external genitalia
    ambiguous, 9–11
    structural defects, 12
external urethral meatus, 16

F
factitious disorders, 158
fallopian tubes, 8
famciclovir, 57
fatty tumours, 205–6
female embryogenesis (Carnegie stages), 2–7,
    2–7
female genital arousal disorder, 162
female genital mutilation, 34, 161–2, 161
    surgical repair, 231–2, 232
female pseudohermaphroditism, 10–11
    reconstruction, 221–2, 222
fenticonazole, 47
Fenton's operation, 227, 228
fetal androgens, 11
fibroblastic tumours, 201–2
fibroepithelial polyps, 169, 170
fibrohistiocytic tumours, 202
fibromyalgia, 155
fibrosarcoma, 202
filariasis, 71
fixed drug eruption, 104, 105
flucloxacillin, 75
fluconazole, 47
5-fluorouracil, 42
focal dermal hypoplasia, 89
folliculitis, 74–5, 75
Fordyce spots, 38, 101
fossa navicularis fissure, 231, 231
fourchette adhesions, 235
Fox–Fordyce disease, 102, 102
furunculosis, 74–5, 75

G
Galli–Galli disease, 90
Gardnerella vaginalis, 44, 48
Gartner's ducts, 7, 12
    cysts, 169
gender identity disorder, 161
genetic disorders, 86–100
genital herpes, 55–7, 56, 78
    children, 80, 80
    in pregnancy, 56
genital papular acantholytic dyskeratosis, 130–1
genital warts, 59
    children, 60–1
    see also human papillomavirus
genitourinary medicine (GUM) clinics, 44–5
germ cell neoplasms, 213

glans clitoris, 14
glomus tumour, 207–8
glucagonoma syndrome, 90–1, 91
Goltz syndrome, 89
gonadal differentiation disorders, 9–10
    ovarian dysgenesis, 9–10
    pure gonadal dysgenesis, 10
    true hermaphroditism, 10
gonorrhoea, 51–2, 51
Gougerot–Carteaud syndrome, 100
graft-versus-host disease, 131
granular cell tumour, 208–9
    malignant, 209

H
haemangioma, 206
Haemophilus ducreyi, 54
Haemophilus influenzae, 80
Hailey–Hailey disease, 87–8, 88
    variants, 88
hair disorders, 102–4
Hand–Schuller–Christian syndrome, 95
Hart's line, 15, 22, 38
hermaphroditism, 10
herpes simplex virus *see* genital herpes
hidradenitis suppurativa, 102–4, 103
hidradenoma papilliferum, 186, 187
HIV infection, 63–4
Hormodendrum compactum, 74
human papillomavirus, 57–61
    vaccines, 61
hymen, imperforate, 12
hymenal caruncle, 15
hymenal fissure, 230–1, 231
hymenorrhaphy, 231
hyperaesthesia, 145
hyperpigmentation, 98–100
    post-inflammatory, 98, 98
hypoactive sexual desires, 162
hypopigmentation, 100
    post-inflammatory, 100, 100
hypospadias, 13

I
ichthyosis linearis circumflexa, 88
IgA pemphigus, 112
iliococcygeus, 18
imaging, 40
imiquimod, 42, 61, 62
immune responsiveness, 28–9
imperforate anus, 13
imperforate hymen, 12
impetigo, 75
infants
    gluteal granuloma, 133
    napkin rash, 132, 132, 133
        psoriasiform, 133, 133
    perianal dermatitis, 133
    vulva, 37–8
    see also children
infections, 71–81
    bacterial, 74–7
    children, 79–81

mycotic, 73–4
nematodes, tapeworms and flukes, 71–2
protozoal, 72–3, 73
sexually transmitted *see* sexually transmitted
    diseases
sources of, 71
viral, 77–9
see also individual conditions
inflammatory bowel disease, 91
inflammatory dermatoses, 110–28
infliximab, 93
inguinofemoral region, 19
intertrigo, 110
investigations, 39–40
    biopsy, 39–40
    blood tests, 40
    cytology, 40
    imaging, 40
    microbiology, 40
    patch tests, 40
    Wood's lamp examination, 40
irritant dermatitis, 106, 107, 112–13
irritant napkin dermatitis, 132
ischiococcygeus, 18
isoconazole, **47**
itraconazole, **47**, 74
ivermectin, 71

J
Jarisch–Herxheimer reaction, 54

K
kala-azar, 72
Kaposi's sarcoma, 207
Kawasaki's disease, 133
keratin, 170, 170
keratinocytes, 23
keratoacanthoma, 171
keratosis follicularis, 86–7, 87
    variants, 88
kidney, abnormalities of, 12
Klebsiella granulomatis, 55

L
labial adhesions, 131–2, 132, 235
    surgical repair, 233, 233
labia majora, 14
labia minora, 8, 14
    hypertrophy, 224–5, 225, 226
    normal variants, 38
    structural defects, 12
Lactobacillus, 44
LAMB syndrome, 99
Langerhans cells, 24
Langerhans cell histiocytosis, 95
laser therapy, surgical repair, 229–30
Laugier–Hunziker syndrome, 99, 210
leiomyoma, 199, 200
leiomyosarcoma, 199–200
leishmaniasis, 72
lentigines, 99
lentigo simplex, 210
leprosy, 76–7

Letterer–Siwe syndrome, 95
leukaemia, 213
lichen planus, 98, 123–7
    aetiology, 123
    clinical features, 123–5, 123–6
    course and potential for malignancy, 125–6
    differential diagnosis, 126
    histology, 126, 126
    management, 127
    surgical intervention, 236–7, 236
lichen sclerosus, 59, 115–23
    aetiology, 116–17
    clinical features, 117–19, 117–20
    differential diagnosis, 120–1
    histology, 119, 120
    history of terminology, 115–16
    and malignancy, 122–3, 122
    management and course, 121–2
    surgical intervention, 233–6, 234–6
lichen simplex, 114–15, 114
ligneous disease, 95, 96
linear IgA disease of children, 108, 109
lipoblastoma-like tumour, 205
lipoma, 205
    spindle cell, 205
liposarcoma, 205–6
Lipschutz ulcer, 78, 78
lupus erythematosus, 96
lymphadenectomy, 247, 248
lymphangioma, 207
lymphatic tumours, 207
lymph nodes
    groin, 250–1
    pelvic, 249–50
    sentinel, 247–9, 248, **249**
lymphogranuloma venereum, 50, 50
lymphoma, 213

M
malacoplakia, 95
Malassezia furfur, 74
malathion, 63
male pseudohermaphroditism, 11
    reconstruction, 222–3, 223
malignant fibrous histiocytomas, 202
malignant melanoma, 211–12, 211, 212
malingering, 158
mammary glands *see* anogenital mammary-like
    glands
management, 40–1
    topical treatment, 41–2, **41**, **42**
maternal androgens, 11
meatal stenosis, 13
mebendazole, 71
medically unexplained symptoms, 157–8
melanocytes, 23–4
melanocytic naevi, 210–11, 210, 211
melanosis, 99, 99
Melkersson–Rosenthal syndrome, 95
menarche, 26
menopause, 28
Merkel cells, 24
    carcinoma, 193, 193

mesenchymal tumours, 199
    of unknown origin, 209–10
mesonephric-like cysts, 169
mesonephric (Wolffian) ducts, 7, 7
mesothelial cysts, 169
metastatic carcinoma, 193–4
metronidazole, 46, 73
Michaelis–Gutmann bodies, 95
miconazole, **47**
microbiology, 40
Microsporum canis, 74
milia, 37
minor vestibular glands, 15–16
Mobiluncus, 48
molluscum bodies, 62
molluscum contagiosum, 61–2, 62
mons pubis, 13–14
mucinous cysts, 168, 168
Mucor, 74
Mullerian ducts, 5–6
multiple hamartoma syndrome, 90
Munchausen's syndrome, 158
mycobacterial infections, 76–7
Mycobacterium
    M. leprae, 76
    M. tuberculosis, 76
Mycoplasma
    M. genitalium, 77
    M. hominis, 44, 77
mycotic infections, 73–4
myofibroblastic tumours, 203–5

N
naevus
    melanocytic, 210–11, 210, 211
    Spitz, 210
    white sponge, 88–9, 89
napkin rash, 132, 132, 133
    psoriasiform, 133, 133
necrolytic migratory erythema, 90–1, 91
necrotizing fasciitis, 77
Neisseria gonorrhoeae, 45, 51, 75
Netherton's syndrome, 88, 91
neural tumours, 208–9
neurofibroma, 208
neurofibromatosis, 89–90
nodular fasciitis, 203
non-epithelial tumours, 199–213
    fibroblastic, 201–2
    fibrohistiocytic, 202
    germ cell neoplasms, 213
    lymphoma and leukaemia, 213
    mesenchymal, 199
        of unknown origin, 209–10
    myofibroblastic, 203–5
    neural, 208–9
    non-mesenchymal, non-epithelial neoplasms,
        210–12
    perivascular cell, 207–8
    smooth muscle, 199–200
    striated muscle, 201
    tumours of fat, 205–6
    tumours of lymphatic origin, 207

vascular tissue, 206–7
    see also individual tumours
non-infective, non-neoplastic lesions, 85–134
    blood and lymphatic vessels, 128–30
    bullous (blistering) diseases, 107–10
    children, 131–4
    classification, 85–6
    conditions associated with systemic disease,
        90–8
    disorders of skin appendages, 100–4
    drug reactions, 104–7
    genetic disorders, 86–90
    inflammatory dermatoses, 110–28
    pigmentary disorders, 98–100
    symptoms, 86
    see also individual lesions
non-mesenchymal, non-epithelial neoplasms,
    210–12
normal variants, 38–9, 39
nymphectomy, 224–5, 225, 226
nystatin, **47**

O
obstetric trauma, surgical repair, 226, 226, 227
oedema, 129–30, 130
old age, 28
Onchocerca volvulus, 71
onchocerciasis, 71
orf, 78
orgasmic dysfunction, 162
ovarian dysgenesis, 9–10
oxyuriasis (threadworms), 71, 80

P
Paget's disease, extramammary, 85, 183–5,
    183, 184, **185**
    primary, 183–5
    secondary, 185
paraganglioma, 209
paragenital haematoma, 28
parvovirus B19, 79, 79
patch tests, 40
pelvic floor muscles, 18–19, 18, 19
pemphigus vulgaris, 109, 109, 110
penicillins, 54
perianal dermatitis of newborn, 133
perianal streptococcal dermatitis *see* cellulitis
perineal erythema, toxin-mediated, 81
perineum, 17, 20
    blood supply, 20
    innervation, 21–2
    lymphatic drainage, 20–1
perivascular cell tumours, 207–8
permethrin, 63
phenothrin, 63
Phthirus pubis, 63, 63
phycomycosis, 74
Piedraia hortae, 74
piedra (trichosporis), 74
pigmentary disorders, 98–100
pilonidal sinus, 102
pinta, 52
piperazine, 71

pityriasis versicolor, 74
plasma cell orificial mucositis, 128
plasmacytosis circumorificialis, 128
podophyllotoxin, **61**, 62
postcoital fissures, surgical repair, 230–1,
    231
praziquantel, 72
pregnancy, 27–8
    genital herpes in, 56
    vulva, 38
premature ovarian failure, 28
prepuberty, 25
prepuce, 8
priapism, 162
prolapse, surgical repair, 226–7, 228
protozoal infections, 72–3, 73
    sexually transmitted, 45–6, 45
pseudohermaphroditism
    female, 10–11
        reconstruction, 221–2, 222
    male, 11
        reconstruction, 222–3, 223
Pseudomonas aeruginosa, 75
pseudoverrucous papules and nodules, 133
pseudoxanthoma elasticum, 89
psoriasis, 110–11, 110
    management, 111
psychiatric interventions, 164–5
psychiatric morbidity, 155–8
    depression and anxiety, 156–7
    medically unexplained symptoms,
        157–8
    psychotic illnesses, delirium and
        drug-induced states, 157
psychological assessment, 163–4
    brief psychological evaluation, 163–4
    communication, 163
psychological interventions, 164–5
psychological morbidity, 158–62
    childhood sexual abuse, 159–60
    chronic vulval pain syndromes, 158–9
    cosmetic procedures, 161
    female genital mutilation, 161–2, **161**
    sexual assault and rape, 160
    surgery, 160–1
psychopharmacological treatments, 164–5
psychotic illness, 157
puberty, 25–6
pubic lice, 63, 63
pubococcygeus, 18–19
puborectalis, 19
pure gonadal dysgenesis, 10
pyoderma gangrenosum, 93–4

R
radiation therapy, 251
rape, 160
Reiter's disease, 111–12
renal agenesis, 12
reproductive years, 26–8
rhabdomyoma, 201
rhabdomyosarcoma, 201
Rikotansky–Kuster–Hauser syndrome, 11

S

sarcoidosis, 94–5, 94
sarcoma
    alveolar soft-part, 210
    epithelioid, 209–10, 209
    Ewing's, 209
    Kaposi's, 207
Sarcoptes scabiei, 62
scabies, 62–3, 63
Schistosoma
    S. haematobium, 72
    S. japonicum, 72
    S. mansoni, 72
schistosomiasis (bilharzia), 72
schwannoma, 208
    malignant, 208
sebaceous gland disorders, 100–1, 101
sebaceous glands, 8–9
seborrhoeic dermatitis, 111, 112
    children, 133
    management, 111
seborrhoeic keratosis, 170, 170
seminal fluid, 29
sentinel node procedures, 247–9, 248, **249**
sexual abuse in children, 134
    psychological effects in adults, 159–60
sexual assault, 160
sexual determination, 1–2
sexual differentiation, 1–2
sexual dysfunction, 162
    female genital arousal disorder, 162
    hypoactive sexual desires, 162
    orgasmic dysfunction, 162
sexually transmitted diseases, 44–64
    bacterial infections, 48–55
    ectoparasite infestation, 62–3, 63
    HIV, 63–4
    protozoal infections, 45–6
    screening for, 44–5
    viral infections, 55–62
    yeast infections, 46–8, 46, 47
Shigella, 80
silver sulphadiazine cream, 42
Sjögren's syndrome, 96
smooth muscle tumours, 199–200
Sneddon–Wilkinson disease, 112
somatoform disorders, 158
spermatozoa, destruction of, 28–9
spindle cell lipoma, 205
spindle cell nodule, postoperative, 203
Spitz naevi, 210
squamous carcinoma
    incidence, 239
    invasive, 176–9, 176–9
squamous papillomas, 170
staging of vulval cancer, 241–2, 242
staphylococcal scalded skin syndrome, 75
Staphylococcus
    S. aureus, 75
    S. epidermidis, 79
steroids, topical, 41–2, 41, 42, 106
    adverse effects, 106–7, 106
Stevens–Johnson syndrome, 104–5, 105

Streptococcus
    S. faecalis, 75
    S. pyogenes, 75
striated muscle tumours, 201
structural defects, 11–13
    external genitalia, 12
    lower reproductive tract, 11–12
    vulval and intestinal abnormalities, 13
    vulval mammary tissue, 13
    vulval and urinary system, 12–13
subcorneal pustulosis, 112
superficial perineal pouch, 19, 20
surgery, 221–37
    bladder exstrophy, 223–4, 224
    female pseudohermaphroditism, 221–2, 222
    labial adhesions, 233, 233
    labia minora hypertrophy, 224–5, 225, 226
    lichen planus, 236–7, 236
    lichen sclerosus, 233–6, 234–6
    male pseudohermaphroditism, 222–3, 223
    psychological morbidity, 160–1
    vulval cancers, 243–9, **243**
    vulval trauma, 225–33, 226–33
    see also individual procedures
Sutton's ulcers, 98
sweat glands
    carcinomas, 189–90
    disorders, 101–2
Sweet's syndrome, 93
syphilis, 52–4, 53
    chancre, 53
    congenital, 80
syringoma, 101, 101, 188, 188

T

tacrolimus, 93
telangiectasia, 106
terbinafine, 74
threadworms, 71, 80
tinea cruris, 73–4, 73
tinea incognito, 106
tinidazole, 46
topical treatment, 41–2, **41, 42**
toxic epidermal necrolysis, 105
toxic shock syndrome, 75
transepidermal water loss, 25
transsexuality, 161
traumatic lesions, 131, 225–33, 226–33
    children, 134
    female genital mutilation, 34, 161–2, **161**, 231–2, 232
    obstetric, 226, 226, 227
    postcoital fissures, 230–1, 231
    surgical, 226–30
        post-Bartholin's abscess drainage, 228–9
        post-laser therapy, 229–30
        postprolapse repair, 226–7, 228
        post-vulvectomy, 227–8, 229, 230
Treponema
    T. carateum, 52
    T. pallidum, 52
    T. pertenue, 52

trichilemmoma, 189
trichloroacetic acid, **61**
trichoepithelioma, 188–9
Trichomonas, 45
    T. vaginalis, 45, 80
trichomoniasis, 45–6, 45
trichomycosis (nodosa), 76
Trichophyton
    T. mentagrophytes, 73
    T. rubrum, 73
Trichosporon beigelii, 74
tuberculosis, 76
tumours
    anogenital mammary-like gland, 187–8
    Bartholin's gland, 190–2
    benign adnexal, 188–9
    benign squamous non-neoplastic, 169–72
    Buschke–Lowenstein, 59
    desmoid, 201
    of fat, 205–6
    fibroblastic, 201–2
    fibrohistiocytic, 202
    glomus, 207–8
    granular cell, 208–9
    lipoblastoma-like, 205
    of lymphatic origin, 207
    mesenchymal, 199, 209–10
    myofibroblastic, 203–5
    neural, 208–9
    perivascular cell, 207–8
    smooth muscle, 199–200
    striated muscle, 201
    vascular tissue, 206–7
    yolk sac, 213
    see also carcinoma; and individual tumours
Turner's syndrome (45X), 1, 10

U

ulcerative colitis, 92
ulcerative lesions, 105–6
ulcers
    aphthous, 97, 97, 98
    Lipschutz, 78, 78
    Sutton's, 98
Ureaplasma urealyticum, 77
ureter, abnormalities of, 12
urethra, 16, 27
    abnormalities, 12–13
urogenital diaphragm, 16, 18
urogenital septum, 4, 6
urogenital triangle, 18

V

vagina, 16–17, 17
    epithelium, 22–4, 22, 23
    normal flora, 44
    reproductive phase, 26–7
    secretions, 26
vaginal agenesis, 11
vaginal atresia, 11
vaginal cysts, 12
vaginal intraepithelial neoplasia (VAIN), 58, 59
vaginal pigmentation, 99

vaginal septa, 11–12
vaginal tenting, 27
valaciclovir, 57
varicella, 77–8, 78
varicose veins, 128, 128
vascular tissue tumours, 206–7
verruciform xanthoma, 170–1, 171
verrucous carcinoma, 179–81, 180
vestibular micropapillomatosis, 169–70
vestibular papillomatosis, 38–9, 39
vestibule, 15
   normal variants, 38
vestibulitis, 146
vestibulodynia, 149
viral infections, 77–9
   sexually transmitted, 55–62
   see also individual conditions
virilization, 9
vitiligo, 100, 100
vulva, 13
   epithelium, 22–4, 22, 23
   infancy and childhood, 37–8
   physiology, 25
   postmenopausal women, 38
   pregnancy, 38
   reproductive phase, 27
vulval cancers, 239–51
   adjuvant treatment, 249–51
      close surgical margins, 249
      pelvic/groin nodes, 249–51
      radiation therapy, 251

chemoradiation, 251
   diagnosis and investigations, 243
   epidemiology and pathogenesis, 239–40
   guidelines for management, 249
   incidence, 239
   staging, 241–2, 242
   surgery, 243–9, 243
   see also individual cancer types
vulval clinics, 34–5
vulval fibroma, prepubertal, 201
vulval intraepithelial neoplasia (VIN), 58,
     59, 172–6
   differentiated, 174–7, 175
   incidence, 239
   undifferentiated, 172–4, 173, 174
vulval mammary tissue *see* anogenital
     mammary-like glands
vulval oedema, 129–30, 130
vulval tears, surgical repair, 226, 226, 227
vulval trauma *see* traumatic lesions
vulvectomy, 160, 227–8, 229, 230
   outcome, **244**
   radical, 246
vulvitis
   cyclic, 146
   Zoon's, 127–8, 128
vulvodynia, 145–51
   complex regional pain syndrome,
     146–7
   generalized unprovoked, 147–8

   history, 145–6, 146
   localized, 149–51, 149, 150
   psychological aspects, 159
vulvoperineoplasty, 233–5, 234
vulvovaginal adenosis, 131
vulvovaginal adhesions, 236–7, 236
vulvovaginal candidiasis, 46–8, 46, 47
   treatment, **47**
vulvovaginitis, 79–80, 146

W
white sponge naevus, 88–9, 89
Wood's lamp examination, 40
Wuchereria bancrofti, 71

X
45X (Turner's syndrome), 1, 10
45X/46XX mosaicism, 10
46XX, 46XY, 10
45X/46XY mosaicism, 10

Y
Y chromosome, sex-determining region, 1
yeast infections, sexually transmitted, 46–8,
   46, 47
yolk sac tumours, 213

Z
Zoon's vulvitis, 127–8, 128
zoster, 77–8, 78